Musculoskeletal Examination and Assessment

For my mother and father (NJP)
For my parents Thomas and Gretta McGovern, my husband Steve and daughters Hannah and Grace (DR)

For Elsevier

Content Strategist: Rita Demetriou-Swanwick
Content Development Specialist: Sally Davies, Nicola Lally
Senior Project Manager: Kamatchi Madhavan
Designer/Design Direction: Maggie Reid
Illustration Manager: Nichole Beard
Illustrator: MPS

Musculoskeletal Examination and Assessment

A HANDBOOK FOR THERAPISTS

Fifth Edition

EDITED BY
NICOLA J. PETTY DPT MSc GradDipPhys FMACP FHEA
Associate Professor, School of Health Sciences, University of Brighton, Eastbourne, UK

DIONNE RYDER MSc (Manipulative Therapy) MMACP FHEA
Senior Lecturer, Department of Allied Health Professions and Midwifery, School of Health and Social Work, University of Hertfordshire, Hatfield, UK

FOREWORD BY
JEREMY LEWIS PhD FCSP
Consultant Physiotherapist, Professor of Musculoskeletal Research, Sonographer and Independent Prescriber, www.LondonShoulderClinic.com; Professor (adjunct) of Musculoskeletal Research, Clinical Therapies, University of Limerick, Ireland; Reader in Physiotherapy, Department of Allied Health Professions and Midwifery, School of Health and Social Work, University of Hertfordshire, Hatfield, Hertfordshire, UK

ELSEVIER   Edinburgh   London   New York   Oxford   Philadelphia   St Louis   Sydney   Toronto   2018

ELSEVIER

© 2018 Elsevier Ltd. All rights reserved.

First edition 1997
Second edition 2001
Third edition 2006
Fourth edition 2011
Fifth edition 2018

ISBN 978-0-7020-6717-4

British Library Cataloguing in Publication Data
A catalogue record for this book is available from the British Library

Library of Congress Cataloging in Publication Data
A catalog record for this book is available from the Library of Congress

Notices

Knowledge and best practice in this field are constantly changing. As new research and experience broaden our understanding, changes in research methods, professional practices or medical treatment may become necessary.

Practitioners and researchers must always rely on their own experience and knowledge in evaluating and using any information, methods, compounds or experiments described herein. In using such information or methods they should be mindful of their own safety and the safety of others, including parties for whom they have a professional responsibility.

With respect to any drug or pharmaceutical products identified, readers are advised to check the most current information provided (i) on procedures featured or (ii) by the manufacturer of each product to be administered, to verify the recommended dose or formula, the method and duration of administration and contraindications. It is the responsibility of practitioners, relying on their own experience and knowledge of their patients, to make diagnoses, to determine dosages and the best treatment for each individual patient and to take all appropriate safety precautions.

To the fullest extent of the law, neither the Publisher nor the authors, contributors or editors, assume any liability for any injury and/or damage to persons or property as a matter of products liability, negligence or otherwise, or from any use or operation of any methods, products, instructions or ideas contained in the material herein.

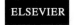 your source for books, journals and multimedia in the health sciences

www.elsevierhealth.com

 Working together to grow libraries in developing countries

www.elsevier.com • www.bookaid.org

The publisher's policy is to use **paper manufactured from sustainable forests**

Printed in China

Last digit is the print number: 9 8 7 6 5 4 3 2 1

CONTENTS

FOREWORD

The science and practice relating to the assessment of people with musculoskeletal problems are constantly evolving. It remains an ongoing challenge to keep up to date with the literature due to the rate at which new research, ideas and philosophical approaches are being published across an ever-increasing landscape of communication services, systems and networks.

If you are entrusted with the exceptional privilege of supporting members of your community who are experiencing musculoskeletal problems, no matter if you are new to your profession or have considerable experience, then this textbook, *Musculoskeletal Examination and Assessment*, will support, augment and enrich the skills you require for the assessment procedures. It brings together 14 highly respected and expert clinicians across 16 chapters and synthesizes their collective knowledge and skills within a biopsychosocial framework. In doing so, it supports clinical practice by bringing together, in one place, an extensive aggregation of knowledge.

The text presents the reader with different clinical reasoning models and skilfully and comprehensively guides the clinician through the assessment process that initially involves discussing pertinent specific and general health issues with the individual, followed by general physical assessment approaches. Each region is presented systematically from the temporomandibular region to the foot and ankle. Each chapter contains a wealth of information and is supported by clear diagrams and explanations guiding the reader through the assessment procedures recommended by the authors.

Musculoskeletal Examination and Assessment is now in its fifth edition. This in itself is a testament to the role it has played in training and educating many generations of clinicians. In the foreword to the first edition, published in 1997, Geoff Maitland commented that the

text was appropriate for all clinical levels. This edition is no different. In the foreword to the third edition, Agneta Lando described how the text takes the reader through a logical sequence of questioning, examination and assessment, and synthesizes the explosive growth in musculoskeletal research. This edition is no different. In the foreword to the fourth edition, Alison Rushton remarked that the text continues to strive to present best current practice to assist development of the process of examination and assessment. This edition is no different. Nicola Petty and Dionne Ryder, in this new updated edition, have continued with the same tradition and have, as editors, constructed, and as authors, contributed, together with the other 12 expert authors, a valuable, informative and important text. The editors and authors of this fifth edition are to be complimented and sincerely thanked for their efforts.

The best clinicians are the ones who recognize that it is the patient who is the most important person in any healthcare system. They are also the clinicians who are constantly learning, reflecting and evolving as they synthesize new knowledge from a multitude of sources. They are continuing to educate themselves. On education, President John F. Kennedy (35th President of the United States) during American Education Week (Proclamation 3422) on 25 July 1961 said, 'Let us think of education as the means of developing our greatest abilities, because in each of us there is a private hope and dream which, fulfilled, can be translated into benefit for everyone'.

Musculoskeletal Examination and Assessment is one of those learning sources that will support your clinical development and education and will make an important contribution to the library of all those involved in assessing musculoskeletal conditions. For many, it will be a constant clinical companion and, without doubt, for those who use it as intended, the book will not remain in the pristine condition it arrived in. It will become well thumbed, with possibly highlighted, pages, possibly with annotations, reference markers and maybe also with questions, thoughts and reflections added by the reader. In doing so you will be using this book as intended: to improve your knowledge and musculoskeletal assessment skills so that you may improve the care you offer to those entrusting you with the range of musculoskeletal conditions that present to you. Providing this care is an honour and a substantial responsibility. Undertake this duty with the seriousness it demands, deliver it in a kind and supportive way and use this book to support you to achieve this goal.

JEREMY LEWIS
2017

PREFACE

This new edition has been significantly updated and benefited from being co-edited with Dionne Ryder. There are nine new contributors to this edition, with only ourselves, Linda Exelby, Colette Ridehalgh and Kieran Barnard from the previous edition and this provides the opportunity to gain fresh perspectives. Each chapter reflects contemporary practice with the addition of new examination and assessment processes and removal of outdated ones. All the contributors have significant experience in managing patients with musculoskeletal conditions and have drawn from their own clinical and academic backgrounds to provide a logical and reasoned approach to examination. We are grateful, not only for the valuable input each contributor has made to the text, but also for their energy and enthusiasm in completing the job under tight timescales.

Thanks must go to Elsevier and, in particular, Rita Demetriou-Swanwick, Sally Davies and Nicola Lally for their guidance and support throughout the publishing process.

The overall aim of the book is to provide a clear and accessible guide to musculoskeletal examination and assessment for pre-registration students. The skills required of the clinician are to work alongside another person and facilitate his or her rehabilitation. When successful, it can bring immense satisfaction and reward; however success is not always easy to achieve with the inherent uncertainty of clinical practice. Each person is a unique blend of physical being, intellect, will, emotion and spirit, living within, and being influenced by, a social and cultural world. Rehabilitation is thus a complex process and requires high levels of clinical expertise. This text aims to provide a comprehensive step-by-step approach to the technical skills and clinical reasoning involved in the examination and assessment of people with musculoskeletal conditions.

NICOLA J. PETTY

DIONNE RYDER

Eastbourne and Hatfield 2016

CONTRIBUTORS

COLLEEN BALSTON, BSc(Hons) MSc MMACP FHEA
Senior Lecturer, Department of Allied Health Professions and Midwifery, School of Health and Social Work, University of Hertfordshire, Hatfield, UK

KIERAN BARNARD, BSc(Hons) MSc MCSP MMACP
Advanced Practitioner Physiotherapist, Hip and Knee Clinical Lead, Sussex MSK Partnership, Brighton, UK; Private Practitioner, Flex Physiotherapy, Horsham, UK

HELEN COWGILL, BSc(Hons) MMACP MCSP
Clinical Director, TMJ Physio, London; Clinical Lead Physiotherapist, Department of Physiotherapy, Kings College Hospital NHS Foundation Trust, London; Invited Lecturer, Kings College London, London; Liverpool University, Liverpool and Coventry University, Coventry, UK

LINDA A. EXELBY, BSc GradDip(Man Ther) FMACP
Clinician at Fontwell and Southbourne Physiotherapy Clinics. Eastergate nr Chichester, UK. Invited Lecturer, Department of Allied Health Professions and Midwifery, School of Health and Social Work, University of Hertfordshire, Hatfield, UK

GAIL FORRESTER-GALE, BSc(Hons) MSc PGCertEd SFHEA MMACP
Senior Lecturer, Physiotherapy Department, School of Health, Faculty of Health and Life Sciences, Coventry University, Coventry, UK

KEVIN HALL, BSc(Hons) MSc MMACP
Advanced Practitioner, Western Sussex Hospitals NHS Foundation Trust, West Sussex; NIHR Clinical Doctoral Fellowship, University of Brighton and Western Sussex Hospitals NHS Foundation Trust, UK

ANDREA MOULSON, BSc(Hons) MA MSc (NMS Physiotherapy) PGCert (Learning and Teaching) MMACP
Senior Lecturer in Physiotherapy, Department of Allied Health Professions and Midwifery, School of Health and Social Work, University of Hertfordshire, Hatfield, UK; Extended Scope Practitioner, Physiotherapy Department, The Hillingdon Hospital Trust, Hillingdon, Middlesex, UK

NICOLA J. PETTY, DPT MSc GradDipPhys FMACP FHEA
Associate Professor, School of Health Sciences, University of Brighton, Eastbourne, UK

COLETTE RIDEHALGH, BSc(Hons) MSc PhD MMACP
Senior Lecturer, School of Health Sciences, University of Brighton, Eastbourne, East Sussex, UK

DIONNE RYDER, MSc(Manipulative Therapy) MMACP PGCert (Learning and Teaching) FHEA
Senior Lecturer, Department of Allied Health Professions and Midwifery, School of Health and Social Work, University of Hertfordshire, Hatfield, UK

BILL TAYLOR, MSc GradDip(Adv Man Ther (Canada))
Director, Taylor Physiotherapy, Edinburgh, UK; Visiting Lecturer, Edinburgh University, Edinburgh, UK

HOWARD TURNER, BSc BAppSc(Phty)
Part-time Teaching Fellow, University of Bath, Bath; Visiting Lecturer, Keele University, Keele, Staffordshire; Private Practitioner, Wilmslow Physiotherapy, Wilmslow, Cheshire, UK

HUBERT VAN GRIENSVEN, BSc DipAc MSc(Pain) PhD
Senior Lecturer in Pain, Department of Allied Health Professions and Midwifery, School of Health and Social Work University of Hertfordshire, Hatfield, UK

CHRIS WORSFOLD, MSc PGDip(Man Phys) MMACP MCSP
Physiotherapist Specializing in Neck Pain, The Tonbridge Clinic, Kent, UK; Visiting Lecturer, School of Health Sciences, University of Brighton, Eastbourne, East Sussex, UK

1

INTRODUCTION

NICOLA J. PETTY ■ DIONNE RYDER

This text aims to provide guidance to the process of examination and clinical reasoning for patients with musculoskeletal dysfunction within a biopsychosocial framework.

The text provides a step-by-step approach to the subjective and physical examination of the various regions in the body. The next chapter (Chapter 2) on subjective examination provides a general guide to the way in which questions might be asked as well as the clinical relevance of questions. Chapter 3, on the physical examination, provides a guide to performing the testing procedures and to understanding the relevance of the tests. Chapter 4 explores clinical reasoning and how to make sense of the findings from the subjective and physical examination. Thus Chapters 2–4 provide an overview of key principles and as such are considered essential reading. Each regional chapter will follow a similar structure but will seek to identify how these principles are applied to each specific region and include; temporomandibular, upper cervical, cervico-thoracic, thoracic, shoulder, elbow, wrist/hand, lumbar, pelvis, hip, knee and foot/ankle. There is some repetition of information from Chapters 2 and 3 in each of the regional chapters to help reinforce the information and avoid excessive page turning.

The division of the body into regions is anatomically, biomechanically, functionally and clinically contrived. More realistic regions might, for example, be the cervico-thoracic-shoulder region and the lumbo-pelvic-hip region. So, while readers are introduced here to the individual regions, they need to maintain an awareness of the wider regional areas that are clinically and functionally relevant for any particular patient.

A word of warning to the novice clinician who may believe what is shown in this text is the only way to do something. What you see in this text is one way of demonstrating an assessment technique favoured by the particular clinician on the particular model at that time. Furthermore, the ability of the photographer to capture the technique will also have affected how the clinician performed it and of course the photographs will only be able to capture handling from one angle. Initially, novices have to start somewhere, and may want to replicate the techniques shown. Once novices understand what they are trying to achieve with a technique, then they would be wise to consider alternative ways of carrying out the technique, making adaptations for themselves and for their patients. They can determine whether or not their adapted technique is effective and efficient by asking themselves:

■ Is it easy and comfortable to perform? A technique is easy and comfortable when posture is carefully considered to produce forces easily; the position of the feet, legs, trunk and arms, as well as the position of the patient and plinth height, will all contribute to the ease with which a technique is carried out. When learning, an easy way of checking whether a technique is easy to do is to prolong your position and force applied for much longer than it needs to be, and see whether it continues to feel easy. If it becomes tiring small alterations may be needed.
■ Is it comfortable for the student model or patient? While learning, it can be helpful for models to imagine they are a patient in pain, so they raise the standard of comfort required and then

provide honest and constructive feedback to their partner.

■ Does it achieve what it intends to achieve? A technique achieves what it intends to achieve when it is comfortable, accurate, specific, controlled and appropriate, and handling is sensitively adapted to the tissue response. Whenever a technique is being carried out, it is helpful to ask whether you think you are achieving what you are intending to achieve, and if not, then adapt your technique. This is not just for novices as they learn techniques; normal everyday clinical practice requires clinicians to adapt their examination procedures to individual patients.

For those learning these examination procedures for the first time, here are some tips on how you might improve your handling which may help make findings from tests more valid and reliable:

■ Practise, practise and practise! There is no substitute for plenty of good-quality practice.

■ When practising, split the task into bite-sized chunks, building up into a whole. For example, practise hand holds, then application of force, then the hand hold and force on different individuals, then the communication needed with your model, then everything all together on different individuals.

■ Imagine what is happening to the tissues when you are carrying out an examination procedure.

■ Tell your model very specifically what you want in terms of feedback; model feedback needs to be honest and constructive.

■ Verbalize out loud to your model what you are doing.

■ When you do a technique, evaluate it and predict the feedback you will receive from your model, so you learn to become independent of your model's feedback.

■ Act as a model and feel what is happening.

■ Act as an observer: if you can see a good technique and feel a good technique then this can help you to perform a good technique.

■ Use a video recorder to observe yourself when working with a peer model.

■ Imagine yourself doing the examination procedures in your mind in any spare moments.

It is perhaps worth mentioning at the outset that the clinician examining patients with a musculoskeletal condition may not be able to identify a particular source of symptoms or ongoing pathological process. In some patients it may be possible – for example, the clinician may suspect a meniscal tear in the knee, or a lateral ligament sprain of the ankle. However, in other patients, particularly those for whom symptoms have persisted, when one integrates current knowledge of pain mechanisms, and considers these effects on the presenting symptoms, the goal of identifying exact pathology is not realistic. When the detailed analysis of movement dysfunction is considered in conjunction with psychosocial factors, the clinician is then in a position to establish a reasoned treatment and management strategy. The reader is referred to the companion text for further information on the principles of treatment and management of patients with musculoskeletal dysfunction (Petty & Barnard 2017).

REFERENCE

Petty, N.J., Barnard, K., 2017. Principles of musculoskeletal treatment and management: a handbook for therapists, third ed. Elsevier, Edinburgh.

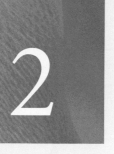

2

SUBJECTIVE EXAMINATION

HUBERT VAN GRIENSVEN ■ DIONNE RYDER

CHAPTER CONTENTS

INTRODUCTION

This chapter and Chapter 3 cover the general principles and procedures for examination of the musculoskeletal system. This chapter is concerned with the subjective examination, during which information is gathered from the patient and from other sources, such as the patient's medical notes, while Chapter 3 covers the objective or physical examination. This examination system provides a framework that can be adapted to fulfil the examination requirements for people with musculoskeletal problems in various clinical settings.

Clinical Reasoning Within Health and Disability

In order to understand a patient's problems fully the clinician must consider all factors that may impact on a person's health (Fig. 2.1) (World Health Organization 2001).

Throughout the subjective examination the clinician looks for cues to identify possible sources of a patient's symptoms and contributing physical and psychosocial factors, so that appropriate management options relevant to the individual patient can be selected.

3

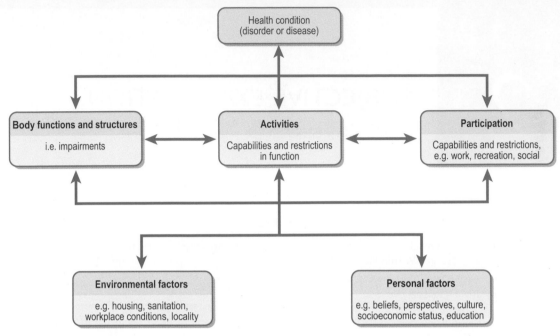

FIG. 2.1 ■ Framework of health and disability. *(From World Health Organization 2001.)*

The process of clinical reasoning also helps to determine whether these factors must be considered in the physical assessment. Clinical reasoning has been defined as:

a process in which the clinician, interacting with significant others (client, caregivers, health care team members), structures meaning, goals and health management strategies based on clinical data, client choices, and professional judgment and knowledge (Higgs & Jones 2000, p. 11).

Research has demonstrated that clinicians use a number of clinical reasoning models, which can be divided broadly into those with a more cognitive/thinking process such as hypothetico-deductive reasoning (Rivett & Higgs 1997), pattern recognition (Barrows & Feltovich 1987) and those utilizing more interactive processes such as narrative or collaborative reasoning (Jones 1995; Edwards et al. 2004, 2006; Jones & Rivett 2004; Jones et al. 2008).

Fig. 2.2 presents the patient-centred collaborative model of reasoning. This model brings together both cognitive and interactive processes, recognizing that

these are intrinsically linked and central to understanding the complexity of the mind–body interaction. To provide a framework to assist in the organization of knowledge and reasoning throughout the subjective and physical examination, hypothesis categories have been proposed (Jones & Rivett 2004) which reflect the framework of health and disability (World Health Organization 2001) (Box 2.1). More detailed information is provided in Chapter 4.

THE SUBJECTIVE EXAMINATION STEP BY STEP

The accuracy of the information gained in the subjective examination depends to a large extent on the quality of the communication between the clinician and patient. The clinician needs to listen carefully to the patient, speak at an easy pace, keep questions short and ask only one question at a time (Hengeveld & Maitland 2014). For further details, please refer to Chapter 9 in Petty and Barnard (2017).

The quality of the information gained in the subjective examination depends to a large extent on the clinician using clinical reasoning skills to ask pertinent

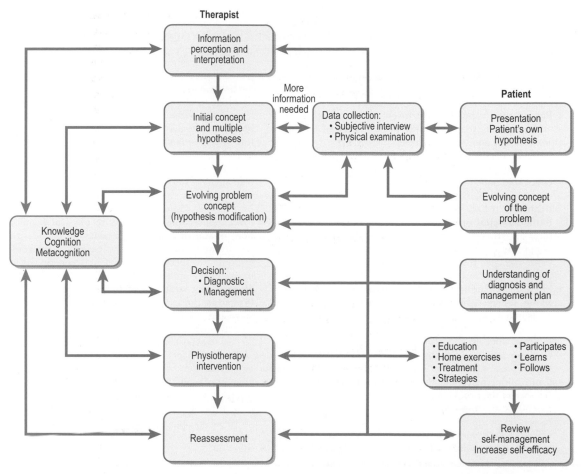

FIG. 2.2 ■ Patient-centred model of clinical reasoning. *(From Jones & Rivett 2004.)*

questions. This chapter aims to provide background information with regard to the questions asked, to enable clinicians to question effectively and obtain relevant information on which to base a patient-centred physical examination. It outlines a very detailed subjective examination, which will not always be required in full. For example, not every question needs to be asked to the same depth – the clinician must tailor the examination to the patient. The most important findings in the subjective examination are highlighted with asterisks (*) for easy reference. They can be used at subsequent treatment sessions to evaluate the effects of treatment intervention.

The aim of the subjective examination is to obtain sufficient information to enable the clinician to identify a primary hypothesis with possible alternative hypotheses on the cause of the patient's symptoms. This information will be used by the clinician to reason clinically and plan a safe, efficient and effective physical examination which seeks to confirm or refute these emerging hypotheses. It also enables the clinician to place the examination and treatment in a patient-centred context. A summary of the subjective examination is shown in Table 2.1.

The Patient's Perspective

Establishing the patient's personal views and expectations is a useful way to open the subjective examination. The clinician can ask an open question about the patient's reason for attending and give the opportunity

---

BOX 2.1
SUBJECTIVE AND PHYSICAL EXAMINATION
HYPOTHESES CATEGORIES (JONES & RIVETT 2004)

- **Activity capability/restriction**: what activities the patient is able and unable to do, e.g. walking, lifting, sitting
- **Participant capability/restriction**: the patient's ability/inability to be involved in life situations, i.e. work, family and leisure activities
- **Patients' perspectives on their experience**: an important category in its own right, as it must be acknowledged that patients' perceptions will have a significant impact on their presentation and response to treatment
- **Pathobiological mechanisms**: the state of the structures or tissues thought to be producing the patient's symptoms in relation to tissue pathology, ongoing tissue damage, the stage of the healing process and the pain mechanisms involved
- **Physical impairments and associated structure/ tissue sources**: the target tissue from where symptoms may be coming, in conjunction with the resulting impairment. Sole identification of specific tissues is often difficult and management directed to the resulting impairment, whilst hypothesizing the pathological processes involved is most effective
- **Contributing factors to the development and maintenance of the problem**: these may be environmental, psychosocial, behavioural, physical or heredity factors. Environmental factors may include a patient's workstation or work environment, home and car. Psychosocial factors may include the patient's belief that

pain or exercise 'will do harm', resulting in fear-avoidant behaviours, or misunderstanding the nature of the problem, resulting in catastrophization. Behavioural factors may include what patients do at work or at home, their level of physical activity, such as they may lead a very sedentary lifestyle. Physical contributing factors include elements such as reduced range of movement and muscle weakness. Heriditary factors play a part in the development of some musculoskeletal conditions, such as ankylosing spondylitis and osteoarthritis (Solomon et al. 2001)

- **Precautions/contraindications to physical examination, treatment and management**: this includes the severity and irritability of the patient's symptoms, response to special questions and the underlying nature of the problem
- **Management strategy and treatment plan**
- **Prognosis**: this can be affected by factors such as the stage and extent of the injury as well as the patient's expectations, personality and lifestyle. Psychosocial (yellow flags) risk factors, patient's perceived stress at work (blue flags) and work conditions, including employment and sickness policy as well as type and amount of work (black flags) are considered to influence the outcome of treatment strongly. Orange flags indicate mental health disorders which will need to be managed by an appropriately trained professional (Main & Spanswick 2000; Jones & Rivett 2004)

---

for the patient to formulate an answer (Gask & Usherwood 2002). The clinician may choose to ask further questions at that time or at a later stage in the examination. For example, the clinician may ask what the patient thinks the problem is, or alternatively what the best explanation is that the patient has had. The patient's ability to provide a robust answer can be as informative as a struggle to formulate one or an admission that the condition is a mystery.

Insight into the patient's perspective can help the clinician to frame the examination within a patient-centred context (Goodrich & Cornwell 2008):

- It makes it clear that the clinician is interested in the patient as a person, and helps to develop rapport between clinician and patient.

- It enables the clinician to adopt a collaborative and patient-centred approach.
- It identifies whether the patient's belief and understanding in relation to the condition are realistic and helpful. This has to be kept in mind when the patient is provided with an explanation. It may need to be addressed through patient education at a later stage (Petty & Barnard 2017, Chapter 8).
- It identifies whether the reason for referral stated in the referral letter corresponds with the patient's reason for attending. For example, a patient may ask for an explanation of the symptoms and not wish to have a treatment.
- It explores to what extent patients' symptoms are problematic to them in their day-to-day activities

TABLE 2.1	
Summary of Subjective Examination	
	Information Gained
Getting to know the patient	Patient expectations, beliefs, identifying their perspective
Social context	Age and gender, home and work situation, dependants and leisure activities
Body chart	Type and area of current symptoms, depth, quality, intensity, abnormal sensation, relationship of symptoms
Behaviour of symptoms	Aggravating factors, easing factors, severity and irritability of the condition, 24-hour behaviour, daily activities, stage of the condition
Special questions on family history	General health, drugs, steroids, anticoagulants, recent unexplained weight loss, rheumatoid arthritis, spinal cord or cauda equina symptoms, dizziness, recent radiographs
Past medical history	Relevant medical history, previous episodes, effect of previous treatment
History of present condition	History of each symptomatic area – how and when it started, how it has changed

Data from Nicholas, M., Linton, S., Watson, P., & Main, C. (2016) Early identification and management of psychosocial risk factors ('Yellow Flags') in patients with low back pain: a reappraisal. Physical Therapy (2016) 91(5):737–753.

and so can assist in identifying what their expectations and goals are of attending for physiotherapy.

In order to identify to what extent patients' symptoms are problematic to them, the therapist may use brief screening questions such as the following (Aroll et al. 2003; Barker et al. 2014):

- In the past month, has your pain been bad enough to stop you doing many of your day-to-day activities?
- In the past month, has your pain been bad enough to make you feel worried or low in mood?

Social History

Social history is often very relevant to the onset and progression of the patient's problem. This includes the patient's age, employment, home situation and details of any leisure activities. In order to treat appropriately, it is important that the condition is viewed within the context of the patient's social and work environment.

Body Chart

A body chart (Fig. 2.3) is an efficient way of recording information about the area and type of symptoms the patient is experiencing. Its completion early on in the examination ensures that the clinician has an appreciation of the type and extent of the patient's symptoms, thereby facilitating more focused questioning and allowing more experienced clinicians to use pattern recognition reasoning. It can also reassure patients that the clinician is interested and listening to their story.

Area of Current Symptoms

The clinician is advised to be exact in mapping out the area of the symptoms. Although the most common symptom of musculoskeletal dysfunction is pain, it must not be assumed to be the only presenting symptom. Patients often report a range of symptoms, e.g. crepitus, clicking, locking. It is important to use the words chosen by patients to identify their symptoms, e.g. an ache, a catch, in order to avoid confusion and reinforce that the clinician is actively listening. A clear demarcation between areas of pain, paraesthesia (abnormal sensation), stiffness and weakness can help to distinguish symptoms and the clinician can then establish how they interrelate. Conversely, no clear pattern may emerge and this may have consequences for the clinician's reasoning and planning of the examination (see Chapter 3 and Petty & Barnard 2017, Chapter 8 Understanding and managing persistent pain).The area of the symptoms does not always identify the structure at fault, since symptoms can be felt in one area but emanate from a distant area. For example, pain felt in the elbow may be locally produced, or may be due to pathology in the cervical spine, the shoulder or the radial nerve (see the section on referred pain, below).

Asking patients to identify which symptom troubles them most (if more than one area) can help to focus the examination to the most important areas and to prioritize treatment.

In addition, patients are asked where they feel the symptoms are coming from: 'If you had to put your

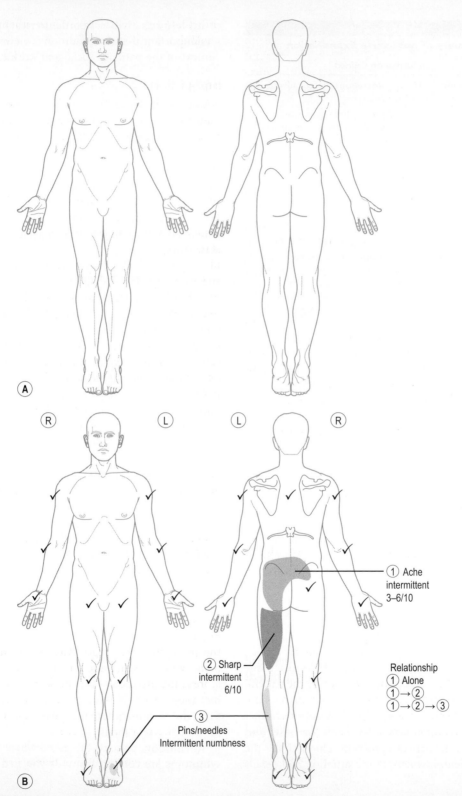

FIG. 2.3 ■ (A) Blank body chart. (B) Example of a completed body chart. *(Redrawn from Grieve 1991, with permission.)*

finger on one spot where you feel it is coming from, where would you put it?' When the patient is able to do this, it can help to pinpoint the source of the symptoms, although careful reasoning is needed in interpreting this information, as it may simply be an area of pain referral.

Areas Relevant to the Region Being Examined

All other relevant areas are checked for the presence of any symptoms and any unaffected areas are marked with ticks (✓) on the body chart. It is important to remember that the patient may describe only the worst symptom, not thinking that it is important to mention lesser or different symptoms, even though this may be highly relevant to the understanding of the patient's condition. The cervical and thoracic spinal segments can, for example, give rise to referred symptoms in the upper limb; and the lumbar spine and sacroiliac joints can give rise to referred symptoms in the lower limb. Quite frequently patients present with classical signs and symptoms of a peripheral condition such as tennis elbow, but on examination the symptoms are found to emanate from the cervical spine, which is confirmed when palpation or other diagnostic tests of the spine either relieve or aggravate the symptoms.

Pain: the Most Common Presenting Symptom

The International Association for the Study of Pain (IASP) defines pain as:

> *An unpleasant sensory and emotional experience associated with actual or potential tissue damage, or described in terms of such damage (IASP 2015).*

This definition highlights the complexity of pain and makes it clear that pain always has an emotional aspect. It also demonstrates that pain does not require tissue damage, even if it is experienced as such by the patient. Pain may be widespread or focal. It may or may not follow an anatomical distribution. It is important that clinicians recognize that pain is a subjective phenomenon that is different for each individual. Pain has many dimensions, as shown in Fig. 2.4. It is therefore difficult to estimate the extent of another person's psychological and emotional experience of pain.

Quality of the Pain

The clinician asks the patient: 'How would you describe your pain?' The adjectives patients use to describe their pain may be of an emotional rather than a physical nature, such as torturous, miserable or terrifying, which may provide insight into the way they experience their pain. Descriptions of the pain, such as burning, sharp, stabbing, can assist identification of the physiological mechanism involved. This, along with the location and behaviour of symptoms, may assist in determining the structures at fault. An understanding of the neurobiological mechanisms responsible for pain can help to formulate a treatment approach specifically targeting these mechanisms (Woolf 2004). Peripheral origins of pain can be either nociceptive or neuropathic, and pain may be enhanced by central sensitization (Box 2.2; see Petty & Barnard 2017, Chapter 8). Please note that numerous factors can cause or influence pain, such as a lesion of the central nervous system, altered activity of the sympathetic nervous system or psychological state. Further information can be found in Chapter 8 of Petty and Barnard (2017).

Recording Pain Intensity

Pain intensity can be measured using numerical or visual analogue rating scales (Hinnant 1994). These are outlined in Fig. 2.5.

To complete the numerical rating scales, the patient is asked to indicate the number which best describes the intensity of their pain. Typically the numbers are presented on an 11-point Likert scale ranging from 0 to 10. The anchor on the left is 0, representing an absence of pain, while 10 on the right represents the worst imaginable pain. For the visual analogue scale (VAS), patients are asked to mark on a 100-mm line the point that best represents the intensity of their pain, with the same anchors at 0 and 100. The VAS score is the distance of the mark from 0. The requirements of a line that is exactly 100 mm long and measurement in millimeters can make a numerical scale more practical for clinical use.

The clinician has to be clear and consistent when asking the patient to fill in a pain score, especially if

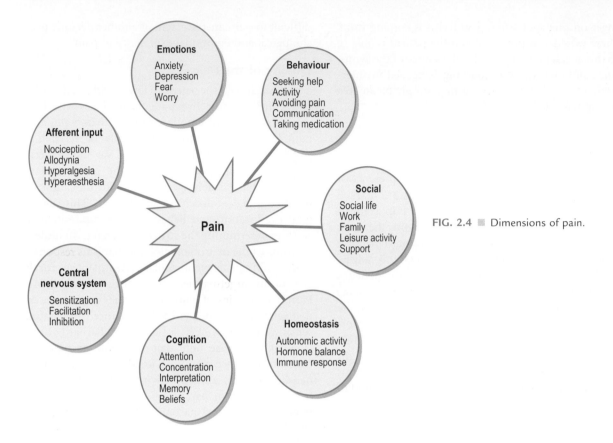

FIG. 2.4 ■ Dimensions of pain.

comparison is to be made at a later date. For example, it must be clear whether the patient is asked about the pain on that day, on average, or at its worst. Some clinicians ask patients to score their pain at its best as well as its worst to establish a range. A set of pain-rating scales developed by the British Pain Society (2014) asks patients to score their pain on the day, but also on average over the last week. The set also includes scales for distress associated with the pain (on the day and on average), the level of interference with activities and the effectiveness of previous treatment. It is available as a free download in multiple languages.

Pain scales are not interchangeable, i.e. someone who marks pain at 80 mm on the VAS will not necessarily give the pain a description of 8 out of 10 on the numerical scale. As a consequence a score can only be compared with another score on the same scale. The pain intensity score can be repeated several times a day or over a period of treatment as part of a pain diary. This can then be used to construct a pain profile from

which the behaviour of pain, or the effectiveness of a treatment for pain, can be judged. There is however recognition that measuring a range of different domains to include condition-specific function, generic health status, work disability, patient satisfaction as well as pain is important in eval2uating interventions in patients with persistent problems (Bombadier 2000; Strong & van Griensven 2013).

Referred Pain

Pain which is felt distant to the tissue in which it originates is known as referred pain. The more proximal the source of the pain, the more extensive is the possible area of referral. For example, the zygapophyseal joints in the lumbar spine can refer symptoms to the foot (Mooney & Robertson 1976), the hip joint typically refers symptoms no further than the knee, whereas the joints of the foot tend to produce local symptoms. Referred pain is thought to be the consequence of the convergence of sensory neurons on to a common

BOX 2.2
PAIN CHARACTERISTICS

NOCICEPTIVE PAIN

Pain that arises from actual or threatened damage to non-neural tissue and is due to the activation of nociceptors (IASP 2015). It can be subdivided into mechanical, inflammatory and ischaemic causes.

Mechanical	Inflammatory	Ischaemic
Localized intermittent pain	Constant/varying pain	Usually intermittent
Predictable consistent response to mechanical stimuli, e.g. stretch, compression or movement	Worsened rapidly by movement	Predictable pattern – aggravated by sustained postures and/ or repetitive activities
	Latent pain	
	Night pain and pain on waking	
	High irritability and severity	
No pain on waking but pain on rising	Movements limited by pain	Eased by change of position or by cessation of a repetitive activity
Usually mild to moderate severity	Responds to non-steroidal anti-inflammatory drugs (NSAIDs)	
Responds to simple painkillers		

(van Griensven 2014)

PERIPHERAL NEUROPATHIC PAIN

Pain caused by a lesion or disease of the somatosensory nervous system (IASP 2015). The mere presence of certain symptoms or signs suggestive of neuropathy (e.g. touch-evoked pain) does not justify the use of the term *neuropathic* (IASP 2015). Please note that neuropathic pain may also be due to a lesion or disease in the central nervous system (for instance, after a spinal cord lesion or stroke), in which case it is called *central* neuropathic pain.

- Neuroanatomical distribution, i.e. along a spinal segment or peripheral/cranial nerve pathway/course
- Typical descriptions include burning, sharp, shooting, electric shock-like, although neuropathic pain can manifest in many different ways
- May manifest as allodynia (pain provoked by stimuli that are normally innocuous), paraesthesia (abnormal sensation), dysaesthesia (painful paraesthesia), hypoaesthesia, hyperaesthesia, possibly a mixture of these
- Provoked by nerve stretch, compression (Phalen's test) or palpation (Tinel's test)
- Possible associated hypoaesthesia or analgesia (partial or complete sensory loss), muscle weakness and autonomic changes

- Poor response to simple analgesia and anti-inflammatory medication
- Response to passive treatment varies

(Hansson & Kinnman 1996; Cook & van Griensven 2013)

CENTRAL SENSITIZATION

Increased responsiveness of nociceptive neurons in the central nervous system to their normal or subthreshold afferent input (IASP 2015). This can develop as part of any persistent pain condition and be a consequence of ongoing nociceptive or neuropathic input: 'The following symptoms may suggest central sensitisation, but have to be interpreted with caution.'

- Widespread, non-anatomical distribution
- Hyperalgesia (increased sensitivity to pain), allodynia evident
- Inconsistent response to stimuli and tests
- Patients have difficulty in locating and describing their pain
- Pain seems to have 'a mind of its own'
- Simple analgesics are ineffective
- Unpredictable or failed response to passive treatments

(Woolf 2012; van Griensven 2015)

AUTONOMIC

Although the sympathetic nervous system is an afferent system, it can have an indirect impact on pain systems through the release of (nor)adrenaline affecting capillary response and indirectly cortisol inhibiting inflammation. Although this is beneficial to the body in a fight-or-flight situation, long-term elevation of levels of (nor)adrenaline and cortisol can lead to poor tissue quality and reduced immune response. Recognition of autonomic system arousal is important so it can be explained to the patient and managed using relaxation techniques, exercise and help with the origins of the patient's stress.

May manifest locally as:
- Discoloration
- Dryness
- Swelling
- Sweating
- Pilo erection

General manifestations may include:
- Palpitations
- Changes in blood pressure
- Hyperhydrosis
- Changes in breathing
- Changes in digestive function
- Muscle tension
- Fatigue
- Poor wound healing

(van Griensven 2005; Hall 2015)

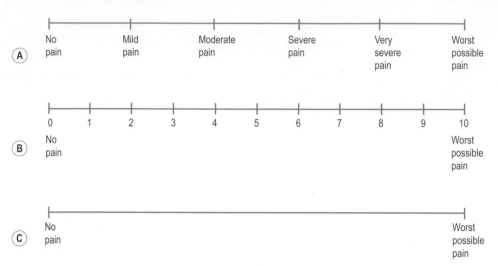

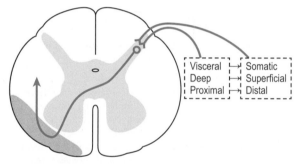

FIG. 2.5 ■ Pain intensity rating scales. (A) Simple descriptive pain intensity scale. (B) 1–10 numerical pain intensity scale. (C) Visual Analogue Scale (VAS). Please note that the VAS must be 100 mm long. *(From Hinnant DW 1994 Psychological evaluation and testing. In Tollison CD (ed.) Handbook of pain management, 2nd edn. Baltimore: Williams & Wilkins. © Williams and Wilkins.)*

FIG. 2.6 ■ Dorsal horn pathways underlying referred pain. Primary neurons from different tissues synapse with a single secondary neuron. Input from the more commonly stimulated neuron (box on the right) is either shared with, or facilitated by, the input from the less commonly stimulated neuron (box on the left) (McMahon 1997). The arrows between the boxes indicate the direction of pain referral.

secondary neuron in the spinal cord (Bogduk 2009). Fig. 2.6 illustrates how afferents from, for instance, viscera or deep somatic structures converge on a secondary neuron which normally receives input mainly from cutaneous regions (McMahon 1997; Arendt-Nielsen et al. 2000). Two theories explain how this may produce pain referral. The *convergence-projection* theory suggests that neurons from both origins stimulate a shared secondary neuron (McMahon 1997). The *convergence-facilitation* theory proposes that the

nociceptive neurons from the visceral or deep somatic tissue do not have a secondary pathway, but that they merely sensitize those that do (McMahon 1997).

Spinal structures such as facet joints, ligaments and discs can also produce somatically referred pain (Bogduk 2009). This type of pain is distinct from either radicular pain, which results from sensitization of the nerve root and has a lancinating quality, and from radiculopathy, in which spinal nerve conduction is blocked (Bogduk 2009). Further questioning about the nature of the pain and neurological symptoms, followed by detailed examination, is essential to distinguish between these types of spinal pain.

Visceral pain may also be referred to somatic tissues, thus generating somatic pain as well as sensitization (Cervero & Laird 2004). Areas of referred symptoms from the viscera are shown in Fig. 2.7 (Lindsay et al. 1997), but it must be remembered that pain from viscera is notoriously diffuse and poorly localized (Al-Chaer & Traub 2002).

Pain is most likely to be referred to tissues innervated by the same segments as pain is 'projected' from the viscera to the area supplied by corresponding somatic afferent fibres (Fig. 2.6). In addition the uterus is capable of referring symptoms to regions innervated by both T10–L2 and S2–S5 (van Cranenburgh 1989). Symptoms referred from the viscera can sometimes be distinguished from those originating in the

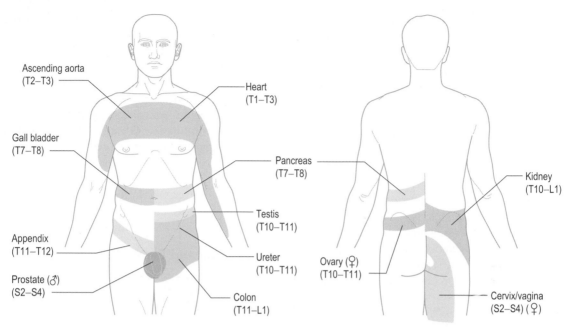

FIG. 2.7 ■ Sites of referred pain from the viscera. *(From Lindsay et al. 1997, with permission.)*

musculoskeletal system when they are not aggravated by activity or relieved by rest, but this is not always the case. The clinician needs to be aware that symptoms can be referred from the spine to the periphery, from the periphery to other peripheral regions or more centrally, from the viscera to the spine, or from the spine to the viscera.

Another potential source of referred musculoskeletal pain is the trigger point, described as an exquisitely tender spot in discrete bands of hardened muscle that produces local and referred pain (Bron & Dommerholt 2012). Although trigger points were originally described as potentially arising in any soft tissue (Travell & Simons 1983), they are now seen as associated with muscle overuse, overactivity or trauma (Dommerholt 2011; Bron & Dommerholt 2012). Commonly found trigger points and their characteristic area of referral can be seen in Fig. 3.36. Examination of suspected trigger points is described in Chapter 3.

Abnormal Sensation

Areas of abnormal sensation are mapped out on the body chart. Abnormal sensations include paraesthesia (abnormal sensation), anaesthesia (complete loss of sensation), hypoaesthesia (reduced touch sensation), hyperaesthesia (heightened perception to touch) and allodynia (pain provoked by stimuli that are normally innocuous). Paraesthesia includes sensations of tingling, pins and needles, swelling, tight bands around part of the body and water trickling over the skin. When painful, it is known as dysaesthesia. Detailed descriptions and definitions can be found on the IASP website (IASP 2015).

The sensory changes listed above can be generated anywhere along a peripheral or cranial nerve, including the nerve root, but also the spinal cord or brain. A common cause for more sensory changes is ischaemia of the nerve, e.g. when part of the brachial plexus is compressed by a cervical rib or when a median nerve compression results in carpal tunnel syndrome. Knowledge of the cutaneous distribution of nerve roots (dermatomes), brachial and lumbosacral plexuses and peripheral nerves enables the clinician to distinguish between the sensory loss resulting from a root lesion and that resulting from a peripheral nerve lesion. Cutaneous innervation areas and dermatomes are shown in Chapter 3 (Figs 3.15–3.18).

Constant or Intermittent Symptoms

The word 'constant' is used here to mean symptoms that are felt unremittingly for 24 hours a day; any relief of symptoms even for a few minutes would mean that the symptoms were intermittent. Some patients describe their pain as constant until asked whether there is time at all when they are without pain. The frequency of intermittent symptoms is important as there may be wide variations, from symptoms being felt once a month to once an hour. Specific details are useful at this stage so that progress can be clearly monitored at subsequent treatment sessions. Constant pain that does not vary is characteristic of serious pathology, e.g. neoplastic disease. Constant pain that varies in intensity may be suggestive of ongoing inflammatory or infective processes. Pain with a consistent response to mechanical forces, for instance as a consequence of certain positions or movements, is suggestive of a nociceptive or tissue-based origin (van Griensven 2014).

Relationship of Symptoms

The question of the relationship of symptomatic areas to each other is very important as it helps to establish links between symptoms and gives clues as to the structure(s) at fault. For example, if posterior leg pain is felt when back pain is made worse, then it suggests that the leg pain and the back pain are being produced by the same structure. If, on the other hand, the symptoms occur separately, so that the patient can have back pain without leg pain and leg pain without back pain, then different structures would be thought to be producing these two symptoms.

This completes the information that can be documented on the body chart. An example of a completed body chart is shown in Fig. 2.3B.

Behaviour of Symptoms

The clinician asks how the symptoms affect the patient's function, e.g. sitting, standing, lying, bending, walking, running, walking on uneven ground, walking up and down stairs, washing, driving, lifting and digging, work, leisure activities and sport, including impact on training. The clinician finds out whether the patient is left- or right-handed/footed as there may be increased stress on the dominant side. Information of how a patient's symptoms behave during normal activities is used to reason the extent of the patient's functional impairment and activity and participation capabilities and restrictions (World Health Organization 2001). The impact on the patient's function and quality of life can be measured using a range of functional outcome measures: some are generic, whilst others are region- or disease-specific, e.g. Roland Morris Questionnaire, Oswestry Disability Index, EQ-5D. Using outcome measures will provide some baseline measures which can be used to measure the impact of any future interventions. Selection of measures must however take into account a range of considerations such as suitability for a particular patient as well as reliability and validity (Kyte et al. 2015).

Aggravating and Easing Factors

Using clinical reasoning to make sense of aggravating and easing information, the clinician can hypothesize the likely underlying reasons for the patient's symptoms, e.g. the structure(s) at fault and judge the severity and irritability of the patient's presentation. This gives valuable information of the extent and the vigour that will be required to reproduce the patient's symptom(s) in the physical examination.

Further questioning can also establish patients' response to their pain and the impact of their coping strategies provides an insight into the relative contribution of personal factors within the framework of functioning, health and disability (World Health Organization 2001).

Aggravating Factors

For each symptomatic area the clinician asks what movements, positions or environmental factors aggravate or reproduce the patient's symptoms. The clinician must analyse in detail the aggravating movement or posture in order to hypothesize what structures may be stressed and possibly causing symptoms. To assist with the clinical reasoning process the clinician can ask the patient about theoretically known aggravating factors for structures that could be hypothesized as a source of the symptoms, e.g. squatting and going up and down stairs for suspected hip and knee problems, and lifting the head to look upwards for cervical spine problems. A list of common aggravating factors for each joint as well as for muscle and neurological tissue can be found in Table 2.2.

TABLE 2.2

Common Aggravating Factors – for Each Region or Structure, Examples of Various Functional Activities and a Basic Analysis of the Activity Are Given

	Functional Activity	Analysis of the Activity
Temporomandibular joint	Yawning	Depression of mandible
	Chewing	Elevation/depression of mandible
	Talking	Elevation/depression of mandible
Headaches	Stress, eye strain, noise, excessive eating, drinking, smoking, inadequate ventilation, odours	
Cervical spine	Reversing the car	Rotation
	Sitting reading/writing	Sustained flexion
Thoracic spine	Reversing the car	Rotation
	Deep breath	Extension
Shoulder	Tucking shirt in	Hand behind back
	Fastening bra	Hand behind back
	Lying on shoulder	Joint compression
	Reaching up	Flexion
Elbow	Eating	Flexion/extension
	Carrying	Distraction
	Gripping	Flexion/extension
	Leaning on elbow	Compression
Forearm	Turning key in a lock	Pronation/supination
Wrist/hand	Typing/writing	Sustained extension
	Gripping	Extension
	Power gripping	Extension
	Power gripping with twist	Ulnar deviation and pronation/supination
	Turning a key	Thumb adduction with supination
	Leaning on hand	Compression
Lumbar spine	Sitting	Flexion
	Standing/walking	Extension
	Lifting/stooping	Flexion
Sacroiliac joint	Standing on one leg	Ipsilateral upward shear, contralateral downward shear
	Turning over in bed	Nutation/counternutation of sacrum
	Getting out of bed	Nutation/counternutation of sacrum
	Walking	Nutation/counternutation of sacrum
Hip	Squat	Flexion
	Walking	Flexion/extension
	Side-lying with painful hip uppermost	Adduction and medial rotation
	Stairs	Flexion/extension
Knee	Squat	Flexion
	Walking	Flexion/extension
	Stairs	Flexion/extension
Foot and ankle	Walking	Dorsiflexion/plantarflexion, inversion/eversion
	Running	Dorsiflexion/plantarflexion, inversion/eversion
Muscular tissue		Contraction of muscle
		Passive stretch of muscle
Nervous tissue		Passive stretch or compression of nervous tissue

How quickly are the patient's symptoms reproduced? The time it takes to bring on the symptoms (or make them worse) indicates how irritable the symptoms are and so how difficult or easy it may be to reproduce the patient's symptoms in the physical examination. For example, knee symptoms that are felt after a 90-minute football match will be harder to reproduce in the clinic than symptoms provoked by climbing a single flight of stairs.

Is the patient able to maintain a position or movement? If symptoms are too severe the patient may report having to stop a particular activity. For example, a patient reporting neurogenic symptoms along the course of the median nerve may be severely limited when using a keyboard due to the mechanosensitivity of the neural tissue.

What happens to other symptoms when this symptom is produced or made worse? This information helps to confirm the relationship between the symptoms. If different symptoms are aggravated by the same position or movement, it suggests that the symptoms are being produced by the same source or structure(s).

Detailed information on each of the above activities is useful in order to help identify functional restrictions and the structure(s) at fault. The most notable functional restrictions are highlighted on the patient's clinical records with asterisks (*), further explored in the physical examination, and can be used as reassessment markers at subsequent treatment sessions to evaluate treatment interventions.

Easing Factors

These are movements, positions and other factors that ease the patient's symptoms.

As with the aggravating factors, the exact movement or posture and the time it takes to ease the symptoms are established. This information helps the clinician judge irritability and therefore how difficult or easy it may be to relieve the patient's symptoms in the physical examination. Symptoms that are readily eased by changes in movement or posture may respond to treatment more quickly than symptoms that are not readily eased. The clinician analyses in detail the easing movement or posture in order to hypothesize which structures are causing the symptoms.

Again, easing factors are determined for each symptomatic area. The effect of the easing of one symptom on the other symptoms is established as this helps to confirm the relationship between symptoms. If different symptomatic areas ease with the same position or movement, it suggests that the symptoms are being produced by the same source or structure.

Coping Strategies

Having established aggravating and easing factors, the clinician must identify whether and how the patient is responding to these in order to manage the condition. For example, the patient may have changed or abandoned activities in response to the symptoms. The clinician must judge whether this accommodation is likely to be helpful or not. Short-term reduction or avoidance of some activities can be an effective strategy to overcome an injury and is therefore known as *adaptive*. On the other hand, avoiding most activities over a longer period of time is recognized as *maladaptive*: it may avoid pain, but also leads to a decline in fitness and functional ability. Maladaptive coping strategies can therefore contribute to and perpetuate the patient's problem and compromise treatment (Harding & Williams 1995; Shorland 1998; Main et al. 2008). Unhelpful coping strategies may include:

■ Activity avoidance, leading to disuse, lack of fitness, strength and flexibility. This may have consequences for the ability to take part in leisure activities and work.
■ Underactivity/overactivity cycles: activity avoidance on days with pain, followed by excessive activity on other days in order to make up for loss of activity. Reduced activity tolerance due to disuse on 'bad' days leads to tissue overload on 'good' days. Over time there may be a gradual increase in pain and decrease in activity.
■ Long-term use of medication may lead to side-effects such as constipation, indigestion, drowsiness. While medication may help to control symptoms, its side-effects are likely to build up over time and interfere with general function and recovery. Moreover, the patient may become drug-dependent.
■ Visiting a range of therapists and specialists in the pursuit of a diagnosis or cure (Butler & Moseley 2003).

■ An unwillingness to take control but persisting with passive and unhelpful coping strategies.

Severity and Irritability of Symptoms

The severity and irritability of symptoms must be determined in order to plan an appropriate, clinically reasoned physical examination (Banks & Hengeveld 2014). Generally, the tests carried out in the physical examination require the patient to move and/or sustain positions that provoke symptoms. Sometimes the intensity of the provoked symptoms is too great for these positions to be sustained, i.e. the patient's symptoms are severe. At other times, the symptoms gradually increase with each movement tested. In this case, the patient's symptoms are said to be irritable and, if not monitored, the physical examination may have to be stopped until the symptoms subside. Before starting the physical examination the clinician must reason whether the patient's symptoms are severe and/or irritable, so that the examination can be carried out in a way that avoids unnecessary exacerbation of the patient's symptoms.

Severity of the Symptoms

The severity of the symptoms is the degree to which symptoms restrict or stop movement and/or function and is related to the intensity of the symptoms (Banks & Hengeveld 2014). For example, the clinician asks a patient with cervical spine symptoms: 'When you are driving your car and you turn your head and you get that sharp pain in your neck, can you stay in that position?' If a movement at a certain point in range provokes symptoms so intense that the movement must be ceased immediately, then the symptoms are defined as severe.

If the symptoms are severe then the patient will not be able to tolerate structures being tested more extensively, such as the application of overpressures or repeated or combined movements. For these patients movements must be performed just short of, or just up to, the first point of symptoms. On the other hand, when symptoms are of low severity the patient will be able to tolerate more extensive testing (Banks & Hengeveld 2014). Severity is often expressed by clinicians as a subjective descriptive measure in terms of being mild, moderate or high.

Irritability of the Symptoms

The irritability of the symptoms refers to the amount of provocation required to produce symptoms, the severity and how long it takes for the provoked symptom to ease (Banks & Hengeveld 2014). When a movement is performed and pain, for example, is produced (or increased) and continues to be present for a period of time, then the symptom(s) are considered to be irritable. Anything more than a few seconds would require a pause between testing procedures, to allow symptoms to return to their resting level. If the symptom disappears as soon as the movement is stopped, then the symptom is considered to be non-irritable.

So the clinician might ask: 'When you turn your head around to the left and feel the sharp pain and then immediately turn your head back, what happens to the sharp pain?' The patient may say the sharp pain eases immediately or report it takes a while to go. If the pain eases immediately, the pain is considered to be non-irritable and physical testing can be more extensive, e.g. all movements could be examined or selected movements could be sustained or repeated. If the symptoms take a few minutes to disappear then the symptoms are irritable and the clinician would, using their clinical reasoning, justify a limited physical examination to avoid making the patient's symptoms worse. The clinician may choose to carry out movements just to the onset of symptom provocation, reduce the number of movements examined and allow a pause for the symptoms to settle after each movement. Alternatively, the clinician may choose to carry out all movements just short of the onset of symptom provocation, so that all movements can be carried out and no pauses are needed.

Occasionally latent irritability may occur, for example, if symptoms are neurogenic in origin, where a movement or position may induce symptoms that are delayed by some minutes and often continue for a considerable length of time. Very clear communication between clinician and patient and careful management are required with these patients to avoid unnecessary exacerbation of their symptoms. Although it is important for clinicians to make a judgement of irritability, it is worth bearing in mind there is an element of subjectivity in this (Barakatt et al. 2009). Patients' symptoms often present as a combination requiring careful reasoning, for example, symptoms may be non-severe but irritable or may be severe but non-irritable or both severe and irritable.

Twenty-Four-Hour Behaviour of Symptoms

Night Symptoms

Questions will be modified depending on the patient's behaviour of symptoms.

- Does the patient have difficulty getting to sleep because of the symptom(s)? Lying may in some way alter the stress on the structure(s) at fault and provoke or ease symptoms. For example, weight-bearing joints such as the spine, sacroiliac joints, hips, knees and ankles have reduced compressive forces in lying compared with upright postures.
- Which positions are most comfortable and uncomfortable for the patient? The clinician can then analyse these positions to help confirm the possible source of symptoms.
- How many and what type of pillows are used by the patient? How are they placed? For example, foam pillows are often uncomfortable for patients with cervical spine symptoms because their size and lack of conformity can create excessive flexed or side-flexed cervical spine resting positions.
- Does the patient use a firm or soft mattress, and has it recently been changed? Alteration in sleeping posture caused by a new mattress is sometimes sufficient to provoke spinal symptoms.
- Is the patient woken by symptoms, and, if so, which symptoms and are they associated with movement, e.g. turning over in bed?
- To what extent do the symptoms disturb the patient at night?
  - How many times in any one night is the patient woken?
  - How many nights in the past week was the patient woken?
  - What does the patient do when woken? For example, can the patient reposition him- or herself or does s/he have to get up?
  - Can the patient get back to sleep?
  - How long does it take to get back to sleep?
- It is useful to be as specific as possible as this information can then be used to judge severity

and irritability as well as consider if lack of sleep may be contributing to the pain state. This information would guide potential treatment priorities and provide a baseline to evaluate response to treatment.

The clinician determines the pattern of symptoms from first thing in the morning through the day and at the end of the day.

Morning Symptoms

What are the patient's symptoms like in the morning immediately on waking before movement? When the patient gets up, what happens to the symptoms? Prolonged morning pain and stiffness that improves minimally with movement suggest an inflammatory process such as rheumatoid arthritis (Magee 2014). Minimal or absent pain with stiffness in the morning is associated with mechanical or degenerative conditions such as osteoarthrosis or cervical spondylosis (Huskisson et al. 1979; Rao et al. 2007).

Evening Symptoms

The patient's symptoms at the beginning of the day are compared with those through to the end of the day. They may depend upon the patient's daily activity levels. Symptoms aggravated by movement and eased by rest generally indicate a mechanical problem of the neuromusculoskeletal system. Symptoms that increase with activity may be due to repeated mechanical stress, an inflammatory process or a degenerative process. Ischaemic symptoms are eased with activity. If symptoms are worse after work compared with when off work, it is important to explore work activities that may be aggravating the symptoms.

Stage of the Condition

Knowing whether the symptoms are getting better, getting worse or remaining static gives an indication of the stage of the condition and helps the clinician to reason a prognosis clinically. Symptoms that are deteriorating tend to take longer to respond to treatment than symptoms that are resolving. It can be helpful to understand the natural history of the conditions under consideration (van Griensven 2005).

Risk Factors for Chronicity

In the first weeks or months, certain aspects of a patient's presentation may suggest that the patient has an increased chance that the acute or subacute pain will become persistent (Box 2.1). These are known as *risk factors* for chronicity. In back pain, psychological and social risk factors have been referred to as *psychosocial yellow flags* (Kendall et al. 1997; Waddell 2004). A list of yellow and other flags is provided in Table 2.3. Risk factors and yellow flags draw the clinician's attention to the possibility of chronicity, but they are not diagnoses or absolute predictors of an individual patient's recovery (Mallen et al. 2007). The clinician is therefore advised to verify whether a patient's risk factors may or may not be relevant to the patient in question. It is equally important not to give up on a patient on the basis of risk factors, but to address the issues that may prevent the patient from making a full recovery.

Systematic reviews have identified risk factors in patients with musculoskeletal pain. Some studies have focused on patients with back pain (Pincus et al. 2002) or back and neck pain (Linton 2000), while others have included all musculoskeletal conditions (Mallen et al. 2007). These studies suggest that the following findings may predict poor recovery or poor response to treatment.

Pain-Related Risk Factors

- high levels of pain
- long pain duration
- high number of pain sites
- in back pain: nerve root pain or specific spinal pathology.

Psychological Risk Factors

- anxiety
- depression
- psychological distress
- belief that pain must be avoided
- belief that the pain is work-related
- patient perception that patient's health is poor
- catastrophizing, or an exaggerated negative 'mental set' associated with the pain experience (Sullivan et al. 2001), consisting of a combination of rumination, magnification and a sense of helplessness (Haythornthwaite 2013).

Social Risk Factors

- high levels of disability
- compensation issues (accident-related claims, application for benefits).

If a patient is thought to be at risk of developing persistent pain, it is important to make every effort to optimize pain control. This may include advice, physiotherapy intervention and liaising with the general practitioner or physician regarding prescription medication. In addition, it is important to provide patients with a realistic explanation for their pain and the reassurance that they are expected to recover (Kendall et al. 1997). Patients must be taught active strategies to cope with their symptoms, rather than passive strategies, such as avoidance of all activity (Kendall et al. 1997).

Special Questions

Special questions must always be asked as they help the clinician to identify certain precautions or contraindications to physical examination and/or

TABLE 2.3
Types of Flags (Based on Waddell 2004; Linton & Shaw 2011)

Flag	Nature	Example
Red	Symptoms suggestive of serious pathology	Severe unintended weight loss, progressive neurological symptoms
Orange	Psychiatric symptoms	Clinical depression, personality disorder
Yellow	Psychological and social predictors of chronicity	Unrealistic beliefs regarding nature of the pain, belief that pain must be avoided, compensation claim
Blue	Perceptions about effect of work on pain or health	Belief that work will cause further injury, belief that manager is not supportive
Black	Obstacles to recovery beyond patient and clinician	Work that cannot be adapted, lack of options to return to work, overly solicitous family members

treatment (Table 2.4). The clinician needs to reason clinically regarding the pathology that may be underlying the patient's condition and screen for any features of the patient's presentation that suggest a non-musculoskeletal origin, for example, visceral or systemic conditions (Goodman & Snyder 2013). This is not easy, as in the early stages serious conditions can manifest as a musculoskeletal condition. For example, aortic aneurysms can masquerade as simple backache (Greenhalgh & Selfe 2010). Certainly it is important for clinicians to be aware of the non-linear course of systemic pathology. There are three identified stages: (1) *subclinical stage,* where there are pathological changes in the absence of signs and symptoms; (2) *prodromal stage,* characterized by vague non-specific symptoms with few signs; and (3) *clinical stage,* more easily identifiable because there will be signs and symptoms. Signs and symptoms suggestive of serious potential pathology, such as tumours, infection, fracture or cord/cauda equina compression, are referred to as *red flags.* Red flags have been identified through clinical observation and retrospective analysis. Evidence for the utility of red flags varies and an understanding of how indicative they are of serious pathologies continues to evolve (Greenhalgh & Selfe 2010) (Table 2.5).

It is important to realize that the presence of a single red flag does not usually indicate the presence of a serious pathology but needs to be considered within the context of the whole person, with the clinician questioning and reasoning patient responses. In addition to red flags, clinicians need to be aware of possible red herrings, where there can be misattribution of symptoms by the patient or clinician, leading to reasoning errors (Greenhalgh & Selfe 2004). The subjective examination is identified as being more useful than the physical examination in identifying serious pathology (Deyo et al. 1992). Further information can be obtained from textbooks, for example, Goodman and Snyder (2013) and Greenhalgh and Selfe (2010).

For all patients, the following information is gathered.

General Health

It is important to ascertain the general health of the patient. The clinician must be aware of the impact of patients' lifestyle choices on their health, such as smoking, alcohol intake, use of recreational drugs and levels of physical activity. The clinician asks about any feelings of general malaise or fatigue, fever, nausea or vomiting, stress, anxiety or depression. Feeling unwell or tired is common with systemic, metabolic or malignant disease (Greenhalgh & Selfe 2010).

Weight Loss

Has the patient noticed any recent weight loss? This may be due to the patient feeling unwell, perhaps with nausea and vomiting, especially if pain is severe. The clinician needs to be alert, especially if the patient reports having lost >10% of body weight over a period of 3–6 months, as this level of loss may be indicative of malignant or systemic diseases such as tuberculosis (TB) and human immunodeficiency virus (HIV) (Greenhalgh & Selfe 2010).

Cancer

It is important to ask specifically about a history of cancer. A family history of the disease may be relevant, as some cancers have a strong family history, e.g. breast cancer (Greenhalgh & Selfe 2010). A history of malignant disease which is in remission does not contraindicate physical examination or treatment, although presenting symptoms must be confirmed as musculoskeletal in origin. If, on the other hand, there is active malignancy, then the primary aim of the physical examination will be to clarify whether the presenting symptoms are being caused by the malignancy or whether there is a separate musculoskeletal disorder. If the symptoms are thought to be associated with the malignancy then this will contraindicate most musculoskeletal interventions.

Tuberculosis

With the incidence of TB on the rise, particularly in deprived socioeconomic groups (Bhatti et al. 1995), asking patients about exposure to TB is relevant. The skeletal system is affected in 1–2% of patients who are HIV-negative and 60% of patients who are HIV-positive (Greenhalgh & Selfe 2010). Most extrapulmonary TB presents in the spine at T10–L1 and patients in the early stages may well present with backache. A previous history will also be noted, as TB can remain dormant for 30–40 years.

TABLE 2.4
Precautions to Spinal and Peripheral Passive Joint Mobilizations and Nerve Mobilizations

Aspects of Subjective Examination	Subjective Information	Possible Cause/Implications for Examination and/or Treatment
Body chart	Constant unremitting pain	Malignancy, systemic, inflammatory cause
	Symptoms in the upper limb below the acromion or symptoms in the lower limb below the gluteal crease	Nerve root compression. Carry out appropriate neurological integrity tests in physical examination
	Widespread sensory changes and/or weakness in upper or lower limb	Compression on more than one nerve root, metabolic (e.g. diabetes, vitamin B_{12}), systemic (e.g. rheumatoid arthritis)
Aggravating factors	Symptoms severe and/or irritable	Care in treatment to avoid unnecessary provocation or exacerbation
Special questions	Feeling unwell	Systemic or metabolic disease
	General health:	
	■ History of malignant disease, in remission	Not relevant
	■ Active malignant disease if associated with present symptoms	Contraindicates musculoskeletal treatment, may do gentle maintenance exercises
	■ Active malignant disease not associated with present symptoms	Not relevant
	■ Hysterectomy	Increased risk of osteoporosis
	Recent unexplained weight loss	Malignancy, systemic
	Diagnosis of bone disease (e.g. osteoporosis, Paget's brittle bone)	Bone may be abnormal and/or weakened
	Diagnosis of rheumatoid arthritis or other inflammatory joint disease	Avoid strong direct force to bone, especially the ribs Avoid accessory and physiological movements to upper cervical spine and care with other joints
	Diagnosis of infective arthritis	In active stage immobilization is treatment of choice
	Diagnosis of spondylolysis or spondylolisthesis	Avoid strong direct pressure to the subluxed vertebral level
	Systemic steroids	Osteoporosis, poor skin condition requires careful handling, avoid tape
	Anticoagulant therapy	Increased time for blood to clot. Soft tissues may bruise easily
	Human immunodeficiency virus (HIV)	Check medication and possible side-effects
	Pregnancy	Ligament laxity, may want to avoid strong forces
	Diabetes	Delayed healing, peripheral neuropathies
	Bilateral hand/feet pins and needles and/or numbness	Spinal cord compression, peripheral neuropathy
	Difficulty walking	Spinal cord compression, peripheral neuropathy, upper motor neuron lesion
	Disturbance of bladder and/or bowel function	Cauda equina syndrome
	Perineum (saddle) Anaesthesia/paraesthesia	Cauda equina syndrome
	For patients with cervicothoracic symptoms: dizziness, altered vision, nausea, ataxia, drop attacks, altered facial sensation, difficulty speaking, difficulty swallowing, sympathoplegia, hemianaesthesia, hemiplegia	Cervical artery dysfunction, upper cervical instability, disease of the inner ear
	Heart or respiratory disease	May preclude some treatment positions
	Oral contraception	Increased possibility of thrombosis – may avoid strong techniques to cervical spine
	History of smoking	Circulatory problems – increased possibility of thrombosis
Recent history	Trauma	Possible undetected fracture, e.g. scaphoid

TABLE 2.5			
Updated Hierarchical List of Red Flags (Greenhalgh & Selfe 2010)			
4 Red Flags	3 Red Flags	2 Red Flags	1 Red Flag
>50 years +	<10 and >51 years	11–19 years	Loss of mobility, trips, falls and problems with stairs
History of cancer +	Medical history: Cancer, TB, HIV, or IV drug use, osteoporosis	Weight loss 5–10% of BW (3–6 months)	'Bothersome legs'
Unexplained weight loss +	Weight loss >10% of BW (3–6 months)	Constant progressive pain	Weight loss <5% of BW (3–6 months)
Failure to improve after 1/12 of conservative treatment	Severe night pain	Band-like pain	Smoking
	Loss of sphincter tone and S4	Abdominal pain and changed bowel habit	Systemically unwell Trauma Bilateral pins and needle
	Bladder and bowel symptoms	Inability to lie supine	Previous failed treatment Thoracic pain
	Positive extensor plantar response	Spasm and disturbed gait	Headache Marked articular stiffness

BW, body weight; HIV, human immunodeficiency virus; IV, intravenous; TB, tuberculosis.

Human Immunodeficiency Virus

What is the patient's HIV status? HIV is an acquired disease, affecting the immune system, leaving infected patients vulnerable to serious illnesses; however, they can remain asymptomatic for up to 10 years. HIV is a neurotrophic virus causing demyelination of the central and peripheral nervous system tissues from the early stages of infection. This can result in patients presenting with myelopathies affecting the spine and/or painful sensory peripheral neuropathies producing symptoms in the patient's hands or feet (Goodman & Snyder 2013).

Inflammatory Arthritis

Has the patient ever been diagnosed as having rheumatoid arthritis or reactive arthritis such as ankylosing spondylitis? The clinician also needs to find out if a member of the patient's family has ever been diagnosed as having this disease, as it is hereditary and the patient may be presenting with the first signs. Symptoms vary between individuals but usually patients report an insidious onset associated with feelings of malaise and fatigue. They may well have been referred with diffuse musculoskeletal pain and on questioning report spontaneous swelling of joints, especially of the hands and feet, and morning stiffness that lasts longer than 45 minutes (Goodman & Snyder 2013). If rheumatoid arthritis is suspected then the patient needs to be referred to a rheumatologist. In patients with existing rheumatoid arthritis then care will need to be taken in the physical examination due to the impact of joint erosion and chronic synovitis, especially affecting ligamentous stability of the upper cervical spine.

Cardiovascular Disease

Does the patient have a history of cardiovascular disease, e.g. hypertension, angina, previous myocardial infarction, stroke? Altered haemodynamics is another red flag as vascular pathologies such as deep-vein thrombosis have pain as an initial feature. Clinicians will therefore need to consider whether the symptoms reported raise suspicion of an underlying vascular pathology. Subjectively patients may report exercise-induced non-dermatomal pain which is described as pulsing or throbbing. They may also report feeling weak or fatigued. If the patient does have a history of cardiovascular disease then the clinician will need to ask in more detail about how this is managed, for example, medication and monitoring. If the patient has a pacemaker fitted then s/he will need to be treated at least 3 metres away from pulse short-wave therapy equipment (Watson 2016). (See also Chapters 6 and

7.) For more detail on altered haemodynamics, the reader is directed to Taylor and Kerry (2015).

Respiratory Disease

Does the patient have any condition which affects breathing? If so, how is it managed? Patients with breathing problems may be unable to lie supine or prone due to breathlessness; also their ability to exercise will be limited. Medications such as steroids prescribed for long-term respiratory conditions such as asthma can affect bone health.

Epilepsy

Is the patient epileptic? What type of seizures does s/he have? Is the condition well controlled, are there any specific triggers and when was the last seizure?

Thyroid Disease

Does the patient have a history of thyroid disease? How well is it managed? Thyroid dysfunction is associated with a higher incidence of musculoskeletal conditions such as adhesive capsulitis, Dupuytren's contracture, trigger finger and carpal tunnel syndrome (Cakir et al. 2003).

Diabetes Mellitus

Has the patient been diagnosed as having diabetes? If so, is the diabetes type 1 or 2? How long since diagnosis? How is the diabetes managed? How well controlled is the condition? Patients with diabetes can present with a range of musculoskeletal conditions, such as carpal tunnel syndrome, frozen shoulder and peripheral neuropathy (Greenhalgh & Selfe 2010). Healing of tissues is likely to be slower in the presence of this disease, so impacting on prognosis (Brem & Tomic-Canic 2007).

Osteoporosis

The clinician will need to ask patients if they have osteoporosis as this would be a precaution to physical testing. Osteoporosis is the most prevalent of the metabolic bone diseases; its incidence increases with age, and is especially common in postmenopausal women. Secondary osteoporosis is also seen in patients with endocrine and metabolic disorders such as hypothyroidism and diabetes. Osteoporosis can also be a side-effect of long-term use of some prescribed medications such as steroids and anticonvulsants. Patients can present with episodic acute thoracic/high lumbar pain associated with compression fractures (Goodman & Snyder 2013). They may not have been diagnosed, so clinicians need to identify risk factors to inform their clinical reasoning and refer on if they have concerns.

Neurological Symptoms

Has the patient experienced any neural tissue symptoms such as tingling, pins and needles, pain, weakness or hypersensitivity? The clinician must clinically reason whether symptoms are likely to be upper motor neuron (UMN) from the central nervous system in origin or lower motor neuron from the peripheral nervous system. For spinal conditions, gathering the following information will assist with reasoning:

▪ Has the patient experienced symptoms of spinal cord compression (i.e. compression of the spinal cord that runs from the foramen magnum to L1)? This can occur at any spinal level, but most commonly occurs in the cervical spine, often as a result of spinal stenosis, resulting in cervical myelopathy. Typical symptoms, including pain, neck stiffness, paraesthesia, weakness, clumsiness, disequilibrium, difficulty with bladder control and functional deficits, and signs, including decreased cervical range of motion, sensory abnormalities, weakness, spasticity and gait disturbance, become more obvious as the disease progresses (Salvi et al. 2006). Metastatic disease may also be a cause of cord compression with severe pain, often described as band-like, around the trunk as a significant presenting feature (Greenhalgh & Selfe 2010). Recent onset of spinal cord compression would require a prompt referral to a medical practitioner. Reporting of these symptoms would indicate neurological integrity tests in the physical examination.

▪ Clinicians screen patients for cauda equina syndrome, usually caused by prolapsed intervertebral disc or metastatic disease. Compression of the conus medullaris at the level of L1–L2 produces sensory and motor neural problems, the most significant of which is irreversible bladder and bowel dysfunction (Greenhalgh &

Selfe 2010). Patients are asked if they have bladder or bowel sphincter disturbance, which could include retention, loss of control (incontinence), hesitancy, urgency or a sense of incomplete evacuation. Does the patient have any altered sensation (anaesthesia/paraesthesia) around the anus, perineum or genitals? Patients may be embarrassed answering such questions, so the clinician may want to explain why this information is important. Patients are asked about bilateral symptoms of their legs such as heaviness and gait disturbance. These symptoms must be clinically reasoned in the light of any associated back pain as well as coexisting conditions and medications such as amitriptyline, which may provide an alternative explanation for alterations in bladder or bowel function. Cauda equina syndrome is relatively rare but if suspected is defined as a surgical emergency, with early spinal decompression producing the most successful outcomes. Clinicians need to remain vigilant and have a pathway protocol in place so that patients can be managed quickly and appropriately (Greenhalgh & Selfe 2010).

Neuropathic Pain Symptoms

Neuropathic pain is pain caused by a lesion or disease of the somatosensory nervous system (IASP 2015). If the clinician suspects that the patient's pain may be of a neuropathic nature, validated neuropathic screening tools may be helpful. These tools enable the clinician to score the patient's signs and symptoms in a systematic way. Commonly used screening tools are the Leeds Assessment of Neuropathic Symptoms and Signs (LANSS), the Neuropathic Pain Questionnaire (NPQ), Douleur Neuropathique en 4 questions (DN4), painDETECT and ID-Pain. For a review of these tools, see Bennett et al. (2007). LANSS and DN4 include a few simple physical tests such as brush allodynia and raised pinprick threshold.

Joint Hypermobility Syndrome (JHS)

Has the patient been diagnosed with JHS? Patients with JHS may present with widespread diffuse pain, whilst also reporting a range of symptoms such as clunking, clicking, stiffness and tiredness (Simmonds

& Keer 2007). If JHS is suspected, five simple questions can help to identify this syndrome subjectively (Hakim & Grahame 2003):

1. Can you now (or could you ever) place your hands flat on the floor without bending your knees?
2. Can you now (or could you ever) bend your thumb to touch your forearm?
3. As a child, did you amuse your friends by contorting your body into strange shapes or could you do the splits?
4. As a child or teenager, did your kneecap or shoulder dislocate on more than one occasion?
5. Do you consider yourself 'double-jointed'?

Positive answers to these questions have to be clinically reasoned in the context of the patient's presenting symptoms and explored in the physical examination.

Cervical Artery Dysfunction

Early features of cervical artery dysfunction can mimic a musculoskeletal pain presentation as patients often present with neck pain and unusual or severe headaches. The clinician needs to screen for cervical artery dysfunction, e.g. vertebral artery insufficiency due to dissection, asking about a history of exposure to trauma or infection (Thomas 2016). Follow-up questions seek detailed information about any features indicating ischaemia, such as visual disturbance, balance or gait disturbance, speech difficulties or limb weakness or paraesthesia. A clinical pattern may emerge just from the subjective history that does not fit a typical musculoskeletal pattern, which will raise the clinician's suspicion of a more serious underlying pathology. For further information the reader is directed to Rushton et al. (2014) and Chapter 6.

Drug Therapy

There are a series of questions about medication that can inform the clinical reasoning process:

1. Has the patient been on long-term medication/steroids? High doses of corticosteroids for a long period of time can weaken the skin and cause osteoporosis. In this case, the patient requires careful handling and avoidance of the use of tape so that the skin is not damaged. Owing to

the raised likelihood of osteoporosis, strong direct forces to the bones may be inadvisable. Long-term use of medication may lead to side-effects such as constipation, indigestion and drowsiness as well as perhaps causing the patient to become drug-dependent. This may interfere with the patient's general function and hinder recovery.

2. Has the patient been taking anticoagulants? If so, care is needed in the physical examination in order to avoid trauma to tissues and consequent bleeding.

3. Has drug therapy been prescribed for the patient's musculoskeletal problem or is the patient self-medicating with over-the-counter preparations? This can give useful information about the pathological process and may affect treatment. For example, the strength of any painkillers may indicate the intensity of the patient's pain. The World Health Organization three-step analgesic ladder recommends suitable analgesia based on the level and underlying mechanism of a patient's pain (Vargas-Schaffer 2010). For a comprehensive account of pain pharmacology the reader is directed to Smith and Muralidharan (2014). Care may be needed if the patient attends for assessment/treatment soon after taking painkillers as the pain may be temporarily masked and assessment/treatment may cause exacerbation of the patient's condition. In addition, the clinician needs to be aware of any side-effects of the drugs taken. The clinician must continue to monitor medication use and be prepared to discuss a patient's medication with medical colleagues.

Radiographs, Medical Imaging and Tests

Has the patient been X-rayed or had any other medical tests? If so, what did they reveal and what does the patient understand about what s/he has been told? Plain radiographs are useful to diagnose fractures, arthritis and serious bone pathology such as infection, osteoporosis or tumour. Imaging can provide useful additional information but the findings must be correlated with the patient's clinical presentation. This is particularly true for spinal radiographs, which may reveal normal age-related degenerative changes of the spine that do not necessarily correlate with the patient's symptoms (Brinjikji et al. 2015). There is evidence that imaging results can negatively affect patients' sense of well-being. Imaging reports can contribute to persistent pain if patients are not also provided within the context of normal epidemiological data (McCullough et al. 2012). For this reason, routine spinal radiographs are no longer considered necessary for non-traumatic spinal pain (NICE guidelines low back pain and sciatica in over 16s assessment and management (2016)). Other imaging techniques include computed tomography, magnetic resonance imaging, myelography, discography, bone scans and arthrography. The results of these tests can help to determine the nature of the patient's condition but are requested only when based on sound reasoning and clinically indicated. Further details of these tests and their diagnostic value can be found in Goodman and Snyder (2013).

In addition, has the patient had any other investigations such as blood tests? Full blood count will provide information on numbers of red and white blood cells and platelets results outside normal ranges could indicate a number of different conditions, so is useful as an initial screening test. This can be followed with more specific tests such as erythrocyte sedimentation rate, a useful indicator of serious pathology, for example, malignant myelomas and TB. A C-reactive protein blood test is commonly used to detect inflammatory diseases and infection (Greenhalgh & Selfe 2010).

Past Medical History

The following information is obtained from the patient and/or medical notes:

■ Details of any medical history such as major or long-standing illnesses, accidents or surgery that are relevant to the patient's condition.

Family History

The clinician asks about any relevant family history that may indicate a patient's predisposition for the development of a condition, as will become evident in the special questions below, as many conditions have a genetic predisposition. In addition, an understanding of the family history may help to explain a patient's perceptions of the problem.

History of the Present Condition

This is often discussed earlier in the initial examination but it is useful to revisit again towards the end of the subjective examination once the clinician has more information about the symptoms the patient is presenting with. For each symptomatic area, the clinician ascertains:

- how long the symptom has been present
- whether there was a sudden or slow onset of the symptom
- whether there was a known or unknown cause that provoked the onset of the symptom, i.e. trauma or change in lifestyle that may have triggered symptoms
- whether the patient has sought any treatment already and, if so, what type of treatment and to what effect
- whether the patient feels the symptoms are getting better, worse or staying the same.

These questions give the clinician information about the possible cause of the patient's presenting symptoms.

- To confirm the relationship of symptoms, the clinician asks when each symptom began in relation to others. If, for example, the low-back pain started 5 weeks ago and increased a week ago when posterior thigh pain developed, this would suggest that the back and thigh pain are associated and that the same structures may well be at fault. If there was no change in the back pain when the thigh pain began, the symptoms may not be related and different structures may be producing the two pain areas.
- History of any previous symptoms, e.g. the number and duration of previous episodes, when they occurred, possible causes and whether the patient fully recovered between episodes. If there have been no previous episodes, has the patient experienced other symptoms such as stiffness which may have been a precursor to the development of pain?
- Has the patient had treatment previously? If so, what type? What was the outcome of any past treatments for the same or a similar problem? Past treatment records, if available, may then be obtained for further information. It may well be the case that a previously successful treatment modality will be successful again, but establishing the possible reasons for a recurrence will need to be explored.

Plan of the Physical Examination

When relevant information has been collected, the subjective examination is complete. It is useful at this stage for the clinician to reconfirm briefly with the patient their understanding of their main complaint, and to offer them the opportunity to add anything that they may not have had the opportunity to raise so far, before explaining to them the purpose and plan for the physical examination. For ease of reference, highlight with asterisks (*) important subjective findings and particularly one or more functional restrictions. These can then be re-examined at subsequent treatment sessions to evaluate treatment intervention.

A summary of this first part of the patient examination can be found in Fig. 2.8.

In order to plan the physical examination, the hypotheses generated from the subjective examination are tested (Fig. 2.9).

- Are there any contraindications to physical examination that need to be explored further, such as red flags, e.g. neurological involvement, cord compression? Are there any precautions to elements of the physical examination, such as recent fracture, trauma, steroid therapy or rheumatoid arthritis?
- Clinically reasoning throughout the subjective examination using distribution of symptoms, pain mechanisms described, behaviour of symptoms, as well as the history of onset, the clinician needs to decide on structures that could be the cause of the patient's symptoms. The clinician needs a prioritized list of working hypotheses based on the most likely causes of the patient's symptoms – a primary working hypothesis. These may include the structures underneath the symptomatic area, e.g. joints, muscles, nerves and fascia, as well as the regions referring into the area. These possible referring regions will need to be examined as a possible cause of symptoms, e.g. cervical spine, thoracic spine, shoulder

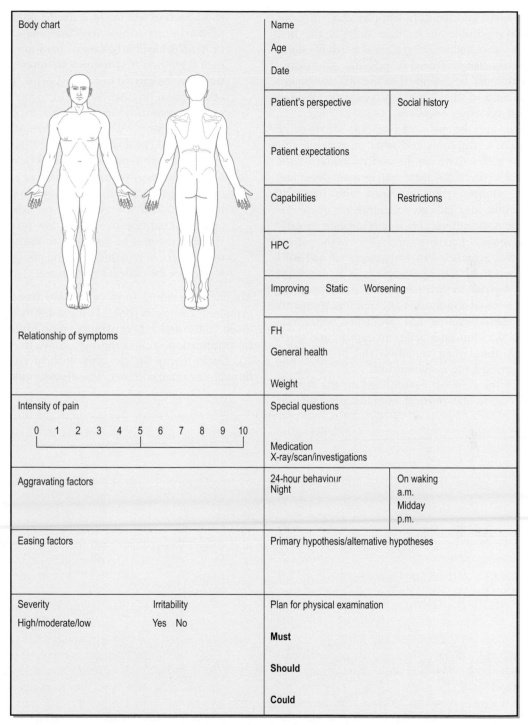

FIG. 2.8 ■ Subjective examination chart. *FH*, family history; *HPC*, history of the present condition.

and wrist and hand. In complex cases it is not always possible to examine fully at the first attendance and so, using clinical reasoning skills, the clinician will need to prioritize and justify what 'must' be examined in the first assessment session, and what 'should' or 'could' be followed up at subsequent sessions.

■ What are the pain mechanisms driving the patient's symptoms and what impact will this information have on an understanding of the problem and subsequent management decisions? For example, pain associated with repetitive activities may indicate inflammatory or neurogenic nociception. This would indicate an early assessment of activities and advice to the patient to pace activities. Patients' acceptance and willingness to be active participants in management will depend on their perspective and subsequent behavioural response to the symptoms. If patients are demonstrating fear avoidance behaviours then the clinician's ability to explain and teach them about their condition will be pivotal to achieving a successful outcome.

■ Once the clinician has decided on the tests to include in the physical examination, the next consideration will be: how do the physical tests need to be carried out? Are symptoms severe and/ or irritable? Will it be easy or hard to reproduce each symptom? If symptoms are severe, physical tests may be carried out to just before the onset of symptom production or just to the onset of symptom production; further stressing of tissues, e.g. overpressures, will not be carried out, as the patient would be unable to tolerate this. If symptoms are irritable, physical tests may be examined to just before symptom production or just to the onset of provocation, with fewer physical tests being examined to allow for rest periods between tests. Alternatively, in cases of low severity and irritability, will it be necessary to use combined movements, or repetitive movements, in order to reproduce the patient's symptoms?

A clinical reasoning form (Fig. 2.10) based on the hypothesis categories (Box 2.1) suggested by Jones and Rivett (2004) and a short planning form for the physical examination, such as the ones shown in Appendix 2.1, can be useful for clinicians to help guide them through the often complex clinical reasoning process.

APPENDIX 2.1 CLINICAL REASONING FORMS

Physical examination planning sheet (short version)

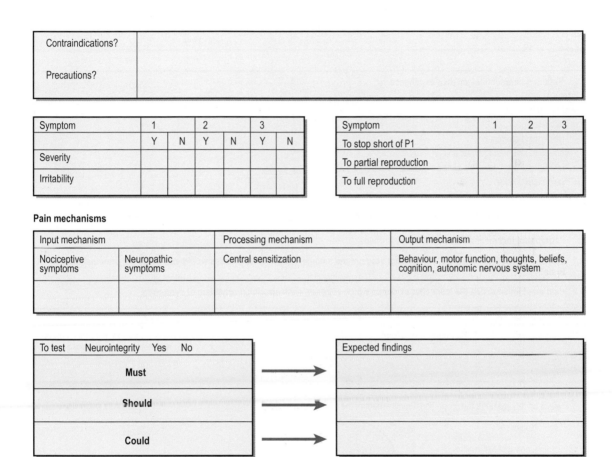

FIG. 2.9 ■ Physical examination planning sheet (short version).

Clinical Reasoning From Using hypothesis categories Jones & Rivett 2004.

1. Activity and participation capabilities/restrictions

Activity capability	Restriction
Participation capability	Restriction

2. Patient's perspectives on their experience
Examples:
- Their understanding
- Their feelings
- Their coping strategies
- Attitude to self-management and physical activity
- Their beliefs/what does this experience mean to them?
- Their expectations
- Their goals

3. Pathobiological mechanisms

3.1 Tissue sources/tissue healing, e.g., at what stage of the inflammatory healing process would you judge the principal disorder to be?

3.2 Pain mechanisms. List the subjective evidence which supports each specific mechanism of symptoms

Input mechanism		Processing mechanism	Output mechanism
Nociceptive symptoms	Neuropathic symptoms	Central sensitization	Behaviour, motor function, thoughts, beliefs, cognition, autonomic nervous system

Reflect on this pie chart the proportional involvement of the pain mechanisms

Nociceptive
Peripheral neuropathic
Central sensitization
Autonomic nervous system

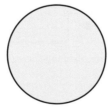

4. The sources of the symptoms
List in order of likelihood the possible structures at fault for each area/component of symptoms

Tissue sources	Symptom 1:	Symptom 2:	Symptom 3:	Symptom 4:
Local				
Referred				
Neurogenic				
Vascular				
Visceral				

FIG. 2.10 Clinical reasoning form.

5.   **Contributing factors**

Examples:
- Physical
- Environmental
- Psychosocial
- Health related

6.   **History of symptoms**

Onset/physical impairment/stage/implications for physical examination

7.   **List for each area of symptoms**

	Aggravating activity	Time to aggravate	Stops the activity	Easing the activity	Time to ease	Irritability Yes/No	Severity Yes/No
Symptoms 1 (P_a)							
Symptoms 2 (P_a)							

8.   **Give an indication of the proportion of inflammatory to mechanical components in this patient's pain presentation, together with the clinical features that support or negate your hypothesis**

Mechanical   Inflammatory

Justification		Justification

9.   **Health considerations, precautions and contraindications to physical examination and management**

9.1   **Does the patient have any health, red flag or precaution to limit your physical examination?**

Consider the following in relation to red flags

9.2   **Is reproduction of symptoms easy or difficult to reproduce? How vigorously would you examine this patient for each area of symptoms?**

Symptom	Short of P_1	To P_1 only	25% reproduction of pain	Full reproduction of pain
P_1				
P_2				
P_3				

9.3   **Will a neurological integrity examination be necessary**

Yes   No
Justify your decision

FIG. 2.10, cont'd

10. Indicate your primary (working) hypothesis (H1) regarding the cause of the patient's complaint and identify evidence to support this decision

Primary hypothesis (H1)	Alternative H2	Alternative H3	Alternative H4	Alternative H5
Evidence:				

To test	Neurointegrity	Yes	No		Expected findings
	Must			→	
	Should			→	
	Could			→	

FIG. 2.10, cont'd

REFERENCES

Al-Chaer, E., Traub, R., 2002. Biological basis of visceral pain: recent developments. Pain 96, 221–225.

Arendt-Nielsen, L., et al., 2000. Referred pain as an indicator for neural plasticity. In: Sandkühler, J., et al. (Eds.), Nervous system plasticity and chronic pain. Elsevier, Amsterdam, pp. 344–356.

Aroll, B., et al., 2003. Screening for depression in primary care with two verbally asked questions: cross sectional study. Br. Med. J. 327, 1144–1146.

Banks, K., Hengeveld, E., 2014. The Maitland concept as a clinical practice framework for neuromusculoskletal disorders. In: Hengeveld, E., Banks, K. (Eds.), Maitland's vertebral manipulation. Churchill Livingstone, Edinburgh (chapter 1).

Barakatt, E., et al., 2009. The reliability of Maitland's irritability judgements in patients with low back pain. J. Man. Manip. Ther. 17, 135–140.

Barker, C., et al., 2014. Problematic pain – redefining how we view pain? Br. J. Pain 8, 9–15.

Barrows, H.S., Feltovich, P., 1987. The clinical reasoning process. Med. Educ. 21, 86–91.

Bennett, M., et al., 2007. Using screening tools to identify neuropathic pain. Pain 127, 199–203.

Bhatti, N., et al., 1995. Increasing incidence of tuberculosis in England and Wales: a study of the likely causes. Br. Med. J. 310, 967–969.

Bogduk, N., 2009. On the definitions and physiology of back pain, referred pain, and radicular pain. Pain 147, 17–19.

Bombadier, C., 2000. Outcome assessments in the evaluation of treatment of spinal disorders: summary and general recommendations. Spine 25, 3100–3103.

Brem, H., Tomic-Canic, M., 2007. Cellular and molecular basis of wound healing in diabetes. J. Clin. Invest. 117, 1219–1222.

Brinjikji, W., et al., 2015. Systematic literature review of imaging features of spinal degeneration in asymptomatic populations. AJNR Am. J. Neuroradiol. 36, 811–816.

British Pain Society, 2014. www.britishpainsociety.org.

Bron, C., Dommerholt, J., 2012. Etiology of myofascial trigger points. Curr. Pain Headache Rep. 16, 439–444.

Butler, D., Moseley, L., 2003. Explain pain. Neuro Orthopaedic Institute, Adelaide.

Cakir, M., et al., 2003. Musculoskeletal manifestations in patients with thyroid disease. Clin. Endocrinol. (Oxf) 59, 162–167.

Cervero, F., Laird, J., 2004. Referred visceral hyperalgesia: from sensations to molecular mechanisms. In: Brune, K., Handwerker, H. (Eds.), Hyperalgesia: molecular mechanisms and clinical implications. IASP Press, Seattle, pp. 229–250.

Cook, N., van Griensven, H., 2013. Neuropathic pain and complex regional pain syndrome. In: van Griensven, H., et al. (Eds.), Pain. A textbook for health professionals, 2nd ed. Churchill Livingstone, Edinburgh, pp. 137–158.

Deyo, R.A., et al., 1992. What can the history and physical examination tell us about low back pain? J. Am. Med. Assoc. 268, 760–765.

Dommerholt, J., 2011. Dry needling – peripheral and central considerations. J. Man. Manip. Ther. 19, 223–237.

Edwards, I., et al., 2004. Clinical reasoning strategies in physical therapy. Phys. Ther. 84, 312–330.

Edwards, I., et al., 2006. The interpretation of experience and its relationship to body movement: a clinical reasoning perspective. Man. Ther. 11, 2–10.

Gask, L., Usherwood, T., 2002. ABC of psychological medicine. The consultation. Br. Med. J. 324, 1567–1569.

Goodman, C., Snyder, T., 2013. Differential diagnosis for physical therapists screening for referral, 5th ed. Elsevier, St Louis.

Goodrich, J., Cornwell, J., 2008. Seeing the person in the patient. The Point of Care review. The King's Fund, London.

Greenhalgh, S., Selfe, J., 2004. Margaret, a tragic case of spinal red flags and red herrings. Physiotherapy 90, 73–76.

Greenhalgh, S., Selfe, J., 2010. Red flags II: a guide to identifying serious pathology of the spine. Elsevier, Edinburgh.

Grieve, G.P., 1991. Mobilisation of the spine, 5th ed. Churchill Livingstone, Edinburgh.

Hakim, A., Grahame, R., 2003. A simple questionnaire to detect hypermobility; and adjunct to the assessment of patients with diffuse musculoskeletal pain. Int. J. Clin. Pract. 57, 163–166.

Hall, J., 2015. Guyton and Hall textbook of medical physiology, 13th ed. Saunders, Edinburgh.

Hansson, P., Kinnman, E., 1996. Unmasking mechanisms of peripheral neuropathic pain in a clinical perspective. Pain Rev. 3, 272–292.

Harding, V., de C. Williams, A.C., 1995. Extending physiotherapy skills using a psychological approach: cognitive-behavioural management of chronic pain. Physiotherapy 81, 681–688.

Haythornthwaite, J., 2013. Assessment of pain beliefs, coping, and function. In: McMahon, S.B., et al. (Eds.), Wall & Melzack's textbook of pain, 6th ed. Saunders, Philadelphia, pp. 328–338.

Henegveld, E., Maitland, G., 2014. Communication in the therapeutic relationship. In: Hengeveld, F., Banks, K. (Eds.), Maitland's vertebral manipulation. Churchill Livingstone, Edinburgh (chapter 3).

Higgs, J., Jones, M. (Eds.), 2000. Clinical reasoning in the health professions, 2nd ed. Butterworth Heinemann, Oxford.

Hinnant, D.W., 1994. Psychological evaluation and testing. In: Tollison, C.D. (Ed.), Handbook of pain management, 2nd ed. Williams & Wilkins, Baltimore.

Huskisson, E.C., et al., 1979. Another look at osteoarthritis. Ann. Rheum. Dis. 38, 423–428.

IASP, 2015. The International Association for the Study of Pain. www.iasp-pain.org.

Jones, M.A., 1995. Clinical reasoning and pain. Man. Ther. 1, 17–24.

Jones, M.A., Rivett, D.A., 2004. Clinical reasoning for manual therapists. Butterworth-Heinemann, Edinburgh.

Jones, M., et al., 2008. Clinical reasoning in physiotherapy. In: Higgs, J., et al. (Eds.), Clinical reasoning in the health professions, 3rd ed. Butterworth Heinemann/Elsevier, Amsterdam, pp. 245–256.

Kendall, N., et al., 1997. Guide to assessing psychosocial yellow flags in acute low back pain. Accident Rehabilitation and Compensation Insurance Corporation and National Advisory Committee on Health and Disability, Wellington, NZ.

Kyte, D., et al., 2015. An introduction to patient reported outcome measures PROMS in physiotherapy. Physiotherapy 101, 119–125.

Lindsay, K.W., et al., 1997. Neurology and neurosurgery illustrated, 3rd ed. Churchill Livingstone, Edinburgh.

Linton, S., 2000. A review of psychological risk factors in back and neck pain. Spine 25, 1148–1156.

Linton, S., Shaw, W., 2011. Impact of psychological factors in the experience of pain. Phys. Ther. 91, 700–711.

Magee, D.J., 2014. Orthopedic physical assessment, 6th ed. Saunders Elsevier, Philadelphia.

Main, C.J., Spanswick, C.C., 2000. Pain management, an interdisciplinary approach. Churchill Livingstone, Edinburgh.

Main, C., et al., 2008. Pain management. Practical applications of the biopsychosocial perspective in clinical and occupational settings, 2nd ed. Churchill Livingstone, Edinburgh.

Mallen, C., et al., 2007. Prognostic factors for musculoskeletal pain in primary care: a systematic review. Br. J. Gen. Pract. 57, 655–661.

McCullough, B., et al., 2012. Lumbar MR imaging and reporting epidemiology: do epidemiologic data in reports affect clinical management? Radiology 262, 941–946.

McMahon, S., 1997. Are there fundamental differences in the peripheral mechanisms of visceral and somatic pain? Behav. Brain Sci. 20, 381–391.

Mooney, V., Robertson, J., 1976. The facet syndrome. Clin. Orthop. Relat. Res. 115, 149–156.

National Institute for Health and Clinical Excellence, 2016. Low back pain and sciatica in the over 16s: Assessment and Management. NICE guideline (NG59).

Petty, N.J., Barnard, K., 2017. Principles of musculoskeletal treatment and management: a handbook for therapists, 3rd ed. Elsevier, Edinburgh.

Pincus, T., et al., 2002. A systematic review of psychological factors as predictors of chronicity/disability in prospective cohorts of low back pain. Spine 27, E109–E120.

Rao, R., et al., 2007. Degenerative cervical spondylosis pathogenesis and management. J. Bone Joint Surg. Am. 89, 1360–1378.

Rivett, D.A., Higgs, J., 1997. Hypothesis generation in the clinical reasoning behavior of manual therapists. J. Phys. Ther. Educ. 11, 40–45.

Rushton, A., et al., 2014. International framework for examination of the cervical region for potential cervical arterial dysfunction prior to orthopaedic manual therapy intervention. Man. Ther. 9, 222–228.

Salvi, F., et al., 2006. The assessment of cervical myelopathy. Spine J. 6, S182–S189.

Shorland, S., 1998. Management of chronic pain following whiplash injuries. In: Gifford, L. (Ed.), Topical issues in pain. Falmouth: Neuro-Orthopaedic Institute UK. pp. 115–134.

Simmonds, J., Keer, R., 2007. Hypermobility and the hypermobility syndrome. Man. Ther. 12, 298–309.

Smith, M., Muralidharan, A., 2014. Pain pharmacology and pharmacological management of pain. In: van Griensven, H., et al. (Eds.), Pain. A textbook for health professionals, 2nd ed. Churchill Livingstone, Edinburgh, pp. 159–180.

Solomon, L., et al., 2001. Apley's system of orthopaedics and fractures, 8th ed. Arnold, London.

Strong, J., van Griensven, H., 2013. Assessing pain. In: van Griensven, H., et al. (Eds.), Pain. A textbook for health professionals, 2nd ed. Churchill Livingstone, Edinburgh, pp. 91–114.

Sullivan, M., et al., 2001. Theoretical perspectives on the relation between catastrophizing and pain. Clin. J. Pain 17, 52–64.

Taylor, A., Kerry, R., 2015. Haemodynamics and clinical practice. In: Jull, G., et al. (Eds.), Grieves modern musculoskeletal physiotherapy, 4th ed. Elsevier, Edinburgh, pp. 347–351.

Thomas, L., 2016. Cervical arterial dissection: an overview and implications for manipulative therapy practice. Man. Ther. 21, 2–9.

Travell, J., Simons, D., 1983. Myofascial pain and dysfunction: the trigger point manual. Williams & Wilkins, Baltimore.

van Cranenburgh, B., 1989. Inleiding in de toegepaste neurowetenschappen, deel 1, Neurofilosofie (Introduction to applied neuroscience, part 1, Neurophysiology), 3rd ed. Uitgeversmaatschappij de Tijdstroom, Lochum.

van Griensven, H., 2005. Pain in practice – theory and treatment strategies for manual therapists. Elsevier, Edinburgh.

van Griensven, H., 2014. Neurophysiology of pain. In: van Griensven, H., et al. (Eds.), Pain. A textbook for health professionals, 2nd ed. Churchill Livingstone, Edinburgh, pp. 77–90.

van Griensven, H., 2015. When pain goes weird: central sensitisation and its implications for physiotherapy practice. In Touch 152, 14–19.

Vargas-Schaffer, G., 2010. Is the WHO analgesic ladder still valid? Twenty-four years of experience. Can. Fam. Physician 56, 514–517.

Waddell, G., 2004. The back pain revolution, 2nd ed. Churchill Livingstone, Edinburgh.

Watson, T. 2016 Electrotherapy on the web. www.electrotherapy.org.

Woolf, C., 2004. Pain: moving from symptom control toward mechanism specific pharmacologic management. Ann. Intern. Med. 140, 441–451.

Woolf, C., 2012. Central sensitisation: implications for the diagnosis and treatment of pain. Pain 152, S2–S15.

World Health Organization, 2001. International classification of functioning, disability and health. World Health Organization, Geneva. http://www.who.int/classifications/icf/en/.

3

PHYSICAL EXAMINATION

DIONNE RYDER ■ HUBERT VAN GRIENSVEN

CHAPTER CONTENTS

INTRODUCTION

The physical examination should not be the indiscriminate application of routine tests, but rather 'should be tailored to each patient's unique presentation' (Jones & Rivett 2004, p. 5).

Following on from the subjective examination the clinician should have already identified a 'must, should and could' plan tailored for the individual patient. Physical testing should be selective, justified through clinical reasoning; the aim being to collect evidence to 'rule in' or 'rule out' possible hypotheses.

The clinician is advised to choose how to approach the physical examination on the basis of the findings of the subjective examination, by considering whether a specific musculoskeletal problem or a broader level of dysfunction is likely to be the main barrier to

recovery. A clear mechanism of injury, consistent behaviour, location of symptoms suggestive of specific physical structures and relatively recent onset favour an approach based on 'ruling in': the clinician focuses on establishing all the tissues and contributing factors involved.

On the other hand, if the problem is widespread, long-standing or has had a significant influence on the patient's overall well-being and function, an approach of 'ruling out' is advocated. In patients with this type of presentation it may not be meaningful to attempt to find a tissue at fault. Not only may persistence and dysfunction have led to a large set of tissues or systems at fault, specific tissue diagnosis may not be helpful in selecting an effective management strategy. The clinician therefore attempts to 'rule out' specific diagnoses suggested by the subjective examination.

35

The aims of the physical examination can be summarized as:

- to determine whether specific structures and/or factors are responsible for producing or maintaining the patient's symptoms
- to get an impression of whether and how function has been affected
- to explore the influence of behavioural aspects of the patient's condition and presentation.

Several factors should be considered in interpreting the findings of physical tests. If symptoms are reproduced (or eased) then there may be an assumption that the test has somehow affected the structures at fault. The word 'structures' is used in its widest sense, and could include anatomical structures or physiological mechanisms. None of the tests stress individual structures in isolation – each test affects a number of tissues, both locally and at a distance. For example, knee flexion will affect the tibiofemoral and patellofemoral intraarticular and periarticular joint structures, surrounding muscles and nerves, as well as joints, muscles and nerves proximally at the hip and spine and distally at the ankle.

If an abnormality is detected in a structure, which theoretically could refer symptoms to the symptomatic area, then that structure is suspected to be a source of the symptoms. Whilst this might be the case, the assessment of referred pain must be demonstrated through the reproduction of local symptoms.

The term 'objective' is sometimes applied to the physical examination. Objective suggests that this part of the examination is not prejudiced and that the tests are valid and reliable, producing robust results. This is certainly misleading as most tests rely on the skill of the clinician to observe, move and palpate the patient.

When interpreting the findings of physical tests it is important to consider the sensitivity and specificity values of the test. This refers to how likely a positive or negative test will rule in or rule out a suspected diagnosis. For example, the sensitivity of the Lachman test to detect tears of the anterior cruciate ligament (ACL) is the proportion of people who will test positive who do have an ACL tear, but some people without a tear may also have a positive response. On the other hand, the specificity of the Lachman test is the ability of the test to identify correctly those without an ACL

tear (true-negative rate). These values relate to the tests alone and not the prevalence of the condition within a given population.

Predictive values can be more valuable than specificity and sensitivity because they predict the likelihood of a positive or negative result within a particular population; for example, sports people playing contact sport are more likely to sustain an ACL tear.

Likelihood ratios (LRs) summarize diagnostic accuracy by combining sensitivity and specificity information. An LR >1 indicates a pathology is present whilst <1 indicates the test result is associated with absence of pathology. Ideally a positive LR of >2 and negative LR <0.5 would indicate a test result is more accurate (Valdes & LaStayo 2013).

The clinician needs to take these factors into account when clinically reasoning a patient's presentation based on the findings of the physical examination. The clinician should collate and clinically reason all the information obtained from the subjective and physical examination in order to make sense of the patient's overall presentation; that is, 'making features fit' (Hengeveld & Banks 2014) and, if features are not fitting a recognized musculoskeletal pattern, then question why that might be. The clinician must therefore keep an open mind to avoid bias, thinking logically throughout the physical examination, reflecting in action using a process of continuous analytical assessment or reasoning. Jumping to conclusions based on the findings of just one or two tests, would result in errors and misattribution of symptoms, resulting in misguided management decisions and poor outcomes.

Key findings of the physical examination are marked with an asterisk (*) as patient-specific reassessment markers to evaluate interventions (Hengeveld & Banks 2014).

For an overview of the physical examination, see Table 3.1.

Clinicians will use their clinical reasoning to alter the order of testing according to the patient and presenting condition. Some tests common to a number of areas of the body, such as posture, muscle tests and neurological examination, are described in this chapter, rather than repeating them in each chapter. More specific regional tests, such as for cervical artery dysfunction, are described in the relevant chapters.

TABLE 3.1
Summary of the Physical Examination

Observation	Informal and formal observation of posture, muscle bulk and tone, soft tissues, gait, function and patient's response
Active physiological movement	Active movements With selective adaptions such as repeated, sustained, in functional/combined positions
Passive physiological movement	Passive movements With selective adaptions such as repeated, sustained, in functional/combined positions Passive physiological accessory movement
Joint integrity tests	For example, knee adduction (varus) and abduction (valgus) stress tests
Muscle tests	Strength, control, length, isometric contraction
Nerve tests	Neurological integrity, neurosensitivity tests, including response to load and nerve palpation
Special tests	Vascular, soft tissue
Palpation	Superficial and deep soft tissues, bone, joint, ligament, muscle, tendon and nerve
Joint tests	Accessory movements to test available glides in a range of directions: anterior/posterior, medial/lateral, caudad/cephalad with selective adaptions to joint position

PHYSICAL EXAMINATION STEP BY STEP

Observation

Initial Observation

The clinician's observation of the patient begins from the moment they first meet. How is the patient moving? A reluctance to move may suggest how the patient is affected both physically and as an individual. Does the patient appear in pain? During the subjective examination, is the patient comfortable or constantly shifting position? It may well be that this informal observation is as informative as the formal assessment, as a patient under such scrutiny may not adopt their usual posture. The clinician can also observe whether the patient is using aids (prescribed or non-prescribed) such as collars, sticks and corsets and whether these aids are being used in an appropriate way.

Informal and formal observation can give the clinician some initial cues:

■ Pathology: for example, local inflammations; e.g. olecranon bursitis produces a localized swelling over the olecranon process.
■ Possible factors that may be contributing to the patient's problem. If a muscle appears wasted on observation then the clinician will need to judge the relevance of this observation to the patient's presenting symptoms and test to confirm any relationship with symptom production.
■ An opportunity to reason collaboratively with the patient to gain her perspective on underlying causes; her willingness to weight bear, for example. So, using questions such as 'How does that feel?' 'What do you make of that?' ensures continued collaboration. The clinician should note whether the patient is demonstrating signs of illness behaviour, i.e. altered behaviour in response to pain, injury or illness (Box 3.1).
■ For example, is a patient bracing or breath holding prior to moving? This may be an indication of an illness behaviour that is appropriate or adaptive in an acute situation or is maladaptive and so may be an ongoing driver of symptoms.

Formal Observation

Observation of Posture. It should be remembered, however, that the posture a patient adopts reflects a multitude of factors, including not only the state of bone, joint, muscle and neural tissue, but also the symptoms experienced and the patient's emotions and view of his own body.

The clinician observes posture by examining the anterior, lateral and posterior views of the patient. There are a number of tools that can be used to measure and record posture, from use of plumb lines to more sophisticated software applications that allow baseline measures to be taken and reassessed at a later date. As with any measures, there are issues of reliability to be considered (Fedorak et al. 2003; May et al. 2006; Herrington 2011). Kendall et al. (2010) describe four types of postural alignment:

BOX 3.1
ILLNESS BEHAVIOURS (KEEFE & BLOCK 1982; WADDELL 2004)

Behaviour has to be interpreted with caution, so the clinician needs to maintain awareness of the following when considering whether the patient demonstrates illness behaviour (Waddell 2004):

- The patient needs to be examined fully
- Be aware of observer bias
- Isolated behavioural symptoms mean nothing; multiple findings are more likely to be relevant
- Illness behaviour does not explain the cause of the patient's pain, nor does it suggest that the patient is not in pain
- Illness behaviour does not mean that there is no physical disease; most patients have both a physical problem and a degree of illness behaviour
- Illness behaviour is not a diagnosis
- Illness behaviour does not mean that the patient is faking or malingering

The following findings may suggest illness behaviour (Waddell 2004):

- Non-anatomical pain drawing
- Pain adjectives and description (see Chapter 2)
- Non-anatomical or behavioural descriptions of symptoms
- Behavioural signs
- Overt pain behaviours:
  - Guarding – abnormally stiff, interrupted or rigid movement while moving from one position to another
  - Bracing – a stationary position in which a fully extended limb supports and maintains an abnormal distribution of weight
  - Rubbing – any contact between hand and back, i.e. touching, rubbing or holding the painful area
  - Grimacing – obvious facial expression of pain that may include furrowed brow, narrowed eyes, tightened lips, corners of mouth pulled back and clenched teeth
  - Sighing – obvious exaggerated exhalation of air, usually accompanied by the shoulders first rising and then falling; the cheeks may be expanded first
- Excessive, inappropriate or ineffective use of walking aids
- Excessive periods of rest ('down time')
- Help with personal care.

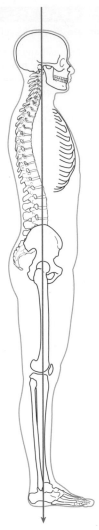

FIG. 3.1 ■ Ideal alignment. *(From Kendall et al. 2010 © Williams and Wilkins.)*

1. Ideal alignment, defined as posture that is most efficient, is summarized in Fig. 3.1.
2. The kyphosis–lordotic posture (Kendall et al. 2010): there is an anteriorly rotated pelvis, an increased lumbar lordosis with a reciprocal thoracic kyphosis and slight flexion of the hips. The neck flexors, upper-back extensors and external obliques will be elongated and weak. The rectus abdominis may be elongated. Hip flexors will be shortened. This is shown in Fig. 3.2.
3. The flat-back posture (Kendall et al. 2010), shown in Fig. 3.3, is characterized by a slightly extended cervical spine, flexion of the upper part of the thoracic spine (the lower part is straight), flattened/straight lumbar spine, a posterior

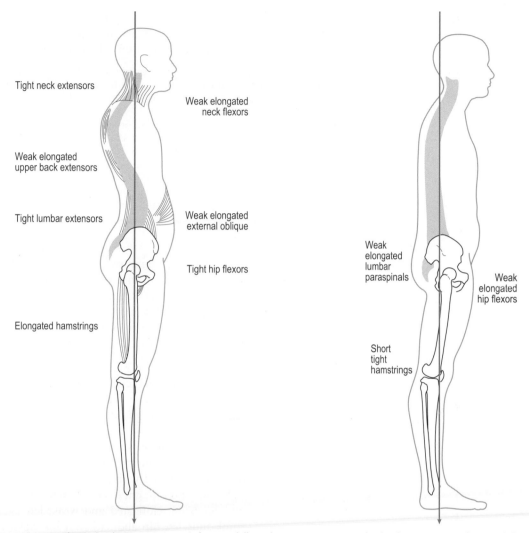

FIG. 3.2 ■ Kyphosis–lordosis posture. *(After Kendall et al. 2010 © Williams & Wilkins.)*

FIG. 3.3 ■ Flat-back posture. *(After Kendall et al. 2010 © Williams & Wilkins.)*

pelvic tilt and extension of the hip joints and slight plantarflexion of the ankle joints. This is thought to be due to elongated and weak hip flexors and short, strong hamstrings.

4. The sway-back posture (Kendall et al. 2010), shown in Fig. 3.4, is characterized by a forward head posture, slightly extended cervical spine, increased flexion and posterior displacement of the upper trunk, flattening of the lumbar spine,

posterior pelvic tilt, hyperextended hip joints with anterior displacement of the pelvis, hyperextended knee joints and neutral ankle joints. This posture is thought to be due to elongated and weak hip flexors, external obliques, upper-back extensors and neck flexors, short and strong hamstrings and upper fibres of the internal oblique abdominal muscles, and strong, but not short, lumbar paraspinal muscles. Individuals

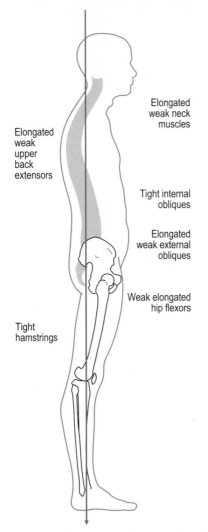

Elongated weak neck muscles

Elongated weak upper back extensors

Tight internal obliques

Elongated weak external obliques

Weak elongated hip flexors

Tight hamstrings

FIG. 3.4 ■ Sway-back posture. *(After Kendall et al. 2010 © Williams & Wilkins.)*

with hypermobility tend to adopt end-of-range postures such as sway or hyperextension of the knees.

Hypermobility

The Beighton score (Box 3.2) is used to determine whether a patient has hypermobility (Beighton et al. 1973).

Hypermobility is diagnosed if the score is at least 4 out of 9. A positive Beighton score is part of the Brighton criteria for joint hypermobility syndrome

> **BOX 3.2**
> **BEIGHTON SCORE**
> **(BEIGHTON ET AL. 1973)**
>
> The Beighton score is a 9-point scale with points awarded for five manoeuvres (1 point for each joint). Patients scoring 4 or more out of 9 are considered to have hypermobility syndrome.
> - Passive dorsiflexion of little fingers beyond 90°
> - Passive apposition of the thumbs to the flexor aspects of the forearm
> - Hyperextension of the elbows beyond 10°
> - Hyperextension of the knees beyond 10°
> - Forward flexion of the trunk with knees straight so that palms rest easily on the floor

(JHS), together with a mixture of other problems such as multiple joint pain, dislocating joints and duration of symptoms (Grahame et al. 2000) (Box 3.3). Please note that hypermobility alone cannot be classed as JHS. For detailed advice on examination, please refer to Keer and Butler (2010).

■ Handedness pattern (Kendall et al. 2010), shown in Fig. 3.5, is characterized, for right-handed individuals, as a low right shoulder, adducted scapulae with the right scapula depressed, a thoracolumbar curve convex to the left, lateral pelvic tilt (high on the right), right hip joint adducted with slight medial rotation, and the left hip joint abducted with some pronation of the right foot. It is thought to be due to the following muscles being elongated and weak: left lateral trunk muscles, hip abductors on the right, left hip adductors, right peroneus longus and brevis, left tibialis posterior, left flexor hallucis longus and left flexor digitorum longus. The right tensor fasciae latae may or may not be weak. There are short and strong right lateral trunk muscles, left hip abductors, right hip adductors, left peroneus longus and brevis, right tibialis posterior, right flexor hallucis longus and right flexor digitorum longus. The left tensor fasciae latae is usually strong and there may be tightness in the iliotibial band. There is the appearance of a longer right leg. Additionally alternative postural patterns may be observed in individuals who participate in specific activities such as rowing or golf.

BOX 3.3
BRIGHTON CRITERIA
(SIMMONDS & KEER 2007)

Diagnostic Criteria for Joint Hypermobility
Syndrome (JHS: Grahame et al. 2000)

MAJOR CRITERIA

1. A Beighton score of 4/9 or greater (either currently or historically)
2. Arthralgia for longer than 3 months in four or more joints

MINOR CRITERIA

1. A Beighton score of 1, 2 or 3/9 (0, 1, 2 or 3 if aged 50+)
2. Arthralgia (for 3 months or longer) in 1–3 joints or back pain (for 3 months or longer), spondylosis, spondylolysis/spondylolisthesis
3. Dislocation/subluxation in more than one joint, or in one joint on more than one occasion
4. Soft-tissue rheumatism: three or more lesions (e.g. epicondylitis, tenosynovitis, bursitis)
5. Marfanoid habitus (tall, slim, span/height ratio 41.03, upper:lower segment ratio less than 0.89), arachnodactyly (positive Steinberg/wrist signs)
6. Abnormal skin striae, hyperextensibility, thin skin, papyraceous scarring
7. Eye signs: drooping eyelids or myopia or antimongoloid slant
8. Varicose veins or hernia or uterine/rectal prolapse

JHS is diagnosed in the presence of two major criteria or one major and two minor criteria or four minor criteria. Two minor criteria will suffice where there is an unequivocally affected first-degree relative. JHS is excluded by the presence of Marfan or Ehlers–Danlos syndromes (EDS) other than the EDS hypermobility type (formerly EDS III).

Note: criteria major 1 and minor 1 are mutually exclusive, as are major 2 and minor 2.

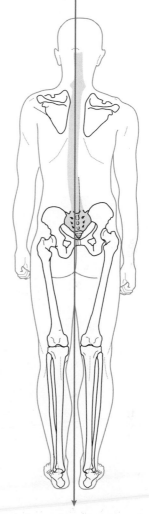

FIG. 3.5 ■ Handedness posture. *(After Kendall et al. 2010 © Williams & Wilkins.)*

Other postural observations may include skin creases at various spinal levels indicating possible regions of 'give' or excessive movement. A common example would be a crease at the midcervical spine indicating a focus of movement at that level; this observation would be followed up later on in the examination with passive accessory intervertebral movement (PAIVM) and passive physiological intervertebral movement (PPIVM), to confirm or refute a hypothesis of hypermobility at this level.

For further details on examination of posture, readers are referred to Magee (2014) and Kendall et al. (2010).

The clinician can also observe the patient in sustained postures and during habitual/repetitive movement where these are relevant to the problem. Sustained postures and habitual movements are thought to have a major role in the development of dysfunction (Sahrmann 2002). Clinically reasoning the relevance of a patient's posture is vital to establish whether it is a driver for the patient's presenting symptoms. Assumptions must not be made and hypotheses should be confirmed. If a patient reports neck pain when sitting then assessment in this position would be most relevant. If on examination this patient was observed to hold the pelvis in posterior pelvic tilt, with an extended cervical spine and forward head posture with a skin crease midcervical spine, then the clinician will need to assess this aggravating position to identify whether it is contributing to the patient's ongoing pain

(Fig. 3.6A). When the clinician encourages a more upright optimal posture, resulting in a reduction in neck pain, then the link between posture and symptoms has been proven and a postural driver can be 'ruled in'. If there is no change in symptoms then posture as a driver is 'ruled out' (Fig. 3.6B).

An example of a habitual movement pattern may be a patient with lumbar spine pain who has pain on bending forwards. The patient may flex predominantly at the lumbar spine, perhaps due to limitation in

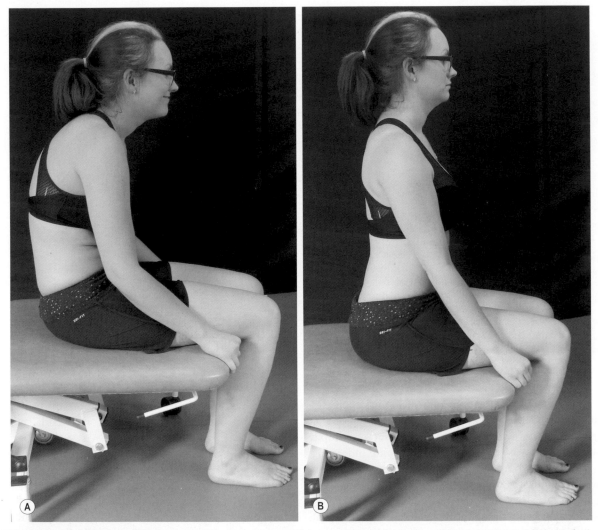

FIG. 3.6 ■ The effect of pelvic tilt on cervical spine posture. (A) In posterior pelvic tilt the cervical spine is extended, producing a forward head posture. (B) When the posterior pelvic tilt is reduced, the cervical spine is in a more neutral position.

hamstring length or hip flexibility (Fig. 3.7A). Controlling this lumbar spine 'give' on flexion and encouraging more flexion through the hips may reduce symptoms (Fig. 3.7B). If movement mainly occurs at the lumbar spine then this region may be found to be hypermobile (tested by PAIVMs and PPIVMs later on in the examination) and the region where movement is least may be found to be hypomobile.

Observation of Muscle Form. The clinician observes the patient's muscle shape, bulk and tone, comparing the left and right sides. It must be remembered that handedness, type, level and frequency of physical activity, including certain sports such as rowing, may produce differences in muscle bulk between sides.

Observation of Soft Tissues. Soft tissues local to symptoms and more generally can be observed, noting colour and texture of the skin, the presence of scars, abnormal skin creases suggesting a possible change in normal biomechanics, swelling of the soft tissues or effusion of the joints. Skin colour and texture can indicate the state of the circulation (a bluish tinge suggesting cyanosis or bruising with redness indicating inflammation), sympathetic changes such as increased sweating, bruising and the presence of other diseases. For example, complex regional pain syndrome type 1 may result in excessive hair growth, shiny skin that has lost its elasticity and nails which may become brittle and ridged. Scars may indicate injury or previous surgery and will be red if recent and white and avascular if old.

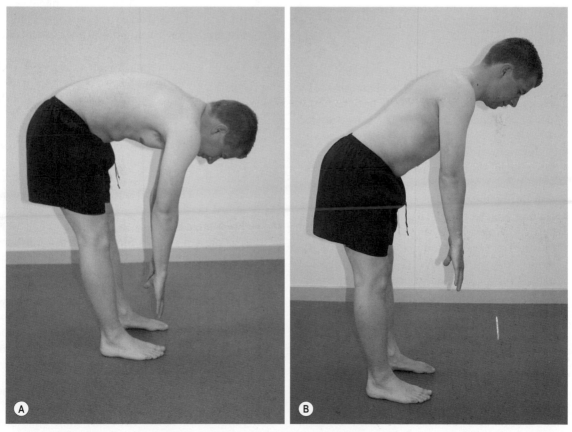

FIG. 3.7 ■ On bending forwards the patient may bend predominantly at the lumbar spine (A) or at the hips (B).

Functional ability may be tested in the observation section, to examine specific activities such as gait, stair climbing, reaching and sit to stand.

Observation of Gait. Gait assessment is often applicable for patients with spinal and lower-limb problems. Normally the patient wears shorts and is assessed without socks or shoes. The clinician observes the patient's gait from the front, behind and from the side, looking at the trunk, pelvis, hips, knees, ankles and feet through both swing and stance phases of the gait cycle from heel strike to toe off. A detailed description of systematic gait observation can be found in Magee (2014). It is also worth considering how the use of video and software applications might enhance this observation process. Common abnormalities of gait include the following:

- An antalgic gait due to pain at the pelvis, hip, knee or foot is characterized by a shortened stance phase of the affected limb, resulting in a shortened swing phase and step length on the unaffected leg.
- An arthrogenic gait, resulting from stiffness or deformity of the hip or knee, is characterized by exaggerated plantarflexion of the opposite ankle and circumduction of the stiff leg to clear the toes.
- A gluteus maximus gait is a result of weakness of this muscle, so that the patient produces a posterior thoracic movement to maintain hip extension during the stance phase.
- Gluteus medius gait (Trendelenburg's sign) is due to weakness of gluteus medius muscle causing an excessive lateral movement of the thorax towards the affected limb, to keep the patient's centre of gravity over the affected limb, during the stance phase of the gait cycle. A positive Trendelenburg sign is where the contralateral hip 'drops' due to gluteus medius weakness on the affected limb.
- A short-leg gait produces a lateral shift of the trunk towards the affected side during the stance phase.
- A drop-foot gait is due to weakness of the ankle and foot dorsiflexors caused by muscle or neural system dysfunction. The patient compensates by

lifting the knee higher on the affected side so that the toes clear the ground. Due to a lack of dorsiflexor control at heel strike there is an audible foot slap.

Functional Ability/Physical Performance Tests

The effects of musculoskeletal problems on global function, can be assessed using standardized and validated physical performance tests. Doing so also provides functional outcome measures that can be used to evaluate progress. The clinician must bear in mind that the outcome of these tests relies on a combination of factors such as strength, flexibility and cardiorespiratory function. For an overview, see Harding et al. (1994) and Galindo (2005). Commonly used outcome measures include:

- Walking tests. The patient walks at her own pace up to a predetermined maximum period, for instance, 5 or 10 minutes. Time, distance and rests are recorded.
- Shuttle walking test (Singh et al. 1992). The patient walks up and down a 10-metre track in increasingly short time intervals. Time and distance are recorded.
- Stand-up tests involve repeated standing up and sitting down over a predetermined period or a maximum number of repetitions.
- Stair-climbing tests. The patient ascends and descends a standard set of stairs for a predetermined period.
- The functional reach test (Duncan et al. 1990). The patient reaches forward along a horizontal ruler at shoulder level, without stepping out or losing balance.

Further assessment of function can be achieved with validated functional questionnaires. Questionnaires may be specific to a pathology or localized body region, but the following cover broad regions and conditions:

- upper limb: QuickDASH (Institute for Work and Health 2006)
- lower limb: Lower Extremity Functional Score (LEFS) (Binkley et al. 1999)

- low back: Roland Morris Disability Questionnaire (RMDQ) or Oswestry Disability Questionnaire (ODQ) (Roland & Fairbank 2000)
- neck: Neck Disability Index (NDI) (Sterling & Rebbeck 2005).

Joint Integrity Tests

These are specific tests to determine the stability of the joint and may be carried out early in the examination in acute presentations, as any instability found will affect, and may contraindicate, further testing. Specific regional tests are described in the relevant chapters.

Active Physiological Movements

An active physiological movement is defined as a movement that can be performed actively. In other words, the patient produces the movement; examples include flexion, extension, abduction, adduction and medial and lateral rotation. These movements test joint range and integrity, nervous system control and range, the muscle system as well as the patient's willingness to move. It is worth mentioning that range of movement is influenced by a number of factors – age, gender, occupation, time of day, temperature, emotional status, effort, medication, injury and disease – and there are wide variations in range of movement between individuals (Gerhardt 1992). The clinician determines what is normal for the patient, e.g. by comparing right and left sides.

The choice of which movements will be assessed should be justified through clinical reasoning, subjective findings, particularly aggravating and easing factors, and based on initial observations.

The order and extent of testing will be guided by the severity and irritability of the patient's presenting symptoms and the clinician's working hypotheses of the underlying cause of symptoms.

The aims of assessing active physiological movements are to:

- determine the pattern, quality, range, resistance and pain response for each movement
- reproduce all or part of the patient's symptoms – the movements that produce symptoms are then analysed and will guide reasoning for further testing

- identify factors that may have predisposed to or arisen from the disorder
- obtain signs on which to assess effectiveness of treatment (reassessment 'asterisks' or 'markers').

The following information can be noted during active movements, and can be depicted on a movement diagram (described later in this chapter):

- the quality of movement
- the range of movement. Joint range can be measured clinically using a goniometer, tape measure or by visual estimation. Readers are directed to other texts on details of joint measurement (American Academy of Orthopaedic Surgeons 1990)
- the presence of resistance through the range of movement and at the end of the range of movement
- pain behaviour (local and referred) through the range
- the occurrence of muscle spasm during the range of movement
- active movement is considered to be normal if there is painless, full active range of movement. Dysfunction is manifested by a reduced (hypomobile) or increased (hypermobile) range of movement, abnormal resistance to movement (through the range or at the end of the range), pain and/or muscle spasm.

The procedure for testing active physiological movement is as follows:

- Resting symptoms prior to each movement should be established so that the effect of the movement on the symptoms can be clearly ascertained.
- The active physiological movement is carried out and the quality of this movement is observed, noting the smoothness and control of the movement, any deviation from a normal pattern of movement, the muscle activity involved and the tissue tension produced through range. Deviations in movement can then be corrected to determine relevance to the symptoms. A relevant movement deviation is one where symptoms are altered when it is corrected; if symptoms do not change on movement correction, this suggests

that the deviation can be 'ruled out' as not relevant to the patient's problem (Van Dillen et al. 1998).

■ Both the quality and quantity of movement can be tested further by modifying the patient's posture during active movements (Sueki et al. 2013). For example, active shoulder movement can be retested with the clinician systematically modifying thoracic, scapular and humeral head positions in order to identify the possible driver of symptoms. Modification should produce a 30% improvement in symptoms and the patient's response to repeated movement should be consistent (Lewis 2009).

■ Active physiological movements test not only the function of joints but also the function of muscles and nerves. This interrelationship is well explained by the movement system balance theory (Sahrmann 2002). It suggests that there is an ideal mode of movement system function and that any deviation from this will be less efficient and more stressful to the components of the system (Comerford & Mottram 2013).

Ideal movement system function is considered to be dependent on:

■ The maintenance of precise movement of rotating parts; in other words, the instantaneous axis of rotation (IAR) follows a normal path. The pivot point about which for example, the vertebrae move constantly changes during physiological movements and its location at any instant is referred to as the IAR. The shape of the joint surfaces and the mobility and length of soft-tissue structures (skin, ligament, tendon, muscle and nerves) are all thought to affect the position of the IAR (Sahrmann 2002).

■ Normal muscle length. As mentioned earlier, muscles can become shortened or lengthened and this will affect the quality and range of movement.

■ Normal motor control, i.e. the precise and coordinated action of muscles.

■ Normal relative stiffness of contractile and non-contractile tissue. It is suggested that the body takes the line of least resistance during movement – in other words, movement will occur where resistance is least. When increased stiffness limits joint range then for normal function to be maintained compensation must occur elsewhere in the movement system. Areas of hypomobility or restriction will often be compensated for by movement at other areas, which then become hypermobile or flexible. With time, these movements become 'learned' and soft tissues around the joint adapt to the new movement patterns; repetitive loading, it is proposed, may result in tissue pathology (Comerford & Mottram 2013).

■ Normal kinetics, i.e. the movement system function of joints proximal and distal to the site of the symptoms.

So it is important to be aware that a movement dysfunction may therefore be due to several factors (Sahrmann 2002):

■ a shortened tissue, which may prevent a particular movement
■ a muscle that is weak and unable to produce the movement
■ a movement 'taken over' by a dominant muscle – this may occur with muscle paralysis, altered muscle length–tension relationship, pain inhibition, repetitive movements or postures leading to learned movement patterns
■ pain on movement.

Behaviour of the pain (both local and referred) throughout the joint range is recorded. The clinician asks the patient to indicate the point in the range where pain is first felt or is increased (if there is pain present before moving) and then how this pain is affected by further movement. The clinician can ask the patient to rate the intensity of pain, as discussed in Chapter 2 and shown in Fig. 2.5. The behaviour of pain through the range can be documented using a movement diagram, which is described later in this chapter.

Muscle spasm observed during movement is noted. Muscle spasm is an involuntary contraction of muscle as a result of nerve irritation or secondary to injury of underlying structures, such as bone, joint or muscle, and occurs in order to prevent movement and further injury.

Overpressure can be applied at the end of a physiological range to explore the extremes of range. If the patient's symptoms allow, i.e. are non-severe, the clinician applies an overpressure passive force to the active movement to assess further the end of range of that movement. In this situation overpressure could be classified as a passive movement; however, normal convention would include overpressure within active movement testing. If the resistance to movement felt by the clinician on applying overpressure is considered to be normal and symptoms are not reproduced then the joint is cleared (Hengeveld & Banks 2014).

Overpressure needs to be carried out carefully if it is to give accurate information; the following guidelines may help the clinician:

- The patient needs to be comfortable and suitably supported and prepared for the test.
- The clinician needs to be in a comfortable position with the couch adjusted to the correct height.
- For accurate/efficient direction of the overpressure force, the clinician's body is positioned in line with the direction of the force.
- The force is applied slowly and smoothly to the end of the available range; the clinician communicates with the patient throughout.
- At the end of the available range, the clinician can then apply small oscillatory movements to feel the resistance at this point in range (Hengeveld & Banks 2014).

There are a variety of ways of applying overpressure; the choice will depend on factors such as the health, age and size of the patient, the joint being overpressed and the size of the clinician. While applying overpressure, the clinician will:

- feel the quality of the movement
- note the range of further movement
- feel the resistance through the latter part of the range and at the end of the range
- note the behaviour of pain (local and referred) through the overpressed range of movement
- feel the presence of any muscle spasm through the range.

Some clinicians do not add overpressure if the movement is limited by pain, and in situations where severity and irritability are high this would be correct. However, it could be argued that when irritability and severity are lower the clinician cannot be certain that the movement is limited by pain unless the clinician explores further. The other reason why it can be informative to apply overpressure in the presence of pain is that one of three scenarios can occur: the overpressure can cause the pain to ease, to stay the same, or to get worse. This information can help the clinician to reason clinically the movement limitation, and may also be helpful in selecting a treatment dose. For example, a rather more provocative movement may be chosen when on overpressure the pain eases or stays the same, compared with when the pain increases. What is vital when applying an overpressure to a movement that appears to be limited by pain is to apply the force extremely slowly and carefully, thereby only minimally increasing the patient's pain.

Normal movement should be painfree, smooth and resistance-free until the later stages of range when resistance will gradually increase until it limits further movement. Less than optimal quality of movement could be demonstrated by the patient's facial expression, e.g. excessive grimacing due to excessive effort or pain, by limb trembling due to muscle weakness or by substitution movements elsewhere due to joint restriction or muscle weakness – for instance, on active hip flexion the clinician may observe lumbar flexion and posterior rotation of the pelvis.

Movement is limited by one or more of a number of factors, such as articular surface contact, limit of ligamentous, muscle or tendon extensibility and apposition of soft tissue, and each of these factors will give a different quality of resistance. For example, wrist flexion and extension are limited by increasing tension in the surrounding ligaments and muscles; knee flexion is limited by soft-tissue apposition of the calf and thigh muscles; and elbow extension is limited by bony apposition. Thus different joints and different movements have different end-feels. The quality of this resistance felt at the end of range has been categorized by Cyriax (1982) and Kaltenborn (2002), as shown in Table 3.2.

The resistance is considered abnormal if a joint does not have its characteristic normal end-feel, e.g. when knee flexion has a hard end-feel or if the resistance is felt too early or too late in what is considered normal range of movement. Additionally, Cyriax describes three abnormal end-feels: empty, springy and muscle spasm (Table 3.3).

The pain may increase, decrease or stay the same when overpressure is applied. This is valuable information as it can confirm the severity of the patient's pain and can help to determine the firmness with which manual treatment techniques can be applied.

As well as overpressure, active range of movement can be explored in a number of ways (Box 3.4), each of which will now be described in more detail.

BOX 3.4

MODIFICATIONS TO THE EXAMINATION OF ACTIVE PHYSIOLOGICAL MOVEMENTS

- Overpressure
- Combined movements
- Repeated movements
- Speed of movement
- Compression or distraction
- Sustained movements
- Injuring movements
- Differentiation tests
- Functional ability

Combined Movements

Combined movements are where movement in one plane is combined with movement in another plane; for example, lumbar flexion combined with lateral flexion or wrist extension with radial deviation. There are a number of reasons why the clinician may choose to combine movements in this way and these include:

- to gain further information of a movement dysfunction
- to mimic in order to explore a functional activity
- to increase the stress of the underlying tissues, particularly the joint.

Following examination of the active movements and various combined movements, the patient can be categorized into one of three patterns (Edwards 1999):

1. Regular stretch pattern. This occurs when the symptoms are produced on the opposite side from that to which movement is directed. An example of this would be a patient with left-sided neck pain which is reproduced on cervical flexion, lateral flexion and rotation to the right, while all other movements are full and painfree.

TABLE 3.2		
Normal End-Feels (Cyriax 1982; Kaltenborn 2002)		
Cyriax	**Kaltenborn**	**Description**
Soft-tissue approximation	Soft-tissue approximation or soft-tissue stretch	Soft end-feel, e.g. knee flexion or ankle dorsiflexion
Capsular feel	Firm soft-tissue stretch	Fairly firm halt to movement, e.g. shoulder, elbow or hip rotation due to capsular or ligamentous stretching
Bone to bone	Hard	Abrupt halt to the movement, e.g. elbow extension

---

TABLE 3.3		
Abnormal End-Feels (Cyriax 1982; Kaltenborn 2002). Abnormality is also Recognized if a Joint Does Not Have its Characteristic End-Feel or if the Resistance is Felt Too Early or Too Late in What is Considered the Normal Range		
Cyriax	**Kaltenborn**	**Description**
Empty feel	Empty	No resistance offered due to severe pain secondary to serious pathology such as fractures, active inflammatory processes and neoplasm
Springy block		A rebound feel at end of range, e.g. with a torn meniscus blocking knee extension
Spasm		Sudden hard end-feel due to muscle spasm

In this case, the patient is said to have a regular stretch pattern. The term 'stretch' is used to describe the general stretch of spinal structures reproducing the patient's symptoms.

2. Regular compression pattern. This occurs when the symptoms are reproduced on the side to which the movement is directed. If left-sided neck pain is reproduced on cervical extension, left lateral flexion and left rotation and all other movements are full and painfree, the patient is said to have a regular compression pattern. The term 'compression' is used to describe the general compression of spinal structures. A recording of the findings of lumbar spine combined movements for a patient with left-sided low-back pain is illustrated in Fig. 3.8.

This demonstrates regular compression pattern with left rotation, extension and left lateral flexion in extension limited to half normal range, with symptoms being produced in the left posterior part of the body.

3. Irregular pattern. Patients who do not clearly fit into a regular stretch or compression pattern are categorized as having an irregular pattern. In this case, symptoms are provoked by a mixture of stretching and compressing movements.

This information, along with the severity and irritability, can help in confirming or refuting a primary hypothesis. The clinician can use this information to inform ongoing testing by positioning the patient in such a way as to increase or decrease the stretching or compression effect. For example, accessory movements can be carried out with the spine at the limit of a physiological movement or in a position of maximum comfort.

To verify further whether the joint is a source of the patient's symptoms, accessory movements may be carried out (see later). The use of combined

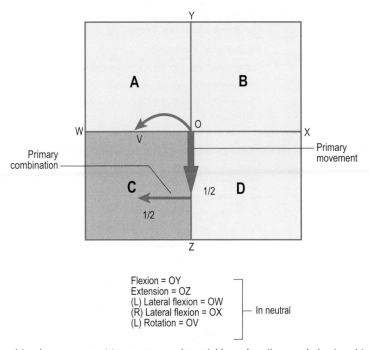

FIG. 3.8 ■ Recording combined movements. Movements can be quickly and easily recorded using this box. It assumes that the clinician is standing behind the patient so that A and B refer to anterior, and C and D to posterior parts of the body; A and C are left side and B and D are right side. The box depicts the following information: left rotation is limited to half range; extension and left lateral flexion in extension range are half normal range. The symptoms are in the left posterior part of the body (represented by the shading). *(From Edwards 1999, with permission.)*

movements and accessory movements together form what are sometimes referred to as 'joint-clearing tests', referred to in this text as 'screening tests'. Normally, if strong end-of-range combined movements and accessory movements do not reproduce the patient's symptoms and reassessment asterisks remain the same, then the joint is not considered to be a source of the patient's symptoms; hence the joint has been screened. If symptoms are produced or there is reduced range of movement, the joint cannot be considered 'normal' and may need further examination. Suggested combined movements to 'clear' each joint are given in Table 3.4 and generally are the more stressful physiological movements.

Repeated Movements

Repeating a movement several times may alter the quality and range of the movement. There may be a gradual increase in range with repeated movements because of the effects of hysteresis on the collagen-containing tissues such as joint capsules, ligaments, muscles and nerves (Threlkeld 1992). If a patient with a Colles fracture who has recently come out of plaster was repeatedly to move his or her wrist into flexion, the range of movement would probably increase. Examining repeated movements may demonstrate muscle fatigue and altered quality of movement. There may be an increase or decrease in symptoms as the movement is repeated.

The change in symptoms with repeated movements has been more fully redefined by the McKenzie method of mechanical diagnosis and therapy (May & Clare 2015). The clinician uses clinical reasoning to select repeated movements that can be tested in standing or lying. Often sagittal movements such as lumbar spine extension in prone lying are tested first. Before testing, symptoms are monitored before sets of 10 movements

TABLE 3.4	
Joint-Clearing Tests	
Joint	**Physiological Movement**
Temporomandibular joint	Open/close jaw, side-to-side movement, protraction/retraction
Cervical spine	Quadrants (flexion and extension)
Thoracic spine	Rotation and quadrants (flexion and extension)
Lumbar spine	Flexion and quadrants (flexion and extension)
Sacroiliac joint	Anterior and posterior gapping
Shoulder girdle	Elevation, depression, protraction and retraction
Shoulder joint	Flexion and hand behind back
Acromioclavicular joint	All movements (particularly horizontal flexion)
Sternoclavicular joint	All movements
Elbow joint	All movements
Wrist joint	Flexion/extension and radial/ulnar deviation
Thumb	Extension carpometacarpal and thumb opposition
Fingers	Flexion at interphalangeal joints and grip
Hip joint	Squat and hip quadrant
Knee joint	All movements
Patellofemoral joint	Medial/lateral glide and cephalad/caudad glide
Ankle joint	Plantarflexion/dorsiflexion and inversion/eversion
Midtarsal joint	Limitation of dorsiflexion, plantarflexion, adduction and medial rotation; abduction and lateral rotation are full range
Metatarsophalangeal joint of the big toe	More limitation of extension than flexion
Metatarsophalangeal joint of the other four toes	Variable; tend to fix in extension with interphalangeal joints flexed

are repeated four to five times. The response to repeated movements allows the clinician to classify patients into mechanical subgroups of derangement, dysfunction, postural syndrome or other. For full operational definitions for this subgrouping the reader is referred to May and Clare (2015). This classification system is used to inform management.

The derangement category constitutes the largest subgroup in patients with spinal pain and is identified where repeated movements produce phenomena known as peripheralization and centralization of symptoms. Centralization is defined as the 'abolition of distal pain in response to therapeutic loading' (May & Clare 2015). It occurs when symptoms arising from the spine and felt laterally from the midline or distally (into arms or legs) are reduced or transferred to a more central position when certain movements are performed. There is evidence that centralization is a good prognostic indicator for physiotherapy intervention (May & Clare 2015). Peripheralization occurs

when symptoms arising from the spine and felt laterally from the midline or distally (into arms or legs) are increased or transferred to a more distal position when certain movements are performed (Fig. 3.9).

If movements cause symptoms at the end of range and repeated movements do not significantly alter the symptoms, the condition is classified as a dysfunction syndrome. This syndrome is thought to be caused by shortening of scar tissue such that, when movement puts the shortened tissue on stretch, pain is produced, but is relieved as soon as the stretch is taken off. It will occur whenever there is inadequate mobility, for example, following trauma or surgery where scar tissue has been laid down during the healing process. Of course, this scenario is commonly seen in the peripheral joints following a period of immobilization, such as after a fracture.

Postural syndrome links pain to static loading and is reduced with postural correction. The subgroup categorized as 'other' accounts for those patients who do not fit into a mechanical syndrome category, such as

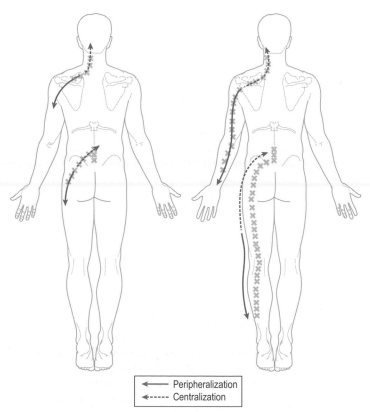

FIG. 3.9 ■ Peripheralization and centralization phenomena.

those with persistent pain, specific spinal conditions such as stenosis and for whom this specific movement approach would not be appropriate.

Speed of the Movement

Movements can be carried out at different speeds, and symptoms are noted. Increasing the speed of movement may be necessary in order to replicate the patient's functional restriction and reproduce the patient's symptoms. For example, a footballer with knee pain may only feel symptoms when running fast and symptoms may only be reproduced with quick movements of the knee, and possibly only when weight bearing. One of the reasons why the speed of the movement can alter symptoms is because the rate of loading of viscoelastic tissues affects their extensibility and stiffness (Threlkeld 1992).

Compression or Distraction

Compression or distraction of the joint articular surfaces can be added during the movement. For example, compression or distraction of the shoulder joint can be applied with passive shoulder flexion. If the lesion is intraarticular then the symptoms are often made worse by compression and eased by distraction (Magee 2014).

Sustained Movements

A movement is held at end of range or at a point in range and the effects on symptoms are noted. In this position, tissue creep will occur, whereby the soft-tissue structures that are being stretched lengthen (Threlkeld 1992). Range of movement would therefore increase in normal tissue. This may be very valuable in assessing patients who have reported that their symptoms are aggravated by sustained postures.

Injuring Movement

The movement carried out at the time of injury can be tested. This may be necessary when symptoms have not been reproduced by the previous movements described above or if the patient has momentary symptoms.

Differentiation Tests

These tests are useful to distinguish between two structures suspected to be a source of the symptoms. A position that provokes symptoms is held constant and then a movement that increases or decreases the stress on one of the structures is added and the effect on symptoms is noted. For example, in the straight-leg raise test, hip flexion with knee extension is held constant, which creates tension on the sciatic nerve and the hip extensor muscles (particularly hamstrings), and cervical flexion is then added. This increases the tension of the sciatic nerve without altering the length of the hip extensors. This can help to differentiate symptoms originating from neural tissue from those of other structures of the lower quadrant.

Passive Physiological Movements

Passive movements allow the clinician to identify all available joint range, which is normally more than can be achieved actively by the patient. The available passive range will vary between individual patients and the clinician must link passive feel with findings on active movement testing. As previously considered in the application of overpressures, the clinician will be feeling for quality of movement, resistance through range, symptom reproduction and end-feel.

A comparison of the response of symptoms to the active and passive movements can help to reason clinically whether the structure at fault is inert, e.g. all tissues that are not contractile or contractile tissue. If the lesion is of inert tissue, such as a ligament, then active and passive movements will be painful and/or restricted in the same direction. For instance, if the anterior joint capsule of the proximal interphalangeal joint of the index finger is shortened, there will be pain and/or restriction of finger extension, whether this movement is carried out actively or passively. If the lesion is in a contractile tissue (i.e. muscle) then active and passive movements are painful and/or restricted in opposite directions. For example, a muscle lesion in the anterior fibres of deltoid will be painful on active flexion of the shoulder joint and on passive extension of the shoulder.

Active physiological movements of the spine are an accumulation of movement at a number of vertebral segments. Spinal passive movement is assessed segmentally using passive physiological intervertebral movement (PPIVMs). To do this, the clinician feels the movement of adjacent spinous processes, articular pillars or transverse processes during physiological movements. An overview of how to perform PPIVMs is given in each relevant chapter and a full description can be found in Hengeveld and Banks (2014). A quick and easy method of recording PPIVMs is shown in Fig. 3.10. This method can also be used for a range of active movements.

Muscle Tests

Comerford and Mottram (2013) state that optimal muscle function requires muscles to be able to:

- shorten concentrically to produce movement – mobility function
- hold isometrically positions and postures – postural control function
- lengthen eccentrically – stability function
- provide proprioceptive feedback to the central nervous system for ongoing coordination and regulation.

However, some muscles are more efficient in terms of a mobility function, whilst others are better suited, due to their anatomy and physiology, to a stability function.

A classification system first applied to the lumbar spine by Bergmark (1989) was further refined by Comerford and Mottram (2001). Muscles are grouped under three broad headings: local stabilizer, global stabilizer and global mobilizer. Generally speaking, the local stabilizer muscles maintain a low, continuous activation in all joint positions regardless of the direction of joint motion and tend to become inhibited in the presence of pain. Examples of stabilizers include vastus medialis obliquus, the deep neck flexors and transversus abdominis. The global stabilizers become activated on specific directions of joint movement, providing eccentric control and rotatory movement, and when dysfunctional tend to become long and weak; examples include gluteus medius, superficial multifidus and internal and external obliques. The global mobilizers when activated produce direction-specific movement, particularly concentric movement, and when dysfunctional tend to become short and overactive; examples include rectus abdominis, hamstrings and sternocleidomastoid (Comerford & Mottram 2013). Further characteristics of each classification are given in Table 3.5.

It is important to remember that muscles do not function in isolation and are dependent on a balance between agonist and antagonists, as well as other local and distant muscle groups. The effect of muscle dysfunction can therefore impact the whole musculoskeletal system.

There is a close functional relationship between agonist and antagonist muscles. Activation of the agonist is associated with reciprocal inhibition of the antagonist. This means that, when a muscle is overactive, this will be associated with inhibition of the

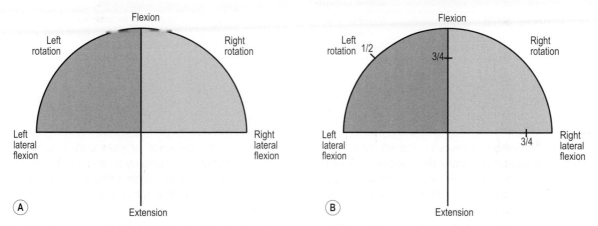

FIG. 3.10 ■ (A) Recording passive physiological intervertebral movements (PPIVMs). (B) Example of a completed PPIVM recording for a segmental level. Interpretation: there is three-quarters range of flexion and right lateral flexion and one-half range of left rotation. There is no restriction of extension.

TABLE 3.5		
Classification of Muscle Function Roles in Terms of Function, Characteristics and Dysfunction (Comerford & Mottram 2013)		
Local Stabilizer	**Global Stabilizer**	**Global Mobilizer**
Examples		
Transversus abdominis	Internal and external obliques	Rectus abdominis
Deep lumbar multifidus	Superficial multifidus	Iliocostalis
Psoas major (posterior fasciculi)	Spinalis	Hamstrings
Vastus medialis oblique	Gluteus medius	Latissimus dorsi
Middle and lower trapezius	Serratus anterior	Levator scapulae
Deep cervical flexors	Longus colli (oblique fibres)	Scalenus anterior, medius and posterior
Function and Characteristics		
Increases muscle stiffness to control segmental movement	Generates force to control range of movement	Generates torque to produce movement
Controls the neutral joint position. Contraction does not produce change in length and so does not produce movement. Proprioceptive function: information on joint position, range and rate of movement	Controls particularly the inner and outer ranges of movement. Tends to contract eccentrically for low-load deceleration of momentum and for rotational control	Produces joint movement, especially movements in the sagittal plane. Tends to contract concentrically. Absorbs shock
Activity is independent of direction of movement	Activity is direction-dependent	Activity is direction-dependent
Continuous activation throughout movement	Non-continuous activity	Non-continuous activity
Dysfunction		
Reduced muscle stiffness, loss of joint neutral position (segmental control). Delayed timing and recruitment	Poor control of inner and outer ranges of movement, poor eccentric control and rotation dissociation. Inner- and outer-range weakness of muscle	Muscle spasm. Loss of muscle length (shortened), limiting accessory and/ or physiological range of movement
Becomes inhibited	Reduced low-threshold tonic recruitment	Overactive low-threshold, low-load recruitment
Local Inhibition	**Global Imbalance**	**Global Imbalance**
Loss of segmental control	Increased length and inhibited stabilizing muscles result in underpull at a motion segment	Shortened and overactive mobilizing muscles result in overpull at a motion segment

antagonist group, which may then become weak. This situation produces what is known as muscle imbalance, i.e. a disruption of the coordinated interplay of muscles. Muscle imbalance can occur where a muscle becomes shortened and alters the position IAR of the joint. This change will result in the antagonist muscle being elongated and weak. Postural positions have been shown to influence trunk muscle activation patterns and altered muscle patterns have been linked to lumbopelvic pain (Dankaerts et al. 2006). For example, in a patient with a kypholordotic posture the erector spinae will be overactive, resulting in an elongated and underactive rectus abdominis. Muscle imbalance can also occur as a result of reflex inhibition of muscle and weakness in the presence of pain and/or injury. To prove a hypothesis of movement dysfunction being a cause of a patient's symptoms, the clinician should correct alignment and/or movement pattern and note the symptom response.

Muscle testing therefore involves examination of the strength and length of both agonist and antagonist muscle groups.

The following tests are commonly used to assess muscle function: muscle strength, muscle control, muscle length, isometric muscle testing and some other muscle tests.

Muscle Strength

This is usually tested manually with an isotonic contraction through the available range of movement and graded according to the Medical Research Council (MRC) scale (Medical Research Council 1976), shown in Table 3.6.

Based on clinical reasoning, for a specific patient muscles can be tested as a group, such as hamstrings, as well as more specifically testing individual muscles, for example, biceps femoris. The strength of a muscle contraction will depend on the age, gender, build and usual level of physical activity of the patient. Details of these tests can be found in Kendall et al. (2010). Some muscles are thought to be prone to inhibition and weakness and are shown in Table 3.7 (Jull &

Janda 1987; Janda 1994, 2002; Comerford & Mottram 2001).

They are characterized by hypotonia, decreased strength and delayed activation, with atrophy over a prolonged period of time (Janda 1993). While the mechanism behind this process is still unclear, it seems reasonable to suggest that the strength of these muscles in particular needs to be examined. Sahrmann (2002) suggests that the postural muscles tend to lengthen as a result of poor posture and that this occurs because the muscle rests in an elongated position. The muscles then appear weak when tested in a shortened position, although their peak tension in outer range is actually larger than the peak tension generated by a 'normal-length' muscle (Fig. 3.11) (Gossman et al. 1982).

Crawford (1973) found that the peak tension of the lengthened muscle in the outer range may be 35% greater than normal muscle. In addition, muscles that lose their length will, over a period of time, become weak. Methods of testing the strength of individual muscles are outlined in Fig. 3.12. The patient is asked to move against the resistance applied by the clinician.

Muscle Control

Muscle control is tested by observing the recruitment and coordination of muscles during active movements. Some of these movements will have already been carried out (under joint tests) but other specific tests will be carried out here. The relative strength, endurance and control of muscles are considered to be more important than the overall strength of a muscle or muscle group (Jull & Janda 1987; Janda 1994, 2002; Jull & Richardson 1994; White & Sahrmann 1994; Sahrmann 2002; Comerford & Mottram

TABLE 3.6

Grades of Muscle Strength

Grade	Muscle Activity
0	No contraction
1	Flicker or trace of contraction
2	Active movement, with gravity eliminated
3	Active movement against gravity
4	Active movement against gravity and resistance
5	Normal strength

From Medical Research Council 1976 Aids to the investigation of peripheral nerve injuries. London: HMSO. Reproduced with kind permission of the Medical Research Council.

TABLE 3.7

**Common Muscle Patterns/Reaction of Muscles to Stress
(Jull & Janda 1987; Janda 1994; Comerford & Mottram 2013)**

Muscles Prone to Become Tight	Muscles Prone to Become Weak
Masseter, temporalis, digastric and suboccipital muscles, levator scapulae, rhomboid major and minor, upper trapezius, sternocleidomastoid, pectoralis major and minor scalenes, flexors of the upper limb, erector spinae (particularly thoracolumbar and cervical parts), quadratus lumborum, piriformis, tensor fasciae latae, rectus femoris, hamstrings, short hip adductors, tibialis posterior, gastrocnemius	Serratus anterior, middle and lower fibres of trapezius, deep neck flexors, mylohyoid, subscapularis, extensors of upper limb, gluteus maximus, medius and minimus, deep lumbar multifidus, iliopsoas, vastus medialis and lateralis, tibialis anterior and peronei

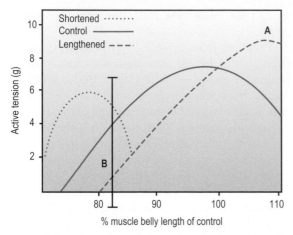

FIG. 3.11 ■ Effects of muscle length on muscle strength. The normal length–tension curve (control) moves to the right for a lengthened muscle, giving it a peak tension some 35% greater than the control (point A). When tested in an inner-range position, however (point B), the muscle tests weaker than normal. *(From Norris 1995, with permission.)*

2013). Relative strength is assessed by observing the pattern of muscle recruitment and the quality of movement and by palpating muscle activity in various positions. It should be noted that this relies on the observational and palpatory skills of the clinician. A common term within the concept of muscle control is recruitment (or activation), which refers to timed onset of muscle activity. For a more indepth description of this concept the reader is directed to Sahrmann (2002) and Comerford and Mottram (2013).

Muscle Length

Muscle length may be tested, in particular for those muscles that tend to become tight and thus lose their extensibility (Comerford & Mottram 2013) (Table 3.7). These muscles are characterized by hypertonia, increased strength and quickened activation time (Janda 1993). Methods of testing the length of individual muscles are outlined in Fig. 3.13.

There are two important comments to make regarding muscle length tests. Firstly, while these tests are described according to individual muscles, it is clear that a number of muscles will be tested simultaneously. This awareness is important when interpreting a test: it cannot be assumed when testing upper trapezius muscle that it is this muscle and no other muscle

that is reduced in length; for example, levator scapulae and scalene muscles may also be contributing to the reduced movement. Secondly, Fig. 3.13 shows some of many muscle length tests; all testing must be justified using reasoning and also be specific to the individual. For example, to test the length of the hamstring muscles fully, the clinician may investigate a number of different components such as hip flexion with some adduction/abduction and/or with some medial/lateral rotation. Similarly, for levator scapulae, the clinician may examine varying degrees of cervical flexion, contralateral lateral flexion and contralateral rotation as well as varying the order of the movements. For further information on fully investigating muscle length tests, see Muscolino (2016).

Muscle length is tested by the clinician stabilizing one end of the muscle and slowly and smoothly moving the body part to stretch the muscle. The following information is noted:

- the quality of movement
- the range of movement
- the presence of resistance through the range of movement and at the end of the range of movement: the quality of the resistance may identify whether muscle, joint or neural tissues are limiting the movement
- pain behaviour (local and referred) through the range.

Reduced muscle length, i.e. muscle shortness or tightness, occurs when the muscle cannot be stretched to its normal length. This state may occur as a result of compensatory changes between agonist and antagonist muscles so the clinician is required to reason muscle length findings within a context of movement analysis.

Isometric Muscle Testing

This may help to differentiate symptoms arising from contractile rather than inert tissues. The joint is put into a resting position (so that the inert structures are relaxed) and the patient is asked to hold this position against the resistance of the clinician. The clinician observes the quality of the muscle contraction to hold this position. The patient may, for example, be unable to prevent the joint from moving or adopting compensatory substitution strategies or may hold with

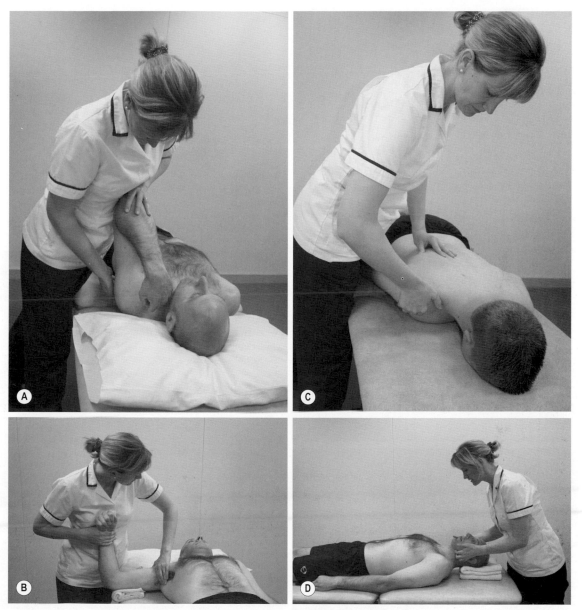

FIG. 3.12 ■ Testing the strength of individual muscles prone to become weak (Jull & Janda 1987; Cole et al. 1988; Janda 1994). (A) Serratus anterior. The patient lies supine with the shoulder flexed to 90° and the elbow in full flexion. Resistance is applied to shoulder girdle protraction. (B) Subscapularis. In supine with the shoulder in 90° abduction and the elbow flexed to 90°. A towel is placed underneath the upper arm so that the humerus is in the scapular plane. The clinician gently resists medial rotation of the upper arm. The subscapularis tendon can be palpated in the axilla, just anterior to the posterior border. There should be no scapular movement or alteration in the abduction position. (C) Lower fibres of trapezius. In prone lying with the arm by the side and the glenohumeral joint placed in medial rotation, the clinician passively moves the coracoid process away from the plinth such that the head of the humerus and body of scapula lie horizontal. Poor recruitment of lower fibres of trapezius would be suspected from an inability to hold this position without substitution by other muscles such as levator scapulae, rhomboid major and minor or latissimus dorsi. (D) Deep cervical flexors. The patient lies supine with the cervical spine in a neutral position and is asked to tuck the chin in. If there is poor recruitment the sternocleidomastoid initiates the movement.

Continued

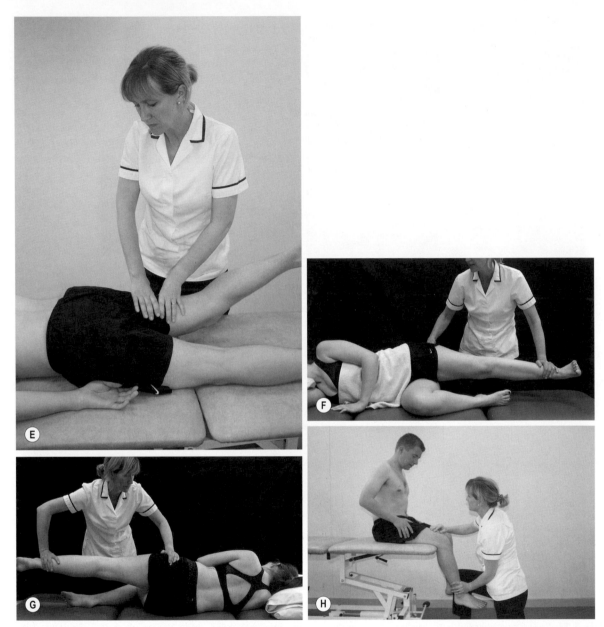

FIG. 3.12, cont'd ■ (E) Gluteus maximus. The clinician resists hip extension. A normal pattern would be hamstring and gluteus maximus acting as prime movers and the erector spinae stabilizing the lumbar spine and pelvis. Contraction of gluteus maximus is delayed when it is weak. Alternatively, the therapist can passively extend the hip into an inner-range position and ask the patient to hold this position isometrically (Jull & Richardson 1994). (F) Posterior gluteus medius. The patient is asked to abduct the uppermost leg actively with the hip in extension and slight lateral rotation. Resistance can be added by the clinician. Use of hip flexors to produce the movement may indicate a weakness in the lateral pelvic muscles. Other substitution movements include lateral flexion of the trunk or backward rotation of the pelvis. Inner-range weakness is tested by passively abducting the hip; if the range is greater than the active abduction movement, this indicates inner-range weakness. (G) Gluteus minimus. The clinician resists abduction of the hip. (H) Vastus lateralis, medialis and intermedius. The clinician resists knee extension.

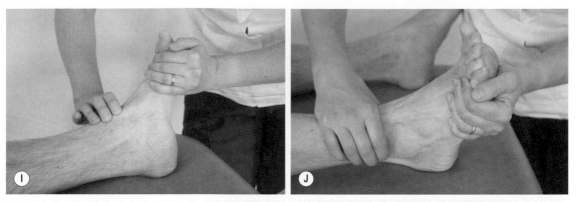

FIG. 3.12, cont'd ■ (I) Tibialis anterior. The clinician resists ankle dorsiflexion and inversion. (J) Peroneus longus and brevis. The clinician resists ankle eversion.

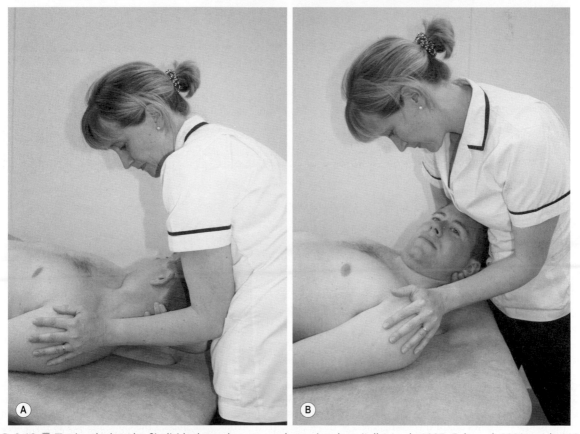

FIG. 3.13 ■ Testing the length of individual muscles prone to becoming short (Jull & Janda 1987; Cole et al. 1988; Janda 1994; Kendall et al. 2010). (A) Levator scapulae. A passive stretch is applied by contralateral lateral flexion and rotation with flexion of the neck and shoulder girdle depression. Restricted range of movement and tenderness on palpation over the insertion of levator scapulae indicate tightness of the muscle. (B) Upper trapezius. A passive stretch is applied by passive contralateral lateral flexion, ipsilateral rotation and flexion of the neck with shoulder girdle depression. Restricted range of movement indicates tightness of the muscle. *Continued*

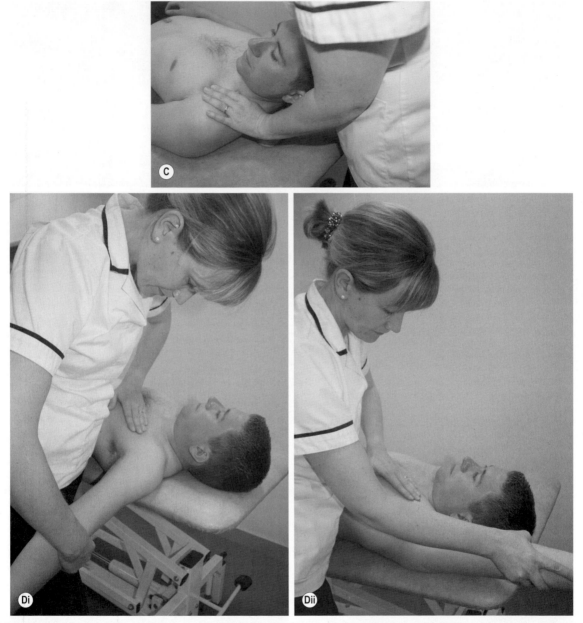

FIG. 3.13, cont'd ■ (C) Sternocleidomastoid. The clinician tucks the chin in and then laterally flexes the head away and rotates towards the side of testing. The clavicle is stabilized with the other hand. (D) Pectoralis major. (Di) Clavicular fibres – the clinician stabilizes the trunk and abducts the shoulder to 90°. Passive overpressure of horizontal extension will be limited in range and the tendon becomes taut if there is tightness of this muscle. (Dii) Sternocostal fibres – the clinician elevates the shoulder fully. Restricted range of movement and the tendon becoming taut indicate tightness of this muscle.

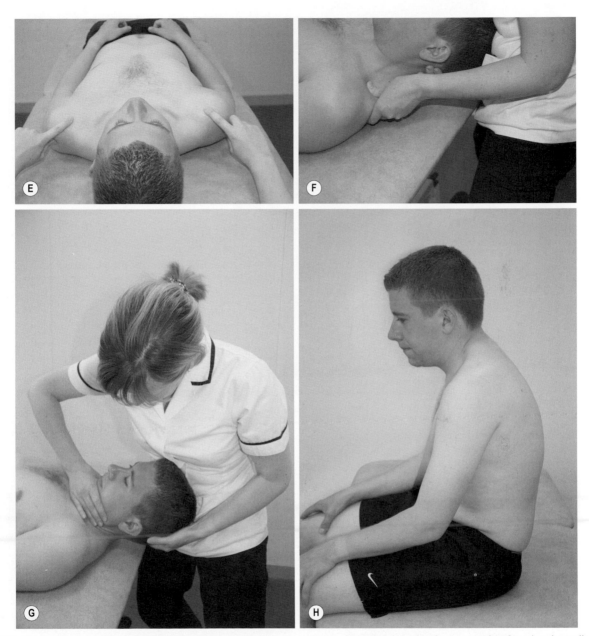

FIG. 3.13, cont'd ■ (E) Pectoralis minor. With the patient in supine and arm by the side, the coracoid is found to be pulled anteriorly and inferiorly if there is a contracture of this muscle. In addition, the posterior edge of the acromion may rest further from the plinth on the affected side. (F) Scalenes. Fixing first and second ribs, the clinician laterally flexes the patient's head away and rotates towards the side of testing for anterior scalene; contralateral lateral flexion tests the middle fibres; contralateral rotation and lateral flexion test the posterior scalene muscle. (G) Deep occipital muscles. The right hand passively flexes the upper cervical spine while palpating the deep occipital muscles with the left hand. Tightness on palpation indicates tightness of these muscles. (H) Erector spinae. The patient slumps the shoulders towards the groin. Lack of flattening of the lumbar lordosis may indicate tightness. *Continued*

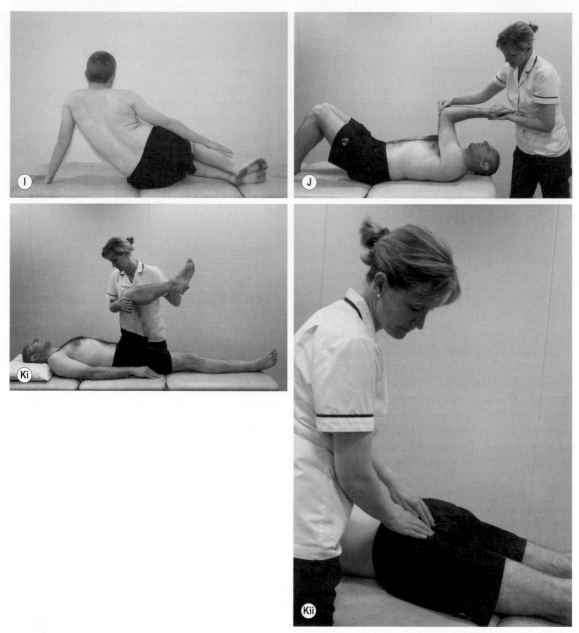

FIG. 3.13, cont'd ■ (I) Quadratus lumborum. The patient pushes up sideways as far as possible without movement of the pelvis. Limited range of movement, lack of curvature in the lumbar spine and/or abnormal tension on palpation (just above the iliac crest and lateral to erector spinae) indicate tightness of the muscle. (J) Latissimus dorsi. With the patient in crook-lying with the lumbar spine flat against the plinth and the glenohumeral joints laterally rotated, the patient is asked to elevate the arms through flexion. Shortness of latissimus dorsi is evidenced by an inability to maintain the lumbar spine in against the plinth and/or inability to elevate the arms fully. (K) Piriformis. (Ki) The clinician passively flexes the hip to 90°, adducts it and then adds lateral rotation to the hip, feeling the resistance to the limit of the movement. There should be around 45° of lateral rota-tion. (Kii) Piriformis can be palpated if it is tight by applying deep pressure at the point at which an imaginary line between the iliac crest and ischial tuberosity crosses a line between the posterior superior iliac spine and the greater trochanter.

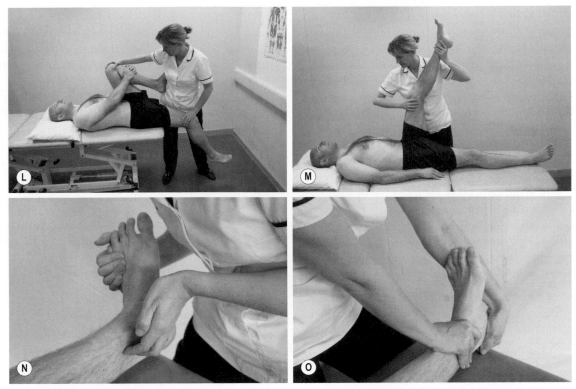

FIG. 3.13, cont'd ■ (L) Iliopsoas, rectus femoris and tensor fasciae latae. The left leg is stabilized against the clinician's side. The free leg will be flexed at the hip if there is tightness of iliopsoas. An extended knee indicates tight rectus femoris. Abduction of the hip, lateral deviation of the patella and a well-defined groove on the lateral aspect of the thigh indicate tight tensor fasciae latae and iliotibial band. Overpressure to each of these movements, including hip abduction for the short adductors, will confirm any tightness of these muscles. (M) Hamstrings. With the patient lying supine, the clinician passively flexes the hip to 90° and then the knee is passively extended. (N) Tibialis posterior. The clinician dorsiflexes the ankle joint and everts the forefoot. Limited range of movement indicates tightness of the muscle. (O) Gastrocnemius and soleus. Gastrocnemius length can be tested by the range of ankle dorsiflexion with the knee extended and then flexed. If the range increases when the knee is flexed, this indicates tightness of gastrocnemius.

excessive muscle activity; all of these circumstances would suggest neuromuscular dysfunction. If symptoms are reproduced on isometric contraction, it could be assumed that symptoms are coming from the muscle; however, it must be appreciated that there will be some shearing and compression of inert structures such as joints. If a more thorough examination of muscle function is reasoned, isometric strength can be tested at various parts of the physiological range.

Cyriax (1982) describes six possible responses to isometric muscle testing, updated as follows:

1. strong and painless – normal
2. strong and painful – suggests minor lesion of muscle or tendon, e.g. lateral epicondylalgia
3. weak and painless – complete rupture of muscle or tendon or disorder of the nervous system
4. weak and painful – suggests gross lesion, e.g. fracture of patella
5. all movements painful – suggests peripheral and/or sensory sensitization
6. painful on repetition – suggests intermittent claudication.

The clinician must bear in mind that pain is a subjective experience, while effort is part-determined by the patient's fear related to effort and pain.

Other Muscle Tests

Specific regional muscle tests will be covered in relevant chapters.

Sensorimotor/Neurological Tests

Inclusion of sensorimotor assessment must be clinically reasoned, based on the patient's presenting symptoms. Symptoms such as weakness, numbness, neuropathic pain along the course of a nerve will all raise the index of suspicion of a neural source. Symptoms indicating possible upper motor neuron (UMN) lesions such as distribution of symptoms bilaterally would prompt the clinician to include additional tests of the central nervous system. The findings of a sensorimotor assessment will assist in confirming or refuting a neural source of symptoms, allow for screening of suspected red flags such as cord compression, as well as facilitate differentiation between UMN and lower motor neuron (LMN) lesions and so help direct appropriate management.

Sensorimotor/neurological examination includes:

- neurological integrity: testing the ability of the nervous system to conduct an action potential:
  - sensory perception
  - coordination
  - tone
  - muscle power
  - reflexes
- tests of neural sensitivity:

  - neurodynamic tests (the response of the nervous system to load/movement)
  - neural palpation.

Integrity of the Nervous System

The most common condition affecting the peripheral nervous system is entrapment neuropathy. Over the last decade there has been increased understanding of the underlying of pathophysiological mechanisms of symptom production (Schmid et al. 2013; Schmid 2015).

The effects of compression of the peripheral nervous system are:

- reduced sensory input
- reduced motor impulses along the nerve
- reflex changes
- pain, usually in the myotome or dermatome distribution
- autonomic disturbance such as hyperaesthesia, paraesthesia or altered vasomotor tone.

Reduced Sensory Input

Sensory changes are due to compression or a lesion of the sensory nerves anywhere from terminal branches in the receptor organ, e.g. joints, skin, to the spinal nerve root. Fig. 3.14 serves to illustrate this.

Knowledge of the cutaneous distribution of nerve roots (dermatomes) and peripheral nerves enables the clinician to distinguish the sensory loss due to a root lesion from that due to a peripheral nerve lesion. The cutaneous nerve distribution and dermatome areas are shown in Figs 3.15–3.18.

It must be remembered, however, that there is a great deal of variability from person to person and an overlap between the cutaneous supply of peripheral nerves (Walton 1989) and dermatome areas (Downs & LaPorte 2011). A sclerotome is the region of bone supplied by one nerve root; the areas are shown in Fig. 3.19 (Inman & Saunders 1944; Grieve 1991).

Reduced Motor Impulses Along the Nerve

A loss of muscle strength is indicative of either a lesion of the motor nerve supply to the muscle(s) – located anywhere from the spinal cord to its terminal branches in the muscle – or a lesion of the muscle itself. If the lesion occurs at nerve root level then all the muscles supplied by the nerve root (the myotome) will be affected. If the lesion occurs in a peripheral nerve then the muscles that it supplies will be affected. A working knowledge of the muscular distribution of nerve roots (myotomes) and peripheral nerves enables the clinician to reason clinically motor loss due to a root lesion from that of a peripheral nerve lesion. The peripheral nerve distribution and myotomes are shown in Table 3.8 and Figs 3.20–3.22. It should be noted that most muscles in the limbs are innervated by more than one nerve root (myotome) and that the predominant segmental origin is given.

Over a period of time of motor nerve impairment there will be muscle atrophy and weakness, as is seen, for example, in the thenar eminence in carpal tunnel syndrome (median nerve entrapment).

Reflex Changes

The deep tendon reflexes test the integrity of the spinal reflex and consist of an afferent or sensory neuron and an efferent or motor neuron. The reflexes test individual nerve roots, as shown in Table 3.8.

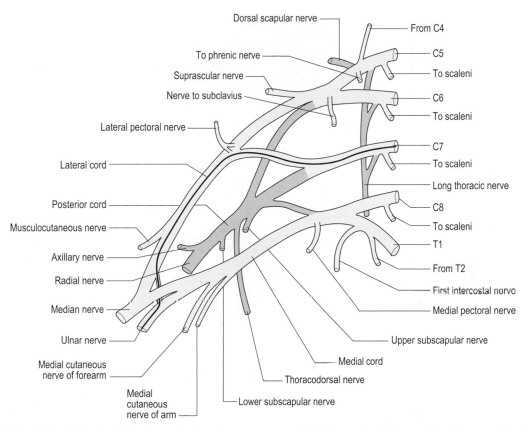

FIG. 3.14 ■ A plan of the brachial plexus showing the nerve roots and the formation of the peripheral nerves. *(From Williams et al. 1995, with permission.)*

Procedure for Examining the Integrity of the Nervous System

In order to examine the integrity of the peripheral nerves, three tests are carried out: skin sensation, muscle strength and deep tendon reflexes.

If a nerve root lesion is suspected, the tests carried out are referred to as dermatomal (area of skin supplied by one nerve root), myotomal (group of muscles supplied by one nerve root) and reflexal.

Testing Sensation. There are five aspects of sensation that can be examined (Fuller 2004; Cook & van Griensven 2013; Gardner & Johnson 2013):

1. light touch: tests patency of $A\beta$ fibres and dorsal column some C fibres may be involved (Schmid 2015).

2. vibration: tests patency of $A\beta$ fibres and dorsal column
3. joint position sense: tests patency of $A\beta$ fibres and dorsal column
4. pinprick: tests patency of $A\delta$ fibres and spinothalamic tract
5. temperature: tests patency of $A\delta$ and C fibres, as well as the spinothalamic tract.

For testing of light touch sensation the patient should be in a relaxed and supported position with the skin exposed. The clinician needs to explain the test and strokes an unaffected area of the skin first so that the patient knows what to expect. For consistency cotton wool is often used to test the ability to feel light touch. The clinician then lightly strokes the cotton wool across the skin of the area being assessed and the patient is asked whether it feels the same as or different

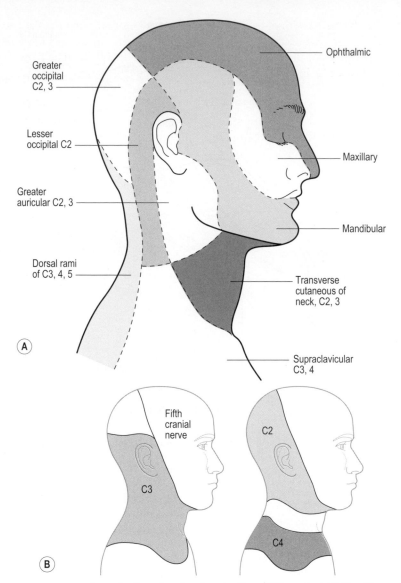

FIG. 3.15 ■ (A) Cutaneous nerve supply to the face, head and neck. *(From Williams et al. 1995, with permission.)* (B) Dermatomes of the head and neck. *(From Grieve 1981, with permission.)*

from the other side. An alternative and more standardized method of assessment of light touch to deep pressure is to use monofilaments (Semmes–Weinstein or West). Each monofilament relates to a degree of pressure, is repeatable and scales from loss of protective sensation through diminished light touch to normal sensation (Bell-Krotoski et al. 1995).

The clinician needs to identify and map out accurately the area of diminished sensation. The next step may be to explore further the area of diminished sensation, by testing pinprick (the ability to feel pain), vibration sensation, temperature sensation, joint position sense (proprioception) and stereognosis (in the hand).

Pinprick sensation can be tested with a disposable Neurotip using a gentle stabbing motion. The patient is told to close their eyes and with the Neurotip the clinician touches many areas, moving from distal to proximal including the trunk. The patient will be asked to confirm when a sharp sensation is felt.

The simplest way to test temperature sensation is with a cold tuning fork or metal teaspoon and compare with one at room temperature. The patient is asked to report what he feels.

Vibration sense can be tested using a 128-Hz tuning fork. With the patient's eyes closed the clinician strikes the fork before placing the flat end of the tuning fork on a bony prominence, testing from distal to proximal, e.g. medial malleolus. The patient is asked to confirm when he feels vibration (Leak 1998; Fuller 2004). The patient confirms when he can no longer feel the vibration and the clinician records the time as the vibration disappearance threshold (O'Connaire et al. 2011): Alternatively, a calibrated Rydel-Seiffer tuning fork can be used (Martina et al. 1998). This is compared with the other limb.

Joint proprioception can be tested by asking the patient to close their eyes, positioning the patient's

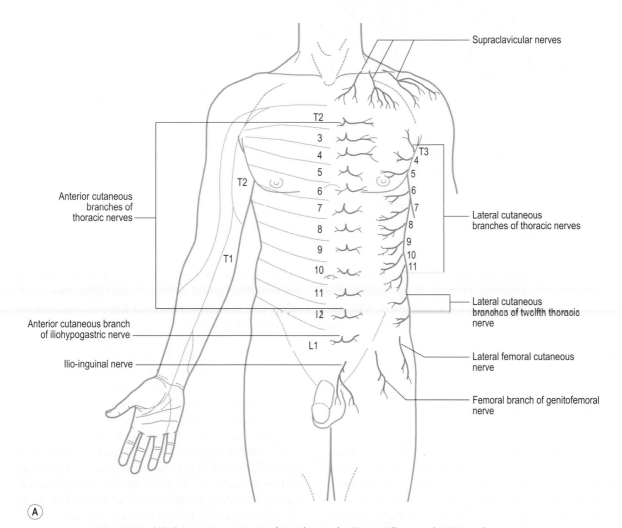

FIG. 3.16 ■ (A) Cutaneous nerve supply to the trunk. *(From Williams et al. 1995, with permission.)*

Continued

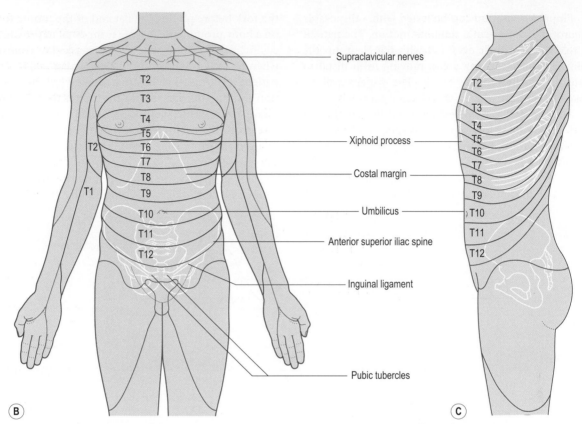

Supraclavicular nerves

Xiphoid process

Costal margin

Umbilicus

Anterior superior iliac spine

Inguinal ligament

Pubic tubercles

FIG. 3.16, cont'd ■ (B) Anterior view of thoracic dermatomes associated with thoracic spinal nerves. (C) Lateral view of dermatomes associated with thoracic spinal nerves. *(From Drake et al. 2005.)*

limb and asking the patient to identify whether it is being moved in a particular direction. Alternatively the patient can be asked to mirror movement with the other limb for example with. With the patient lying prone the clinician flexes the patient's right knee and the patient has to copy the movement with the left knee.

Areas of sensory abnormality should be documented on the body chart. Mapping out an area needs to be accurate, as a change, particularly an increase in the area, indicates a worsening neurological state and may require the patient to be referred to a medical practitioner. For this reason, sensation is often reassessed at each appointment, until it is established that the diminished sensation is stable.

Testing Muscle Strength. Muscle strength testing consists of resisting an isometric contraction of a muscle group over a few seconds. The patient must be in a supported position to minimize substitution strategies. The muscle is placed in midposition and the patient is asked to hold the position against the resistance of the clinician. The resistance is applied slowly and smoothly to enable the patient to give the necessary resistance, and the amount of force applied must be appropriate to the specific muscle group and to the patient. Myotome testing is shown in Figs 3.23 and 3.24. If a peripheral nerve lesion is suspected, the clinician may test the strength of individual muscles supplied by the nerve using the MRC scale, as mentioned earlier. Further details of peripheral nerve injuries are beyond the scope of this text, but they can be found in standard orthopaedic and neurological textbooks.

Reflex Testing. The deep tendon reflexes are elicited by tapping the tendon a number of times. The

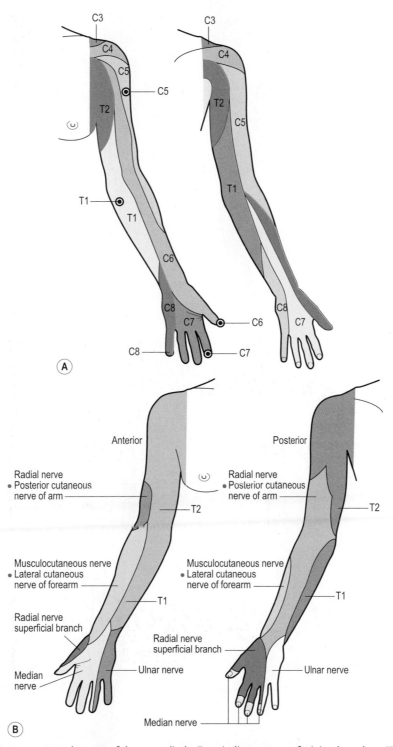

FIG. 3.17 ■ (A, B) Dermatomes and nerves of the upper limb. Dots indicate areas of minimal overlap. *(From Drake et al. 2005.)*

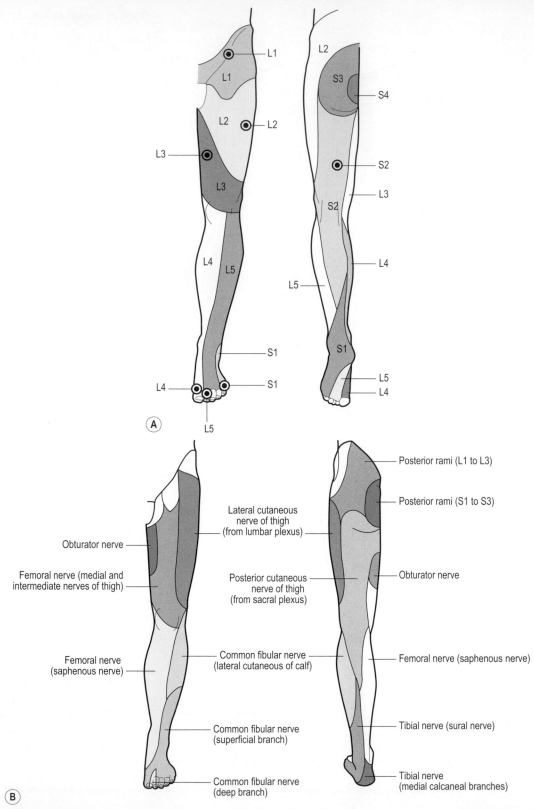

FIG. 3.18 ■ (A, B) Dermatomes and major nerves of the lower limb. Dots indicate areas of minimal overlap. *(From Drake et al. 2005.)*

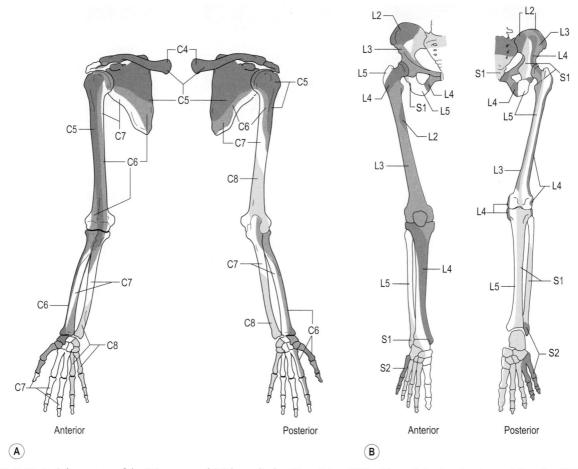

FIG. 3.19 ■ Sclerotomes of the (A) upper and (B) lower limbs. *(From Grieve 1991, with permission based on Inman & Saunders 1944.)*

commonly used deep tendon reflexes are the biceps brachii, triceps, patellar and tendocalcaneus (Fig. 3.25).

The reflex response may be graded and recorded as follows:

– or 0: absent
– or 1: diminished
+ or 2: average
++ or 3: exaggerated
+++ or 4: clonus.

If a reflex is difficult to elicit then the clinician can try testing again using a reinforcement Jendrassik manoeuvre which will facilitate motor neuron activity in the spinal cord. For example, in upper limbs ask the patient to clench the jaw or in lower limbs ask the patient to lock the hands together and try to pull them apart just before the tendon is struck.

A diminished reflex response can occur if there is a lesion of the sensory and/or motor pathways. Reflexes are commonly decreased in the elderly.

Reflex changes alone, without sensory or motor changes, do not necessarily indicate nerve root involvement. Zygapophyseal joints injected with hypertonic saline can abolish ankle reflexes, which can then be restored by a steroid injection (Mooney & Robertson 1976). For this reason, reflex changes alone may not be a relevant clinical finding.

An exaggerated reflex response suggests an upper motor lesion response, such as multiple sclerosis. This

TABLE 3.8
Myotomes (Grieve 1991)

Root	Joint Action	Reflex
V cranial (trigeminal nerve)	Clench teeth, note temporalis and masseter muscles	Jaw
VII cranial (facial nerve)	Wrinkle forehead, close eyes, purse lips, show teeth	
XI cranial (accessory nerve)	Shoulder girdle elevation and sternocleidomastoid	
C1	Upper cervical flexion	
C2	Upper cervical extension	
C3	Cervical lateral flexion	
C4	Shoulder girdle elevation	
C5	Shoulder abduction	Biceps jerk
C6	Elbow flexion	Biceps jerk
C7	Elbow extension	Triceps jerk and brachioradialis
C8	Thumb extension; finger flexion	
T1	Finger abduction and adduction	
T2–L1	No muscle test or reflex	
L2	Hip flexion	
L3	Knee extension	Knee jerk
L4	Foot dorsiflexion	Knee jerk
L5	Extension of the big toe	
S1	Eversion of the foot	Ankle jerk
	Contract buttock	
	Knee flexion	
S2	Knee flexion	
Toe standing		
S3–S4	Muscles of pelvic floor, bladder and genital function	

would prompt further UMN testing, but it should also be realized that all tendon reflexes can be exaggerated by tension and anxiety.

If a UMN lesion is suspected the plantar response should also be tested. This is the most valid test for early detection of UMN lesions. This involves stroking the lateral plantar aspect of the foot and observing the movement of the toes. The normal response is for all the toes to flex, while an abnormal response consists of extension of the great toe and abduction of the remaining toes, which is known as the extensor or Babinski response.

Clonus is associated with exaggerated reflexes and is characterized by rapid, strong oscillating muscular contractions produced by sustained stretching of a muscle. It is most commonly tested in the lower limb, where, with the patient's knee semiflexed and supported, the clinician sharply dorsiflexes the patient's foot.

Additionally tone, defined as resistance to movement, can be tested. Rigidity and spasticity indicating UMN can be reliably screened for using two quick upper-limb tests:

1. wrist: move patient's hand up and down, left and right while holding the wrist (Donaghy 1997)
2. pronator catch: abruptly supinate patient's wrist (Donaghy 1997).

Coordination. Quick screening tests include finger to nose for the upper limb and heel/shin test for lower limb, assessing for tremor, overshooting and 'trick' movements.

Neural Sensitization Tests

Mechanosensitivity of the nervous system is examined by carrying out what are known as neurodynamic tests (Butler 2000). Some of these tests have been used by

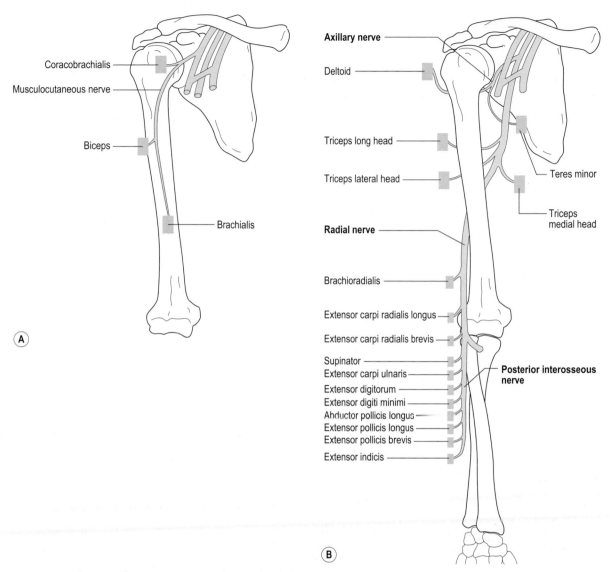

FIG. 3.20 ■ The musculocutaneous (A), axillary and radial (B) nerves of the upper limb and the muscles that each supplies. *(From Medical Research Council 1976 Aids to the investigation of peripheral nerve injuries. London: HMSO. Reproduced with kind permission of the Medical Research Council.)*

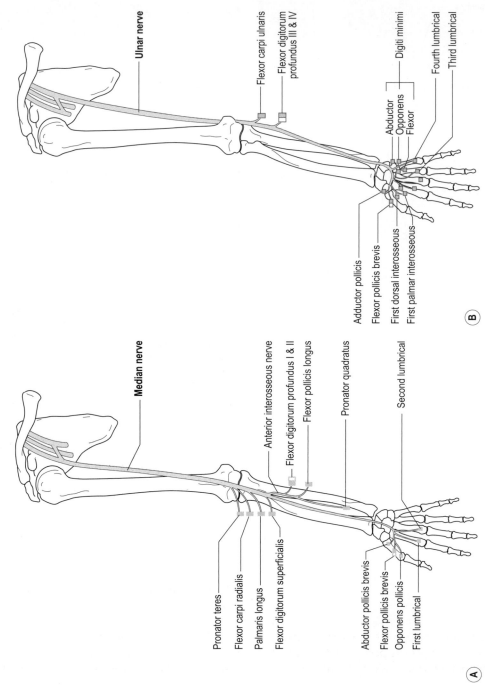

Ulnar nerve

Flexor carpi ulnaris

Flexor digitorum profundus III & IV

Abductor
Opponens
Flexor

Digiti minimi

Fourth lumbrical

Third lumbrical

Adductor pollicis

Flexor pollicis brevis

First dorsal interosseous

First palmar interosseous

B

Median nerve

Anterior interosseous nerve

Flexor digitorum profundus I & II

Flexor pollicis longus

Pronator quadratus

Second lumbrical

Pronator teres

Flexor carpi radialis

Palmaris longus

Flexor digitorum superficialis

Abductor pollicis brevis

Flexor pollicis brevis

Opponens pollicis

First lumbrical

A

FIG. 3.21 ■ Diagram of the (A) median and (B) ulnar nerves of the upper limb and the muscles that each supplies. *(From Medical Research Council 1976 Aids to the investigation of peripheral nerve injuries. London: HMSO. Reproduced with kind permission of the Medical Research Council.)*

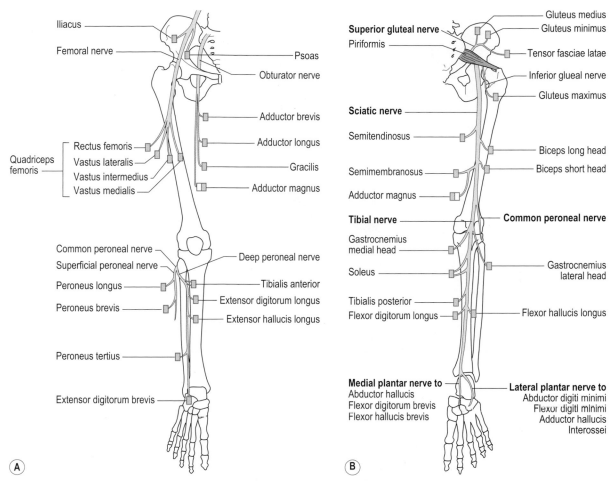

FIG. 3.22 ■ Diagram of the nerves on the (A) anterior and (B) posterior aspects of the lower limb and the muscles that they supply. *(From Medical Research Council 1976 Aids to the investigation of peripheral nerve injuries. London: HMSO. Reproduced with kind permission of the Medical Research Council.)*

the medical profession for over 100 years (Dyck 1984), but they have been an integral part of physiotherapy assessment for the last 30 years (Elvey 1985; Butler 2000; Maitland et al. 2001). Research is ongoing in further understanding and refining the tests (Coppieters & Nee 2015; Ridehalgh et al. 2015). A summary of the tests is given here, but further details of the theoretical aspects of these tests and how they are performed can be found in Butler (2000) and Shacklock (2005). In addition to the sensitization tests described below, the clinician can palpate peripheral nerves with and without the nerves being under tension; details are given under palpation in relevant chapters. Other common tests of mechanosensitivity of the peripheral

nerve include percussion (Tinel's sign) and compression (Phalen's), which will be covered where relevant in regional chapters.

Neurodynamic testing procedures follow the same format as those of joint movement.

Thus, resting symptoms are established prior to any testing movement and then the following information is noted:

- the quality of movement
- the range of movement
- the resistance through the range and at the end of the range
- pain (local and referred) through the range.

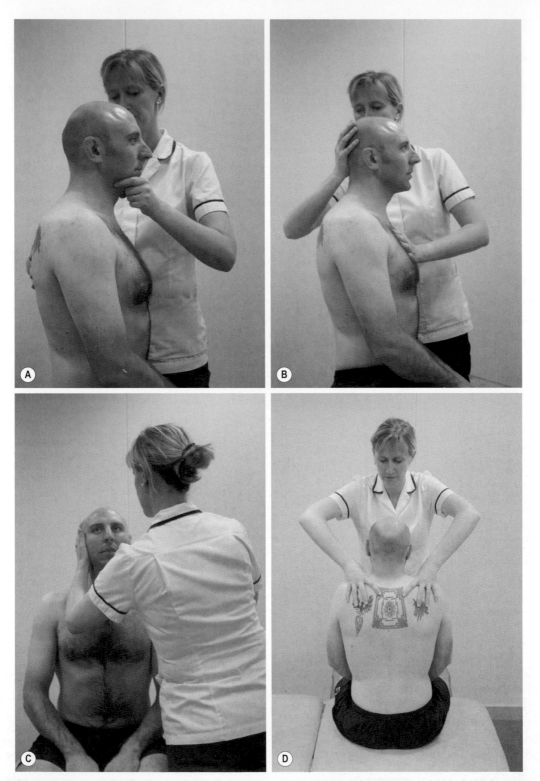

FIG. 3.23 ■ Myotome testing for the cervical and upper thoracic nerve roots. The patient is asked to hold the position against the force applied by the clinician. (A) C1, upper cervical flexion. (B) C2, upper cervical extension. (C) C3, cervical lateral flexion. (D) C4, shoulder girdle elevation.

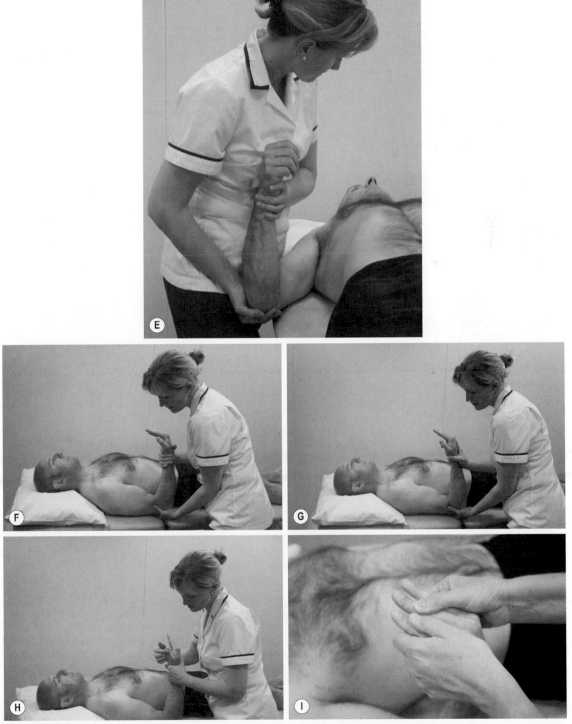

FIG. 3.23, cont'd ■ (E) C5, shoulder abduction. (F) C6, elbow flexion. (G) C7, elbow extension. (H) C8, thumb extension. (I) T1, finger adduction.

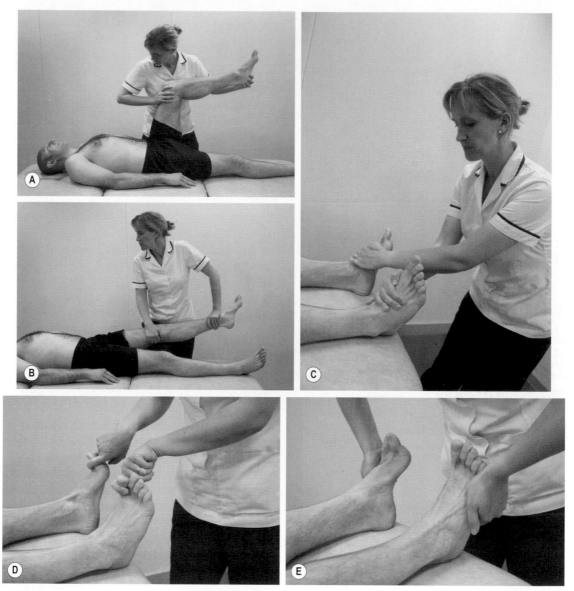

FIG. 3.24 ■ Myotome testing for the lumbar and sacral nerve roots. (A) L2, hip flexion. (B) L3, knee extension. (C) L4, foot dorsiflexion. (D) L5, extension of the big toe. (E) S1, foot eversion.

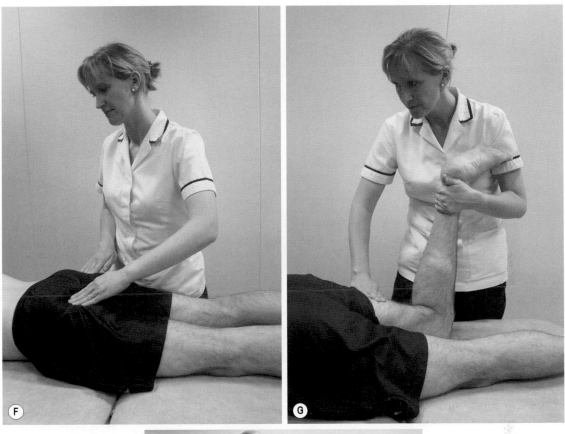

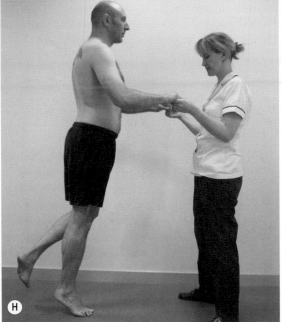

FIG. 3.24, cont'd ■ (F) S1, contract buttock. (G) S1 and S2, knee flexion. (H) S2, toe standing.

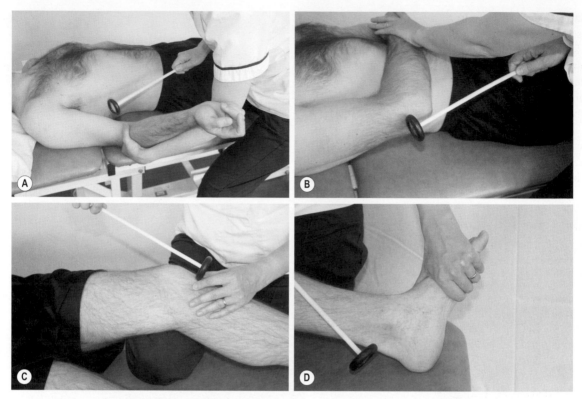

FIG. 3.25 ■ Reflex testing. (A) Biceps jerk (C5 and C6). (B) Triceps jerk (C7). (C) Knee jerk (L3 and L4). (D) Ankle jerk (S1).

A test is considered positive if all or part of the patient's symptoms have been reproduced and the symptoms change with the addition/removal of a sensitizer.

As with all examination techniques, the tests selected should be justified through sound clinical reasoning. Baseline neural integrity tests should be done prior to applying these tests. The joints involved in the test should be checked for available range.

Butler (2000) provides guidelines for the performance of the test:

- In very sensitive and acute disorders it will not be necessary to perform the entire test (e.g. in severe leg pain that does not allow the patient to lie flat, flex the opposite knee before testing the straight-leg raise to allow a little more lateral migration of neural tissue in the spinal and intervertebral canals).
- Test the least affected side first.
- Use reasoning to wind up the test in different orders but remember to be consistent each time (e.g. pillow under the neck)

- Carefully note symptom response, including area and nature of the symptom.
- Do not just symptom hunt; rather, handle the limb with care, feeling for tissue resistance.

The purpose of the test is explained to patients and they are asked to tell the clinician what they feel during the test. Continuous monitoring of symptoms through the test is crucial to obtain useful subjective data. Single movements in one plane are then slowly added, gradually taking the upper or lower limb through a sequence of movements. The order of the test movements will influence tissue response (Coppieters et al. 2006). Taking up tension in the region of symptoms will test nerve tissue more specifically as it will be held on tension for longer. For example, in a chronic ankle sprain with a possible peroneal nerve component, plantarflexion and inversion may be moved first, adding in straight-leg raise with additional sensitizers at the hip afterwards. If a patient's symptoms are very irritable, then adding local components first may prove to be too provocative. What matters is consistency in sequencing at each time of testing. Each movement is added on slowly and carefully and the clinician monitors the patient's symptoms continuously. If the patient's symptoms are reproduced then the clinician moves a part of the spine, or limb that is far away from where the symptoms are, to increase the overall length of the nervous system (sensitizing movement), also known as a tensioner technique, or to decrease the overall length of the nervous system (desensitizing movement) or to examine the nerve's relationship with its interface and its ability to 'slide'. In order for the test to be valid all other body parts are kept still. The clinician may assume a positive test if a desensitizing movement eases the patient's symptoms or a sensitizing movement increases the patient's symptoms. For example, for a patient in supine with the addition of hip flexion with knee extension producing posterior thigh pain, the clinician may then add cervical flexion. If the thigh pain is increased with cervical flexion positive test and suggests a neurodynamic component to the thigh pain.

Neurodynamic tests include the following:

- passive neck flexion
- straight-leg raise
- prone knee bend
- femoral nerve slump test
- saphenous nerve test
- slump
- obturator nerve test
- upper-limb neurodynamic tests (ULNT 1, 2a, 2b and 3).

Passive Neck Flexion. In the supine position, the head is flexed passively by the clinician (Fig. 3.26). The normal response would be painfree full-range movement. Sensitizing tests include the straight-leg raise or one of the upper-limb tension tests. Passively flexing the neck produces movement and tension of the spinal cord and meninges as well as upper cervical extensor muscles and joints (Breig 1978; Tencer et al. 1985).

Straight-Leg Raise. The patient lies supine. The way in which the straight-leg raise is carried out depends on where the patient's symptoms are. The basic component movements of the straight-leg raise are hip

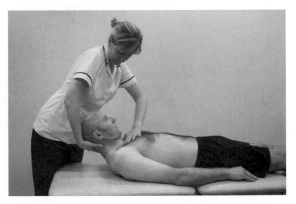

FIG. 3.26 ■ Passive neck flexion.

adduction, hip medial rotation, hip flexion and knee extension (to bias the sciatic nerve). The foot can be positioned to bias different nerves; ankle dorsiflexion/forefoot eversion would sensitize the tibial nerve, ankle plantarflexion/forefoot inversion, the common peroneal nerve and dorsiflexion/inversion the sural nerve. Additional movements of the forefoot may be used to bias the medial and lateral plantar nerves, which may be useful if symptoms are in the foot (Alshami et al. 2008). Neck flexion can be used to affect the spinal cord, meninges and sciatic nerve, and/ or trunk lateral flexion to lengthen the spinal cord and sympathetic trunk on the contralateral side.

The straight-leg raise moves and tensions the nervous system (including the sympathetic trunk) from the foot to the brain (Breig 1978). The normal response to hip flexion/adduction/medial rotation with knee extension and foot dorsiflexion would be a strong feeling of tension or tingling in the posterior thigh, posterior knee and posterior calf and foot (Miller 1987; Slater 1994). The clinician identifies what is normal for individual patients by comparing both limbs (Fig. 3.27).

Prone Knee Bend. Traditionally, this test is carried out in the prone position, as the name suggests, with the test being considered positive if, on passive knee flexion, symptoms are reproduced. This does not, however, differentiate between neural tissue (femoral nerve) and anterior thigh muscles and fascia, which are also being stretched. Normal range is between 110 and 150°, with both limbs being compared. This test

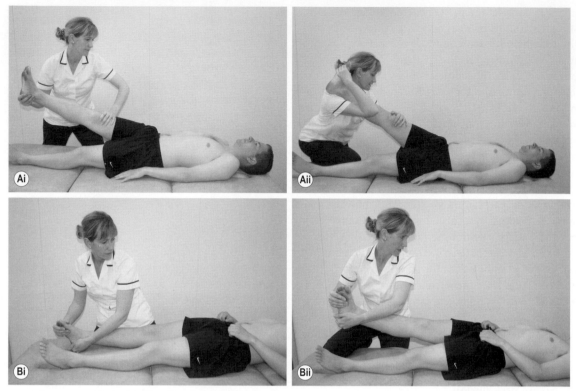

FIG. 3.27 ■ (A) Straight-leg raise if, for example, symptoms are in the posterior thigh. (Ai) Hip adduction, medial rotation and then flexion to the onset of patient's posterior thigh symptoms. (Aii) The clinician then adds ankle dorsiflexion and forefoot eversion. If the posterior thigh symptoms are increased (or decreased) with the dorsiflexion/eversion, this would be a positive test. (B) Straight-leg raise if, for example, symptoms are over lateral calf brought on with ankle plantarflexion and forefoot inversion. (Bi) Passive ankle plantarflexion and forefoot inversion to the onset of the patient's lateral calf symptoms. (Bii) The clinician then adds hip adduction, medial rotation and flexion. If the lateral calf symptoms are increased (or decreased) with the addition of hip movements, this would be a positive test.

has been shown to apply tension to midlumbar nerve roots (L2–L4) and evidence suggests it is a good indicator of lateral discal pathology (L3–L5) (Butler 2000; Nadler et al. 2001; Kobayashi et al. 2003).

Femoral Nerve Slump Test. The femoral nerve can be more selectively tested with the patient in side-lying with the head and trunk flexed, allowing cervical extension to be used as a desensitizing test (Fig. 3.28). The test movements are as follows:

- The clinician determines any resting symptoms and asks the patient to say immediately if any of the symptoms are provoked during any of the movements.

- The patient is placed in side-lying with the symptomatic side uppermost with a pillow under the head (to avoid lateral flexion/rotation of the cervical spine). The patient is asked to hug both knees up on to the chest.

- The patient releases the uppermost knee to the clinician, who flexes the knee and then passively extends the hip, making sure the pelvis and trunk remain still. The clinician may need to add hip medial or lateral rotation and/or hip abduction/adduction movement to produce the patient's symptoms.

- At the point at which symptoms occur the patient is then asked to extend the head and neck slightly

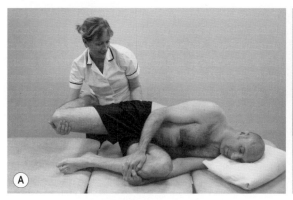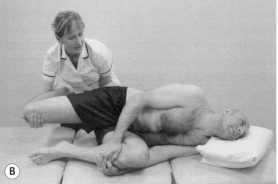

FIG. 3.28 ■ Femoral nerve slump test (in side-lying). (A) With knee flexion, the clinician passively extends the hip to the point of onset of the patient's anterior thigh symptoms. (B) Patient extends the cervical spine. If the anterior thigh symptoms are reduced (or increased) with the neck movement, this would be a positive test.

while the clinician maintains the trunk and leg position. A typical positive test would be for cervical extension to ease the patient's anterior thigh pain. However, if cervical extension increases the patient's anterior thigh pain, this is also a positive test.

Saphenous Nerve Test. The patient lies prone and the hip is placed in extension and abduction with the knee extended. The clinician then passively adds lateral rotation of the hip, dorsiflexion and inversion of the foot (Fig. 3.29A). Shacklock (2005) suggests internal rotation of the hip because of the position of the sartorius muscle but advocates trying different positions. Butler (2000) suggests external rotation of the hip based on a study of saphenous nerve entrapments in adolescents (Nir-Paz et al. 1999). The clinician can sensitize the test by, for example, moving the foot into plantarflexion if symptoms are above the knee (Fig. 3.29B) or by moving the hip into medial rotation if symptoms are below the knee, or by contralateral side flexion of the spine.

Slump. This test is fully described by Maitland et al. (2001) and Butler (2000) and is shown in Fig. 3.30.

The slump test can be carried out as follows:

- The clinician establishes the patient's resting symptoms and asks the patient to say immediately if any of the symptoms are provoked.

- The patient sits with thighs fully supported at the edge of the plinth with hands behind the back.
- The patient is asked to flex the trunk by 'slumping the shoulders towards the groin'.
- The clinician monitors trunk flexion.
- Active cervical flexion is carried out.
- The clinician monitors cervical flexion.
- Active knee extension is carried out on the asymptomatic side.
- Active foot dorsiflexion is carried out on the asymptomatic side.
- Return the foot and knee back to neutral.
- Active knee extension is carried out on the symptomatic side.
- Active foot dorsiflexion is carried out on the symptomatic side.
- Return the foot and knee back to neutral.
- Active bilateral foot dorsiflexion is carried out.
- Active bilateral knee extension is carried out.
- Return the foot and knee back to neutral.

Now that all the combinations of lower-limb movements have been explored, the clinician chooses the most appropriate movement to add a sensitizing movement. This would commonly be as follows:

- Active knee extension on the symptomatic side is carried out.
- Active foot dorsiflexion on the symptomatic side is carried out.

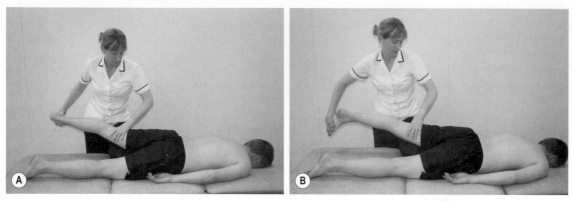

FIG. 3.29 ■ Saphenous nerve test. (A) With the hip in extension, abduction and lateral rotation and the knee extended, the clinician moves the foot into dorsiflexion and eversion. (B) If symptoms are above the knee the clinician can then move the foot into plantarflexion and inversion. If the symptoms are reduced (or increased) with foot movement, this would be a positive test.

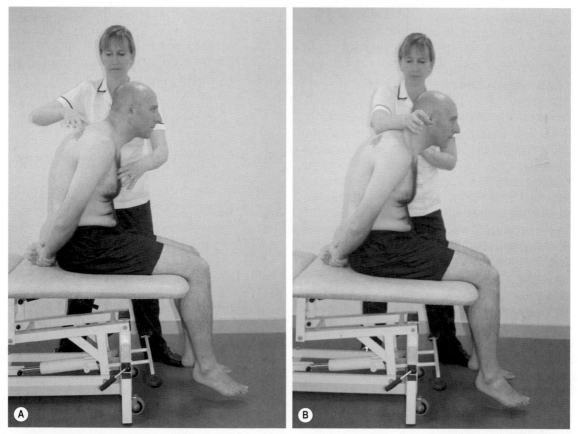

FIG. 3.30 ■ Slump test. Demonstrated for a patient with left posterior thigh pain. (A) Active trunk flexion with arms behind back. (B) Monitoring trunk flexion.

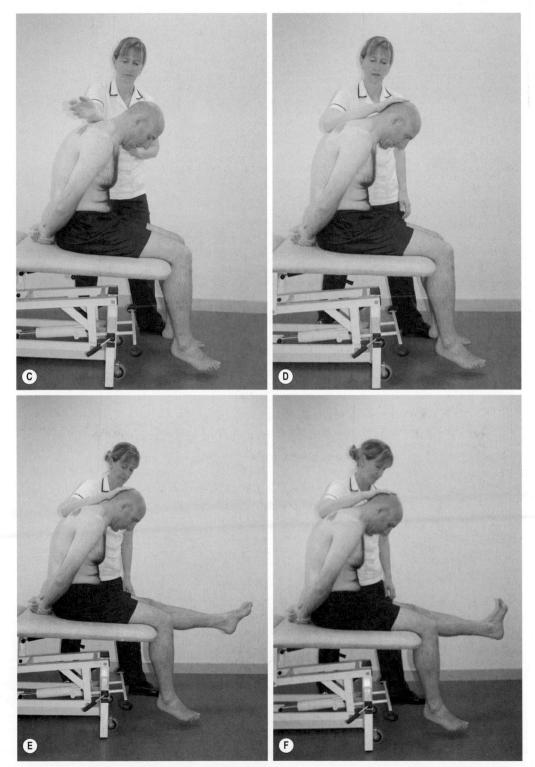

FIG. 3.30, cont'd ■ (C) Active cervical flexion. (D) Monitoring of cervical flexion. (E) Left leg: knee extension. (F) Left leg: dorsiflexion.   *Continued*

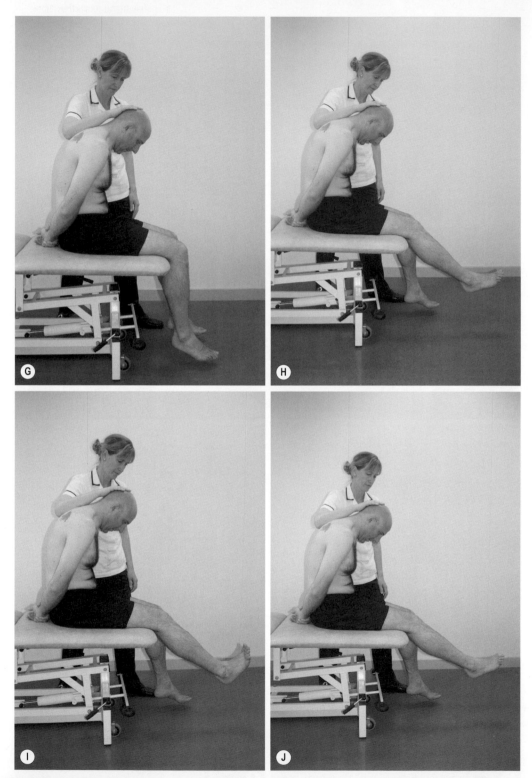

FIG. 3.30, cont'd ▪ (G) Return to start position. (H) Right leg: knee extension (reduced range due to onset of right thigh pain). (I) Right leg: knee extension (reduced range due to onset of left thigh pain); addition of dorsiflexion increases right thigh pain. (J) Right leg: release of dorsiflexion reduces right thigh pain.

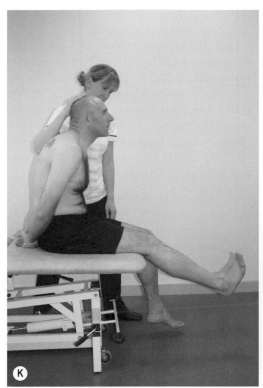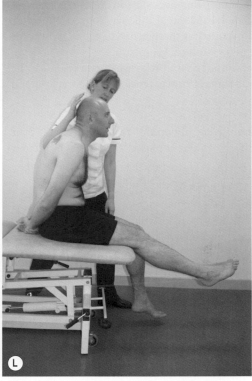

FIG. 3.30, cont'd ■ (K) Active cervical extension. If cervical extension reduces (or increases) the patient's right posterior thigh pain, this would be a positive test. (L) Active cervical extension may produce an increase in range which would increase further on release of dorsiflexion.

■ The patient is asked to extend the head to look upwards and report on any change in the symptoms. It is vital that there is no change in position of the trunk and lower limbs when the cervical spine is extended. A reduction in symptoms on cervical extension would be a typical positive test indicating a neurodynamic component to the patient's symptoms, but an increase in symptoms would also indicate a neurodynamic component.

The normal response might be:

■ pain or discomfort in the midthoracic area on trunk and neck flexion
■ pain or discomfort behind the knees or in the hamstrings in the trunk and neck flexion and knee extension position; symptoms are increased with ankle dorsiflexion
■ some restriction of knee extension in the trunk and neck flexion position

■ some restriction of ankle dorsiflexion in the trunk and neck flexion and knee extension position; this restriction should be symmetrical
■ a decrease in pain in one or more areas with release of the neck flexion
■ an increase in the range of knee extension and/ or ankle dorsiflexion with release of the neck flexion.

The desensitizing test is cervical extension. Sensitizing tests can include cervical rotation, cervical lateral flexion, hip flexion, hip adduction, hip medial rotation, thoracic lateral flexion, altering foot and ankle movements as for the straight-leg raise test, or one of the upper-limb tension tests.

Obturator Nerve Test. The slump position can be used further to differentiate muscle or nerve dysfunction as a cause of groin strain. By positioning the patient in sitting and abducting the hip to the onset of symptoms, slump and neck flexion are then added and if symptoms are increased this may suggest obturator nerve involvement; if there is no change in symptoms this may suggest a local groin strain.

Greater emphasis on the sympathetic chain can be tested by adding cervical extension and thoracic lateral flexion.

Upper-Limb Neurodynamic Tests. There are four tests, each of which is biased towards a particular nerve:

1. ULNT 1 – median nerve
2. ULNT 2a – median nerve
3. ULNT 2b – radial nerve
4. ULNT 3 – ulnar nerve.

The test movements are outlined below. The following tests are described with the assumption that the symptoms are in the upper limb. The order of the movements has been chosen so that the last movement is the easiest for the clinician to estimate by eye. The area of the patient's symptoms will help the clinician to select the most appropriate ULNT. For example, where symptoms are mainly in the distribution of the radial nerve, ULNT 2b would be carried out.

ULNT 1: MEDIAN NERVE BIAS (Fig. 3.31). The following sequence of movements would be appropriate, if, for example, the patient has symptoms in the upper arm or below (in the anterior forearm and hand):

1. neutral position of body on couch
2. contralateral lateral flexion of the cervical spine
3. shoulder girdle depression
4. shoulder abduction
5. wrist and finger extension
6. forearm supination
7. lateral rotation of the shoulder
8. elbow extension
9. ipsilateral lateral flexion of the cervical spine.

If symptoms are over the upper fibres of trapezius then:

10. wrist flexion would be used, instead of ipsilateral lateral flexion of the cervical spine.

The movement of ipsilateral lateral flexion of the cervical spine is used to test whether or not there is a neurodynamic component to the patient's symptoms.

If there was a neurodynamic component, the patient's symptoms would be expected to be produced at some stage during the arm movements from 2 to 8, and these symptoms would be reduced (or increased) by ipsilateral lateral flexion of the cervical spine.

ULNT 2A: MEDIAN NERVE BIAS (Fig. 3.32). This test is useful in cases where the patient has restricted glenohumeral range. The following sequence of movements would be appropriate if, for example, the patient has symptoms in the upper arm or below (in the anterior forearm and hand):

1. neutral position of body on couch, but with shoulder girdle overhanging the edge
2. contralateral lateral flexion of the cervical spine
3. shoulder girdle depression
4. wrist, finger and thumb extension
5. forearm supination
6. elbow extension
7. shoulder lateral rotation
8. shoulder abduction
9. desensitizing movement of ipsilateral lateral flexion of the cervical spine.

If symptoms were near the cervical spine, for example, over the upper fibres of trapezius, then the movement of wrist flexion, for example, could be used as the desensitizing movement.

ULNT 2B: RADIAL NERVE BIAS (Fig. 3.33). The following sequence of movements would be appropriate if, for example, the patient has symptoms in the upper arm or below (in the posterior forearm and hand):

1. neutral position of body on couch, but with shoulder girdle overhanging the edge
2. contralateral lateral flexion of the cervical spine
3. shoulder girdle depression
4. wrist, finger and thumb flexion
5. shoulder medial rotation
6. elbow extension
7. desensitizing movement of ipsilateral lateral flexion of the cervical spine

or

8. wrist extension if symptoms are near the cervical spine, for example, over the upper fibres of trapezius.

ULNT 3: ULNAR NERVE BIAS (Fig. 3.34). The following sequence of movements would be appropriate if,

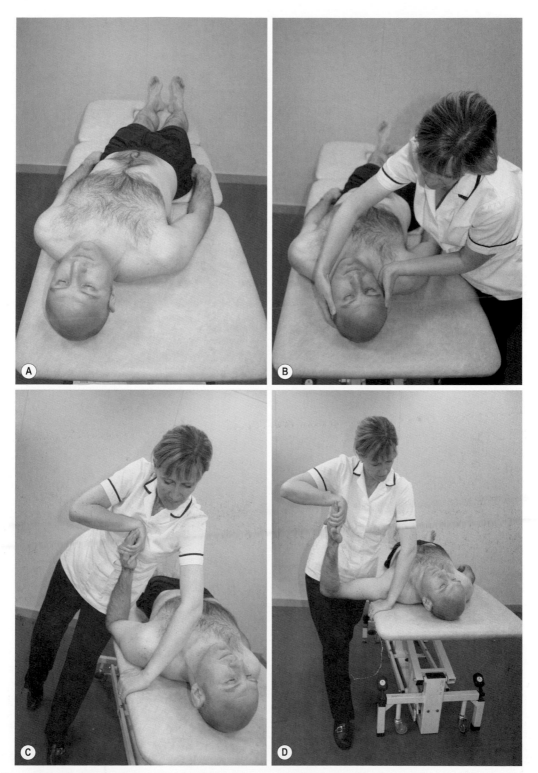

FIG. 3.31 ■ Upper-limb neurodynamic test (ULNT 1). (A) Neutral start position. (B) Contralateral lateral flexion of the cervical spine. (C) Shoulder girdle depression. (D) Shoulder abduction.   *Continued*

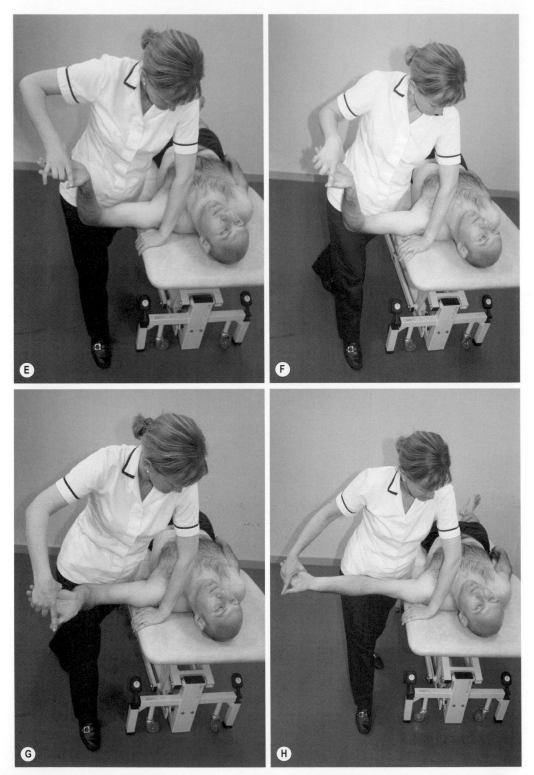

FIG. 3.31, cont'd ■ (E) Wrist and finger extension. (F) Forearm supination. (G) Shoulder lateral rotation. (H) Elbow extension.

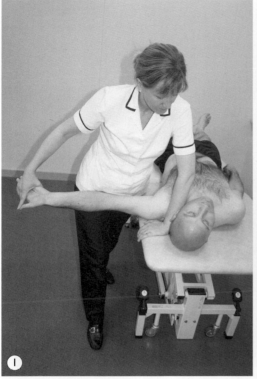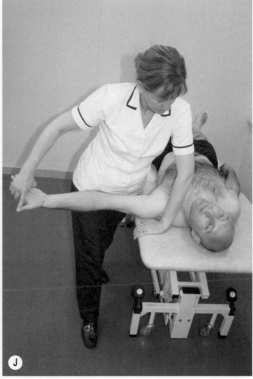

FIG. 3.31, cont'd ▪ (I) Ipsilateral lateral flexion of the cervical spine if symptoms are in the arm. If ipsilateral lateral flexion reduces (or increases) the patient's symptoms, this would be a positive test. (J) Wrist flexion may be used to desensitize the movement, if the patient's symptoms are close to the cervical spine such as over the upper fibres of trapezius. If wrist flexion reduces (or increases) the patient's neck symptoms this would be a positive test.

for example, the patient has symptoms in the upper arm or below (in the medial forearm and hand):

1. neutral position of body on couch
2. contralateral lateral flexion of the cervical spine
3. shoulder girdle stabilized
4. wrist and finger extension
5. forearm pronation
6. elbow flexion
7. shoulder abduction
8. shoulder lateral rotation
9. further shoulder abduction
10. desensitizing movement of ipsilateral lateral flexion of the cervical spine

or

11. wrist flexion if symptoms are near the cervical spine, for example, over the upper fibres of trapezius.

Normal responses to ULNT 1 (Kenneally et al. 1988) are a deep ache or stretch in the cubital fossa extending to the anterior and radial aspects of the forearm and hand, tingling in the thumb and first three fingers, and a stretching feeling over the anterior aspect of the shoulder. Contralateral cervical lateral flexion increased symptoms while ipsilateral cervical lateral flexion reduced the symptoms.

Normal responses to ULNT 2b (Yaxley & Jull 1993) on asymptomatic subjects are a feeling of stretching pain over the radial aspect of the proximal forearm; these symptoms are usually increased with the addition of contralateral cervical lateral flexion.

ULNT 3 normal responses are a stretching pain and pins and needles over the hypothenar eminence, and the ring and little fingers (Butler 2000).

Additional tests for the upper-limb tension test include placing the other arm in a ULNT position and

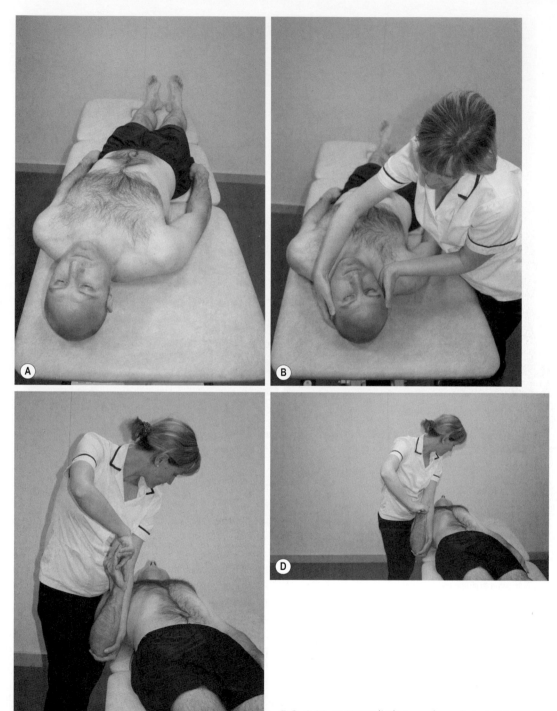

FIG. 3.32 ■ Upper-limb neurodynamic test (ULNT) 2a. (A) Neutral position of body on couch, but with shoulder girdle overhanging the edge. (B) Contralateral lateral flexion of the cervical spine. (C) Shoulder girdle depression. (D) Wrist, finger and thumb extension.

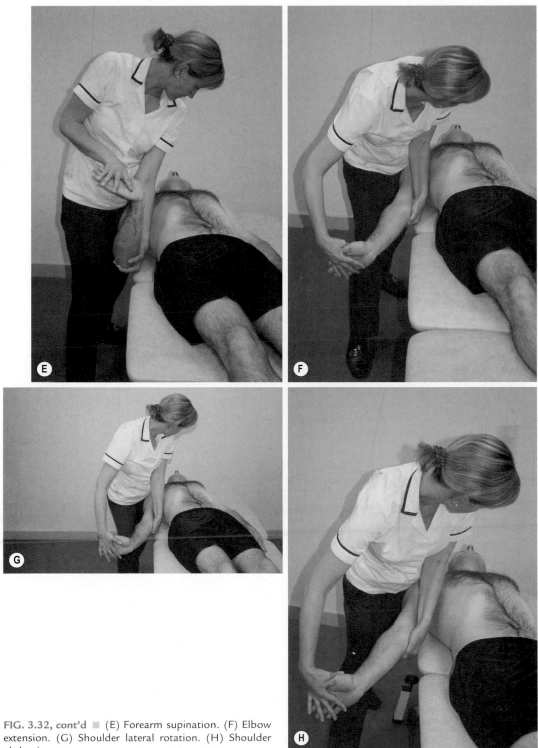

FIG. 3.32, cont'd ■ (E) Forearm supination. (F) Elbow extension. (G) Shoulder lateral rotation. (H) Shoulder abduction.

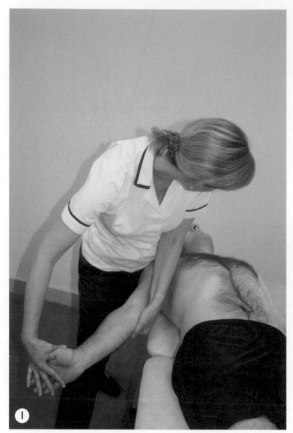

FIG. 3.32, cont'd ■ (I) Desensitizing movement of ipsilateral lateral flexion of the cervical spine.

adding in either the straight-leg raise or the slump test. The tests can also be carried out with the subject in other starting positions; for instance, the ULNT can be performed with the patient prone, which allows accessory movements to be carried out at the same time. Other upper-limb movements can be carried out in addition to those suggested; for instance, pronation/supination or radial/ulnar deviation can be added to ULNT 1.

Nerve Tissue Palpation

Clinicians can further confirm neural tissue involvement through palpation of the nerves directly where they are superficial, and indirectly in and out of tension positions (Walsh & Hall 2009). Palpation of nerves can be expected to elicit a variety of sensations. Where a nerve contains more fascicles and connective tissue it

will be more difficult to elicit a neural response, e.g. common peroneal nerve as it winds around the head of the fibula – protected by connective tissue. Normally nerves feel hard and round and are likened to guitar strings. When a nerve is under tension or if the nerve is adhered to the surrounding interface structures, transverse movement will be reduced. At an entrapment site the nerve may feel hard, swollen and thickened.

For further information on nerve palpation the reader is referred to Butler (2000) and region-specific chapters in this text.

Other Neurological Tests

These tests include various tests for spinal cord and peripheral nerve damage and are discussed in the relevant chapters.

Miscellaneous Tests

These can include vascular tests, and tests of soft tissues (such as meniscal tears in the knee). These tests are all discussed in detail in the relevant chapters.

Palpation

The clinician must be aware of the psychological impact of touch for a patient. Palpation will have a neurophysiological effect and this may produce a change in the patient's symptoms. Clear communication is required to ensure the patient is comfortable.

During the palpation of soft tissues and skeletal tissues, the following should be noted:

- the temperature of the area (increase is indicative of local inflammation)
- localized increased skin moisture (indicative of autonomic disturbance)
- the presence of oedema and effusion
- mobility and feel of superficial tissues, e.g. ganglions, nodules
- the presence or elicitation of muscle spasm
- tenderness of bone, ligament, muscle, tendon, tendon sheath, trigger point and nerve
- increased or decreased prominence of bones
- joint effusion or swelling of a limb can be measured using a tape measure, comparing left and right sides
- pain provoked or reduced on palpation.

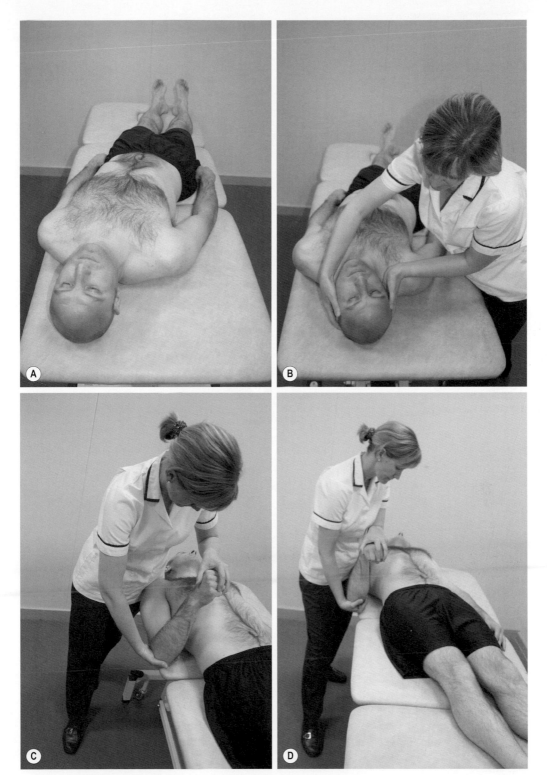

FIG. 3.33 ■ Upper-limb neurodynamic test (ULNT) 2b. (A) Neutral position of body on couch, but with shoulder girdle overhanging the edge. (B) Contralateral lateral flexion of the cervical spine. (C) Shoulder girdle depression. (D) Wrist, finger and thumb flexion.

Continued

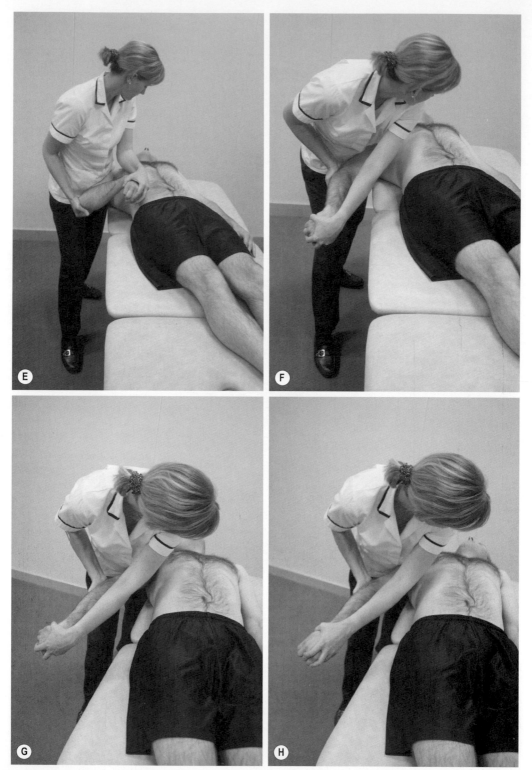

FIG. 3.33, cont'd ■ (E) Shoulder medial rotation. (F) Elbow extension. (G) Desensitizing movement of ipsilateral lateral flexion of the cervical spine, or (H) wrist extension would be used as a desensitizing movement if symptoms are near the cervical spine, for example over the upper fibres of trapezius.

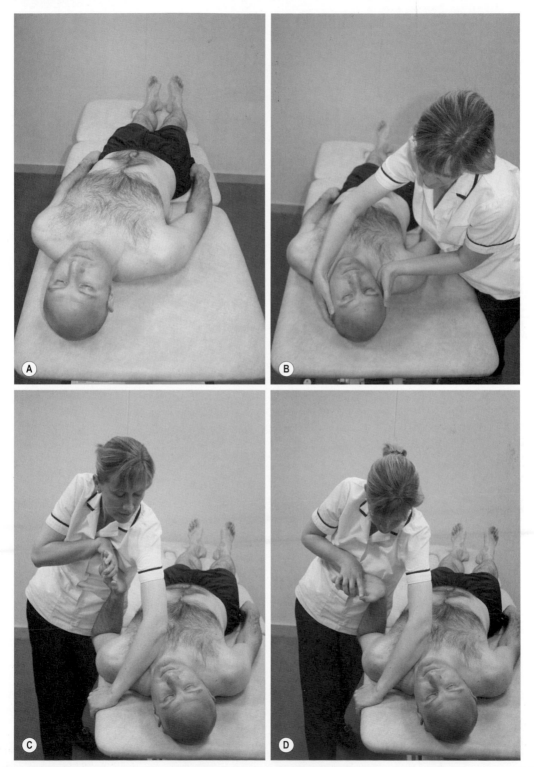

FIG. 3.34 ■ Upper-limb neurodynamic test (ULNT) 3 (ulnar nerve bias). (A) Neutral position of body on couch. (B) Contralateral lateral flexion of the cervical spine. (C) Shoulder girdle stabilized. (D) Wrist and finger extension.   *Continued*

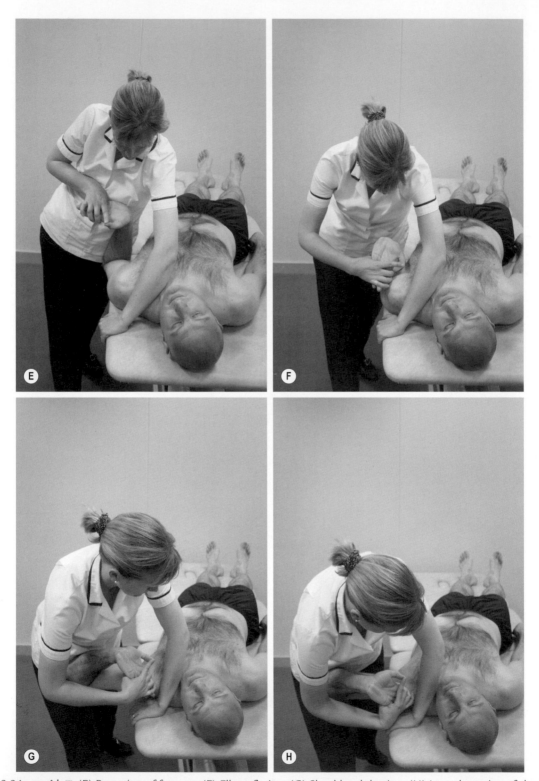

FIG. 3.34, cont'd ■ (E) Pronation of forearm. (F) Elbow flexion. (G) Shoulder abduction. (H) Lateral rotation of shoulder.

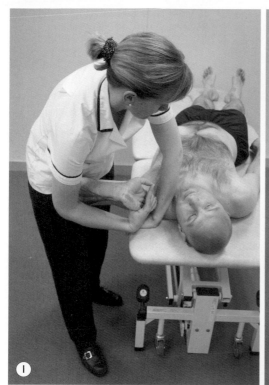

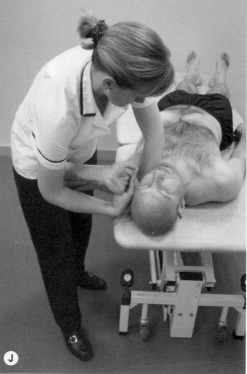

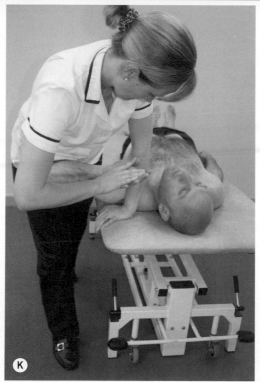

FIG. 3.34, cont'd ■ (I) Further shoulder abduction. (J) Desensitizing movement of ipsilateral lateral flexion of the cervical spine (if symptoms are in the forearm or hand), or (K) wrist flexion if symptoms are near the cervical spine or shoulder.

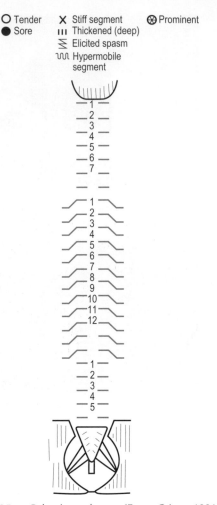

FIG. 3.35 ■ Palpation chart. *(From Grieve 1991, with permission.)*

Hints on the method of palpation are given in Box 3.5. Further guidance on palpation of the soft tissues can be found in Hunter (1998). Palpation can be used to inform clinicians about tissue states. The diagnostic use of palpation has been questioned and, due to its subjectivity, there are issues of reliability as well as validity; however, within a clinically reasoned examination it can yield useful information, especially when skilfully applied. Palpation findings can be recorded on a body chart (see Fig. 2.3) and/or palpation chart for the vertebral column (Fig. 3.35).

Trigger Points (Fig. 3.36)

Trigger points are described in Chapter 2. Trigger points may be either latent or active and can produce allodynia and referred pain. In a latent trigger point this is only when evoked, for instance by palpation, while an active trigger point produces symptoms spontaneously (Dommerholt 2011). In order to examine for a trigger point, the muscle is put on a slight stretch and the clinician applies pressure with the fingers over the muscle. A trigger point can be considered active if it is a small area with marked sensitivity in comparison with surrounding tissues and reproduces the patient's symptoms (Dommerholt 2011). This includes reproduction of referred pain if present.

Accessory Movements

Accessory movements are defined as those movements which a person cannot perform actively but which can be performed on that person by an external force (Maitland et al. 2001). They take the form of gliding (sometimes referred to as translation or sliding) of the joint surfaces (medially, laterally, anteriorly or posteriorly), distraction and compression of the joint surfaces and, in some joints, rotation movements where this movement cannot be performed actively, e.g. rotation at the metacarpal and interphalangeal joints of the fingers. These movements are possible because all joints have a certain amount of play or 'slack' in the capsule and surrounding ligaments (Kaltenborn 2002).

Limitation in physiological range of movement may be due to a limitation of the accessory range of movement at the joint. Application of biomechanical models proposing the concave convex rule (Fig. 3.37)

Sternocleidomastoid

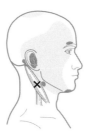

Splenius capitis

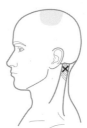

Temporalis

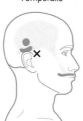

Masseter

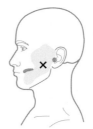

Upper trapezius

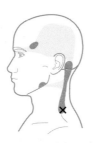

Upper trapezius

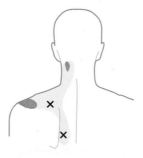

Levator scapulae

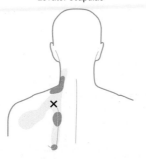

Multifidus

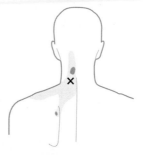

(A)   Trigger area ✕   Pain pattern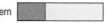

FIG. 3.36 ■ (A–D) Myofascial trigger points (*Trp*).

Continued

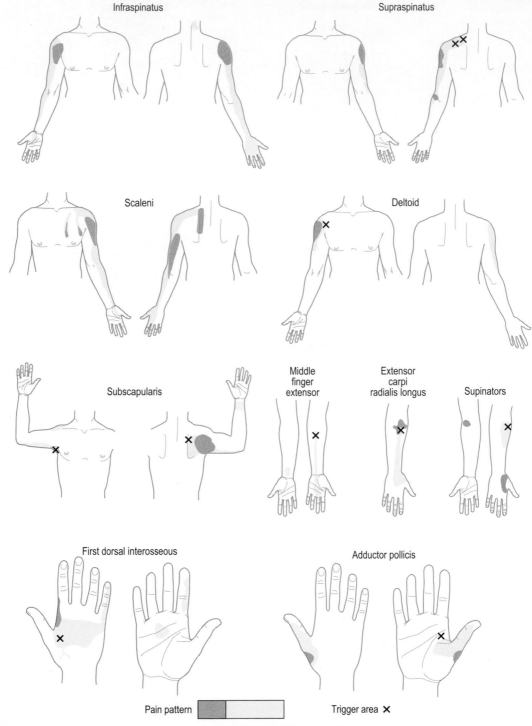

FIG. 3.36, cont'd

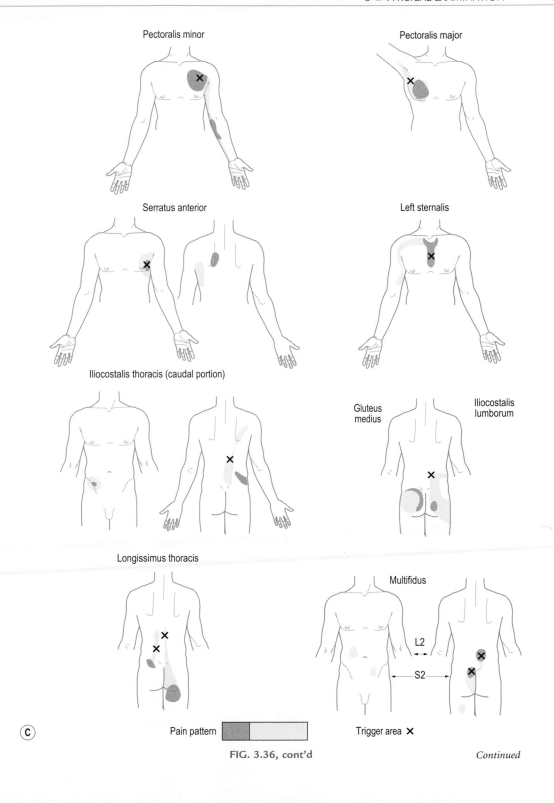

Pectoralis minor

Pectoralis major

Serratus anterior

Left sternalis

Iliocostalis thoracis (caudal portion)

Gluteus medius

Iliocostalis lumborum

Longissimus thoracis

Multifidus

L2

S2

Pain pattern

Trigger area ✕

©

FIG. 3.36, cont'd

Continued

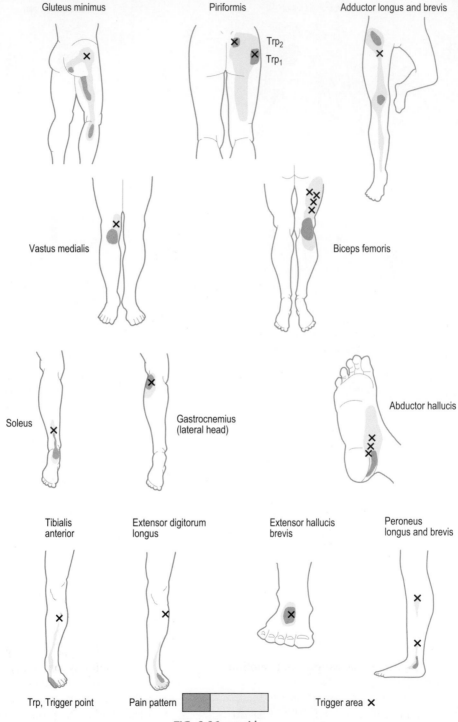

Gluteus minimus

Piriformis

Trp₂
Trp₁

Adductor longus and brevis

Vastus medialis

Biceps femoris

Soleus

Gastrocnemius
(lateral head)

Abductor hallucis

Tibialis
anterior

Extensor digitorum
longus

Extensor hallucis
brevis

Peroneus
longus and brevis

D   Trp, Trigger point   Pain pattern   Trigger area ✕

FIG. 3.36, cont'd

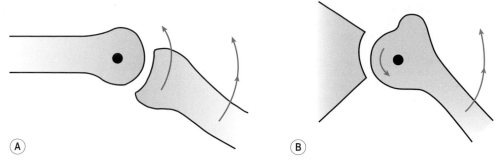

FIG. 3.37 ■ (A, B) Movement of articular surfaces during physiological movements. The single arrow depicts the direction of movement of the articular surface and the double arrow depicts the physiological movement. *(From Kaltenborn 2002, with permission.)*

for assessment of peripheral joints and theories of spinal coupling have had to be adapted in recent years as evidence would suggest that joint surfaces move differently than these theoretical models would suggest in the presence of pathology (Schohmacher 2009). So, whilst models of movement can be useful, careful examination of patients is key to identifying the cause of symptoms.

Indeed, evidence supporting a purely biomechanical basis for testing is limited. An increased understanding of the neurophysiological effects of accessory movement testing has broadened reasoning and thinking to appreciate the complex interactions that occur within the central nervous system (Bialosky et al. 2009). These effects are also psychological as the patient's response to hands-on testing will be influenced by the patient's mood, expectation and conditioning (Bialosky et al. 2011). This means clinicians must be aware of the context within which testing takes place, reasoning all aspects of the complex interaction between body and mind.

Accessory assessment can provide information on:

- the patient's response to localized movement
- identifying and localizing a symptomatic joint
- defining the nature of a joint motion abnormality
- identifying associated areas of joint motion abnormality
- altering local muscle and nerve tissues and identifying either the source of the patient's symptoms or a contributing factor to the patient's condition

- providing a basis for the selection of treatment techniques.

Pressure is applied to a bone close to the joint line and the clinician increases movement progressively through the range and notes the:

- quality of the movement
- range of the movement
- pain behaviour (local and referred) through the range, which may be provoked or reduced
- resistance through range and at the end of the range
- muscle spasm elicitation.

Hints on performing an accessory movement are given in Box 3.6. Findings can include the following:

- undue skeletal prominence
- undue tenderness
- thickening of soft tissues
- decreased mobility of soft tissues, such as periarticular tissues, muscles and nerves
- a point in the range of the accessory movement where symptoms are increased or reduced
- an indication as to the irritability of a problem (see Chapter 2)
- evidence of joint hypermobility
- evidence of joint hypomobility
- elicitation of muscle spasm
- joints that are not affected by the present problem
- the location(s) of the problem(s)
- the relationship of the problems to each other
- the possible indication of structures involved

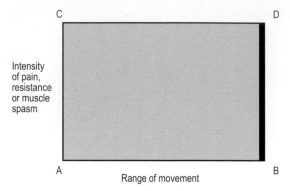

FIG. 3.38 ■ A movement diagram. The baseline AB is the range of movement of any joint and the vertical axis AC depicts the intensity of pain, resistance or muscle spasm.

The vertical axis AC depicts the intensity of quality, nature or intensity of the factors being plotted, such as pain, resistance or muscle spasm. Point A is the absence of any pain, resistance or spasm. Point C is the maximum intensity that the clinician is prepared to provoke. The clinician would need to judge irritability and the underlying cause of the patient's symptoms to assist in reasoning appropriate levels of provocation.

Procedure for Drawing a Movement Diagram

To Draw Resistance (Fig. 3.39). The clinician moves the joint and the first point at which firm resistance is felt is called R_1 and is marked on the baseline AB. A normal joint, when moved passively, has the feel of being well oiled and friction-free until nearer the end of range, when some resistance is felt that increases to limit passive range of movement. As mentioned previously, the resistance to further movement is due to bony apposition, increased tension in the surrounding ligaments and muscles or soft-tissue apposition.

The joint is then taken to the limit of range and the point of limitation is marked by L on the baseline AB. If resistance limits the range, the point of limitation is marked by R_2 vertically above L on the CD line to indicate that it is resistance that limits the range. R_2 is the point beyond which the clinician is not prepared to push. A line is drawn linking R_1 and R_2 to depict the behaviour of the resistance.

If, on the other hand, pain limits the range of movement, an estimate of the intensity of resistance is made at the end of the available range and is plotted vertically above L as R'. The behaviour of the resistance

■ what is limiting the movement and the relationship of pain, resistance or muscle spasm within the available range of movement. A movement diagram can be used to depict this information.

Movement Diagrams

The movement diagram is a useful tool when learning how to examine joint movement and is also a quick and easy way of recording information on joint movements. It was initially described by Maitland (1977) and, for full details of compiling a movement diagram with clinical examples, refer to Hengeveld and Banks (2014).

A movement diagram is a graph representing the behaviour of pain, resistance and muscle spasm, showing the intensity and position in range at which each is felt during a passive accessory or passive physiological movement of a joint (Fig. 3.38).

The baseline AB is the range of movement of any joint. Point A represents the starting point of movement and can be anywhere in range and point B is the end of the passive range of movement.

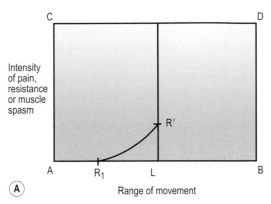

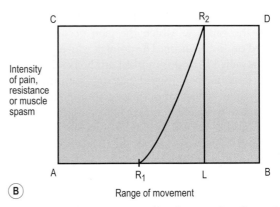

FIG. 3.39 ■ Resistance depicted on a movement diagram for physiological movements. (A) The diagram describes a joint movement that is limited (L) to half range. Resistance is first felt at around one-quarter of full range (R_1) and increases a little at the end of the available range (R'). (B) The diagram describes a joint movement that is limited (L) to three-quarters range. Resistance is first felt at around half of full range (R_1) and gradually increases to the limit range of movement (R_2).

between R_1 and R' is then described by drawing a line between the two points.

The resistance curve of the movement diagram, during physiological movements, is essentially a part of the load–displacement curve of soft tissue (Panjabi 1992; Lee & Evans 1994) and is shown in Fig. 3.40. In a normal joint, the initial range of movement has minimal resistance and this part is known as the toe region (Lee & Evans 1994) or neutral zone (Panjabi 1992). As the joint is moved further into range, resistance increases; this is known as the linear region (Lee & Evans 1994) or elastic zone (Panjabi 1992). R_1 is the point at which the clinician perceives an increase in the resistance and it will lie somewhere between the toe region/neutral zone and the linear region/elastic zone. The ease with which a clinician can feel this change in resistance might be expected to depend on the range of joint movement and the type of movement being examined. It seems reasonable to suggest that it would be easier to feel R_1 when the range of movement is large and where there is a relatively long toe region, such as elbow flexion.

By contrast, accessory movements may only have a few millimetres of movement and no clear toe region (Petty et al. 2002); in this case R_1 may be perceived at the beginning of the range. For this reason, resistance occurs at the beginning of the range of movement for accessory movements, shown in Fig. 3.41. A further complication in finding R_1 occurs with spinal accessory movements, because the movement is not localized to

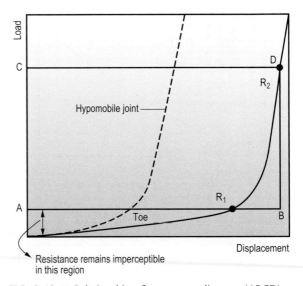

FIG. 3.40 ■ Relationship of movement diagram (ABCD) to a load–displacement curve. *(From Lee & Evans 1994, with permission.)*

any one joint but produces a general movement of the spine (Lee & Svensson 1990).

To Draw Pain Provocation (Fig. 3.42). In this case, the clinician must establish whether the patient has any resting pain before moving the joint.

The joint is then moved passively through range, asking the patient to report any discomfort immediately. Several small oscillatory movements are carried out, gradually moving further into range up to the point where the pain is first felt, so that the exact position in the range at which the pain occurs can be recorded on the diagram. The point at which pain first occurs is called P_1 and is marked on the baseline AB.

The joint is then moved passively beyond P_1 to determine the behaviour of the pain through the available range of movement. If pain limits range, the point of limitation is marked as L on the baseline AB. Vertically above L, P_2 is marked on the CD line to indicate that it is pain that limits the range. The behaviour of the pain between P_1 and P_2 is now drawn.

If, however, it is resistance that limits the range of movement, an estimate of the intensity of pain is made at the end of range and is plotted vertically above L as P'. The behaviour of the pain between P_1 and P' is then described by drawing a line between the two points.

To Draw Muscle Spasm (Fig. 3.43). The joint is taken through range and the point at which resistance due to muscle spasm is first felt is marked on the baseline AB as S_1.

The joint is then taken to the limit of range. If muscle spasm limits range, the point of limitation is marked as L on the baseline AB. Vertically above L, S_2 is marked on the CD line to indicate that it is muscle spasm that limits the range. The behaviour of spasm is then plotted between S_1 and S_2. When spasm limits range, it always reaches its maximum quickly and is

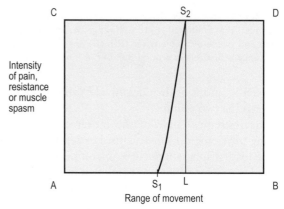

FIG. 3.43 ■ Muscle spasm depicted on a movement diagram. The diagram describes a joint movement that is limited to three-quarters range (L). Muscle spasm is first felt just before three-quarters of full range (S_1) and quickly increases to limit the range of movement (S_2).

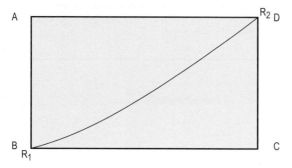

FIG. 3.41 ■ A movement diagram of an accessory movement, where R_1 starts at the beginning of range (at A).

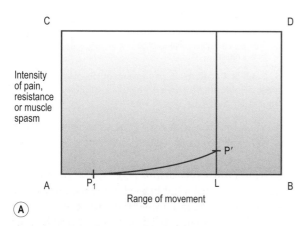

(A)

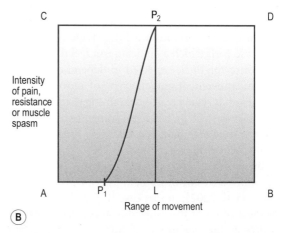

(B)

FIG. 3.42 ■ Pain depicted on a movement diagram. (A) The diagram describes a joint movement that is limited to three-quarters range (L). Pain is first felt at around one-quarter of full range (P_1) and increases a little at the end of available range (P'). (B) The diagram describes a joint movement that is limited to half range (L). Pain is first felt at around one-quarter of full range (P_1) and gradually increases to limit the range of movement (P_2).

more or less a straight line almost vertically upwards. The resistance from muscle spasm varies depending on the speed at which the joint is moved – as the speed increases, so the resistance increases.

Examples of completed movement diagrams are given in Fig. 3.44.

A few examples of movement diagrams for comparison are shown in Fig. 3.45.

Modifications to Accessory Movement Examination

Accessory movements can be modified by altering the:

- speed of applied force; pressure can be applied slowly or quickly and it may or may not be oscillated through the range
- direction of the applied force

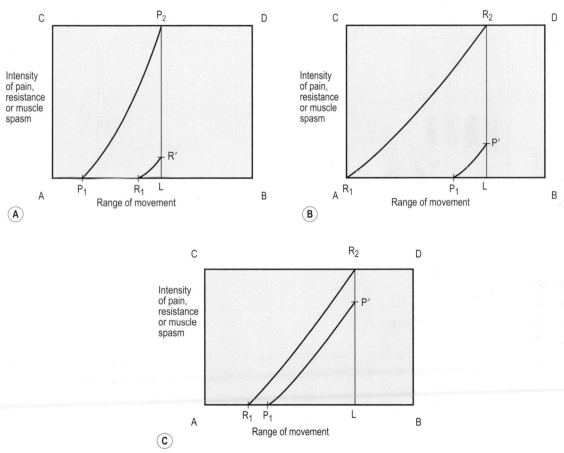

FIG. 3.44 ■ Examples of completed movement diagrams. (A) Shoulder joint flexion. Interpretation: shoulder joint flexion is limited to just over half range (L). Pain first comes on at about one-quarter of full range (P_1) and increases to limit the range of movement (P_2). Resistance is first felt just before the end of the available range (R_1) and increases a little (R'). The movement is therefore predominantly limited by pain. (B) Central posteroanterior pressure on L3. Interpretation: the posteroanterior movement is limited to three-quarters range (L). Resistance is felt immediately, at the beginning of range (R_1), and increases to limit the range of movement (R_2). Pain is first felt just before the limit of the available range (P_1) and increases slightly (P'). The movement is therefore predominantly limited by resistance. (C) Left cervical rotation. Interpretation: left cervical rotation is limited to three-quarters range (L). Resistance is first felt at one-quarter of full range (R_1) and increases to limit range of movement (R_2). Pain is felt very soon after resistance (P_1) and increases (P') to an intensity of about 8/10 (where 0 represents no pain and 10 represents the maximum pain ever felt by the patient). Cervical rotation is therefore limited by resistance but pain is a significant factor.

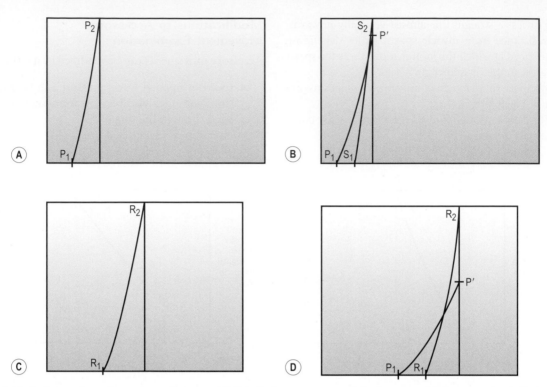

FIG. 3.45 ■ Comparison of movement diagrams. (A) Pain limits movement early in the range. (B) Spasm and pain limit movement early in the range. (C) Resistance limits movement halfway through the range. (D) Limitation of movement to three-quarters range because of resistance, with some pain provoked from halfway through the range.

- point of application of the applied force
- resting position of the joint.

The joint can be placed in any number of start positions. The clinician should use clinical reasoning to select an appropriate start position for the patient based on known aggravating and easing factors and judgements of irritability and severity. For example, accessory movements on the patella can be applied with the knee anywhere between full flexion and full extension, and accessory movements to any part of the spine can be performed with the spine in flexion, extension, lateral flexion or rotation, or indeed, any combination of these positions. The effect of this positioning alters the effect of the accessory movement. For example, central posteroanterior pressure on C5 causes the superior articular facets of C5 to slide upwards on the inferior articular facets of C4, a movement similar to cervical extension; this upward

movement can be enhanced with the cervical spine positioned in extension. This would be appropriate for a patient who has low irritability and severity of symptoms provoked on cervical spine extension.

Accessory movements are carried out on each joint suspected to be a source of the symptoms. After each joint is examined in this way, all relevant patient specific reassessment markers * are reassessed to determine the effect of the accessory movements on the signs and symptoms. For example, in a patient with cervical spine, shoulder and elbow pain, it may be found that, following accessory movements to the cervical spine, there is an increase in range and reduction in pain in both the cervical spine and the shoulder joint but that there is no change in elbow movement. Accessory movements to the elbow joint, however, may be found to improve the elbow range of movements. Such a scenario suggests that the cervical spine is giving rise to the pain in the cervical spine and the

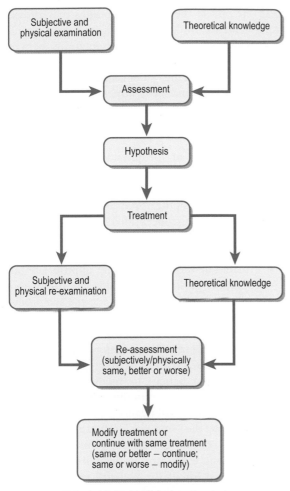

FIG. 3.46 ■ Analytical assessment.

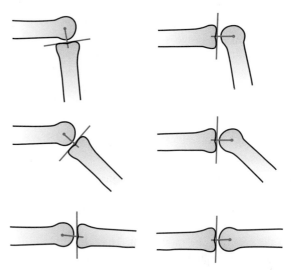

FIG. 3.47 ■ The treatment plane is indicated by the line and passes through the joint and lies 'in' the concave articular surface. *(From Kaltenborn & Evjenth 1989, with permission.)*

shoulder, and the local tissues around the elbow are responsible for producing the pain at the elbow. This process had been termed the 'analytical assessment' by Maitland et al. (2001) and is shown in Fig. 3.46.

Accessory movements have been described by various authors (Cyriax 1982; Grieve 1991; Kaltenborn 2002, 2003; Maitland, cited in Hengeveld & Banks 2014; Mulligan, cited in Hing et al. 2015). This text will deal mainly with those described by Maitland, Kaltenborn and Mulligan and they will be covered in the relevant chapters.

Developed from Kaltenborn's work (Kaltenborn 2002, 2003), the Mulligan concept is both an assessment and management approach to movement

dysfunction (Hing et al. 2015). As mentioned earlier, during normal physiological movements there is a combination of rolling and gliding of bony surfaces at the joint. The Mulligan approach proposes that movement dysfunction results from minor positional faults of a joint restricting movement, and thus restoring the glide component of the movement facilitates full painfree movement at the joint. During examination, the clinician moves the bone parallel (translation) or at right angles (distraction/separation) to the treatment plane. The treatment plane passes through the joint and lies 'in' the concave articular surface (Fig. 3.47). During the application of these accessory movements, it is the relief of symptoms that implicates the joint as the source of symptoms, since the technique aims to facilitate movement. The examination tests can be used as a treatment technique; for details of these, the reader is referred to Hing et al. (2015).

Natural Apophyseal Glides (NAGs)

These are midrange passive oscillatory rhythmic mobilizations applied centrally or unilaterally in the cervical and upper thoracic spine (between C2 and T3). They are carried out in a weight-bearing position and the direction of the force is along the facet treatment plane (anterosuperiorly). They should eliminate the pain provoked during the movement.

Sustained Natural Apophyseal Glides (SNAGs)

These are end-range sustained mobilizations, which are combined with active movements and can be used for all areas of the spine. Like natural apophyseal glides, they are carried out in a weight-bearing position with the direction of the force along the facet treatment plane. They should eliminate the pain provoked during the movement.

Mobilizations With Movement (MWMs)

These are sustained mobilizations carried out with active or passive movements or resisted muscle contraction and are used for the peripheral joints. They are generally applied close to the joint at right angles to the plane of the movement. They should eliminate the pain provoked during the movement. It is proposed that the mobilization affects and corrects a bony positional fault, which produces abnormal tracking of the articular surfaces during movement (Exelby 1996; Mulligan 1999).

Spinal Mobilization With Limb Movement (SMWLMs)

These can be useful differentiation tools where there is lower- or upper-limb movement restriction resulting from spinal or neurodynamic dysfunction. These complement other assessment approaches already described, i.e. symptom referral, active physiological lower-limb movements, PPIVMs and PAVIMs. These transverse glides can be applied to the spine in weight- and non-weight-bearing positions with the addition of upper/lower-limb movements.

COMPLETION OF THE PHYSICAL EXAMINATION

On completion of the physical examination it is important to record the examination accurately and vital at this stage to highlight with an asterisk (*) important findings from the examination (Hengeveld & Banks 2014). These findings must be reassessed at, and within, subsequent treatment sessions to evaluate the effects of treatment on the patient's condition. An outline examination chart that summarizes the physical examination is shown in Fig. 3.48.

The physical testing procedures which specifically indicate joint, nerve or muscle tissues, as a source of the patient's symptoms, are summarized in Table 3.9.

At one end of the scale the findings may provide strong evidence, and, at the other end, may provide weak evidence. A variety of presentations between these two extremes may, of course, be found. For further information the reader is directed to Chapter 4.

Clinicians may find the treatment and management planning form shown in Fig. 3.49 helpful in guiding them through what is often a complex clinical reasoning process.

On completion of the physical examination the clinician:

- gives the patient the opportunity to ask any questions. Any misconceptions patients may have regarding their symptoms should be discussed here
- explains to the patient, using appropriate language, the findings of the physical examination and how these findings relate to the symptoms
- warns the patient of possible exacerbation up to 24–48 hours following the examination. With severe and/or irritable conditions, the patient may have increased symptoms following examination
- requests the patient to report details on the behaviour of the symptoms following examination at the next attendance
- evaluates the findings, reflecting using the clinical reasoning forms to refine the primary hypothesis, writes up a problem list, i.e. a concise numbered list of the patient's problems at the time of the examination. For example, signs and symptoms of patellofemoral dysfunction, could include pain over the knee and difficulty ascending and descending stairs, inhibition of vastus medialis oblique, tightness of the iliotibial band and hamstring muscle group, and lateral tilt and external rotation of the patella. Reasoning should also include contributing factors such as general fitness, poor ergonomics and lack of sleep as these will all impact on the patient's symptoms
- in collaboration with the patient identifies and agrees the long- and short-term goals. Short-term goals for the above example might be relief of some of the knee pain on climbing stairs through application of tape to correct patella alignment, increased contraction of vastus medialis oblique,

Observation	Isometric muscle testing
Joint integrity tests	Other muscle tests
Active and passive physiological movements	Neurological integrity tests
	Neurodynamic tests
	Other nerve tests
	Miscellaneous tests
Muscle strength	Palpation
Muscle control	
Muscle length	Accessory movements and reassessment of each relevant region

FIG. 3.48 ■ Physical examination chart.

TABLE 3.9

Physical Tests which, if Positive, Indicate Joint, Nerve and Muscle as a Source of the Patient's Symptoms

Test	Strong Evidence	Weak Evidence
Joint		
Active physiological movements	Reproduces patient's symptoms	Dysfunctional movement: reduced range, excessive range, altered quality of movement, increased resistance, decreased resistance
Passive physiological movements	Reproduces patient's symptoms; this test is the same as for active physiological movements	Dysfunctional movement: reduced range, excessive range, increased resistance, decreased resistance, altered quality of movement
Accessory movements	Reproduces patient's symptoms	Dysfunctional movement: reduced range, excessive range, increased resistance, decreased resistance, altered quality of movement
Palpation of joint	Reproduces patient's symptoms	Tenderness
Reassessment following therapeutic dose of accessory movement	Improvement in tests which reproduce patient's symptoms	No change in physical tests which reproduce patient's symptoms
Muscle		
Active movement	Reproduces patient's symptoms	Reduced strength Poor quality
Passive physiological movements	Do not reproduce patient's symptoms	
Isometric contraction	Reproduces patient's symptoms	Reduced strength Poor quality
Passive lengthening of muscle	Reproduces patient's symptoms	Reduced range Increased resistance Decreased resistance
Palpation of muscle	Reproduces patient's symptoms	Tenderness
Reassessment following therapeutic dose of muscle treatment	Improvement in tests which reproduce patient's symptoms	No change in physical tests which reproduce patient's symptoms
Nerve		
Passive lengthening and sensitizing movement, i.e. altering length of nerve by a movement at a distance from patient's symptoms	Reproduces patient's symptoms and sensitizing movement alters patient's symptoms	Reduced length Increased resistance
Palpation of nerve	Reproduces patient's symptoms	Tenderness

increased extensibility of the iliotibial band and hamstrings, the patient returning to sport as a longer term goal.

■ through discussion with the patient devises an initial treatment plan in order to achieve the short- and long-term goals. This includes the modalities and frequency of treatment and any patient education required. In the patellofemoral example, this might be treatment which may include passive stretches to the iliotibial band and hamstrings; passive accessory movements to the patella; taping to correct the patella malalignment; specific exercises with biofeedback to alter the timing and intensity of vastus medialis oblique contraction in squat standing, progressing to steps and specific functional exercises and activities.

By the end of the physical examination the clinician will be able to revisit and further develop the hypotheses categories initiated in the subjective examination (adapted from Jones & Rivett 2004) (Fig. 3.50):

List the patient's subjective reassessment asterisks (*) you will use	
Subjective	Physical

What outcome measures will you use to evaluate management interventions?

Indicate your primary hypothesis (H1) regarding the cause of the patient's complaint and identify evidence to support this decision

Primary hypothesis (H1)	Alternative	Alternative	Alternative	Alternative
Evidence				

List the positive and negative factors (from both subjective and physical examination findings) in considering the patient's prognosis

Positive	Negative

Management options

1.1. Based on your primary hypothesis briefly outline a clinically reasoned treatment programme

1.2. What would your management be on day 1? Why was this chosen over other options?

1.3. What is your expectation of the patient's response over the next 24 hours?

If the patient returned better, how would you modify your treatment?

If the patient returned the same, how would you modify your treatment?

If the patient returned worse, how would you modify your treatment?

Comment on this patient's prognosis. (Include your estimation of the % improvement for this patient, the number of treatments required to achieve this and the time period over which it will occur)

FIG. 3.49 ■ Management planning form (to be completed after the physical examination). *(After Maitland 1985.)*

1. Activity and participation capabilities/restrictions

Activity capability	Restriction
Participation capability	Restriction

2. Patient's perspectives on their experience
Examples:
− Their understanding
− Their feelings
− Their coping strategies
− Attitude to self-management and physical activity
− Their beliefs/what does this experience mean to them?
− Their expectations
− Their goals

3.   Pathobiological mechanisms

3.1   Tissue sources/tissue healing, e.g., at what stage of the inflammatory/healing process would you judge the principal disorder to be?

3.2   Pain mechanisms. List the subjective evidence which supports each specific mechanism of symptoms

Input mechanism		Processing mechanism	Output mechanism
Nociceptive symptoms	Neuropathic symptoms	Central sensitization	Behaviour, motor function, thoughts, beliefs, cognition, autonomic nervous system

Reflect on this pie chart the proportional involvement of the pain mechanisms

Nociceptive
Peripheral neuropathic
Central sensitization
Autonomic nervous system

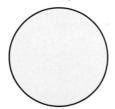

4.   The sources of the symptoms
List in order of likelihood the possible structures at fault for each area/component of symptoms

Tissue sources	Symptom 1:	Symptom 2:	Symptom 3:	Symptom 4:
Local				
Referred				
Neurogenic				
Vascular				
Visceral				

FIG. 3.50 ■ Clinical reasoning form revisited.   *Continued*

5. **Contributing factors**

Examples:
- Physical
- Environmental
- Psychosocial
- Health related

6. **History of symptoms**

Onset/physical impairment/stage/implications for physical examination

7. **List for each area of symptoms**

	Aggravating activity	Time to aggravate	Stops the activity	Easing the activity	Time to ease	Irritability Yes/No	Severity Yes/No
Symptoms 1 (P_a)							
Symptoms 2 (P_a)							

8. **Give an indication of the proportion of inflammatory to mechanical components in this patient's pain presentation, together with the clinical features that support or negate your hypothesis**

Mechanical	Inflammatory
Justification	Justification

9. **Health considerations, precautions and contraindications to physical examination and management**

9.1 **Does the patient have any health, red flag or precaution to limit your physical examination?**

Consider the following in relation to red flags

9.2 **Is reproduction of symptoms easy or difficult to reproduce? How vigorously would you examine this patient for each area of symptoms?**

Symptom	Short of P_1	To P_1 only	25% reproduction of pain	Full reproduction of pain
P_1				
P_2				
P_3				

9.3 **Will a neurological integrity examination be necessary**

Yes   No

Justify your decision

FIG. 3.50, cont'd

10. Indicate your primary (working) hypothesis (H1) regarding the cause of the patient's complaint and identify evidence to support this decision

Primary hypothesis (H1)	Alternative H	Alternative H	Alternative H	Alternative H
Evidence:				

To test Neurointegrity Yes No		Expected findings
Must	→	
Should	→	
Could	→	

FIG. 3.50, cont'd

- activity capability/restriction/participant capability/restriction
- patients' perspectives on their experience
- pathobiological mechanisms, including the structure or tissue that is thought to be producing the patient's symptoms and the nature of the structure or tissues in relation to both the healing process and the pain mechanisms
- physical impairments and associated structures/tissue sources
- contributing factors to the development and maintenance of the problem; there may be environmental, psychosocial, behavioural, physical or heredity factors
- precautions/contraindications to treatment and management; these include the severity and irritability of the patient's symptoms and the nature of the patient's condition
- management strategy and treatment plan
- prognosis – this can be affected by factors such as the stage and extent of the injury as well as the patient's expectations, personality and lifestyle.

For further information on treatment and management of patients with musculoskeletal dysfunction, please see the companion to this text, *Principles of Musculoskeletal Treatment and Management* (Petty & Barnard 2017).

REFERENCES

Alshami, A.M., et al., 2008. A review of plantar heel pain of neural origin: differential diagnosis and management. Man. Ther. 13, 103–111.

American Academy of Orthopaedic Surgeons, 1990. Joint motion. Method of measuring and recording, third ed. Churchill Livingstone, New York.

Beighton, P.H., et al., 1973. Articular mobility in an African population. Ann. Rheum. Dis. 32, 413–418.

Bell-Krotoski, J.A., et al., 1995. Threshold detection and Semmes-Weinstein monofilaments. J. Hand Ther. 8, 155–162.

Bergmark, A., 1989. Stability of the lumbar spine. A study in mechanical engineering. Acta Orthop. Scand. 230 (Suppl.), 20–24.

Bialosky, J., et al., 2011. Placebo response to manual therapy: something out of nothing? J. Man. Manip. Ther. 19, 11–19.

Bialosky, J., et al., 2009. The mechanisms of manual therapy in the treatment of musculoskeletal pain. A comprehensive model. Man. Ther. 14, 531–538.

Binkley, J., et al., 1999. The Lower Extremity Functional Scale (LEFS): scale development, measurement properties, and clinical application. Phys. Ther. 79, 371–383.

Breig, A., 1978. Adverse mechanical tension in the central nervous system. Almqvist and Wiksell, Stockholm.

Butler, D.S., 2000. The sensitive nervous system. Adelaide: Neuro Orthopaedic Institute.

Cole, J.H., et al., 1988. Muscles in action: an approach to manual muscle testing. Churchill Livingstone, Edinburgh.

Comerford, M., Mottram, S., 2001. Movement and stability dysfunction – contemporary developments. Man. Ther. 6, 15–26.

Comerford, M., Mottram, S., 2013. Kinetic control: the management of uncontrolled movement. Churchill Livingstone Elsevier, Edinburgh, pp. 23–42.

Cook, N., van Griensven, H., 2013. Neuropathic pain and complex regional pain syndrome. In: van Griensven, H., et al. (Eds.), Pain. A textbook for health professionals, second ed. Churchill Livingstone, Edinburgh, pp. 137–158.

Coppieters, M.W., et al., 2006. Strain and excursion of the sciatic, tibial and plantar nerves during a modified straight leg raising test. J. Orthop. Res. 24, 1883–1889.

Coppieters, M., Nee, R., 2015. Neurodynamic management of the peripheral nervous system. In: Jull, G., et al. (Eds.), Grieve's modern musculoskeletal physiotherapy, fourth ed. Elsevier, Edinburgh, pp. 287–297.

Cyriax, J., 1982. Textbook of orthopaedic medicine – diagnosis of soft tissue lesions, eighth ed. Baillière Tindall, London.

Dankaerts, W., et al., 2006. Differences in sitting postures are associated with nonspecific chronic low back pain disorders when patients are subclassified. Spine 31, 698–704.

Dommerholt, J., 2011. Dry needling – peripheral and central considerations. J. Man. Manip. Ther. 19, 223–237.

Donaghy, M., 1997. Neurology. Oxford University Press, Oxford.

Downs, M., LaPorte, C., 2011. Conflicting dermatome maps: educational and clinical implications. J. Orthop. Sports Research Ther. 41, 427–434.

Drake, R.L., et al., 2005. Gray's anatomy for students. Churchill Livingstone, Philadelphia.

Duncan, P., et al., 1990. Functional reach: a new clinical measure of balance. J. Gerontol. 45, 192–197.

Dyck, P., 1984. Lumbar nerve root: the enigmatic eponyms. Spine 9, 3–6.

Edwards, B.C., 1999. Manual of combined movements: their use in the examination and treatment of mechanical vertebral column disorders, second ed. Butterworth-Heinemann, Oxford.

Elvey, R.L., 1985. Brachial plexus tension tests and the pathoanatomical origin of arm pain. In: Glasgow, E.F., et al. (Eds.), Aspects of manipulative therapy, second ed. Churchill Livingstone, Melbourne, p. 116.

Exelby, L., 1996. Peripheral mobilisations with movement. Man. Ther. 1, 118–126.

Fedorak, C., et al., 2003. Reliability of visual assessment of cervical and lumbar lordosis. How good are we? Spine 28, 1857–1859.

Fuller, G., 2004. Neurological examination made easy. Churchill Livingstone, Edinburgh.

Galindo, H., 2005. Assessment of function. In: van Griensven, H. (Ed.), Pain in practice: theory and treatment strategies for manual therapists. Butterworth Heinemann, Edinburgh, pp. 153–180.

Gardner, E., Johnson, K., 2013. Sensory coding. In: Kandel, E., Schwartz, J.H., et al. (Eds.), Principles of neural science, fifth ed. McGraw-Hill, New York, pp. 449–474.

Gerhardt, J.J., 1992. Documentation of joint motion, third ed. Isomed, Oregon.

Gossman, M.R., et al., 1982. Review of length-associated changes in muscle. Phys. Ther. 62, 1799–1808.

Grahame, R., et al., 2000. The revised (Brighton 1998) criteria for the diagnosis of benign joint hypermobility syndrome (BJHS). J. Rheumatol. 27, 1777–1779.

Grieve, G.P., 1981. Common vertebral joint problems. Churchill Livingstone, Edinburgh.

Grieve, G.P., 1991. Mobilisation of the spine, fifth ed. Churchill Livingstone, Edinburgh.

Harding, V.R., et al., 1994. The development of a battery of measures for assessing physical functioning in chronic pain patients. Pain 58, 367–375.

Hengeveld, E., Banks, K. (Eds.), 2014. Maitland's vertebral manipulation. Churchill Livingstone, Edinburgh, pp. 433–443.

Herrington, L., 2011. Assessment of the degree of pelvic tilt within a normal asymptomatic population. Man. Ther. 16, 646–648.

Hing, W., et al., 2015. The mulligan concept of manual therapy. Churchill Livingstone, Sydney.

Hunter, G., 1998. Specific soft tissue mobilization in the management of soft tissue dysfunction. Man. Ther. 3, 2–11.

Inman, V.T., Saunders, de C.M., 1944. Referred pain from skeletal structures. J. Nerv. Ment. Dis. 90, 660–667.

Institute for Work and Health, 2006. The QuickDASH outcome measure. A faster way to measure upper-extremity disability and symptoms. Information for users. Toronto: Institute for Work and Health.

Janda, V., 1993. Muscle strength in relation to muscle length, pain and muscle imbalance. In: Harms-Ringdahl, K. (Ed.), Muscle strength. Churchill Livingstone, Edinburgh, p. 83.

Janda, V., 1994. Muscles and motor control in cervicogenic disorders: assessment and management. In: Grant, R. (Ed.), Physical therapy of the cervical and thoracic spine, second ed. Churchill Livingstone, Edinburgh, p. 195.

Janda, V., 2002. Muscles and motor control in cervicogenic disorders. In: Grant, R. (Ed.), Physical therapy of the cervical and thoracic spine, third ed. Churchill Livingstone, New York, p. 182.

Jones, M.A., Rivett, D.A., 2004. Clinical reasoning for manual therapists. Butterworth-Heinemann, Edinburgh.

Jull, G.A., Janda, V., 1987. Muscles and motor control in low back pain: assessment and management. In: Twomey, L.T., Taylor, J.R. (Eds.), Physical therapy of the low back. Churchill Livingstone, Edinburgh, p. 253 (Chapter 10).

Jull, G.A., Richardson, C.A., 1994. Rehabilitation of active stabilization of the lumbar spine. In: Twomey, L.T., Taylor, J.R. (Eds.), Physical therapy of the low back, second ed. Churchill Livingstone, Edinburgh, p. 251.

Kaltenborn, F.M., 2002. Manual mobilization of the joints, vol. I, sixth ed. The extremities. Olaf Norli, Oslo.

Kaltenborn, F.M., 2003. Manual mobilization of the joints, vol. II, fourth ed. The spine. Olaf Norli, Oslo.

Kaltenborn, F.M., Evjenth, O., 1989. Manual mobilization of the upper extremity joints: basis of examination and treatment techniques, fourth ed. Olaf Norlis Bokandel, Universitetsgaten, Sydney.

Keefe, F.J., Block, A.R., 1982. Development of an observation method for assessing pain behavior in chronic low back pain patients. Behav. Ther. 13, 365–375.

Keer, R., Butler, K., 2010. Physiotherapy and occupational therapy in the hypermobile adult. In: Hakim, A., et al. (Eds.), Hypermobility, fibromyalgia and chronic pain. Churchill Livingstone, Edinburgh.

Kendall, F.P., et al., 2010. Muscles testing and function in posture and pain, fifth ed. Williams & Wilkins, Baltimore.

Kenneally, M., et al., 1988. The upper limb tension test: the SLR test of the arm. In: Grant, R. (Ed.), Physical therapy of the cervical and thoracic spine. Churchill Livingstone, Edinburgh, p. 167.

Kobayashi, S., et al., 2003. Changes in nerve root motion and intra-radicular blood flow during intraoperative femoral nerve stretch test. J. Neurosurg. Spine 99, 298–305.

Leak, S., 1998. Measurement of physiotherapists' ability to reliably generate vibration amplitudes and pressures using a tuning fork. Man. Ther. 3, 90–94.

Lee, R., Evans, J., 1994. Towards a better understanding of spinal posteroanterior mobilisation. Physiotherapy 80, 68–73.

Lee, M., Svensson, N.L., 1990. Measurement of stiffness during simulated spinal physiotherapy. Clin. Phys. Physiol. Meas. 11, 201–207.

Lewis, J., 2009. Rotator cuff tendinopathy/subacromial impingement syndrome: is it time for a new method of assessment? Br. J. Sports Med. 43, 259–264.

Magee, D., 2014. Orthopedic physical assessment, sixth ed. Elsevier Saunders, Missouri.

Maitland, G., 1977. Maitland's vertebral manipulation, fourth ed. Butterworths, London.

Maitland, G.D., 1985. Passive movement techniques for intra-articular and periarticular disorders. Aust. J. Physiother. 31, 3–8.

Maitland, G.D., et al., 2001. Maitland's vertebral manipulation, sixth ed. Butterworth-Heinemann, Oxford.

Martina, I., et al., 1998. Measuring vibration threshold with a graduated tuning fork in normal aging and in patients with Polyneuropathy. J. Neurol. Neurosurg. Psychiatry 65, 743–747.

May, S., Clare, H., 2015. The McKenzie method of mechanical diagnosis and therapy – an overview. In: Jull, G., et al. (Eds.), Grieve's modern musculoskeletal physiotherapy, fourth ed. Elsevier, Edinburgh, pp. 460–462.

May, S., et al., 2006. Reliability of procedures used in the physical examination of non-specific low back pain: a systematic review. Aust. J. Physiother. 52, 91–102.

Medical Research Council, 1976. Aids to the investigation of peripheral nerve injuries. London: HMSO.

Miller, A.M., 1987. Neuro-meningeal limitation of straight leg raising. In: Dalziel, B.A., Snowsill, J.C. (Eds.), Manipulative Therapists Association of Australia, 5th biennial conference proceedings. Melbourne, pp. 70–78.

Mooney, V., Robertson, J., 1976. The facet syndrome. Clin. Orthop. Relat. Res. 115, 149–156.

Mulligan, B.R., 1999. Manual therapy 'NAGs', 'SNAGs', 'MWMs' etc, fourth ed. Plane View Services, New Zealand.

Muscolino, J., 2016. The muscle bone palpation manual, second ed. Elsevier Mosby, Missouri.

Nadler, S., et al., 2001. The crossed femoral nerve stretch test to diagnose diagnostic sensitivity for the high lumbar radiculopathy: 2 case reports. Arch. Phys. Med. Rehabil. 82, 522–523.

Nir-Paz, R., et al., 1999. Saphenous nerve entrapment in adolescence. Paediatrics 103, 161–163.

Norris, C.M., 1995. Spinal stabilisation, muscle imbalance and the low back. Physiotherapy 81, 127–138.

O'Connaire, E., et al., 2011. The assessment of vibration sense in the musculoskeletal examination: moving towards a valid and reliable quantitative approach to vibration testing in clinical practice. Man. Ther. 16, 296–300.

Panjabi, M.M., 1992. The stabilising system of the spine: part II. Neutral zone and instability hypothesis. J. Spinal Disord. 5, 390–396.

Petty, N.J., Barnard, K. (Eds.), 2017. Principles of musculoskeletal treatment and management: a handbook for therapists, third ed. Elsevier, Edinburgh.

Petty, N.J., et al., 2002. Manual examination of accessory movements – seeking R1. Man. Ther. 7, 39–43.

Ridehalgh, C., et al., 2015. Sciatic nerve excursion during a modified passive straight leg raise test in asymptomatic participants and participants with spinally referred leg pain. Man. Ther. 20, 564–569.

Roland, M., Fairbank, J., 2000. The Roland-Morris Disability Questionnaire and the Oswestry Disability Questionnaire. Spine 25, 3115–3124.

Sahrmann, S.A., 2002. Diagnosis and treatment of movement impairment syndromes. Mosby, St Louis.

Schmid, A., 2015. The peripheral nervous system and its compromise in entrapment neuropathies. In: Jull, G., et al. (Eds.), Grieve's modern musculoskeletal physiotherapy, fourth ed. Elsevier, Edinburgh, pp. 78–89.

Schmid, A., et al., 2013. Reappraising entrapment neuropathies – mechanisms, diagnosis and management. Man. Ther. 18, 449–457.

Schohmacher, J., 2009. The convex–concave rule and the lever law. Man. Ther. 14, 579–582.

Shacklock, M., 2005. Clinical neurodynamics. Churchill Livingstone, Edinburgh.

Simmonds, J.V., Keer, R.J., 2007. Hypermobility and the hypermobility syndrome. Man. Ther. 12, 298–309.

Singh, S., et al., 1992. Development of a shuttle walking test of disability in patients with chronic airways obstruction. Thorax 47, 1019–1024.

Slater, H., 1994. cited in Butler D.S., 2000 The sensitive nervous system. Neuro Orthopaedic Institute: Adelaide.

Sterling, M., Rebbeck, T., 2005. The Neck Disability Index (NDI). Aust. J. Physiother. 51, 271.

Sueki, D.G., et al., 2013. A regional interdependence model of musculoskeletal dysfunctions: research mechanisms and clinical implications. J. Man. Manip. Ther. 21, 90–102.

Tencer, A.F., et al., 1985. A biomechanical study of thoracolumbar spine fractures with bone in the canal: part III. Mechanical properties of the dura and its tethering ligaments. Spine 10, 741–747.

Threlkeld, J., 1992. The effects of manual therapy on connective tissue. Phys. Ther. 72, 893–902.

Valdes, K., LaStayo, P., 2013. The value of provocative tests for the wrist and elbow. A literature review. J. Hand Ther. 26, 32–43.

Van Dillen, L.R., et al., 1998. Reliability of physical examination items used for classification of patients with low back pain. Phys. Ther. 78, 979–988.

Waddell, G., 2004. The back pain revolution, second ed. Churchill Livingstone, Edinburgh.

Walsh, J., Hall, T., 2009. Reliability, validity and diagnostic accuracy of palpation of the sciatic, tibial and common peroneal nerves in the examination of low back related leg pain. Man. Ther. 14, 623–629.

Walton, J.H., 1989. Essentials of neurology, sixth ed. Churchill Livingstone, Edinburgh.

White, S.G., Sahrmann, S.A., 1994. A movement system balance approach to musculoskeletal pain. In: Grant, R. (Ed.), Physical therapy of the cervical and thoracic spine, second ed. Churchill Livingstone, Edinburgh, p. 339.

Williams, P.L., et al. (Eds.), 1995. Gray's anatomy, thirty-eighth ed. Churchill Livingstone, Edinburgh.

Yaxley, G.A., Jull, G.A., 1993. Adverse tension in the neural system. A preliminary study of tennis elbow. Aust. J. Physiother. 39, 15–22.

4

CLINICAL REASONING AND ASSESSMENT: MAKING SENSE OF EXAMINATION FINDINGS

DIONNE RYDER

CHAPTER CONTENTS

INTRODUCTION

The previous chapters describe, step by step, a clinically reasoned subjective and physical examination. This chapter aims to revisit some of the information included within the preceding two chapters to explore how data is interpreted by the clinician. It is hoped that, taken together, the three chapters will provide an overview of the broad clinical reasoning processes that underpin effective/robust treatment and management decisions.

CLINICAL REASONING

Clinical reasoning is the process by which the clinician interprets subjective information along with physical examination findings, in order to identify the most appropriate management decisions for individual patients. However, this seemingly straightforward explanation belies the complexity of reasoning. Successful reasoning requires the ability to interpret and process multiple pieces of information concurrently, whilst prioritizing patients' needs within a healthcare framework. Effective communication skills are required to gather information to negotiate and collaborate with the patient in exploring possible solutions. Advanced cognitive skills are necessary to incorporate a range of knowledge and, where available, evidence to support thinking. Interactions with patients do not take place within a vacuum so an ability to identify the patient's human context and reflect how clinical practice is shaped and influenced by the clinician's own life experiences is also central to effective reasoning (Higgs & Jones 2008).

*Clinical reasoning is the foundation of effective patient care. It is through this process of critical thinking, incorporating the best available evidence and reflecting on the process, that collaborative decisions are made with the patient about the most appropriate care for each individual patient (**Higgs & Jones 2008**).*

The complex process of clinical reasoning has been studied and presented in the form of a number of theoretical models (Jones 1995; Gifford 1998; Edwards et al. 2004; Jones & Rivett 2004; Danneels et al. 2011) which have developed over time in response to new knowledge, so allowing clinical practice to evolve.

Whilst these models seek to represent how clinicians function in practice, research has shown that clinicians, whether expert or novice, often use a number of different reasoning strategies in parallel (Doody & McAteer 2002). Experienced clinicians have been identified as using pattern recognition reasoning early on in a patient encounter. It is thought that they use their well-organized and extensive knowledge base to search quickly for familiar patterns to forward or inductively reason. It is thought that using illness scripts to create patterns they are able to identify quickly presenting features of frequently encountered conditions (Feltowich & Barrows 1984) (Fig. 4.1).

Although pattern recognition allows for fast and efficient inductive reasoning, it is vulnerable to errors whereby the clinician may seek to make the features fit (Maitland et al. 2005). This can result in the bias sifting of information, whereby data supporting a favoured or familiar pattern are accepted, whilst contradictory data are rejected. This was the first of three types of reasoning errors identified by Grant (2008), the others being errors in interpreting the meaning and misjudging the relevance of information.

Due to the high risk of error, clinicians do not rely entirely on pattern recognition but seek to explore/test further initial hypotheses generated by pattern recognition. This testing is referred to as hypothetico-deductive reasoning, also identified as backward reasoning, and has been identified as a reasoning strategy primarily adopted by novice practitioners because of their limited experience. Using this deductive reasoning initial or working hypotheses are confirmed or refuted through gathering data by further questioning and selected physical examination testing. Although more time consuming than pattern recognition, the hypothetico-deductive reasoning process is considered more robust. However it is dependent on the ability of clinicians to interpret subjective and physical findings. How clinicians interpret the information gathered will depend on their propositional and non-propositional knowledge base. Propositional knowledge is identified as scientific/theoretical knowledge derived from the literature. Non-propositional knowledge can be further subdivided into professional craft knowledge, accumulated through experience or from formal teaching opportunities, and personal knowledge, encompassing the frame of reference for all individual clinicians, their beliefs and values shaped by their experiences (Higgs & Titchen 1995) (Fig. 4.2).

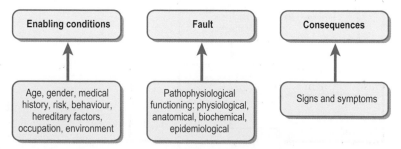

FIG. 4.1 ■ Illness scripts. Experts will have an illness script for each condition/disease they know. How complete they are will depend on how often they have encountered patients with the condition. *(From Feltowich & Barrows 1984, with permission.)*

Pattern recognition and hypothetico-deductive reasoning are considered forms of diagnostic reasoning and do not encompass the cognitive, psychological, social and intellectual context in which care is being given (Kerry 2010). Through interpretive reasoning

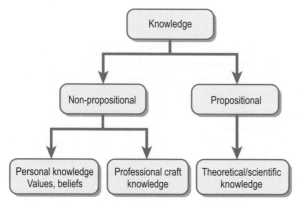

FIG. 4.2 ■ Knowledge flow diagram. *(From Higgs & Titchen 1995, with permission).*

the clinician seeks to interpret and understand the patient's problem through the use of narrative reasoning by listening to the patient's story (Edwards et al. 2006). A good example of this evolution in clinical reasoning is the patient-centred model included at the beginning of Chapter 2 (see Fig. 2.2).

In contrast to the previous versions of this model, originally presented by Jones (1995) (Fig. 4.3), the patient is included as an integral part of the decision-making process.

The revised model acknowledges that the patient's thoughts and beliefs are integral to the process of reasoning and so should be incorporated through interpretive reasoning in order to encompass patient-centred care (Cooper et al. 2008).

Clinical expertise should not be measured in terms of years qualified but on how effective reflection is on the development of dialectical reasoning skills which encompass both diagnostic and interpretive paradigms (Terry & Higgs 1993; Jones & Rivett 2004;

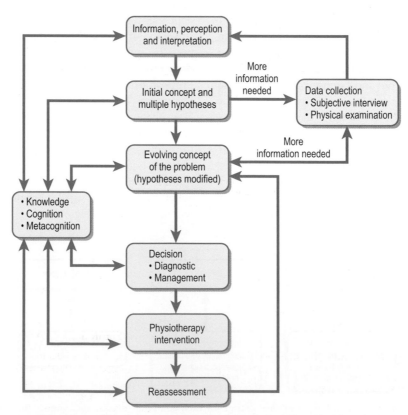

FIG. 4.3 ■ Clinical reasoning process. *(From Jones 1995, with permission.)*

Wainwright et al. 2011). Recognizing that clinical reasoning and expert practice is an ongoing journey that supports the importance of continuing professional development through self-reflection (Higgs & Jones 2008). A powerful tool for developing reflective skills is through engagement with case studies, peer coaching, completion of clinical reasoning templates or the development of mind maps. The reader is directed to section six of Higgs and Jones (2008) book, Clinical reasoning in the health professions, for an in-depth exploration of strategies to develop clinical reasoning skills.

DEVELOPMENTS IN DECISION MAKING

Many of the developments in clinical reasoning within musculoskeletal physiotherapy have been driven by the volume of evidence emerging, particularly in relation to a greater understanding of pain (Wright 1995; Melzack 2001; Bialosky et al. 2009; Woolf 2012). The pressures of the health economy have also been a driver for change, with clinicians being increasingly accountable to service commissioners to provide the most cost-effective care. This has resulted in the development of a whole series of adjuncts to clinical reasoning, such as clinical guidelines, clinical prediction rules (CPRs), treatment protocols and diagnostic/treatment classification systems.

Clinical guidelines seek to synthesize what is a potentially overwhelming evidence base to identify best practice. In 1994 the Clinical Standards Advisory Group developed guidelines on the management of low-back pain aimed at reducing the burden of persistent low-back pain on health services and the economy. The 2016 National Institute for Health and Care Excellence (NICE) guidelines on the management of low-back pain are used by commissioners in the UK to purchase musculoskeletal services.

In a similar way, CPRs have been developed to inform clinical decision making. CPRs are tools that use a combination of patient history and physical examination findings to identify the likelihood of a particular condition being present (diagnostic) or to predict a particular outcome (prognostic) or to select the most effective management option (prescriptive). CPRs have been developed from practice through patient profiling or subgrouping of patients. An example of a diagnostic CPR is the Ottawa ankle rules (Stiell et al. 1993). These rules help clinicians to exclude the likelihood of a fracture in patients presenting with an ankle sprain. The decision to refer for an X-ray is based on specific areas of bony tenderness and the patient's ability to weight bear. The rules have been found to be accurate in excluding fractures of the ankle and midfoot, in patients over 18 years of age, with a sensitivity of 100% and also offer economic and patient benefits by reducing unnecessary radiographs by 30–40% (Bachmann et al. 2003).

A prognostic CPR for management of acute non-specific low-back pain was developed by Flynn et al. (2002). This is an example of a rule whereby it has been found that patients fitting a profile matching four out of five criteria were identified as being most likely to respond favourably to spinal manipulation (Table 4.1).

The prediction rule included within these criteria a psychological measure, the fear avoidance belief questionnaire (FABQ). Fear avoidance has been recognized as a poor prognostic indicator: patients demonstrating fear avoidance behaviours were less likely to respond to a specific manual therapy intervention (Leeuw et al. 2007). Of course CPRs should be evaluated critically for example it can be argued that a single intervention such as manipulation does not reflect practice, whereby manual therapy is integrated within a package of care, usually including functionally relevant exercises, education and advice (Moore & Jull 2010).

Whilst CPRs have been identified as useful adjuncts in clinical reasoning, there is concern that their indiscriminate use could harm patients if clinicians no longer rely on their own clinical reasoning skills (Learman et al. 2012).

TABLE 4.1
Criteria for Clinical Prediction Rules of Spinal Manipulation (Flynn et al. 2002)
Less than a 16-day symptom duration
A score of 19 or less on the fear avoidance beliefs questionnaire
Lumbar hypomobility
Hip internal rotation range of >35° motion
No symptoms distal to the knee

There are examples of more complex classification systems, such as the McKenzie method of mechanical diagnosis and therapy, based on repeated movements (May & Clare 2015) (see Chapter 3). As implied in the title, this classification is biomechanically based and so will be suitable for some patients, though not all. In contrast, classification-based cognitive functional therapy for people with persistent non-specific low-back pain, first proposed by O'Sullivan (2005), classifies patients into groups based on the primary driver of their symptoms. Patients are assessed across a range of different domains, including physical impairment, pain, functional loss, activity limitation and psychological adaptation. This classification system continues to be developed into a clinical reasoning framework for the targeted assessment and management of low-back pain (O'Sullivan et al. 2015) and acknowledges that, for those with persistent symptoms and psychological factors, such as fear and anxiety, these factors will result in behaviours that will be the primary driver of their symptoms. These psychological drivers will require acknowledgement and management if successful outcomes are to be achieved (McCarthy et al. 2004).

The recognition that patients with the same complaint, such as persistent non-specific low-back pain, will present differently and therefore need different management approaches is now widely accepted. Stratifying patients into more specific subgroups is evident in the development of the STarT back tool (Hill 2011). This algorithm categorizes patients with low-back pain into one of three groups. Those identified by an initial questionnaire as being at 'low risk' of developing persistent pain receive advice; those at 'medium risk' are referred for standard musculoskeletal care and those identified as 'high risk' receive psychologically informed care.

Whilst all of these approaches inform practice, the challenge for individual clinicians is the decision making that is required to incorporate them into their reasoning so that they are able to offer safe, evidence-informed, patient-centred care.

It is evident from developments in clinical reasoning theories that practice continues to evolve. There has been a shift from a biomedical approach, seeking a diagnosis based on underlying pathobiological processes, to incorporate the psychosocial paradigms with the recognition that body and mind cannot be separated (Chapman et al. 2008) (Fig. 4.4).

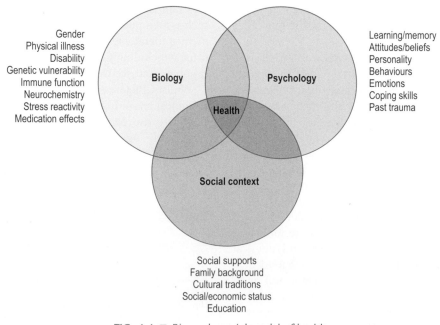

Gender
Physical illness
Disability
Genetic vulnerability
Immune function
Neurochemistry
Stress reactivity
Medication effects

Biology

Psychology

Learning/memory
Attitudes/beliefs
Personality
Behaviours
Emotions
Coping skills
Past trauma

Health

Social context

Social supports
Family background
Cultural traditions
Social/economic status
Education

FIG. 4.4 ■ Biopsychosocial model of health.

So how do clinicians make sense of all the data collected in the subjective and physical examination to identify 'wise action' for their patients? The World Health Organization (2001) *International Classification of Functioning, Disability and Health* (ICF), introduced in Chapter 2 (see Fig. 2.1) provides a useful starting point, as this framework incorporates all factors capable of impacting on an individual's health and well-being (Atkinson & Nixon-Cave 2011).

Building on this framework are the reasoning categories developed by Jones et al. (2002), also introduced in Chapter 2 (see Box 2.1) and revisited at the end of Chapter 3.

These reasoning categories are included in the clinical reasoning documentation at the end of Chapter 3. The planetary model of reasoning (Danneels et al. 2011) is a vertical representation of the World Health Organization (2001) ICF framework showing the continuum of the influence of pain and psychosocial factors as orbiting planets around other components of the ICF framework (Fig. 4.5).

This chapter will use these reasoning categories as a framework to review some of the data gathered within the previous two chapters in order to explore how the information guides clinical reasoning.

CLINICAL REASONING IN THE SUBJECTIVE EXAMINATION

The primary aim of the subjective examination is for the clinician to enter into a therapeutic relationship by building a rapport with the patient (Roberts et al. 2013). The clinician will ask the patient why she has come for assessment and what her goals and expectations are for the initial session (Chester et al. 2014). Open questions, such as, 'What would be a successful outcome for you?' can be helpful in identifying what the patient may be seeking. Usually the patient will indicate having some functional or physical difficulty often, though not always, as a result of pain. This early discussion provides the clinician with very useful insights into the patient's lifestyle, level of physical

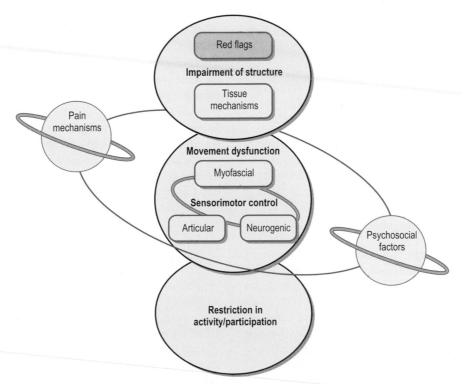

FIG. 4.5 ■ Planetary model. *(From Danneels et al. 2011, with permission.)*

activity and the impact of the condition on their life. (Opsommer & Schoeb 2014). It offers the patient an opportunity to tell her story and for the clinician to engage in narrative reasoning with the patient (Fleming & Mattingly 2008). This type of reasoning will require the clinician to demonstrate active listening using cues such as head nodding, eye contact, making use of pauses and asking reflective questions (Maguire & Pitceathly 2002). The role of communication is explored more fully in the companion text (see Chapter 9, Petty & Barnard 2017).

The clinician will have the opportunity to indicate what can be offered in terms of the diagnosis and treatment of movement dysfunctions and wider healthcare management, with the focus on restoring function and promoting healthy living (Chartered Society of Physiotherapy 2008; Middleton 2008; Banks & Hengeveld 2014). An appreciation of the patient's expectations at the outset will help foster a collaborative partnership between patient and clinician. Offering treatment choice and setting agreed goals are thought to enhance a patients motivation and compliance. Patients who share in decision making take greater responsibility for their own management and are more likely to achieve better outcomes (Jones et al. 2008; Main et al. 2010).

ACTIVITY AND PARTICIPATION CAPABILITIES AND RESTRICTIONS

Using the World Health Organization (2001) framework the clinician explores the impact of the patient's condition on her life by considering her level of activity, what the patient is able and unable to do, e.g. walking, lifting, sitting and her ability/inability to participate in life situations, i.e. work, family and leisure activities.

From the outset the clinician should be reasoning from a biopsychosocial perspective, initially using forward or inductive reasoning of the possible causes for the patient's symptoms (Rivett & Jones 2004). This will assist in developing hypotheses on possible tissues/structures, to examine in the physical examination that may be restricting the patient's activities or participation in life. Alternatively, psychological factors may be limiting the patient, as a result of fear-avoidant, hyper-vigilant behaviours. Identification of these at this point

would provide a cue for the clinician to modify his language, seeking not to dismiss fears but to interpret and understand the patient's beliefs about her symptoms (Barker et al. 2009; Darlow et al. 2013). At this stage the clinician may begin to formulate management strategies in terms of initial advice and education aimed at promoting normal activity and participation. Educating patients may enhance the therapeutic relationship as they become active participants in their own care. Answering patients' specific questions and tailoring information to suit their situation will encourage empowerment, a vital component of patient-centred care (Moseley et al. 2004; Caladine & Morris 2015).

Similarly, information about the patient's ability to participate in everyday activities will be very relevant; for example, the financial pressures of being self-employed and unable to work, or the social isolation that may result from being unable to participate in leisure activities (Froud et al. 2014). The implications of loss on the individual and family can be significant and should be acknowledged (Nielsen 2014).

Seeking information on what patients are still capable of doing is equally important. Gifford (2005) labelled these 'pink flags'. He argued that there can be a preoccupation, on the part of the clinician, to focus on what patients cannot do in the desire to problem solve. He promoted identifying positively all the things they are able to do, for example, encouraging patients to continue to work, using normal activity to promote recovery. The assessment of activity and participation capabilities offers an opportunity for the clinician to encourage activity and deliver a positive message of hope, reducing the potential for medicalizing patients (MacKereth et al. 2014).

PATIENTS' PERSPECTIVES ON THEIR PAIN EXPERIENCE

Patients usually seek treatment because of pain and so seeking to understand what pain may mean from the patient's perspective will increase the likelihood of achieving a therapeutic rapport.

Pain is 'an unpleasant sensory and emotional experience associated with actual or potential tissue damage, or described in terms of such damage' (IASP 2015).

A patient's response to pain is unique and is influenced by beliefs, cultural and social constructs, and memories of past experience (Main et al. 2010). Patients beliefs are learned and are considered modifiable, with evidence demonstrating that pain education can be effective in reframing the patient's pain experience (Moseley et al. 2004; Louw et al. 2011). It is also recognized that persistent pain may influence mood, with more widespread symptoms increasing the likelihood of depression. The patient's response to simple screening questions such as:

- In the past month, has your pain been bad enough to stop you doing many of your day-to-day activities?
- In the past month, has your pain been bad enough to make you feel worried or low in mood (Aroll et al. 2003; Barker et al. 2014)?

will assist the clinician in reasoning whether the patient should be referred to an appropriately trained mental health professional, to offer additional support, alongside musculoskeletal management (Main & Spanswick 2000; Kent et al. 2014).

It is acknowledged that pain and beliefs will influence a patient's behaviour. In the acute stages avoidance strategies, referred to as adaptive, can assist in protecting tissues from further harm, allowing tissue healing to take place. However, in patients with persistent pain, avoidance behaviours are unhelpful and defined as maladaptive. Maladaptive movement patterns and altered loading may result in proprioceptive deficits and altered body schema (Luomajoki & Moseley 2011). Changes in muscle activity associated with guarding or deconditioning are thought to be responsible for pain production beyond the original symptomatic tissue. Using their knowledge of tissue healing, clinicians can reason whether behaviours are adaptive or maladaptive and use this to inform assessment and management decisions (Diegelmann & Evans 2004). Increasingly, physiotherapy clinicians are being trained to integrate psychological therapy techniques such as cognitive behavioural therapy and acceptance commitment therapy within their practice to manage maladaptive behaviours (Henschke et al. 2010).

Adopting psychological therapy approaches will require the clinician to appreciate the emotional dimension of clinical reasoning. The clinician's reasoning of pain will also be influenced by his own constructs, which may be quite different to those expressed by the patient (Langridge et al. 2016). Much has been written on how faulty beliefs, such as pain equals harm, can be a barrier to patient recovery, but beliefs held by clinicians can also negatively influence clinical reasoning. Evidence indicates that clinicians holding negative beliefs are less likely to adopt best-practice clinical guidelines (Darlow et al. 2012; Nijs et al. 2013). Recognition of the existence of these beliefs will require clinicians to be self-reflective enough to recognize how their own attitudes and beliefs will impact on the decisions they make (Bishop et al. 2008; Nijs et al. 2013). Within the patient-centred model of reasoning (see Fig. 2.2), such reflection is termed metacognition and is essential if clinicians are to remain open-minded to allow their practice to evolve.

PATHOBIOLOGICAL MECHANISMS

Although there has been a shift in emphasis from a purely biomedical focus, as indicated above, clinicians are still rightly concerned with what is happening at tissue level. Pathobiological mechanisms can be considered in two parts: (1) tissue responses and healing; and (2) pain mechanisms.

Tissue Responses and Healing

Clinicians can use their knowledge of tissue healing to stage conditions as acute, subacute or chronic/persistent. For example, in an acute ankle sprain, the clinician would initially seek to unload injured tissue, perhaps prescribing crutches, advising a regime of protection, rest, ice, compression and elevation (PRICE), whilst encouraging movement within pain tolerance, before moving towards a progressive loading programme (Bleakley et al. 2010; Kerkhoffs et al. 2012). However a patient who presents following an ankle sprain with persistent pain beyond normal tissue-healing timeframes and a continued reluctance to weight bear would, after having been screened to exclude other causes, be encouraged to 'trust' the ankle with a graded loading intervention aimed at restoring normal function (Woods & Asmundson 2008).

Reasoning will also be influenced by the underlying health of the patient's tissues with comorbidities such as diabetes mellitus and lifestyle choices such as smoking potentially negatively impacting on the tissue-healing process. Comorbidities may slow recovery, so reasoning about tissue health is specific to the individual patient. This reasoning will guide advice given, and assist in the selection of interventions and staging of rehabilitation strategies.

Pain Mechanisms

Identifying ongoing pain mechanisms will also inform what is happening at tissue level. Clinical reasoning of pain mechanisms using Gifford's mature organism model of reasoning (Fig. 4.6) will allow the clinician to consider pain in terms of inputs from peripheral tissues, including nociception, which can be identified as mechanical, inflammatory or ischaemic, depending on characteristics (see Box 2.2) or as peripheral neuropathic, generated by somatosensory tissues such as nerve roots.

These pain mechanisms are amenable to 'hands-on' management approaches. Alternatively, the clinician may reason the patient's symptoms no longer have a peripheral tissue source, indicating abnormal processing within the central nervous system. This central processing of pain is amplified by feelings of anxiety and beliefs that pain is harmful. It is evident that patients with persistent pain can become trapped in

a vicious cycle (Main et al. 2010). In an effort to seek a tissue diagnosis, for example, lumbar disc, patients may consult numerous practitioners navigating the 'sea of endless professionals' (Butler & Moseley 2003). This can further complicate the patient's pain journey, as the patient is left juggling numerous different diagnoses and opinions. Directing treatment to localized tissue is likely to be unsuccessful even though the problem may have originated peripherally. So it can be reasoned for these patients that their management focus will include a psychological approach to reduce abnormal central processing and impact on centrally mediated pain alongside other physical interventions.

Pain also results in output mechanisms resulting in altered motor responses, linked to maladaptive movement or suboptimal movement patterns, for example, due to increased muscle tone.

Autonomic system activation is linked with upregulation and protective mechanisms in the presence of pain, resulting in neuroendocrine changes such as raised cortisol levels. Raised cortisol over an extended period has been linked to depression, poor tissue healing and loss of sleep (Hannibal & Bishop 2014). So when patients report they are not sleeping then this information needs to be linked to their stress biology (Sapolsky 2004).

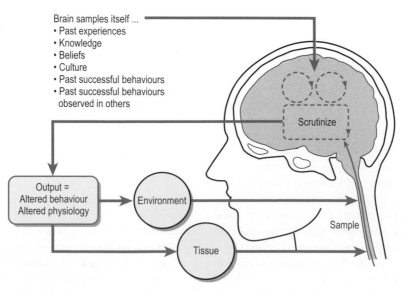

FIG. 4.6 ■ Mature organism model. *(From Gifford 1998, with permission.)*

To reason aspects of a patient's presentation successfully, clinicians will require sound physiological knowledge of body systems and how they interact and impact on one another.

PHYSICAL IMPAIRMENTS AND ASSOCIATED STRUCTURE/TISSUE SOURCES

Patients' descriptions and location of their symptoms will assist in reasoning symptomatic underlying tissue. Whilst completing the body chart the clinician will be using anatomical and pain mechanism knowledge to consider all the structures lying beneath and capable of referring into symptomatic areas (Woolf 2004; Bogduk 2009). This information, matched with reported limitations in activity, will be explored in an analysis of the aggravating and easing factors reported by the patient. These cues in the subjective will provide justification for the 'musts, should and could' lists in planning the physical examination. Based on this, the clinician will prioritize testing, seeking to confirm or refute primary working hypotheses. In order to deliver effective treatment the clinician will hypothesize on the possible target tissues capable of producing the patient's symptoms.

From the outset the clinician will be developing hypotheses of the likely cause of the patient's symptoms. These hypotheses are then tested using hypothetico-deductive reasoning and refined through further subjective and physical examination data collection. The clinician will be making judgements about the existence of tissue pathology based on information from the history of the present condition. If the patient can identify a specific mechanism of injury, such as an ankle inversion injury, this allows for hypothesis generation of tissue trauma. This would include all structures likely to be stressed and capable of producing the lateral ankle symptoms reported by the patient and mapped on to the body chart. This hypothesis would also include consideration of the extent of injury, for example, the likelihood of a fracture. This would prompt follow-up questions about the velocity of the fall, the ability of the patient to weight bear afterwards (Stiell et al. 1993) and the extent of swelling. This is an example of how clinicians might use pattern recognition or forward reasoning of a familiar condition such as an ankle sprain.

As already discussed in Chapter 3, physical tests are often not tissue-specific and will require the clinician to use diagnostic reasoning to synthesize responses from a number of physical tests in order to identify the possible source of symptoms. If meaningful conclusions are to be drawn the clinician will need to weigh up the sensitivity and specificity of tests selected, as well as critically reflect on the accuracy of his own handling skills (Christensen et al. 2008).

Further medical investigations may or may not be the solution to identifying specific tissue sources of symptoms. Blood tests can confirm the existence of an inflammatory condition such as rheumatoid arthritis or can be used to exclude sinister pathologies. Imaging is helpful where clinically reasoned, for example, an X-ray if a fracture is suspected or to confirm a diagnosis; for example, an ultrasound to identify a Morton neuroma, for which a further intervention may be appropriate (Bignotti et al. 2015). Patients with persistent pain may believe that scans will indicate tissue faults and so diagnose the cause of their pain; however, there is often poor correlation between what is reported on scans and how patients may present in the clinic (Brinjikji et al. 2015). This can be difficult for patients to accept. Indeed, evidence has shown that magnetic resonance imaging results, given without the epidemiological data of what is found in a normal asymptomatic population, increase dependence on narcotic medication in patients with persistent non-specific low-back pain (McCullough et al. 2012). Requests for investigations should be based on very sound clinical reasoning, with the clinician providing clear justification.

In some patients it is possible to identify specific tissue sources; for example, reactive Achilles tendinopathy presents with a recognized pattern of localized pain and swelling and is usually linked to specific provocative activities (Kountouris & Cook 2007). The underlying pathological processes of tissue healing can be hypothesized using the available evidence to stage the condition (Cook et al. 2016). The clinician reasons why the tissue has become symptomatic.

- Is it related to a change in activity? This should be detected in the patient's history of the present complaint such as a change in load or training.
- Is there a problem elsewhere in the kinetic chain increasing load on the tendon? Perhaps a

previous injury has restricted range or strength, resulting in altered loading patterns (Cook & Purdam 2012)?

■ Are the patient's gender, age and lifestyle choices factors? Achilles tendinopathy is more common in males and is associated with activity (Cook et al. 2007; Gaida et al. 2010).

Using a knowledge of tissue healing, to clinically reason all possible factors contributing to the development of tissue symptoms, will assist the clinician in the selection of appropriate management strategies.

CONTRIBUTING FACTORS TO THE DEVELOPMENT AND MAINTENANCE OF THE PROBLEM

Throughout the subjective examination the clinician is seeking to identify factors contributing to the development and/or persistence of the patient's symptoms, e.g. environmental, behavioural, physical.

Consideration of the patient's environment has been highlighted as an important aspect in disability (World Health Organization 2011), so it is often useful to explore this early in the subjective examination.

■ How does the patient function at home?
■ Does the patient have family support? Is this helpful or unhelpful?
■ What does the patient's job involve?
■ Could work be a cause of tissue stress?
■ How adaptable is the patient's work situation?

This information will assist the clinician in selecting management options that are realistic and patient-specific. See also black flags in Table 2.3 (Waddell 2004; Linton & Shaw 2011). Related to this will be patients' perception of their work. Patients may believe work has been the cause of their symptoms, or that their colleagues or managers are unsympathetic or unsupportive. These thoughts could impact on their motivation to return to work if signed off sick. In order to offer patient-centred advice the clinician may need to ask additional questions, such as:

■ Are you concerned that the physical demands of your job might delay your return to work?
■ Do you expect your work could be modified temporarily so you could return to work sooner? (Nicholas et al. 2011)

Psychosocial factors may also contribute to symptom development or persistence and these are identified as yellow flags (see Table 2.3). These are summarized under seven headings, ABCDEFW with examples for each:

■ Attitudes: guarding or fear of movement, catastrophizing, external locus of control
■ Behaviours: rest, reduced activity, poor pacing – boom–bust cycle
■ Compensation issues: history of claims, no incentive to return to work, long-term sick leave
■ Diagnosis and treatment: conflicting diagnosis, seeking a cure, passive recipient of care
■ Emotion: fear, anxiety, feeling of hopelessness, low mood
■ Family: overprotective or lacking in support
■ Work: low-skilled manual work, belief work is harmful, shift work, job dissatisfaction.

It is important that the clinician is aware that different psychological flags may be significant at different points in the patient's journey. This should prompt regular reassessment of these factors through narrative reasoning. Clinicians can use their intuition, supported through information from the subjective examination, to assess for yellow flags (Beales et al. 2016). In addition, use of brief validated questionnaires such as STarT back tools (Hill 2011) or Orebro musculoskeletal pain questionnaire (Linton & Boersma 2003) can help confirm the clinician's judgements. Screening tools can produce false positives and false negatives whereby patients without psychological risk factors may be identified as high-risk or vice versa (Nicholas et al. 2011). Screening is not diagnostic but rather a predictor of chronicity. Results from screening tools should be viewed and reasoned in the context of the full examination (Beales et al. 2016) and used to inform rather than direct clinical reasoning.

Psychological factors have the potential to drive behaviours that can impact on physical function. These behaviours can lead to possible avoidance of activity resulting in deconditioning at one end of the spectrum or, in the case of those endurance copers, suppressing thoughts, result in overconditioning at the other end (Hasenbring et al. 2012).

Resulting physical factors may contribute to symptoms. The clinician will use their knowledge of normal movement in order to clinically reason the impact of altered muscle activation patterns on movement dysfunction. Observations along with reported aggravating and easing factors will inform the examination of selected active movements. Muscle lengths, strength and control tests will further inform the clinician's thinking. Testing of passive movements will examine the involvement of associated articular components as the clinician feels for available range and tissue response. However it should not be assumed that areas judged to be hyper- or hypomobile are a cause of the patient's symptoms as these may be incidental findings. Cause and effect should be supported with modification or mini treatments producing a change in the patient's symptoms. One such approach is the shoulder symptom modification procedure. This involves a systematic assessment of the influence of thoracic posture, scapular position and humeral head position on shoulder symptoms (Lewis 2016). An alternative example is assessment of repeated movements using the concept advocated by McKenzie whereby clinicians use their clinical reasoning to select repeated movements. The patient's response to repeated movements allows the clinician to classify low-back pain patients into subgroups; derangement, dysfunction, postural syndrome or other (May & Clare 2015). In this example the clinician will be seeking to confirm or refute a hypothesis of physical impairment.

It is worth noting that a patient's response to hands-on testing may be influenced by placebo which will depend on the patient's mood, expectation and conditioning (Bialosky et al. 2011). This means clinicians must be aware of the context within which testing takes place in order to reason all aspects of the complex interaction between body and mind. For further details the reader is directed to Chpt 8 Understanding and Managing Persistent Pain by Hubert Van Griensven in the companion text (Petty and Barnard 2017).

PRECAUTIONS/CONTRAINDICATIONS TO PHYSICAL EXAMINATION, TREATMENT AND MANAGEMENT

In order to ensure wise action for patients, clinicians must be able to reason clinically when assessment and treatment are contraindicated and when precautions require modification in the extent and vigour of the physical examination.

As autonomous practitioners, clinicians must be able to screen their patients for red flags, identified as indicators of serious pathology, such as neoplasms. This is more than asking a standard list of questions but requires associated reasoning to identify the relative weight and suspected index of suspicion (Goodman & Snyder 2013). The context in which these screening questions are asked is also significant; clinicians need to be mindful not to alarm patients. Clear explanations are required as patients will be reasoning alongside the clinician and may subconsciously or consciously withhold information that they may feel is not relevant (Greenhalgh & Selfe 2004).

The red-flag system continues to evolve over time (see Table 2.5 for an updated list; Greenhalgh & Selfe 2010) and clinicians must continue to update their knowledge base on how serious pathologies present. Clinicians also need to be aware of 'red herrings' due to misattribution of symptoms, biomedical masqueraders and overt illness behaviour that may lead to reasoning errors.

To inform reasoning and screen for precautions and contraindications clinicians will also seek information about family history asking about cancer, for example. Heredity factors play a part in the development of some musculoskeletal conditions, such as ankylosing spondylitis and rheumatoid arthritis. A diagnosis of inflammatory joint disease such as rheumatoid arthritis would contraindicate accessory and physiological movements to the upper cervical spine and care is needed in applying forces to other joints.

Identifying specific pathologies can assist in identifying the need for caution. Fractures are probably the most straightforward example. How vigorously techniques are applied will depend on the stage of fracture healing. The patient's general health and the presence of comorbidities such as osteoporosis will impact on the quality and healing timeframes (Gandhi et al. 2005; Marsell & Einhorn 2011). Osteoporosis can be caused by a number of factors, including long-term use of steroids, early menopause or hysterectomy so careful questioning is required (NICE 2012).

Diabetes can also cause delayed healing; especially if poorly controlled, diabetes is also associated with peripheral neuropathies (Brem & Tomic-Canic 2007). Patients may complain of bilateral pins and needles or numbness in both hands and/or both feet, leading to reduced mobility. There are many reasons why a patient may report sensory changes or have difficulty walking. Of concern would be the possibility of red flag pathologies such as spinal cord, cauda equine compression or an upper motor neurone lesion such as a stroke.

Early features of cervical artery dysfunction can mimic a musculoskeletal pain presentation, as patients often present with neck/occipital pain and unusual or severe headaches. In order to make a differential diagnosis, follow-up questions should seek details of risk factors, information about any features indicating ischaemia or bleeding, such as visual disturbance, balance or gait disturbance, speech/swallowing difficulties or limb weakness or paraesthesia (Rushton et al. 2014). (See Chapter 6 for more indepth discussion of this topic area.)

The presence of spinal spondylolysis or spondylolisthesis would contraindicate strong direct pressure to the affected vertebral level as this might compromise neural tissue.

If a patient is pregnant or postpartum, hormonal changes may cause a reduction in joint stiffness and an increase in range of joint movement, particularly around the pelvis, so contraindicating excessive forces being applied (Calguneri et al. 1982; Stuber et al. 2012). Excessive forces would be contraindicated too in hypermobile patients such as those with Ehlers–Danlos syndrome (Simmonds & Keer 2008).

Anticoagulant therapy causes an increase in the time for blood to clot; so the clinician would need to be aware that this may cause soft tissues to bruise when force is applied. Conversely, oral contraceptives and smoking are associated with an increased risk of thrombosis.

Heart or respiratory disease may preclude some treatment positions; for example, the patient may not tolerate lying flat.

In order to reason safely, clinicians require a knowledge of a wide range of pathological conditions, their clinical presentation as well as a working knowledge of the side-effects of commonly prescribed medications. The reader is referred to a pathology textbook (Goodman & Snyder 2013) for further information.

SEVERITY AND IRRITABILITY

The clinician's judgement of the severity and irritability for each symptom, as defined in Chapter 2, will also guide the extent and vigour of the physical examination.

Whether the symptoms are constant or intermittent, they are deemed to be severe if the patient reports that a single movement, which increases pain, is so severe that the movement has to be stopped. Severe symptoms may limit the extent of the physical examination. The clinician would, in this situation, aim to examine the patient as fully as possible, but within the constraints of the patient's symptoms and so will have decided how much of the symptoms to provoke, e.g. to stop short of the point of pain (P_1) (see Fig. 3.42).

The effect of severe pain on active and passive movement testing is given below as an example of how a physical test is adapted.

Active movements would involve the patient moving to a point just before the onset of (or increase in) the symptom, or just to the point of onset (or increase), and would then immediately return to the starting position. No overpressures would be applied. This requires the clinician to give clear instructions to the patient.

For passive movements, patients may be asked to say as soon as they think they are about to feel their symptom (intermittent), or, if their symptom is constant, are about to feel an increase in their symptom. In both cases, pain is avoided. Alternatively, the patient may be able to tolerate movement just to the onset (or increase) of the symptom. The clinician would carry out the passive movement and, under the instruction of the patient, take the movement to only the first point of pain – and then immediately move away from the point of symptom reproduction. In both situations the clinician should give clear instructions to the patient. The clinician must be able to control the movement and carry it out very slowly. This is necessary in order to avoid causing unnecessary symptoms and to obtain an accurate measure of the range of movement for reassessment purposes (Box 4.1).

The irritability of symptoms is the time taken for symptoms to increase with provocation and subside once the provocation is stopped. When a movement is performed, and pain is provoked, for example, and this provoked pain continues to be present for a length of time, even though the movement is stopped then the pain is said to be irritable. In the context of a physical examination, any period of time that is required for

BOX 4.1
COMMUNICATION SUGGESTIONS WHEN ASSESSING A PATIENT WITH SEVERE CONDITIONS

Active Movements

For example, if active shoulder flexion is being examined the clinician may instruct the patient in the following way (emphasis is in italics):

Intermittent severe symptom: 'Lift your arm up in front of you, *and as soon as you think you are about to get your arm pain, bring your arm down again*' or 'Lift your arm up in front of you, *and as soon as you get your arm pain, bring your arm down again*'.

Constant severe symptom: 'Lift your arm up in front of you, *and as soon as you think your arm pain is going to increase, bring your arm down again*' or 'Lift your arm up in front of you, *and as soon as your arm pain increases, bring your arm down again*'

Passive Movements

For example, for passive shoulder flexion, the clinician may instruct the patient in the following way (emphasis is in italics):

Intermittent severe symptoms: 'I want to move your arm, but I want you to tell me *as soon as you think you are about to get your arm pain*, and I'll bring your arm down'.

'I want to move your arm, but I want you to tell me *as soon as you get your arm pain*, and I will bring your arm down'.

Constant severe symptoms: 'I want to move your arm, but I want you to tell me *as soon as you think you are about to get more of your arm pain*, and I'll bring your arm down'.

'I want to move your arm up, but I want you to tell me *as soon as you get more of your arm pain*, and I will bring your arm down'

BOX 4.2
COMMUNICATION SUGGESTIONS WHEN ASSESSING A PATIENT WITH IRRITABLE CONDITIONS

Active Movement

Intermittent symptoms (emphasis is in italics): 'Lift your arm up in front of you, and *as soon as you think you are about to get your arm pain*, bring your arm down again'.

Constant symptoms: 'Lift your arm up in front of you and *as soon as you think your arm pain is going to increase*, bring your arm down again'

Passive Movement

For example, for passive shoulder flexion, the clinician may instruct the patient in the following way (emphasis is in italics):

Intermittent symptoms: 'I want to move your arm, but I want you to tell me *as soon as you think you are about to get your arm pain*, and I'll bring your arm down'.

Constant symptoms: 'I want to move your arm, but I want you to tell me *as soon as you think you are about to get more of your arm pain*, and I'll bring your arm down'

symptoms to return to their resting level is classified as irritable. If symptoms are provoked and require a pause before the examination can recommence in order to settle sufficiently, this will increase the appointment time, which may be a problem in a busy department. As well as this, repeatedly provoking symptoms and then waiting for them to settle will add little to the clinician's understanding of the patient's condition and result in a bad experience for the patient. For this reason, an alternative strategy is used whereby movements are carried out within the symptom-free range; irritable symptoms are not provoked at all.

For the examination of active movements for a patient with intermittent symptoms, the patient would move to a point just before the onset of the symptoms and then immediately return to the start position. In this way, symptoms are not provoked and therefore there will be no lingering symptoms. For passive movements, patients may be asked to say as soon as they think they are about to feel the symptom (intermittent), or feel that it is about to increase (constant). In both cases, further pain provocation is avoided. The clinician must give clear instructions to the patient (Box 4.2).

For irritable symptoms, whether intermittent or constant, it is particularly important that the clinician clarifies after each movement the patient's resting symptoms, to avoid exacerbating symptoms. In patients where symptoms are severe but not irritable the clinician will identify the tolerable level of symptom reproduction with the patient and so may seek to reproduce 25% of symptoms (see Fig. 3.42).

The clinician's reasoning of underlying pain mechanisms will also inform the assessment of severity and irritability. For patients reasoned to have a neuropathic presentation with high levels of pain, tissues are likely to be irritable (Butler 2000). To confirm a hypothesis of a neuropathic pain driver the clinician would use subjective and physical examination findings (see Box 2.2 for typical characteristics) (Hansson & Kinnman 1996; Cook & van Griensven 2013). The clinician could confirm a hypothesis of neuropathic pain through application of validated screening tools and the use of sensorimotor tests to assess the baseline conductivity of the system (Bennett et al. 2007). Neuropathic pain states would cue the clinician to handle with care, requiring careful assessment of severity and irritability. Strategies to reduce rather than reproduce symptoms would further confirm a neuropathic hypothesis. Unloading positions to ease neural tissue sensitivity would reassure the patient and inform reasoning of management decisions (Butler 2000).

MANAGEMENT STRATEGY AND TREATMENT PLANNING

Management options will be formulated on the basis of reasoning all strands of the subjective and physical examinations and can be considered in two phases: the initial appointment on day 1 and follow-up appointments.

The first step in this process occurs between the subjective and physical examinations. In the subjective examination, in seeking to make sense of the patient's symptoms, a primary hypothesis and other possible alternative hypotheses are formulated. Using hypothetico-deductive reasoning these hypotheses will be confirmed, refined or refuted during the physical examination (Jones et al. 2008). The process then involves putting the possible structures at fault in priority order to develop a 'must, should and could' plan for the physical examination whilst also taking into account any precautions or contraindications.

The aims of the physical examination are to:

■ confirm, if necessary, any precautions or contraindications
■ identify the most likely source of the patient's symptoms
■ explore further, if relevant, any factors contributing to the patient's condition.

In order to identify the source of the symptoms the clinician uses the information from the subjective examination to forward reason the findings of the physical examination. This includes:

■ the structures thought to be at fault
■ which tests are likely to reproduce/alter the patient's symptoms
■ how the tests need to be performed to reproduce/alter the patient's symptoms; for example, which combined movements may be required
■ what other structures need to be examined in order to disprove them as a source of the symptoms.

The physical testing procedures which specifically indicate joint, nerve or muscle tissues as a source of the patient's symptoms are summarized in Table 4.2.

At one end of the scale the findings may provide strong evidence, and at the other end they may provide weak evidence. Of course there may be a variety of presentations between these two extremes.

The strongest evidence that a joint is the primary source of the patient's symptoms is that active and passive physiological movements, passive accessory movements and joint palpation all reproduce the patient's symptoms, and that, following a joint-based treatment, reassessment identifies an improvement in the patient's signs and symptoms. For example, let us assume a patient has lateral elbow pain caused by a radiohumeral joint dysfunction. In the physical examination there are limited elbow flexion and extension movements with some resistance due to the reproduction of the patient's elbow pain. Active movement is very similar to passive movement in terms of range, resistance and pain reproduction. Accessory movement examination of the radiohumeral joint reveals limited posteroanterior and anteroposterior glide of the radius due to reproduction of the patient's elbow pain with some resistance. Following the application of accessory movements, reassessment of the elbow physiological movements is improved, in terms of range and pain. This scenario would indicate that there is a dysfunction at the radiohumeral joint – first, because elbow movements, both active and passive physiological, and accessory movements, reproduce the patient's symptoms, and, second, because,

TABLE 4.2		
Physical Tests Which, if Positive, Indicate Joint, Nerve and Muscle as a Source of the Patient's Symptoms		
Test	Strong Evidence	Weak Evidence
Joint		
Active physiological movements	Reproduces patient's symptoms	Dysfunctional movement: reduced range, excessive range, altered quality of movement, increased resistance, decreased resistance
Passive physiological movements	Reproduces patient's symptoms; this test same as for active physiological movements	Dysfunctional movement: reduced range, excessive range, increased resistance, decreased resistance, altered quality of movement
Accessory movements	Reproduces patient's symptoms	Dysfunctional movement: reduced range, excessive range, increased resistance, decreased resistance, altered quality of movement
Palpation of joint	Reproduces patient's symptoms	Tenderness
Reassessment following therapeutic dose of accessory movement	Improvement in tests which reproduce patient's symptoms	No change in physical tests which reproduce patient's symptoms
Muscle		
Active movement	Reproduces patient's symptoms	Reduced strength
		Poor quality
Passive physiological movements	Patient's symptoms not reproduced	
Isometric contraction	Reproduces patient's symptoms	Reduced strength
		Poor quality
Passive lengthening of muscle	Reproduces patient's symptoms	Reduced range
		Increased resistance
		Decreased resistance
Palpation of muscle	Reproduces patient's symptoms	Tenderness
Reassessment following therapeutic dose of muscle treatment	Improvement in tests which reproduce patient's symptoms	No change in physical tests which reproduce patient's symptoms
Nerve		
Passive lengthening and sensitizing movement, i.e. altering length of nerve by a movement at a distance from patient's symptoms	Reproduces patient's symptoms and sensitizing movement alters patient's symptoms	Reduced range
		Increased resistance
Palpation of nerve	Reproduces patient's symptoms	Tenderness

following accessory movements, the active elbow movements are improved. Even if the active movements are made worse, this would still suggest a joint dysfunction because it is likely that the accessory movements would predominantly affect the joint, with much less effect on nerve and muscle tissues around the area. Collectively, this evidence would suggest that there is primarily a joint dysfunction.

The strongest evidence that a muscle is the primary source of a patient's symptoms is if active movements, an isometric contraction, passive lengthening and palpation of a muscle all reproduce the patient's symptoms, and that, following a treatment, reassessment identifies an improvement in the patient's signs and symptoms. For example, let us assume that a patient has lateral elbow pain caused by lateral epicondylalgia.

In this case reproduction of the patient's lateral elbow pain is found on active wrist and finger extension, isometric/isotonic/eccentric contraction of the wrist extensors and/or finger extensors and passive lengthening of the extensor muscles to the wrist and hand. These signs and symptoms are found to improve following soft-tissue mobilization examination, sufficient to be considered a treatment dose. Collectively, this evidence would suggest that there is a muscle dysfunction, as long as this is accompanied by negative joint and nerve tests.

The strongest evidence that a nerve is the source of the patient's symptoms is when active and/or passive physiological movements reproduce the patient's symptoms, which are then increased or decreased with an additional neurally sensitizing movement, at a distance from the patient's symptoms. In addition, there is reproduction of the patient's symptoms on palpation of the nerve, and following treatment directed at neural tissue an improvement in the above signs and symptoms occurs. For example, let us assume this time that the lateral elbow pain is caused by a neurodynamic dysfunction of the radial nerve supplying this region. The patient's lateral elbow pain is reproduced during the component movements of the upper-limb neurodynamic test (ULNT) 2b and is eased with ipsilateral cervical lateral flexion desensitizing movement. There is tenderness over the radial groove in the upper arm and, following testing of the ULNT 2b, sufficient to be considered a treatment dose, an improvement in the patient's signs and symptoms. Collectively, this evidence would suggest that there is a neurodynamic dysfunction, as long as this is accompanied by negative joint and muscle tests.

It can be seen that the common factor for identifying joint, nerve and muscle dysfunction as a source of the patient's symptoms is reproduction of the patient's symptoms, an alteration in the patient's signs and symptoms following targeted treatment and a lack of evidence from other potential sources of symptoms. It is assumed that if a test reproduces a patient's symptoms then it is somehow stressing the structure at fault. As mentioned earlier, each test is not purely a test of one structure – every test, to a greater or lesser degree, involves other structures. For this reason, it is imperative that, whatever treatment is given, it is proved to be of value by altering the patient's signs and

symptoms. The other factor common in identifying joint, nerve or muscle dysfunction is the lack of positive findings in the other possible tissues; for example, a joint dysfunction is considered when joint tests are positive and muscle and nerve tests are negative. Thus the clinician collects evidence to implicate tissues and evidence to negate tissues – both are equally important.

An ongoing analysis of the evidence as indicated above facilitates the clinician in reasoning the main driver underlying the patient's symptoms so that treatment can be correctly targeted. For example, the source of symptoms may be a hypermobile motion segment of the lumbar spine which may be symptomatic as a result of a neighbouring hypomobile segment. In this instance it could be hypothesized that treatment directed at the hypomobile segment should improve symptoms. This analysis would also need to be accompanied by consideration of other components of the movement system such as muscle activity, normal movement patterns and associated behaviours.

The clinician's primary hypothesis can be summarized in a statement of a clinical diagnosis or clinical impression. Rather than identifying a particular structure this statement will include detail on presenting symptoms, associated movement dysfunction, underlying pain mechanism, psychosocial considerations and key physical examination findings. For example:

A 15-year-old hockey player presents with non-severe/non-irritable mechanical nociceptive anterior knee pain, secondary to a tight lateral retinaculum tracking the patella laterally during eccentric control of knee flexion. Pain is eased with a medial glide of the patella.

A 45-year-old female dentist presents with right C4–C5 zygapophyseal joint dysfunction, inflammatory and mechanical, nociceptive pain, right side of the neck and lateral upper arm, not severe and not irritable. There are regular compression pattern cervical movements plus a positive ULNT 2a, biasing the median nerve.

Alternatively, read the clinical impression statements below. Although both cases have sustained the same injury, treatment priorities, treatment and goals will differ markedly. This shows that one size does not fit all.

CASE 1:

Clinical Impression

A 28-year-old female track and field athlete has a 3-week history of mechanical and inflammatory nociceptive pain of left lateral ankle origin, anterior talofibular ligament, following a grade 2 inversion injury. Reduced talocrural dorsiflexion/inversion, active and passive range with proprioceptive and strength deficits. Keen to resume training as soon as possible.

CASE 2:

Clinical Impression

A 45-year-old policeman, deconditioned, body mass index 27, has a left ankle inversion injury. Six-month history, persistent discomfort over the lateral aspect, reduced talocrural dorsiflexion/inversion, active and passive range proprioceptive, strength deficits, reluctant to move, deconditioned and anxiety about upcoming fitness test.

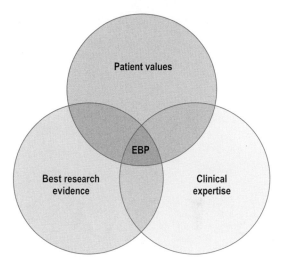

FIG. 4.7 ■ Evidence-based practice (EBP). *(From Sackett et al. 2000, with permission).*

S	Specific
M	Measurable
A	Attainable
R	Relevant
T	Time-bound

FIG. 4.8 ■ SMART goals

Through procedural reasoning the clinician will use the identification of functional problems to offer the patient choice on possible management strategies (Fleming 1991). Interventions offered should be evidence-based and justified (Sackett et al. 2000) (Fig. 4.7). Knowledge of how tissues respond to injury and disease underpins the explanation of the mechanism by which treatment will have an effect.

The clinician will need to be competent in skilful application of the agreed intervention (Banks & Hengeveld 2014) and all options should be presented to the patient so that an agreed plan can be negotiated in order to achieve agreed SMART goals – specific, measurable, attainable, relevant and time-bound (Fig. 4.8).

Achievement of treatment goals will also be dependent on the patient's ability to engage in the process fully. Treatment may be unsuccessful if the patient is not ready to change behaviours that may be barriers to recovery. The stages-of-change model described by Prochaska and DiClemente (1982) can be used to help people make changes that will have a positive impact on their well-being, for example, being more physically active, taking on board advice (Fig. 4.9 and Table 4.3).

Is the patient contemplating change but not yet ready to move on to the action stage? The patient's level of confidence or self-efficacy in achieving behaviour change to reach agreed goals is also a factor in engagement (Nicholas 2007; Menezes Costa et al. 2011). Management should ideally be tailored to promoting self-efficacy, accommodating the patient's degree of motivation, interest and stage of readiness if the benefits of interventions are to be maximized (Rollnick et al. 1993).

Clinical reasoning continues to refine hypotheses about the cause of the patient's symptoms throughout

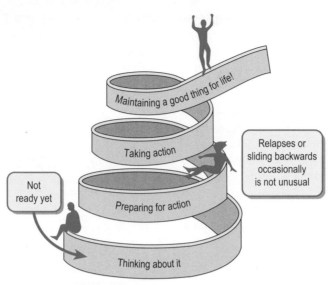

FIG. 4.9 ■ Stages-of-change model. *(Data from Prochaska, J.O. DiClemente, C.C. (1982) Transtheoretical therapy: toward a more integrative model of change. Psychotherapy (1982) 19(3):276–288.)*

the management of the patient in what Maitland termed 'analytical assessment' (Banks & Hengeveld 2014 p. 33). Following treatment, both within and between treatment sessions, the clinician will critically evaluate responses to treatment through the reassessment of subjective and physical markers or asterisks (Maitland used the term comparable signs), seeking to identify change. These individual markers/* used for reassessment come from the subjective examination and can relate to symptoms on the body chart, functional deficits, evaluation of severity and irritability and the volume of medication required to manage symptoms. Physical examination markers (*) indicate retesting of functional activities, active and passive movement, muscle reassessment, neural responses to tests.

An improvement in subjective asterisks seems to be fairly strong evidence that there has been a change. For example, a patient who is able to increase the time ironing or walking, or is able to sleep better, for example, although the response will depend, in part, on the patient's attitude to the problem, to the clinician and towards treatment, which may positively or negatively affect the patient's response. Further questioning of any change is always needed to clarify that it is the condition that has improved and not something

TABLE 4.3	
Stages of Change (Prochaska et al. 1992)	
Precontemplation	The person is not considering change – this is the 'ignorance is bliss' stage
Contemplation	The person appears ambivalent about change – the individual is 'sitting on the fence'
Preparation	The person has had some experience with change and is trying to change. The individual is 'testing the waters'
Action	The person has taken steps towards changing behaviour and has made changes to his or her lifestyle to work towards the desired outcome
Maintenance	The person is working to stay on track and avoid relapse. Positive experience is reaffirming that the person can succeed
Relapse	Although not part of the original model, this refers to a person falling back into old harmful behaviours after going through the other stages

else. For example, if sleeping has improved, the clinician checks the details of the nature of that improvement, and whether there is any other explanation, such as a new mattress or a change in analgesia that may explain the improvement.

Changes in physical findings also need careful and unbiased reasoning by the clinician. A test must be carried out in a reliable way for the clinician to consider that a change in the test is a real change. Clearly, some of the tests carried out are easier to replicate than others. For example, a change in an active movement is rather easier to quantify than the clinician's 'feel' of a passive physiological intervertebral movement. Clinicians will do well to evaluate critically their reassessment asterisks and consider carefully how much weight they can place upon them when they interpret a change.

Reassessment of both subjective and physical aspects includes a combination of the patient's and the clinician's views to increase validity (Cook et al. 2015). These markers provide individual patient-specific outcomes measures that can be linked to validated outcome tools to measure the impact of interventions on the patient, and the patient's health and well-being

(Banks & Hengeveld 2014). Outcomes that measure across a range of domains, such as function, generic health status, work disability, patient satisfaction, as well as pain, are best placed to capture the multidimensional nature of patients attending for musculoskeletal treatment (Bombadier 2000).

At each attendance, the clinician obtains a detailed account of the effect of the last treatment on the patient's signs and symptoms. This will involve the immediate effects after the last treatment, the relevant activities of the patient since the last treatment and enquiring how the patient is presenting on the day of treatment. Patients who say they are worse since the last treatment should be questioned carefully, as this may be due to some activity they have been involved with, rather than any treatment that has been given. Patients who say they are better also need to be questioned carefully, as the improvement may not be related to treatment. If the patient remains the same, following the subjective and physical reassessment, the clinician may consider altering the treatment approach and then seeing whether this alteration has been effective. The process of assessment, treatment and reassessment is depicted in Fig. 4.10.

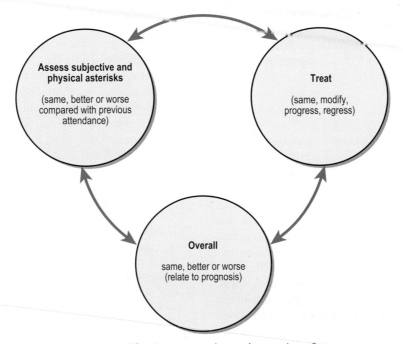

FIG. 4.10 ■ Modification, progression and regression of treatment.

Retrospective assessment at regular intervals allows the clinician the opportunity to reflect and clinically reason with the patient on overall progress, comparing the subjective and physical markers, at a follow-up appointment with the findings at the initial assessment. Reflective reasoning taking into account the patient's view of what has worked and the progress made towards agreed goals will allow the clinician to consider whether additional interventions are required. This continuous analytical assessment would identify when improvement has plateaued, prompting a collaborative review on why this might be. Is there a fault with the selection of reassessment parameters? What is the patient's view? Has treatment been directed towards the right source? Is there an issue with self-management strategies? Is there an indication for additional medical interventions? For further information, the reader is referred to Banks and Hengeveld (2014).

Finally, analysis at the end of a course of treatment will consider overall what has been learned by the clinician but also by the patient. What is the possibility of recurrent problems in the future? Is it likely that the patient will be able to self-manage any remaining functional deficits? This will depend on the patient's level of participation and empowerment to take ownership. Increasingly clinicians should also consider the contribution their intervention has made on the future healthy life expectancy of their patients (Middleton 2008).

PROGNOSIS

Having agreed a clinically reasoned management plan, patients will often ask how long it will take them to recover and how often they will need to attend for treatment.

A number of positive and negative factors from both the subjective and physical examination will assist the clinician in reasoning a predictive response to these questions. Factors to consider might include the patient's age; general health; lifestyle; levels of self-efficacy; personality; expectations and psychosocial factors such as their attitude towards their condition, towards themselves and towards the clinician, as well as pain drivers; severity and irritability of the symptoms; extent of tissue damage; the natural history and

progression of the condition. Physical factors predicting prognosis may include predominant pain mechanisms, extent of physical limitation, number of systems involved; response to movement and manual assessment and proprioceptive awareness.

By considering all of these individual factors, the clinician is then able to predict to what extent, in percentage terms, symptoms will respond to treatment and the anticipated number of treatment sessions required to achieve this improvement. At discharge, it is useful for the clinician to compare the final outcome with the predicted outcome, as this reflection will help clinicians to learn and enhance their ability to hypothesize about prognoses in the future.

CONCLUSION

This chapter has sought to explore clinical reasoning through the subjective and physical examination processes using the hypotheses categories (Jones & Rivett 2004). The continued development of clinical reasoning skills is dependent on reflective practice and a commitment to continued professional development. Much of the evidence cited in this chapter is extrapolated from the non-specific low-back pain literature. The challenge for the future is for clinicians to adapt to the currently incomplete and constantly developing evidence base in order to contribute to the improved health of their patients. This will require the ability to reflect on each and every interaction in order to continue to reason, question and learn from patients through effective communication.

For consideration of the treatment and management approaches the reader is directed to the companion text (Petty & Barnard 2017).

ACKNOWLEDGEMENTS

The author would like to thank Professor Karen Beeton PhD, MPhty, BSc(Hons) FCSP, FMACP for her ongoing support.

REFERENCES

Aroll, B., et al., 2003. Screening for depression in primary care with two verbally asked questions: cross sectional study. Br. Med. J. 327, 1144–1146.

Atkinson, H., Nixon-Cave, K., 2011. A tool for clinical reasoning and reflection using the international classification of functioning disability and health ICF framework and patient management model. Phys. Ther. 91, 416–430.

Bachmann, L.M., et al., 2003. Accuracy of Ottawa ankle rules to exclude fractures of the ankle and mid-foot: systematic review. Br. Med. J. 326, 417.

Banks, K., Hengeveld, E., 2014. The Maitland concept as a clinical practice framework for neuromusculoskeletal disorders. In: Hengeveld, E., Banks, K. (Eds.), Maitland's peripheral manipulation. Churchill Livingstone, Edinbugh (Chapter 1).

Barker, K., et al., 2009. Divided by a lack of common language? A qualitative study exploring the use of language by health professionals treating back pain. BMC Musculoskelet. Disord. 10, 123.

Barker, C., et al., 2014. Problematic pain – redefining how we view pain? Br. J. Pain 8, 9–15.

Beales, D., et al., 2016. Association between the 10 item Orebro musculoskeletal pain screening questionnaire and physiotherapists' perception of the contribution of biopsychosocial factors in patients with musculoskeletal pain. Man. Ther. 23, 48–55.

Bennett, M., et al., 2007. Using screening tools to identify neuropathic pain. Pain 127, 199–203.

Bialosky, J., et al., 2009. The mechanisms of manual therapy in the treatment of musculoskeletal pain. A comprehensive model. Man. Ther. 14, 531–538.

Bialosky, J., et al., 2011. Placebo response to manual therapy: something out of nothing? J. Man. Manip. Ther. 19, 11–19.

Bignotti, B., et al., 2015. Ultrasound versus magnetic resonance imaging for Morton neuroma: systematic review and meta-analysis. Eur. Radiol. 25, 2254–2262.

Bishop, A., et al., 2008. How does the self-reported clinical management of patients with low back pain relate to the attitudes and beliefs of health care practitioners? A survey of UK general practitioners and physiotherapists. Pain 135, 187–195.

Bleakley, C., et al., 2010. Management of acute soft tissue injury using protection rest ice compression and elevation: recommendations from the Association of Chartered Physiotherapists in Sports and Exercise Medicine. ACPSM. Available online at: http://www.physiosinport.org/media/wysiwyg/ACPSM_Physio_Price_A4.pdf.

Bogduk, N., 2009. On the definitions and physiology of back pain, referred pain, and radicular pain. Pain 147, 17–19.

Bombadier, C., 2000. Spine focus issue introduction: outcome assessments in the evaluation of treatment of spinal disorders. Spine 25, 3097–3099.

Brem, H., Tomic-Canic, M., 2007. Cellular and molecular basis of wound healing in diabetes. J. Clin. Invest. 117, 1219–1222.

Brinjikji, W., et al., 2015. SR of imaging features of spinal degeneration in asymptomatic populations. AJNR Am. J. Neuroradiol. 36, 811–816.

Butler, D., 2000. The sensitive nervous system. NOI Group Publications, Adelaide.

Butler, D., Moseley, L., 2003. Explain pain. NOI Group Publications, Adelaide.

Caladine, L., Morris, J., 2015. Patient education: a collaborative approach. In: Jull, G., et al. (Eds.), Grieve's modern musculoskeletal physiotherapy, fourth ed. Elsevier, Edinburgh, pp. 250–253.

Calguneri, M., et al., 1982. Changes in joint laxity occurring during pregnancy. Ann. Rheum. Dis. 41, 126–128.

Chapman, R., et al., 2008. Pain and stress in a systems perspective: reciprocal neural, endocrine and immune interactions. J. Pain 9, 122–145.

Chartered Society of Physiotherapy, 2008. Scope of physiotherapy practice. Available online at: http://www.clinicaledge.com.au/app/webroot/uploads/pd001_scope_of_practice_2008.pdf (accessed 30 January 2017).

Chester, E., et al., 2014. Opening clinical encounters in an adult musculoskeletal setting. Man. Ther. 19, 306–310.

Christensen, N., et al., 2008. Dimensions of clinical reasoning capability. In: Higgs, J., et al. (Eds.), Clinical reasoning in the health professions. Elsevier Butterworth-Heinemann, Oxford, pp. 101–110.

Clinical Standards Advisory Group (CSAG), 1994. Report on low back pain. HMSO, London.

Cook, J.L., et al., 2007. Hormone therapy is associated with smaller Achilles tendon diameter in active post-menopausal women. Scand. J. Med. Sci. Sports 17, 128–132.

Cook, C., et al., 2015. The relationship between chief complaint and comparable sign in patients with spinal pain: an exploratory study. Man. Ther. 20, 451–455.

Cook, J., Purdam, C., 2012. Is compressive load a factor in the development of tendinopathy? Br. J. Sports Med. 46, 163–168.

Cook, J.L., et al., 2016. Revisiting the continuum model of tendon pathology: what is its merit in clinical practice and research? Br. J. Sports Med. doi:10.1136/bjsports-2015-095422.

Cook, N., van Griensven, H., 2013. Neuropathic pain and complex regional pain syndrome. In: van Griensven, H., et al. (Eds.), Pain. A textbook for health professionals, second ed. Churchill Livingstone, Edinburgh, pp. 137–158.

Cooper, K., et al., 2008. Patient-centredness in physiotherapy from the perspective of the chronic low back pain patient. Physiotherapy 94, 244–252.

Danneels, L., et al., 2011. A didactical approach for musculoskeletal physiotherapy: the planetary model. Journal of Musculoskeletal Pain 19, 218–222.

Darlow, B., et al., 2013. The enduring impact of what clinicians say to people with low back pain. Ann. Fam. Med. 11, 527–534.

Darlow, B., et al., 2012. The association between health care professional attitudes and beliefs and the attitudes and beliefs, clinical management, and outcomes of patients with low back pain: a systematic review. Eur. J. Pain 16, 3–17.

Diegelmann, R., Evans, M., 2004. Wound healing: an overview of acute fibrotic and delayed healing. Front. Biosci. 9, 283–289.

Doody, C., McAteer, M., 2002. Clinical reasoning of expert and novice physiotherapists in an outpatient orthopaedic setting. Physiotherapy 88, 258–268.

Edwards, I., et al., 2004. Clinical reasoning strategies in physical therapy. Phys. Ther. 84, 312–330.

Edwards, I., et al., 2006. The interpretation of experience and its relationship to body movement: a clinical reasoning perspective. Man. Ther. 11, 2–10.

Feltowich, P.J., Barrows, H.S., 1984. Issues of generality in medical problems solving. In: Schmidt, H.G., Volder, M.I. (Eds.), Tutorials in problem based learning: a new direction in teaching the health professional. van Gorcum, Assen, the Netherlands, pp. 128–141.

Fleming, M.H., 1991. The therapist with the three track mind. Am. J. Occup. Ther. 45, 1007–1014.

Fleming, M., Mattingly, C., 2008. Action and narrative: two dynamics of clinical reasoning. In: Higgs, J., et al. (Eds.), Clinical reasoning in the health professions, third ed. Butterworth Heinemann, Elsevier, Amsterdam (Chapter 5).

Flynn, T., et al., 2002. A clinical prediction rule to identify patients with low back pain most likely to benefit from spinal manipulation: a validation study. Spine 27, 2835–2843.

Froud, R., et al., 2014. A systematic review and meta-synthesis of the impact of low back pain on people's lives. BMC Musculoskelet. Disord. 15, 50.

Gaida, J., et al., 2010. Asymptomatic Achilles tendon pathology is associated with central fat distribution in men and a peripheral fat distribution in women: a cross sectional study of 298 individuals. BMC Musculoskelet. Disord. 11, 14.

Gandhi, A., et al., 2005. The effects of insulin delivery on diabetic fracture healing. Bone 37, 482–490.

Gifford, L., 1998. Pain the tissues and the nervous system. A conceptual model. Physiotherapy 84, 27–36.

Gifford, L.S., 2005. Editorial. Now for pink flags! PPA News 22, 3–4.

Goodman, C., Snyder, T., 2013. Differential diagnosis for physical therapists; screening for referral, fifth ed. Elsevier, St Louis.

Grant, J., 2008. Using open and distance learning to develop clinical reasoning skills. In: Higgs, J., et al. (Eds.), Clinical reasoning in the health professions. Elsevier Butterworth-Heinemann, Oxford, pp. 441–450.

Greenhalgh, S., Selfe, J., 2004. Margaret, a tragic case of spinal red flags and red herrings. Physiotherapy 90, 73–76.

Greenhalgh, S., Selfe, J., 2010. Red flags II: a guide to identifying serious pathology of the spine. Elsevier, Edinburgh.

Hannibal, K., Bishop, M., 2014. Chronic stress, cortisol dysfunction, and pain: a psychoneuroendocrine rationale for stress management in pain rehabilitation. Phys. Ther. 94, 1816–1825.

Hansson, P., Kinnman, E., 1996. Unmasking mechanisms of peripheral neuropathic pain in a clinical perspective. Pain Reviews 3, 272–292.

Hasenbring, M., et al., 2012. Pain-related avoidance versus endurance in primary care patients with subacute back pain: psychological characteristics and outcome at a 6-month follow-up. Pain 153, 211–217.

Henschke, N., et al., 2010. Behavioural treatment for chronic low-back pain. Cochrane Database Syst. Rev. (7), CD002014.

Higgs, J., Jones, M., 2008. Clinical decision making and multiple problem spaces. In: Higgs, J., et al. (Eds.), Clinical reasoning in the health professions. Elsevier Butterworth-Heinemann, Oxford, pp. 3–18.

Higgs, J., Titchen, A., 1995. The nature, generation and verification of knowledge. Physiotherapy 81, 521–530.

Hill, J., 2011. Psychosocial influences on low back pain, disability and response to treatment. Phys. Ther. 91, 712–721.

IASP, 2015. The International Association for the Study of Pain. Available online at: www.iasp-pain.org (accessed 2 November 2016).

Jones, M.A., 1995. Clinical reasoning and pain. Man. Ther. 1, 17–24.

Jones, M., et al., 2002. Conceptual models for implementing biopsychosocial theory in clinical practice. Man. Ther. 7, 2–9.

Jones, M., et al., 2008. Clinical reasoning in physiotherapy. In: Higgs, J., et al. (Eds.), Clinical reasoning in the health professions, third ed. Butterworth Heinemann/Elsevier, Amsterdam, pp. 245–256.

Jones, M.A., Rivett, D.A., 2004. Clinical reasoning for manual therapists. Butterworth-Heinemann, Edinburgh.

Kent, P., et al., 2014. The concurrent validity of brief screening questions for anxiety depression social isolation catastrophization and fear of movement in people with LBP. Clin. J. Pain 4, 479–489.

Kerkhoffs, G., et al., 2012. Diagnosis, treatment and prevention of ankle sprains: an evidence-based clinical guideline. Br. J. Sports Med. 46, 854–860.

Kerry, R., 2010. The theory of clinical reasoning in combined movement therapy. In: McCarthy, C. (Ed.), Combined movement theory: rational mobilization and manipulation of the vertebral column. Churchill Livingstone, Edinburgh, pp. 19–47.

Kountouris, A., Cook, J., 2007. Rehabilitation of Achilles and patellar tendinopathies. Clin. Rheumatol. 21, 295–316.

Langridge, N., et al., 2016. The role of clinician emotion in clinical reasoning: balancing the analytical process. Man. Ther. 21, 277–281.

Learman, K., et al., 2012. Does the use of a prescriptive clinical prediction rule increase the likelihood of applying inappropriate treatments? A survey using clinical vignettes. Man. Ther. 17, 538–543.

Leeuw, M., et al., 2007. The fear avoidance model of musculoskeletal pain current state of scientific evidence. J. Behav. Med. 30, 77–94.

Lewis, J., 2016. Rotator cuff related shoulder pain: assessment management and uncertainties. Man. Ther. 23, 57–68.

Linton, S., Boersma, K., 2003. Early identification of patients at risk of developing a persistent back problem: the predictive validity of the Örebro musculoskeletal pain questionnaire. Clin. J. Pain 19, 80–86.

Linton, S., Shaw, W., 2011. Impact of psychological factors in the experience of pain. Phys. Ther. 91, 700–710.

Luomajoki, H., Moseley, G.L., 2011. Tactile acuity and lumbopelvic motor control in patients with back pain and healthy controls. Br. J. Sports Med. 45, 437–440.

MacKereth, P., et al., 2014. Complementary therapy approaches to pain. In: van Griensven, H., et al. (Eds.), Pain. A textbook for health professionals, second ed. Churchill Livingstone, Edinburgh, pp. 237–253.

Maguire, P., Pitceathly, C., 2002. Key communication skills and how to acquire them. Br. Med. J. 325, 697–700.

Main, C.J., Spanswick, C.C., 2000. Pain management, an interdisciplinary approach. Churchill Livingstone, Edinburgh.

Main, C., et al., 2010. Addressing patients' beliefs in the consultation. Best Pract. Res. Clin. Rheumatol. 24, 219–225.

Maitland, G.D., et al., 2005. Maitland's vertebral manipulation, seventh ed. Butterworth-Heinemann, London, p. 57.

Marsell, R., Einhorn, T., 2011. Biology of fracture healing. Injury. Injury 42, 551–555.

May, S., Clare, H., 2015. The McKenzie method of mechanical diagnosis and therapy – an overview. In: Jull, G., et al. (Eds.), Grieve's modern musculoskeletal physiotherapy, fourth ed. Elsevier, Edinburgh, pp. 460–462.

McCarthy, C.J., et al., 2004. The bio-psycho-social classification of non-specific low back pain: a systematic review. Phys. Ther. Rev. 9, 17–30.

McCullough, B.J., et al., 2012. Lumbar MR imaging and reporting epidemiology: do epidemiologic data in reports affect clinical management? Radiology 262, 941–946.

Melzack, R., 2001. Pain and the neuromatrix in the brain. J. Dent. Educ. 65, 1378–1382.

Menezes Costa, L., et al., 2011. Self-efficacy is more important than fear of movement in mediating the relationship between pain and disability in chronic low back pain. Eur. J. Pain 15, 213–219.

Middleton, K., 2008. Framing the contribution of allied health professionals delivering high quality health care. UK Department of Health, London, pp. 1–38.

Moore, A., Jull, G., 2010. The primacy of clinical reasoning and clinical practical skills. Man. Ther. 15, 513.

Moseley, G.L., et al., 2004. A randomised controlled trial of intensive neurophysiology education in chronic low back pain. Clin. J. Pain 20, 324–330.

National Institute for Health and Clinical Excellence (NICE), 2009. Guidelines on the management of low back pain. Available online at: https://www.nice.org.uk/.

National Institute for Health and Care Excellence (NICE), 2012. Osteoporosis: assessing the risk of fragility fracture. Available online at: https://www.nice.org.uk/.

Nicholas, M.K., 2007. The pain self efficacy questionnaire. Taking pain into account. Eur. J. Pain 11, 153–163.

Nicholas, M.K., et al., 2011. 'Decade of the Flags' working group. Early identification and management of psychological risk factors ('yellow flags') in patients with low back pain: a reappraisal. Phys. Ther. 91, 737–753.

Nielsen, M., 2014. The patient's voice. In: van Griensven, H., et al. (Eds.), Pain. A textbook for health professionals, second ed. Churchill Livingstone, Edinburgh, pp. 9–20.

Nijs, J., et al., 2013. Thinking beyond muscles and joints: therapists' and patients' attitudes and beliefs regarding chronic musculoskeletal pain are key to applying effective treatment. Man. Ther. 18, 96–102.

Opsommer, E., Schoeb, V., 2014. 'Tell me about your troubles': description of patient–physiotherapist interaction during initial encounters. Physiother. Res. Int. 19, 205–221.

O'Sullivan, P., 2005. Diagnosis and classification of chronic low back pain disorders. Maladaptive movement and motor control impairment as underlying mechanism. Man. Ther. 10, 242–255.

O'Sullivan, P., et al., 2015. Multidimensional approach for targeted management of low back pain. In: Jull, G., et al. (Eds.), Grieve's modern musculoskeletal physiotherapy, fourth ed. Edinburgh, Edinburgh, pp. 465–470.

Petty, N.J., Barnard, K., 2017. Principles of musculoskeletal treatment and management: a handbook for therapists, third ed. Elsevier, Edinburgh.

Prochaska, J.O., DiClemente, C.C., 1982. Transtheoretical theory toward a more integrative model of change. Psychotherapy: Theory, Research and Practice 19, 276–287.

Prochaska, J.O., et al., 1992. In search of how people change: applications to addictive behaviors. Am. Psychol. 47, 1102.

Rivett, D., Jones, M., 2004. Improving clinical reasoning in manual therapy. In: Higgs, J., et al. (Eds.), Clinical reasoning in the health professions, third ed. Butterworth Heinemann/Elsevier, Amsterdam, pp. 403–419.

Roberts, L., et al., 2013. Measuring verbal communication in initial physical therapy encounters. Phys. Ther. 93, 479–491.

Rollnick, S., et al., 1993. Methods of helping patients with behaviour change. Br. Med. J. 307, 188–190.

Rushton, A., et al., 2014. International framework for examination of the cervical region for potential cervical arterial dysfunction prior to orthopaedic manual therapy intervention. Man. Ther. 9, 222–228.

Sackett, D.L., et al., 2000. Evidence-based medicine: how to practice and teach. EBM, second ed. Churchill Livingstone, Edinburgh.

Sapolsky, R., 2004. Why zebras don't get ulcers. St Martin's Press, New York.

Simmonds, J.V., Keer, R.J., 2008. Hypermobility and the hypermobility syndrome, part 2: assessment and management of hypermobility syndrome: illustrated via case studies. Man. Ther. 13, e1–e11.

Stiell, I.G., et al., 1993. Decision rules for the use of radiography in acute ankle injuries. J. Am. Med. Assoc. 269, 1127–1132.

Stuber, K., et al., 2012. Adverse events from spinal manipulation in the pregnant and postpartum periods: a critical review of the literature. Chiropr. Man. Therap. 20, 8.

Terry, W., Higgs, J., 1993. Developing educational programmes to develop clinical reasoning skills. Aust. J. Physiother. 39, 47–51.

Waddell, G., 2004. The back pain revolution, second ed. Churchill Livingstone, Edinburgh.

Wainwright, S.F., et al., 2011. Factors that influence the clinical decision making of novice and experienced physical therapists. Phys. Ther. 91, 87–101.

Woods, M.O., Asmundson, G.J., 2008. Evaluating the efficacy of graded in vivo exposure for the treatment of fear in patients with chronic low back pain: a randomized control trial. Pain 136, 271–280.

Woolf, C., 2004. Pain: moving from symptom control toward mechanism specific pharmacologic management. Ann. Intern. Med. 140, 441–451.

Woolf, C., 2012. Central sensitisation: implications for the diagnosis and treatment of pain. Pain 152, S2–S15.

World Health Organization, 2001. International classification of functioning, disability and health. World Health Organization, Geneva.

World Health Organization, 2011. World report on disability. World Health Organization, Geneva.

Wright, A., 1995. Hypoalgesia post-manipulative therapy: a review of a potential neurophysiological mechanism. Man. Ther. 1, 11–16.

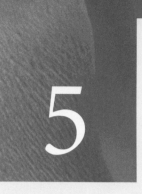

5

EXAMINATION OF THE TEMPOROMANDIBULAR REGION

HELEN COWGILL

CHAPTER CONTENTS

INTRODUCTION

The masticatory system is primarily responsible for chewing, speaking and swallowing. The temporomandibular joint (TMJ) plays an integral role within the masticatory system and is one of the most complex and used joints of the body (Okeson 2013; Magee 2014). The right and left TMJ, along with their associated ligaments and muscles, create a bilateral articulation between the U-shaped mandible and the temporal bone of the cranium (Pertes & Gross 1995). The articulation of these two bones is separated by the intraarticular disc into upper and lower articular compartments, which gives the TMJ the capability to perform a variety of complex movements involving a combination of sliding and hinging movements (Pertes & Gross 1995; Okeson 2013).

Movement of the mandible bone occurs as a series of rotational and translatory movements and is reliant on the combined simultaneous movement of both TMJs (Pertes & Gross 1995). Therefore, movement of one joint cannot occur in isolation or without influence from the other and hence movements are considered as one functional unit. Problems with the mobility of the intraarticular disc can be a major source of pain, limitation of movement and dysfunction. It is critical, during examination, that both TMJs are evaluated to determine the dysfunctional side as pain is not always associated with the side of dysfunction (Cowgill 2014). It is the only joint in the body where limitation of movement is restricted by the teeth and some consider the TMJs along with the teeth as a trijoint complex (Magee 2014). Therefore dental occlusion or bite is paramount when assessing the TMJ. For further information regarding the anatomy and biomechanics of the TMJ, the reader is directed to the textbook by Okeson (2013) which is devoted to temporomandibular dysfunction (TMD) and its management and the relevant chapter in Magee (2014).

TMD is a collective term that encompasses pain arising from the muscles of mastication along with disorders of the TMJ, including capsulitis, degenerative joint disease and internal derangement (Schiffman et al. 1990, 2014; Dimitroulis 1998). The aetiology of TMD is not clearly understood; however, it appears to be multifactorial and reflects an interaction between physical, functional and psychosocial factors (Hotta et al. 1997). Aetiological factors such as trauma, emotional stress, orthopaedic instability and muscle hyperactivity are significant.

Like all other joints, the TMJ has the capacity to adapt to functional demand and depends on many factors, such as loading of the joint, systemic disease and age. Any damage to the TMJ structures may interfere with normal function and thus cause dysfunction. TMD may be caused by macrotrauma due to an acute single event, or chronic microtrauma involving frequent low-grade events to the TMJ over time. Parafunctional habits, including clenching and bruxism (nocturnal grinding), are examples of microtrauma (Okeson 2013). Any force that overloads the joint complex may cause damage to joint structures or disturb the normal functional relationship between the condyle, disc and articular eminence of the temporal bone, resulting in pain, dysfunction or both. Dysfunction of the TMJ can present in a variety of ways, such as restricted movement, joint sounds and lateral deviation of the mandible during mouth opening, and is related to mandibular movement (Pertes & Gross 1995; Okeson 2013; Magee 2014). It is important to remember that normal movements of

the TMJ can be performed without any pain or excessive joint noise.

To appreciate the causes of potential dysfunction and clinical presentation of arthrogenic TMD, it is important to understand the disc–condylar relationship. Displacement of the articular disc is characterized by an abnormal relationship between the articular disc, mandibular condyle and articular eminence of the temporal bone. The two main types of disc displacement are with or without reduction.

- Disc displacement with reduction occurs when the disc is displaced in an anterior or anteromedial position when the mouth is closed and returns to a more normal position relative to the condyle on mouth opening.
- Disc displacement without reduction is characterized by displacement of the disc permanently and the condyle does not recapture or recentre under the disc during mandibular movement (Pertes & Gross 1995).

CLASSIFICATION OF TMD

Broadly, TMD can be classified using the diagnostic criteria published by Schiffman et al. (2014) and the most common disorders are outlined in Table 5.1. For further taxonomic classification for TMD, the reader is directed to Schiffman et al. (2014).

TABLE 5.1
Most Common Pain and Intraarticular Temporomandibular Dysfunction (TMD) (Schiffman et al. 2014)

Most Common Pain-Related TMD	Most Common Intraarticular TMD
Myalgia ■ Local myalgia ■ Myofascial pain ■ Myofascial pain with referral ■ Arthralgia ■ Headache attributed to TMD	■ Disc displacement with reduction ■ Disc displacement with reduction with intermittent locking ■ Disc displacement without reduction with limited opening ■ Disc displacement without reduction without limited opening ■ Degenerative joint disease ■ Subluxation

The above classification system highlights the importance of an accurate diagnosis when treating TMD due to its complex and multifactorial nature. This is because, frequently, a patient does not fit into one classification and can present with more than one disorder. This may make treatment and management of TMD complicated, as frequently patients with TMD are treated simultaneously and referred to more than one specialty (Ahmed et al. 2014). It is important to identify the primary and secondary diagnoses, and any contributing factors which may be driving the patient's pain or disorder.

Craniofacial pain is often caused by TMJ dysfunction; however, pain and TMJ disorders are also associated with the upper cervical spine (C0–C3). The upper cervical spine can refer pain to the same areas as the TMJ, i.e. the frontal, retroorbital, temporal and occipital areas of the head. The TMJ may also refer pain into the pre- or intraauricular area, or along the mandible (Feinstein et al. 1954; Rocabado 1983). Symptoms in these areas can be mediated by both the upper cervical spine and the TMJ due to neural convergence in the trigeminocervical nucleus in the brainstem (Bogduk & Bartsch 2008; Bogduk & Govind 2009). This association is supported by assessing the effects of manual therapy of the cervical spine on the TMJ (Mansilla-Ferragut et al. 2009). Therefore, it is important that examination of the TMJ is always accompanied by examination of the upper cervical spine.

It is vital always to have a differential diagnosis as part of a comprehensive clinical reasoning process. Diseases which may be of vascular origin, e.g. arteritis, or neural origin, e.g. trigeminal neuralgia, as well as craniocervical disorders and ear, nose and throat pathology may mimic TMD and can coexist with TMD, therefore full examination and reproduction of a patient's symptoms are paramount. Where a diagnosis is unclear and non-musculoskeletal, an onward referral to an appropriate specialist is indicated.

Further details of the questions asked during the subjective examination and the tests carried out during the physical examination can be found in Chapters 2 and 3, respectively. This chapter focuses on the TMJ, therefore the subjective assessment will be tailored towards this.

The order of the subjective questioning and the physical tests described below can be altered as appropriate for the patient being examined.

SUBJECTIVE EXAMINATION

Patients' Perspective on Their Experience

It is important to develop a good therapeutic relationship from the moment the clinician meets the patient. Simply starting the assessment process by asking some questions such as age, occupation and potential hobbies can make the patient immediately feel at ease and can help to direct the subjective assessment and the threat and/or meaning of the problem to the patient. For general questions to explore patients' perspectives on their condition, the reader is directed to Chapter 2. Factors from this information may indicate direct and/or indirect mechanical influences on the TMJ. The patient's occupation should be determined and its relevance to the patient's presentation, including psychosocial aspects, needs to be considered. Occupations that are commonly associated with TMD are singers or actors, telephonists and musicians, especially those playing instruments involving the use of a mouthpiece. Students of all ages need to be considered due to the stress associated with examinations and assessments.

It is well established that patients' individual cognitive, behavioural and emotional responses in relation to their pain are independent of the actual source of their pain (Schiffman et al. 2014). Instead the degree of pain experienced is correlated with patients' perception of the threat (in their sensory cortex) of the injury and the attention that they give to the injury (Okeson 2013). This can be related to the homunculus in the sensory cortex. It is estimated that 45% of the homunculus in the sensory cortex is dedicated to the face, mouth and throat (Okeson 2013) and therefore may amplify the patient's experience and meaning given to the pain experienced with TMD. TMD does have significant psychosocial associations and contributing factors and the clinician may ask the types of question to elucidate psychosocial factors that are outlined in Chapter 2. It is useful to use appropriate outcome measures to review any potential psychological factors which are prevalent with patients with TMD (Kraus 2014). Readers are referred to the diagnostic criteria axis II for further information regarding useful outcome measures (Schiffman et al. 2014).

Body Chart

The following information concerning the area and type of current symptoms can be recorded on a body chart (see Fig. 2.3) and it is recommended that a separate facial chart is used to be precise when recording head and facial symptoms.

Area of Current Symptoms

Be exact when recording the area of the symptoms. Symptoms associated with TMD include pain located in the ears, eyes and teeth and possibly radiating into the mandibular and temporal regions (Feinstein et al. 1954; Rocabado 1983), neck pain and headaches (Kraus 2014). Jaw-related symptoms may include pain, limited mouth opening (trismus) or difficulty moving the jaw, crepitus, clicking (on opening and/or closing), popping sounds and joint locking (Kraus 2014). It is recommended that the clinician asks the patient to point with one finger to the area of worst pain; generally those located directly over the TMJ are indicative of intraarticular dysfunction. Other symptoms include bruxism, non-migraine headaches, ear symptoms (including pain, ringing, fullness and subjective hearing loss) and dizziness (Magee 2014). The clinician always needs to check for red flags and precautions to assessment of the affected area (see Table 2.4, Table 6.2 and Box 6.1).

Ask whether the patient has ever experienced disequilibrium, dizziness or other symptoms associated with cervical arterial dysfunction (CAD) or vertebrobasilar insufficiency (Kerry 2013). If these symptoms are a feature described by the patient, the clinician needs to determine what factors aggravate and ease the symptoms, their duration and severity, and ultimately how likely these symptoms are to be related to serious neurovascular pathology. Suspicious presentations need to be referred for medical investigation (Bogduk 1994; Kerry & Taylor 2006). For further reading on this subject the reader is directed to the Taylor and Kerry (2010) masterclass.

Areas Relevant to the Region Being Examined

All other relevant areas need to be checked for symptoms. Due to the close anatomical (Rocabado 1983; Ayub et al. 1984; Darling et al. 1987) links between the TMJ and the cervical spine, the clinician needs to consider carefully any symptoms in the cervical spine. It is important to ask about pain or even stiffness, as this may be relevant to the patient's main symptom. Mark unaffected areas with ticks (✓) on the body chart.

Quality of Pain

Establish the quality of the pain. This is important information when attempting to determine the primary source of pain during differentiation between intra-/extraarticular, retrodiscal or muscular structures.

Intensity of Pain

The intensity of pain can be measured using, for example, a visual analogue scale, as shown in Fig. 2.5. A pain diary (see Chapter 2) may be useful for patients with chronic TMD, cervical spine pain and/or headaches, to determine pain patterns and triggering factors over a period of time.

Abnormal Sensation

Check for any altered sensation locally over the temporomandibular region and face and, if appropriate, over the cervical spine, upper thoracic spine or upper limbs (see Chapter 3).

Constant or Intermittent Symptoms

Ascertain the frequency of the symptoms, and whether they are constant or intermittent. If symptoms are constant, check whether there is variation in the intensity of the symptoms, as constant unremitting pain is indicative of neoplastic disease (Greenhalgh & Selfe 2010).

Relationship of Symptoms

Determine the relationship between the symptomatic areas – do they come together or separately? For example, the patient may have pain over the jaw without neck pain, or the pains may always be present together. This can assist with clinical reasoning as to whether the neck pain is independent of the jaw pain and can assist with planning the physical examination.

Behaviour of Symptoms

Aggravating Factors

The clinician asks the patient about theoretically known aggravating factors for structures that could be a source of the symptoms. Common aggravating factors for the temporomandibular region are mouth opening, prolonged talking, yawning, singing, shouting and chewing challenging foods such as nuts, meat, raw fruit, crusty bread and vegetables. Aggravating factors for other regions, which may need to be queried if they are suspected to be a source of the symptoms, are shown in Table 2.2.

For each symptomatic area, establish what specific movements and/or positions aggravate the patient's symptoms and the relationship between the symptoms described. For example, establish what brings them on or worsens constant symptoms and whether this aggravating movement/activity can be maintained; these factors help indicate severity. It is common for patients with TMD to describe chewing as an aggravating factor; however, it is important to determine whether they can only eat a soft diet, if they are avoiding challenging food groups, have an inability to chew and can chew through the pain. Also, consider that patients with a limitation of mouth opening may be physically unable to get the food into their mouth and may be on a softer or liquid diet as a result. It is also important to question patients about which side they chew on. Usually food will be distributed between the right and left side when chewing. If a patient is chewing unilaterally, understanding why can assist in the clinician's analysis of the patient's symptoms and the implications of chewing unilaterally, including the impact on joint loading and muscle activation.

Determine what happens to other symptoms when this symptom is produced or aggravated and, importantly, how long it takes for symptoms to ease on cessation of the aggravating movement, which will indicate irritability and assist with assessment planning. For further information regarding severity, irritability and nature with regard to assessment planning, the reader is directed to Chapter 2.

The clinician ascertains how the symptoms affect function and how function affects symptoms; for example, a forward head posture will change the resting position of the mandible, which is relevant in office workers. Patients may lean their hand on their jaw to support the head when reading or writing, which would unilaterally compress the TMJ.

Detailed information on each of the above activities gives useful insight to help determine the structure(s)

at fault and to identify functional restrictions. This information can be used to determine the aims of treatment and prognosis. The most notable functional restrictions are highlighted with asterisks (*), explored in the physical examination, and reassessed at subsequent treatment sessions to evaluate treatment intervention (Kerry 2013).

Easing Factors

For each symptomatic area, the clinician asks what movements and/or positions ease the patient's symptoms, how long it takes to ease them and what happens to other symptoms when this symptom is relieved. These questions help to confirm the relationship between the symptoms and also the irritability of the symptoms.

The clinician asks the patient about theoretically known easing factors for structures that could be a source of the symptoms. For example, symptoms from the TMJ may be eased by placing the joint in a particular position, whereas symptoms from the upper cervical spine may be eased by supporting the head or neck. The clinician can then analyse the position or movement that eases the symptoms, to help determine the structure at fault (Kerry 2013).

Parafunctional Habits

Activities of the muscles of mastication can be broadly divided into two main types: functional activities such as chewing and talking and parafunctional activities such as grinding or clenching the teeth, which are non-functional activities (Okeson 2013). Parafunctional habits can occur in the daytime and also during sleep and can be either in single activities (clenching) or rhythmic contractions (bruxing). They can occur in isolation or together and can be hard to separate, and therefore termed as bruxing events. Clinical signs which indicate bruxism and/or excessive functional or parafunctional activity are tongue scalloping, frictional keratosis or linea alba of the buccal mucosa and tooth wear on the posterior molars or canines observed on intraoral examination (Okeson 2013). Examples of common parafunctional habits are detailed in Table 5.2.

Twenty-Four-Hour Behaviour

The clinician determines the 24-hour behaviour of symptoms by asking questions about night, morning

TABLE 5.2	
Common Functional and Parafunctional Habits	
Functional Habits	**Parafunctional Habits**
Mastication or chewing food	Grinding
Swallowing	Clenching
Speech	Chewing gum excessively
	Tongue thrusting
	Sucking cheeks
	Biting nails
	Biting the lip or cheek
	Excessive positional clicking of the joint (party tricks)

and evening symptoms. The reader is referred to Chapter 2 for a full list of subjective questioning about diurnal variation. The following additional questions may be useful with patients with TMD.

Night Symptoms

- Do you grind or clench your teeth at night? Usually the patient will be unaware of bruxism and their partner may be able to provide this information.
- Do you suffer with sleep apnoea?
- Do you currently wear or have you ever worn a splint at night? If so, then the following questions need to be considered:
  - What effect did it have on your symptoms?
  - Current state of the splint (where possible, view the splint for signs of wear).
  - When was the last time it was replaced? This can indicate how strong the patient's bruxist tendency is.
- In patients undergoing orthodontic treatment: Do you use elastic bands overnight or a plastic retainer?

Morning and Evening Symptoms. The clinician determines the pattern of the symptoms first thing in the morning, through the day and at the end of the day. Patients who grind their teeth at night may wake up with a headache and/or facial, jaw or tooth symptoms (Kraus 1994). However, if patients have strong parafunctional habits, they may have pain during the day which can worsen as the day progresses. If stress or the work/study environment is thought to be a

contributing factor, it is worthwhile exploring the pattern of symptoms on a working/study vs. non-working/study day.

Stage of the Condition

In order to determine the stage of the condition, the clinician asks whether the symptoms are getting better, getting worse or remaining unchanged. This will also assist with prognosis.

Special Questions and Red-Flag Screening

Special questions must always be asked, as they may identify certain precautions or contraindications to the physical examination and/or treatment (see Table 2.4). Chapter 2 outlines the special questions that must be considered in order to differentiate between conditions that are suitable for conservative treatment and systemic, neoplastic and other non-musculoskeletal conditions, which require referral to a medical practitioner. Readers are referred to Greenhalgh and Selfe (2010) and Chapter 2 for details of various serious pathological processes that can mimic musculoskeletal conditions and Table 6.2 for specific red flags for the cervical spine.

The following additional special questions need to be considered for TMJ patients.

Clicking

Clicking is usually associated with abnormal disc–condylar mechanics (Okeson 2013; Magee 2014) and establishing the nature of a click can assist diagnosis and prognosis. A click may be heard on auscultation with a disc displacement with reduction when the mandibular condyle pushes under the posterior disc to regain a normal disc–condylar relationship on mouth opening and a reciprocal closing click may be heard as the condyle slips off the posterior disc. Disc displacement without reduction may or may not be associated with a click (Pertes & Gross 1995; Magee 2014).

It is important to remember that anatomical evidence of disc displacement is not always associated with patient symptoms. More often than not, disc displacement is accompanied by a clicking sound and restriction in mandibular movement; however, a painless click is not always indicative of a joint dysfunction. There are variations in the causes of clicks and the reader is directed to the diagnostic criteria

(Okeson 2013; Magee 2014; Schiffman et al. 2014) regarding joint noises and potential presentations.

Bruxism

The extent and nature of teeth grinding need to be established, and its relationship to the present condition considered. The mechanical forces produced during grinding can contribute to TMJ dysfunction. Bruxism is often a manifestation of stress and as such it is important to consider associated psychological factors which may be causing, contributing to and/or mediating the present condition.

Clenching

Clenching can occur at night and also during the day. The normal resting position for the mandible is with the posterior teeth slightly apart and the tip of the tongue in the roof of the mouth. Clenching causes overactivity in the muscles of mastication responsible for this action and can lead to myogenic pain.

Dental Disorders

The association between upper and lower tooth contact (occlusion) and forces through the TMJ should be considered. A thorough history of all dental disorders, including surgery, tooth extraction, orthodontic history, tooth fractures (may indicate bruxism) and prolonged opening during dental examination/ treatment, should be noted. Note should be taken if the patient has any loose dentition or wears dentures as this will be relevant when planning the objective examination. Asymmetrical occlusion or the absence of teeth can have an effect on TMJ loading and the muscles of mastication (Magee 2014), which may lead to pathomechanical changes within and around the TMJ.

Trismus

Trismus, or a limitation of mouth opening, is common with TMD. It should be noted that it can also be a primary presenting sign of malignancy (Beddis et al. 2014).

Cranial Nerve Disorders

Signs and symptoms associated with TMJ dysfunction can be similar to those arising from frank cranial nerve disorders. It is therefore essential to establish whether or not there are cranial nerve disorders present which would require further medical investigation. Alternatively, known cranial nerve disorders may result in, or contribute to, TMJ dysfunction, and vice versa. The relevance of any disorder needs to be established, for example:

- pain and/or altered sensation in the forehead and face needs to be differentiated from trigeminal (cranial nerve [CN] V) neuralgia
- for difficulties in opening and closing, consideration should be given to the trigeminal nerve innervation of masticating muscles
- facial asymmetries need to be differentiated from facial nerve (CN VII) palsies
- aural symptoms should be differentiated from vestibulocochlear nerve (CN VIII) palsies, which may be related to serious neoplastic pathology
- swallowing problems should be differentiated from glossopharyngeal (CN IX) and vagus (CN X) nerve palsies
- tongue asymmetries should be differentiated from hypoglossal nerve (CN XII) disorder (Kerry 2013). Table 6.6 details cranial nerve assessment.

Cervical Arterial Dysfunction

The clinician identifies symptoms suggestive of vasculopathy related to either the vertebral arteries (e.g. vertebrobasilar insufficiency) or the internal carotid arteries. Pathology of these vessels can mimic craniofacial signs and symptoms associated with TMJ dysfunction (see Chapter 6). Symptoms include: disequilibrium, dizziness, altered vision (including diplopia), nausea, ataxia, drop attacks, altered facial sensation, difficulty speaking, difficulty swallowing, sympathoplegia, hemianaesthesia and hemiplegia (Bogduk 1994; Kerry & Taylor 2006). Ptosis (drooping eyelid) is associated with internal carotid artery pathology and may be mistaken for facial asymmetry. Specifically, jaw claudication related to carotid pathologies can mimic mechanical TMJ dysfunction. If present, the clinician determines in the usual way the aggravating and easing factors. Similar symptoms can also be related to upper cervical instability and diseases of the inner ear. It is important to remember that, in their pre-ischaemic stage, cervical vasculopathies can present with just upper cervical and head pain (Kerry

& Taylor 2006; Bogduk & Govind 2009), as shown in Fig. 6.6. Awareness of predisposing factors to vascular injury and information regarding the patient's blood pressure can assist in the diagnosis (Kerry & Taylor 2006, 2008, 2009). See Table 6.3 for screening associated with CAD and Chapter 6 for guidance on testing for CAD. For presentations of temporofrontal headache, the clinician needs also to consider temporal arteritis as a differential diagnosis (Kerry 2013).

Ear Symptoms

Tinnitus is a common complaint alongside TMJ symptoms. Inner-ear ache, blocking and problems with hearing are associated with TMD (Magee 2014) and may be due to the close proximity of the TMJ and auditory canal. Any concerns that the TMJ is not the source of ear symptoms should prompt an onward referral to the appropriate specialist.

Headaches

Headaches are commonly associated with TMD; however, it is important to establish whether the headache is of cervical or TMJ origin. TMD-related headaches are usually located in the temple region and are aggravated by jaw movement, function and/or parafunction and provocation of the masticatory system can reproduce the headache (Schiffman et al. 2014).

History of the Present Condition

A detailed section on general questions to be asked for history of the present condition can be found in Chapter 2. Patients with TMD usually present with pain and a limitation of mouth opening or trismus. For each symptomatic area, the clinician needs to discover how long the symptom has been present, whether there was a sudden or slow onset and whether there was a known cause that provoked the onset of the symptom, such as trauma, stress, surgery or occupation. If the onset was slow, the clinician needs to find out if there has been any change in the patient's lifestyle, e.g. a new diet, recent dental treatment or other factors. Onset of symptoms may be insidious, due to a specific event, trauma, including whiplash, direct trauma to the jaw, prolonged dental treatment or surgery (Kraus 2014). It is important to find out about previous consultations with other healthcare professionals as it has been reported that patients with

TMD on average will have consulted with 3.2 healthcare professionals prior to their initial physiotherapy consultation (Kraus 2014).

Past Medical History

The following information is obtained from the patient and/or dental/medical notes:

- The details of any relevant dental/medical history, particularly involving the teeth, jaw, cranium or cervical spine.
- The history of any previous attacks: how many episodes? When were they? What was the cause? What is the frequency? What was the duration of each episode? Did the patient fully recover between episodes? If there have been no previous attacks, has the patient had any episodes of stiffness in the TMJ or cervical spine? Check for a history of trauma or recurrent minor trauma.
- Ascertain the results of any past treatment for the same or a similar problem.
- Is the patient taking any medication or trialled medication for the problem and what is its effect on symptoms?
- Has the patient had any recent aesthetic cosmetic work completed which may be relevant, such as facial fillers? Fillers can move during the physical assessment, so the clinician needs to clarify where the facial filler has been injected and avoid this area.

PLAN OF THE PHYSICAL EXAMINATION

When all this information has been collected, the subjective examination is complete. It is useful at this stage to highlight with asterisks (*), for ease of reference, important findings and particularly one or more functional restrictions. These can then be reexamined at subsequent treatment sessions to evaluate treatment intervention. The reader is referred to Chapter 2 for general considerations of planning the physical examination, such as consideration of order of testing and contraindications. In addition to these points, the clinician may want to consider the primary and differential diagnosis and may consider using a must/could/should list. Alternatively, a planning form can be useful to help guide clinicians through the often complex clinical reasoning process (see Fig. 2.10).

The information from the subjective examination helps the clinician to plan an appropriate physical examination. The severity, irritability and nature of the condition are the major factors that will influence the choice and priority of physical testing procedures. The first and overarching question the clinician might ask is: 'Is this patient's condition suitable for me to manage as a therapist?' For example, a patient presenting with obvious cranial nerve palsy may only need neurological integrity testing, prior to an urgent medical referral. The nature of the patient's condition will have a major impact on the physical examination. The second question the clinician might ask is: 'Does this patient have a musculoskeletal dysfunction that I may be able to help?' To answer that, the clinician needs to carry out a full physical examination; however, this may not be possible if the symptoms are severe and/or irritable. The reader is referred to Chapter 2 for modification of physical examination in response to severity, irritability and nature.

Points to consider when planning the physical examination specific to the temporomandibular region:

- TMJ examination should always be accompanied by an examination of the upper cervical spine. Therefore, the upper cervical spine will always be on the must list.
- Are there any precautions and/or contraindications to elements of the physical examination that need to be explored further, such as vertebrobasilar insufficiency, neurological involvement, recent fracture, trauma, steroid therapy or rheumatoid arthritis? There may also be contraindications to further examination and treatment, e.g. symptoms of cord compression. Consider precautions such as loose dentition, dentures or fear of the dentist as the examination will include intraoral assessment. Consider medical history, including epilepsy, as it would not be recommended to assess accessory movements due to hand positioning which may be dangerous during an epileptic fit where the teeth may be heavily clenched.

- Be aware of any recent aesthetic cosmetic work such as facial fillers to avoid movement during the physical examination.

PHYSICAL EXAMINATION

Each significant physical test that either provokes or eases the patient's symptoms is highlighted in the patient's notes by an asterisk (*) for easy reference. The highlighted tests are often referred to as 'asterisks' or 'markers'.

The order and detail of the physical tests described below should be appropriate to the patient being examined; some tests will be irrelevant, some tests will be carried out briefly, while others will need to be investigated fully. It is important that readers understand that the techniques shown in this chapter are some of many; the choice depends mainly on the relative size of the clinician and patient, as well as the clinician's preference. For this reason, novice clinicians may initially want to copy what is shown, but then quickly adapt to what is best for them (Kerry 2013). The clinician should always gain consent from the patient and explain the physical examination, including intraoral examination.

OBSERVATION

Informal Observation

Informal observation will have begun from the moment the clinician begins the subjective examination, for example, observing articulation during speech or parafunctional habits present, and observation will continue to the end of the physical examination. Chapter 3 provides further information regarding informal observation.

Formal Observation

The clinician needs to observe the patient in dynamic and static situations; the quality of cervical and jaw movement is noted, as are the postural characteristics and facial expression.

Observation of Posture

The clinician observes the general posture and cervical posture. The myofascial relationships between the neck and the jaw mean that postural dysfunction in one may influence the other. For craniofacial observation, the clinician observes facial symmetry using the anatomical landmarks shown in Fig. 5.1.

Check whether optic, bipupital, otic and occlusive lines of the face are parallel (Fig. 5.1). Additionally, the length (posterior–anterior) of the mandible can be measured from the TMJ line to the anterior notch of the chin, and any side-to-side differences noted. The clinician notes any paralysis such as drooping of the mouth, which may indicate Bell's palsy.

The clinician checks the bony and soft-tissue contours of the face and TMJ. The clinician observes the resting position of the mandible, also known as the upper postural position of the mandible. In the resting position of the mandible the back teeth are slightly apart, the mandible is in a relaxed position and the tip of the tongue lies against the palate just posterior to the inner surface of the upper central incisors. The clinician checks the intercuspal position, in which the back teeth are closed together, and observes the patient's teeth for malocclusion, such as:

- underbite (mandibular teeth anterior to maxillary teeth) or class III occlusion (Okeson 2013)
- overbite (maxillary teeth anterior to mandibular teeth – 2 mm of overbite is normal) or class II (Okeson 2013). If overbite is apparent, the degree of overjet (how far the maxillary incisors close

down over the mandibular incisors) is measured with a ruler and noted (Magee 2014)
- crossbite (deviation of the mandible to one side – use the interincisor gap between the two central incisors as reference points on both mandibular and maxillary sets).

Malocclusion and occlusal interference are noted, and usually seen when teeth are missing, poorly formed, or when a dental brace, dentures or implants are being worn.

Observation of Muscle Form

The main muscles of mastication are the masseter, temporalis, medial pterygoid and lateral pterygoid and of these muscles, only the masseter and temporalis are visible and may be enlarged or atrophied. If there is postural abnormality that is thought to be due to a muscle imbalance, then the muscles around the cervical spine and shoulder girdle may need to be inspected.

Observation of the Intraoral Environment

The clinician looks at the health of the patient's gums and also inspects the intraoral environment for any signs of clenching or bruxism. The three common clinical signs which indicate bruxism or bruxing events are:

1. linea alba or frictional keratosis of the buccal mucosa (ridging of the inner cheek) (Fig. 5.2)
2. deterioration of the wear facets on the posterior molars (Fig. 5.2)
3. tongue scalloping (indentations of the teeth on the tongue) (Fig. 5.3).

A torch and tongue depressor are helpful when observing the intraoral environment, but not essential. Clinical signs seen on intraoral examination may indicate excessive functional or parafunctional activity (Okeson 2013). If patients have a diurnal variation to their symptoms, it is important to establish if their parafunctional habits are nocturnal or are continuing during the day by asking them to observe the clinical signs on waking, at midday and in the evening. If the excessive functional or parafunctional habits are continuing during the day, patients can become consciously aware to reduce the effect of these habits on their TMD.

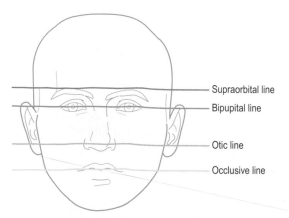

Supraorbital line

Bipupital line

Otic line

Occlusive line

FIG. 5.1 ■ Symmetry of the face can be tested comparing the supraorbital, bipupital, otic and occlusive lines, which should be parallel. *(From Magee 2014, with permission.)*

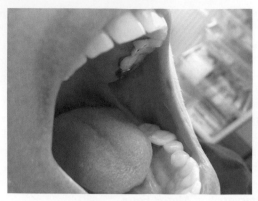

FIG. 5.2 ■ Linea alba (frictional keratosis of the buccal mucosa) of the inner cheek and deterioration or flattening of the wear facets on the posterior molars can be noted on intraoral examination. These are indicative of bruxing events.

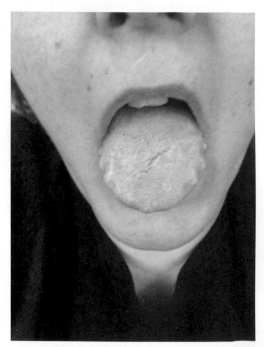

FIG. 5.3 ■ Tongue scalloping can be noted on intraoral examination which is indicative of bruxing events or tongue thrusting.

Observation of Soft Tissues

The clinician observes the colour of the patient's skin and any swelling over the TMJ, face or gums, and takes cues for further examination. The clinician observes the lymph glands and nodes and when palpated, if an abnormality is felt or suspected, refers on appropriately.

Observation of the Patient's Attitudes and Feelings

The age, gender and ethnicity of patients and their cultural, occupational and social backgrounds will all affect their attitudes and feelings towards themselves, their condition and the clinician. The clinician needs to be aware of and sensitive to these attitudes, and empathize and communicate appropriately in order to develop a rapport with the patient and thereby enhance the therapeutic relationship and also the patient's compliance with the treatment (Kerry 2013).

ACTIVE PHYSIOLOGICAL MOVEMENTS

For active passive physiological movements, the clinician should take note of the common procedures and considerations noted in Chapter 3. In addition, the clinician needs to consider the following in relation to TMD:

- Evaluate the quality of movement: minor subluxation, crepitus or a click on opening and/or closing the mouth.
- Assess the range of movement: excessive range, particularly opening, may indicate hypermobility of the TMJ.
- Observe any overactivity of the anterior cervical muscles, particularly with mouth opening.
- Observe for any alteration in the opening pathway:
  - Deviation is where the mandible deviates during mouth opening, but returns to normal midline relationship at maximum mouth opening (Okeson 2013).
  - Deflection is where the mandible is shifted to one side on opening and does not return to the normal midline relationship (Okeson 2013).

TMJ movements can be measured with a ruler; the distance between the incisal edges of the anterior teeth is measured as shown in Fig. 5.4. Painfree mouth opening as measured by the interincisal distance has proven reliability and validity (de Wijer et al. 1995; Beltran-Alacreu et al. 2014) and acceptable interrater

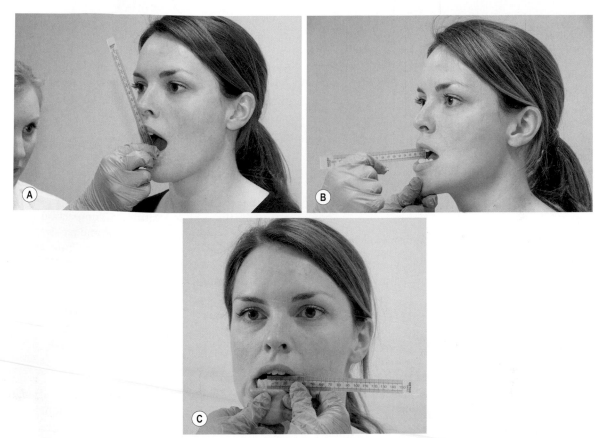

FIG. 5.4 ■ Measuring mouth movement and temporomandibular joint active range of motion with a ruler. (A) Maximal comfortable and maximal mouth or incisal opening. The patient is asked to open the mouth just before pain is felt and is termed maximal comfortable opening. This measurement is the distance between the incisal edges of the anterior teeth. This is repeated with the patient opening as wide as she can even in the presence of pain, which is termed maximal mouth opening. (B) Protrusion. (C) Lateral deviation.

reliability when measured in millimeters (Dworkin et al. 1990; Walker et al. 2000).

TMJ movements can be recorded as shown in Fig. 5.5 or in an active range of motion chart. The active movements of opening/closing, protraction/retraction and lateral deviation with overpressure listed in Table 5.3 are shown in Fig. 5.6 and can be tested with the patient sitting (Kerry 2013) or lying supine. The clinician establishes the patient's symptoms at rest and prior to each movement, and corrects any movement deviation to determine its relevance to the patient's symptoms. Palpation of the movement of the condyles during active movements can be useful to feel the quality of the movement and also to appreciate the biomechanics of the joint, with the first 20–25 mm

mouth opening being a rotational movement, followed by a translatory movement. Excessive anterior movement of the lateral pole of the mandibular condyle may indicate TMJ hypermobility. Auscultation of the joint during jaw movements enables the clinician to listen to any joint sounds, including clicking or crepitus, as shown in Fig. 5.7.

Movements of the TMJ and the possible modifications are given in Table 5.3. Various differentiation tests (Rocabado 2004; Hengeveld & Banks 2014; Magee 2014) can be performed; the choice depends on the patient's signs and symptoms.

Other regions may need to be examined to determine their relevance to the patient's symptoms; they may be the source of the symptoms, or they may be

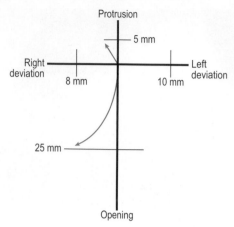

FIG. 5.5 ■ Example of recording movement findings for the temporomandibular joint. Normally opening is around 35–45 mm. The joint mechanics normally function in a 4 : 1 ratio, i.e. 4 mm of opening to every 1 mm of lateral deviation/protrusion. *(From Rocabado 2004.)*

TABLE 5.3
Summary of Active Movements and Their Possible Modification

Active Movements	Modifications to Active Movements
Temporomandibular joint	Repeated
Depression (opening)	Speed altered
Elevation (closing)	Combined, e.g.
Protraction	■ Opening then lateral deviation
Retraction	■ Lateral deviation then opening
Depression in retracted position	■ Protraction then opening
Left lateral deviation	■ Retraction then opening
Right lateral deviation	Sustained
?Upper cervical spine movements	Differentiation tests
Injuring movement	Functional ability
?Cervical spine movement	
?Thoracic spine movements	

contributing to the symptoms. The regions most likely are the upper cervical spine and cervical spine. The joints within these regions can be tested fully (see Chapters 6 and 7) or partially with the use of screening tests (see Chapter 3).

Some functional ability has already been tested by the general observation of jaw movement as the patient has talked during the subjective examination. Any further testing can be carried out at this point in the examination. Clues for appropriate tests can be obtained from the subjective examination findings, particularly the aggravating factors.

PASSIVE PHYSIOLOGICAL MOVEMENTS

The clinician can move the TMJ passively with the patient in the supine position. A comparison of the response of symptoms to the active and passive movements can help to determine the structure at fault. Passive physiological movements can also determine the side of dysfunction, which may not always be the symptomatic side. Other regions may need to be examined to determine their relevance to the patient's symptoms.

MUSCLE TESTS

Muscle tests include examining muscle strength, control, endurance and isometric contraction.

Muscle Strength

The clinician may test muscle groups that depress, elevate, protract, retract and laterally deviate the mandible, as shown in Fig. 5.8, and, if applicable, the cervical musculature. Kraus (1994), however, considers mandibular muscle weakness to be rare in TMJ disorders and difficult to determine manually. It is important to consider the lateral pterygoid muscle, which has attachments to the anterior disc and mandibular condyle, which may cause pain or spasm in patients with disc dysfunction.

Muscle Control

Excessive masticatory muscle activity is thought to be a factor in TMJ conditions. The muscles of the cervical spine, and in particular the deep neck flexors, should be tested. Exercises for the cervical spine and posture have been shown to reduce muscle pain and improve jaw function in patients with TMD (McNeely et al. 2006).

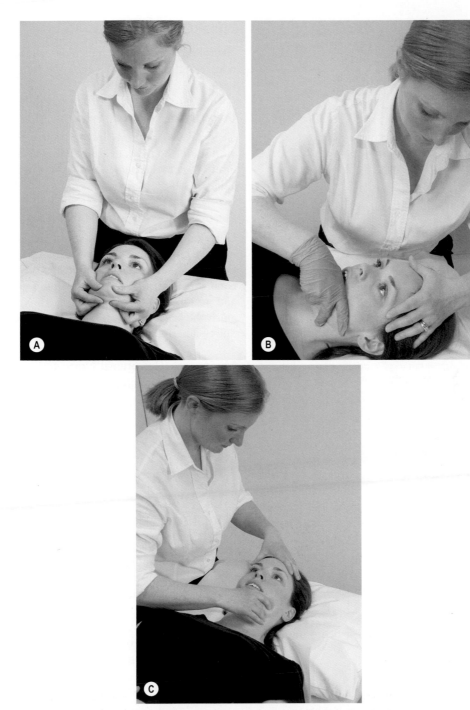

FIG. 5.6 ■ Overpressures to the temporomandibular joint. (A) Depression (opening) and elevation (closing). The fingers and thumbs of both hands gently grasp the mandible to depress and elevate the mandible. (B) Protraction and retraction. A gloved thumb is placed just inside the mouth on the posterior aspect of the bottom front teeth. Thumb pressure can then protract and retract the mandible. (C) Lateral deviation. The left hand stabilizes the head while the right hand cups around the mandible and moves the mandible to the left and right.

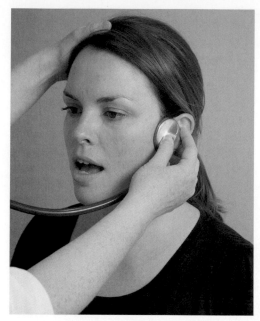

FIG. 5.7 ■ Auscultation of temporomandibular joint (TMJ) noises. The clinician places the stethoscope over the TMJ and listens during TMJ active range of motion, mouth opening/closing, protrusion and lateral deviation, listening for clicking or crepitus.

Isometric Muscle Testing

Test the muscle groups that depress, elevate, protract, retract and laterally deviate the mandible in the resting position, as shown in Fig. 5.8, and, if indicated, in various parts of the physiological ranges. Also, if applicable, test the cervical musculature. In addition the clinician observes the quality of the muscle contraction necessary to hold this position (this can be done with the patient's eyes shut). The patient may, for example, be unable to prevent the joint from moving or may hold with excessive muscle activity; either of these circumstances would suggest a neuromuscular dysfunction (Kerry 2013).

Endurance Testing

Here the clinician can test the muscle with repeated movement with or without resistance and observe the quality of movement and the distance. This is particularly important in patients who are constantly using their TMJ, such as singers and actors.

NEUROLOGICAL TESTS

Neurological examination includes neurological integrity testing, neurodynamic tests and some other nerve tests.

Integrity of Nervous System

Generally, if symptoms are localized to the upper cervical spine and head, neurological examination can be limited to cranial nerves and C1–C4 nerve roots (see Table 6.6).

Dermatomes/Peripheral Nerves

Light touch and pain sensation of the face, head and neck are tested using cotton wool and pinprick respectively, as described in Chapter 3. Knowledge of the cutaneous distribution of nerve roots (dermatomes) and peripheral nerves enables the clinician to distinguish the sensory loss due to a root lesion from that due to a peripheral nerve lesion.

Myotomes/Peripheral Nerves

The following myotomes are tested and are shown in Chapter 3 and Table 3.8:

- trigeminal (CN V)
- facial (CN VII)
- accessory (CN XI)
- C1–C2
- C2
- C3
- C4 and CN XI.

A working knowledge of the muscular distribution of nerve roots (myotomes) and peripheral nerves enables the clinician to distinguish the motor loss due to a root lesion from that due to a peripheral nerve lesion.

Reflex Testing

The jaw jerk (CN V) is elicited by applying a sharp downward tap on the chin with a reflex hammer with the mouth slightly open. A slight jerk is normal; excessive jerk suggests a bilateral upper motor neuron lesion.

Neurodynamic Tests

The following neurodynamic tests may be carried out if indicated, in order to ascertain the degree to which

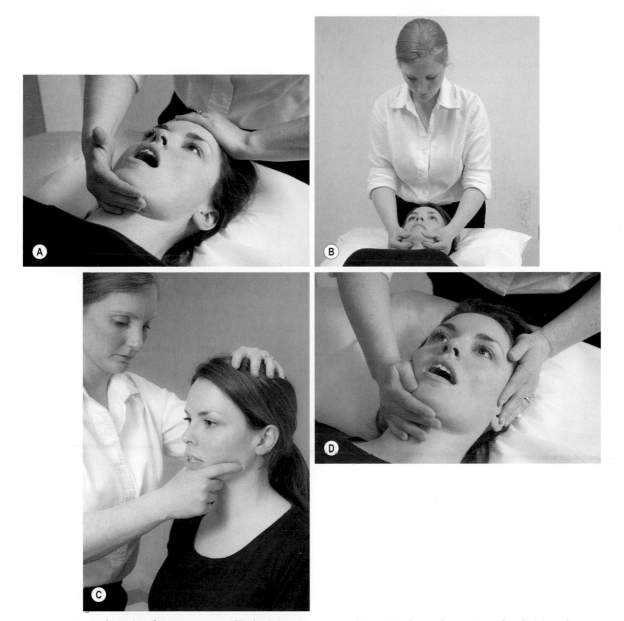

FIG. 5.8 ■ Strength testing for temporomandibular joint movements. (A) Resisted mouth opening. The clinician places one hand under the chin to provide resistance and the other hand stabilizes the head. (B) Resisted mouth closing. The clinician places both hands over the chin and resists the patient closing her mouth. (C) Resisted protrusion. The clinician places the web space of her hand over the patient's chin and resists a forward movement of the chin into protrusion. (D) Resisted lateral deviation. The clinician places one hand over the mandible and the other hand stabilizes the head; the lateral movement of the mandible is resisted.

neural tissue is responsible for the production of the patient's symptom(s):

- passive neck flexion
- upper-limb neurodynamic tests
- straight-leg raise
- slump.

These tests are described in detail in Chapter 3.

Lingual Mandibular Reflex (CN V)

The tongue is actively placed against the soft palate and a normal response is relaxation of masticatory muscles. Loss of this reflex is not necessarily serious, but rather an indication of sensorimotor dysfunction related to the TMJ/upper cervical dysfunction (Kerry 2013).

MISCELLANEOUS TESTS

To facilitate differential diagnosis, further testing may be undertaken as follows:

- Vertebral and carotid arterial examination (Kerry & Taylor 2006, 2009) (see Chapter 6).
- Palpation of the temporal artery for suspected temporal arteritis. A positive finding is a painful and exaggerated pulse (Kerry 2013).
- Further cranial nerve examination. Refer for medical investigation if frank nerve pathology is suspected (see Chapter 6).

Palpation

The TMJ and the upper cervical spine (see Chapter 6) are palpated. It is useful to record palpation findings on a body chart (see Fig. 2.3) and/or palpation chart (see Fig. 3.35).

The clinician is referred to Chapter 3 for general palpation considerations and guidelines (see Box 3.5). In addition to this general palpation, the following is specific to the TMJ region:

- position and prominence of the mandible and TMJ
- the presence or elicitation of any muscle spasm in the muscles of mastication
- tenderness of bony landmarks (zygomatic arch, mandibular ramus and condyle), ligament, muscle (masseter, temporalis, medial and lateral

pterygoids, splenius capitis, suboccipital muscles, trapezius, sternocleidomastoid, digastric) and tendons. Check for tenderness of the hyoid bone and thyroid cartilage. Test for the relevant trigger points shown in Fig. 3.36
- the tendon of the temporalis as it inserts on to the coronoid process of the mandible, as shown in Fig. 5.9
- the medial pterygoid can also be palpated intraorally; however this is very uncomfortable in the normal population
- lymph glands for any enlargement
- there is controversy as to whether the lateral pterygoid can be palpated. It is believed to be palpated indirectly intraorally (Rocabado & Iglarsh 1991).

Accessory Movements

It is useful to use the palpation chart and movement diagrams (or joint pictures) to record findings. These are explained in detail in Chapter 3. The clinician is referred to Chapter 3 for general considerations when performing accessory movements. Consideration of the following is specific to the TMJ region in addition to general considerations.

TMJ accessory movements are listed in Table 5.4 and shown in Fig. 5.10, and are as follows:

- anteroposterior (not commonly assessed due to compression of the highly innervated retrodiscal

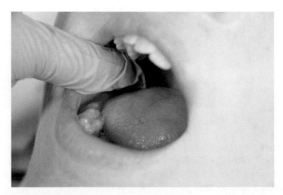

FIG. 5.9 ■ Palpation of the coronoid process for the insertion of the tendon of temporalis muscle on intraoral examination. The clinician's finger is moved up the anterior border of the ramus until the coronoid process and tendon of the temporalis are felt.

TABLE 5.4		
Accessory Movements, Choice of Application and Reassessment of the Patient's Asterisks		
Accessory Movements	**Choice of Application**	**Identify Any Effect of Accessory Movements on Patient's Signs and Symptoms**
Temporomandibular joint	Start position, e.g. with the mandible depressed, elevated, protracted, retracted, laterally deviated or a combination of these positions	Reassess all asterisks
↕ Anteroposterior		
↕ Posteroanterior	Speed of force application	
➝ Med Medial transverse	Direction of the applied force	
➝ Lat Lateral transverse	Point of application of applied force	
➝ Caud Longitudinal caudad		
➝ Ceph Longitudinal cephalad		
?Upper cervical spine	As above	Reassess all asterisks
?Cervical spine	As above	Reassess all asterisks
?Thoracic spine		Reassess all asterisks

area) – see Kerry (2013) for positioning for this test

■ posteroanterior
■ medial transverse
■ lateral transverse
■ longitudinal caudad
■ longitudinal cephalad.

Accessory movements can be performed in supine, as shown in Fig. 5.10, or in a semi-sitting position, as demonstrated by Kerry (2013). Following accessory movements to the TMJ, the clinician reassesses all the physical asterisks (movements or tests that have been found to reproduce the patient's symptoms) in order to establish the effect of the accessory movements on the patient's signs and symptoms. Accessory movements can then be tested for other regions suspected to be a source of the symptoms.

Other Tests for the Temporomandibular Joint

Dynamic Loading and Distraction

The clinician places a cotton roll between the upper and lower third molars on one side only and the patient is asked to bite on to the roll, noting any pain produced. Pain may be felt on the left or right TMJ as there will be distraction of the TMJ on the side of the cotton roll and compression of the TMJ on the contralateral side (Hylander 1979).

Bite Test (Biting on a Tongue Depressor Test) for Loading

When the patient bites unilaterally on a tongue depressor, the interarticular pressure is reduced in the TMJ of the side of the tongue depressor and raised in the contralateral TMJ. This can help determine whether the TMJ pain is articular or myogenic (Rocabado & Iglarsh 1991; Okeson 2013) (Fig. 5.11).

Palpation via External Auditory Meatus

The TMJ can be palpated slightly anterior to the tragus and posteriorly via the external auditory meatus (De Wijer & Steenks 2009), as shown in Fig. 5.12. The TMJ can be palpated during mandibular movement and the clinician feels whether there is equal rotation and translation of each condyle and whether there is equal movement on the return to a resting position (Magee 2014). Correlation with the normal movement parameters and biomechanics needs to be made. This can also be used as a mini-treatment by using a posteroanterior glide to the mandibular condyle with mouth opening (mobilization with movement) if indicated.

COMPLETION OF THE EXAMINATION

Having carried out the above tests, the examination of the temporomandibular region is now complete. The subjective and physical examinations produce a large

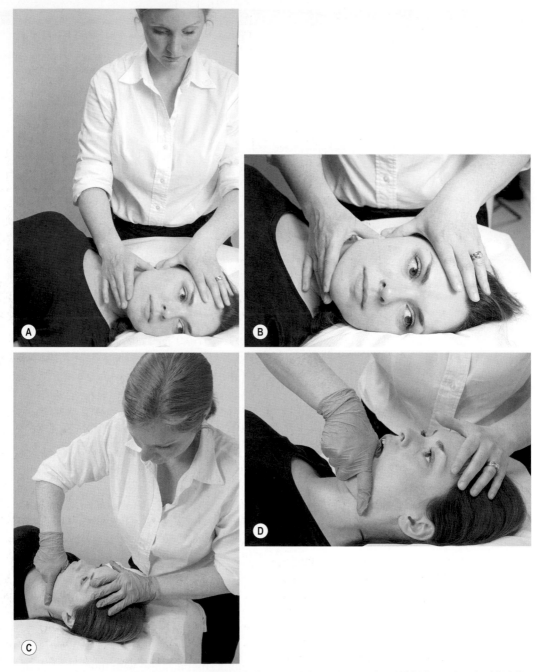

FIG. 5.10 ▪ Accessory movements to the temporomandibular joint. (A) Posteroanterior. With the patient in side-lying, thumbs apply a posteroanterior pressure to the posterior aspect of the head of the mandible. (B) Medial transverse. With the patient in side-lying, thumbs apply a medial pressure to the lateral aspect of the head of the mandible. (C) Lateral transverse. The one hand supports the head while the gloved hand is placed inside the mouth so that the thumb rests along the medial surface of the mandible (inside aspect of the lower teeth). Thumb pressure can then produce a lateral glide of the mandible. (D) Longitudinal cephalad and caudad. With the patient supine and the one hand supporting the head, the gloved hand is placed inside the mouth so that the thumb rests on the top of the lower back teeth. The thumb and outer fingers then grip the mandible and apply a downward pressure (longitudinal caudad) and an upward pressure (longitudinal cephalad).

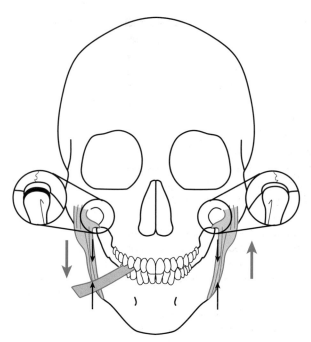

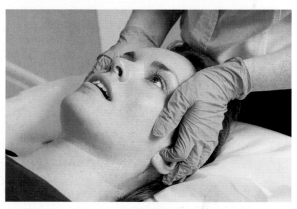

FIG. 5.12 ■ Palpation of mandibular condyle via the auditory canal. The temporomandibular joint is palpated laterally slightly anterior to the tragus and posteriorly via the external meatus, with the mouth open or closed, and during opening and closing movements.

FIG. 5.11 ■ Asking the patient to bite on a tongue depressor. When the bite is unilateral on a hard substance, the joint on the bite side has a sudden reduction in interarticular pressure, with the opposite happening to the contralateral side. This can help determine the problematic articular side. *(Modified from Okeson 2013, with permission.)*

amount of information, which needs to be recorded accurately and quickly. An outline examination chart may be useful for some clinicians and one is suggested in Fig. 3.50. It is important, however, that the clinician does not examine in a rigid manner, simply following the suggested sequence outlined in the chart. Each patient presents differently and this needs to be reflected in the examination process. It is vital at this stage to highlight with an asterisk (*) important findings from the examination. These findings are reassessed at, and within, subsequent treatment sessions to evaluate the effects of treatment on the patient's condition.

The physical testing procedures which specifically indicate joint, nerve or muscle tissues as a source of the patient's symptoms, are summarized in Table 3.9. The reader is referred to Chapter 3 for general guidance on completion of the physical examination, including correlating findings with clinical reasoning. For guidance on treatment and management

principles, the reader is directed to the companion textbook (Petty & Barnard 2017).

VALIDITY OF CLINICAL TESTS

Generally individual tests for TMD have poor validity (Chaput et al. 2012; Julsvoll et al. 2016). However, a cluster of positive tests can assist with diagnosis of an anterior disc displacement without reduction with an accuracy of 71% (Julsvoll et al. 2016), sensitivity of 0.71 and specificity of 0.91 for diagnosis of anterior disc displacement without reduction (Julsvoll et al. 2016). However, Schiffman et al. (2014) in the diagnostic criteria for TMD recommend that sensitivity should be 0.80 or higher and specificity 0.91 or higher for examination of anterior disc displacement without reduction, which questions the validity of the cluster test described by Julsvoll et al. (2016). The best single test was the dental stick or bite test with equal sensitivity as the cluster, although with lower specificity. It is, however, still recommended that imaging is requested for a definitive diagnosis of TMJ-related problems (Schiffman et al. 2014).

MULTIDISCIPLINARY TEAM APPROACH TO TMD

It is essential when assessing and managing patients with TMD that a multidisciplinary team approach is considered due to the multifactorial nature of TMD and its associations. No single cause accounts for all the signs and symptoms of TMD described by a patient, therefore there is no one single treatment strategy that can be recommended for patients with TMD. A multimodal and multidisciplinary approach is proposed, which has been shown as the most effective way to manage TMD (Medlicott & Harris 2006; Ahmed et al. 2014).

An initially conservative approach for management of TMD (Dimitroulis 1998; Lyons 2008; Wright & North 2009) includes physiotherapy, education, drug treatment and the use of a bite guard (occlusal splint). Surgical intervention, including arthrocentesis or arthroscopy of the TMJ (Guo et al. 2009), is indicated in a limited number of patients. Manual therapy for mechanical TMJ presentations and multimodal treatment approaches has been shown to be effective in a number of studies (Cleland & Palmer 2004; McNeely et al. 2006; Medlicott & Harris 2006; Shin et al. 2007; Martins et al. 2016). Therefore, physiotherapists are ideally placed to provide a comprehensive assessment and effective management of patients with TMD.

REFERENCES

Ahmed, N., et al., 2014. Temporomandibular joint multidisciplinary team clinic. Br. J. Oral Maxillofac. Surg. 52, 827–830.

Ayub, E., et al., 1984. Head posture: a case study of the effects on the rest position of the mandible. J. Orthop. Sports Phys. Ther. 5, 179–183.

Beddis, H.P., et al., 2014. Temporomandibular disorders, trismus and malignancy: development of a checklist to improve patient safety. Br. Dent. J. 217, 351–355.

Beltran-Alacreu, H., et al., 2014. Intra-rater and inter-rater reliability of mandibular range of motion measures considering a neutral craniocervical position. J. Phys. Ther. Sci. 26, 915–920.

Bogduk, N., 1994. Cervical causes of headache and dizziness. In: Boyling, J.D., Palastanga, N. (Eds.), Grieve's modern manual therapy, second ed. Churchill Livingstone, Edinburgh, p. 317.

Bogduk, N., Bartsch, T., 2008. Cervicogenic headache. In: Silberstein, S.D., et al. (Eds.), Wolff's headache, eighth ed. Oxford University Press, New York, pp. 551–570.

Bogduk, N., Govind, J., 2009. Cervicogenic headache: an assessment of the evidence on clinical diagnosis, invasive tests, and treatment. Lancet Neurol. 8, 959–968.

Chaput, E., et al., 2012. The diagnostic validity of clinical tests in temporomandibular internal derangement: a systematic review and meta-analysis. Physiother. Can. 64, 116–134.

Cleland, J., Palmer, J., 2004. Effectiveness of manual physical therapy, therapeutic exercise, and patient education on bilateral disc

displacement without reduction of the temporomandibular joint: a single case design. J. Orthop. Sports Phys. Ther. 34, 535–548.

Cowgill, H., 2014. Physiotherapy management of temporomandibular disorders. In Touch 146, 18–23.

Darling, D.W., et al. 1987 Relationship of head posture and the rest position of the mandible. Tenth International Congress of the World Confederation for Physical Therapy 203–206.

de Wijer, A., Steenks, M.H., 2009. Clinical examination of the orofacial region in patients with headache. In: Cesar Fernandez-de-las-Penas, C., et al. (Eds.), Tension-type and cervicogenic headache – physiology, diagnosis, and management. Jones & Bartlett, Sudbury, MA, pp. 197–206.

de Wijer, A., et al., 1995. Reliability of clinical findings in temporomandibular disorders. J. Orofac. Pain 9, 181–191.

Dimitroulis, G., 1998. Temporomandibular disorders: a clinical update. Br. Med. J. 317, 190–194.

Dworkin, S.F., et al., 1990. Assessing clinical signs of temporomandibular disorders: reliability of clinical examiners. J. Prosthet. Dent. 63, 574–579.

Feinstein, B., et al., 1954. Experiments on pain referred from deep somatic tissues. J. Bone Joint Surg. Am. 36A, 981–997.

Greenhalgh, S., Selfe, J., 2010. Red flags II: a guide to identifying serious pathology of the spine. Elsevier, Edinburgh.

Guo, C., et al., 2009. Arthrocentesis and lavage for treating temporomandibular joint disorders. Cochrane Database Syst. Rev. (4), CD004973.

Hengeveld, E., Banks, K., 2014. Maitland's peripheral manipulation, fifth ed. Elsevier, Churchill Livingstone.

Hotta, T.H., et al., 1997. Involvement of dental occlusion and trigeminal neuralgia: a clinical report. J. Prosthet. Dent. 77, 343–345.

Hylander, W.L., 1979. An experimental analysis of temporomandibular joint reaction forces in macaques. Am. J. Phys. Anthropol. 51, 433.

Julsvoll, E.H., et al., 2016. Validation of clinical tests for patients with long-standing painful temporomandibular disorders with anterior disc displacement with reduction. Man. Ther. 21, 109–119.

Kerry, R., 2013. Examination of the temporomandibular region. In: Petty, N.J. (Ed.), Neuromusculoskeletal examination and assessment. Churchill Livingstone, Edinburgh, pp. 169–187.

Kerry, R., Taylor, A.J., 2006. Cervical arterial dysfunction assessment and manual therapy. Man. Ther. 11, 243–253.

Kerry, R., Taylor, A.J., 2008. Arterial pathology and cervicocranial pain – differential diagnosis for manual therapists and medical practitioners. Int. Musculoskelet. Med. 30, 70–77.

Kerry, R., Taylor, A.J., 2009. Cervical arterial dysfunction: knowledge and reasoning for manual physical therapists. J. Orthop. Sports Phys. Ther. 39, 378–387.

Kraus, S.L., 1994. Physical therapy management of TMD. In: Kraus, S.L. (Ed.), Temporomandibular disorders, second ed. Churchill Livingstone, Edinburgh.

Kraus, S., 2014. Characteristics of 511 patients with temporomandibular disorders referred to physical therapy. Oral Surg. Oral Med. Oral Pathol. Oral Radiol. 118, 432–439.

Lyons, M.F., 2008. Current practice in the management of temporomandibular disorders. Dent. Update 35, 314–318.

Magee, D.J., 2014. Orthopedic physical assessment, sixth ed. W.B. Saunders, Philadelphia.

Mansilla-Ferragut, P., et al., 2009. Immediate effects of atlanto-occipital joint manipulation on active mouth opening and pressure pain sensitivity in women with mechanical neck pain. J. Manipulative Physiol. Ther. 32, 101–106.

Martins, W.R., et al., 2016. Efficacy of musculoskeletal manual approach in the treatment of temporomandibular disorder: a systematic review with meta-analysis. Man. Ther. 21, 10–17.

McNeely, M.L., et al., 2006. A systematic review of the effectiveness of physical therapy interventions for temporomandibular disorders. Phys. Ther. 86, 710–725.

Medlicott, M.S., Harris, S.R., 2006. A systematic review of the effectiveness of exercise, manual therapy, electrotherapy, relaxation training, and biofeedback in the management of temporomandibular disorders. Phys. Ther. 86, 955–973.

Okeson, J.P., 2013. Management of temporomandibular disorders and occlusion, seventh ed. Elsevier, St Louis, MO.

Pertes, R.A., Gross, S.G., 1995. Clinical management of temporomandibular disorders and orofacial pain. Quintessence, Chicago.

Petty, N.J., Barnard, K., 2017. Principles of musculoskeletal treatment and management: a handbook for therapists, third ed. Elsevier, Edinburgh.

Rocabado, M., 1983. Biomechanical relationship of the cranial, cervical and hyoid regions. Cranio. 1, 62–66.

Rocabado, M., 2004. A university student with chronic facial pain. In: Jones, M.A., Rivett, D.A. (Eds.), Clinical reasoning in manual therapy. Butterworth Heinemann, Edinburgh, pp. 243–260.

Rocabado, M., Iglarsh, A., 1991. Musculoskeletal approach to maxillofacial pain. J.B. Lippincott, Philadelphia, PA.

Schiffman, E.L., et al., 1990. The prevalence and treatment needs of subjects with temporomandibular disorders. J. Am. Dent. Assoc. 1, 295–303.

Schiffman, E., et al., 2014. Diagnostic criteria for temporomandibular disorders (DC/TMD): for clinical and research applications: recommendations of the international RDC/TMD consortium network and orofacial pain special interest group. J. Oral Facial Pain Headache 28, 6–27.

Shin, B.C., et al., 2007. Effectiveness of combining manual therapy and acupuncture on temporomandibular dysfunction: a retrospective study. Am. J. Chin. Med. 35, 203–208.

Taylor, A.J., Kerry, R., 2010. A 'systems based' approach to risk assessment of the cervical spine prior to manual therapy. Int. J. Osteopath. Med. 13, 85–93.

Walker, N., et al., 2000. Discriminant validity of temporomandibular joint range of motion measurements obtained with a ruler. J. Orthop. Sports Phys. Ther. 30, 484–492.

Wright, E.F., North, S.L., 2009. Management and treatment of temporomandibular disorders: a clinical perspective. J. Man. Manip. Ther. 17, 27–54.

6

EXAMINATION OF THE UPPER CERVICAL REGION

GAIL FORRESTER-GALE

CHAPTER CONTENTS

INTRODUCTION

The occiput, atlas (C1), axis (C2) and the surrounding soft tissues are collectively referred to as the craniocervical spine (CCS). It is an anatomically and biomechanically unique region and the most mobile area of the spine. There are no intervertebral discs between the occiput and C1 or between C1 and C2. The C1 vertebra lacks a spinous process; it resembles a bony ring and is often referred to as a 'washer' between the occiput and C2 (Bogduk 2002). C2 has a vertical bony growth called the odontoid peg, which provides stability and facilitates mobility. Together with C3 these vertebrae form a unique complex of joints, referred to as:

- C0–C1: the atlantooccipital joint (A-O joint)
- C1–C2: the atlantoaxial joint (A-A joint)
- C2–3 facet joints.

The A-O joint is a bicondyloid joint with long, thin congruent joint surfaces oriented in an anterior–posterior direction. This arrangement facilitates movements in the sagittal plane of upper cervical flexion and extension, also referred to as retraction and protraction, which resemble a head-on-neck nodding movement (Bogduk & Mercer 2000; Amiri et al. 2003; Chancey et al. 2007). The A-A segment consists of three joints: a central pivot joint between the odontoid peg and the osseoligamentous ring, which is formed by the transverse ligament and the anterior arch of the atlas, and two biconvex, horizontally oriented facet joints bilaterally. This triad of articulations facilitates rotation, which is the largest movement in the CCS and indeed in the entire spine, with approximately 38–56° rotation occurring to each side (Ishii et al. 2004; Salem et al. 2013) (Fig. 6.1). Owing to the configuration of the occipitoatlantoaxial joint surfaces, movements of rotation and side flexion are not pure; they are coupled. Rotation in the upper cervical spine (UCS) is consistently coupled with contralateral side flexion (Salem et al. 2013).

CCS stability is provided through a combination of mechanical restraint from the ligamentous system and sensorimotor control from the neuromuscular system. The principal ligaments providing stability in this region are generally recognized as the transverse ligament (Fig. 6.2A) and the alar ligaments, with a number of other ligaments including the tectorial membrane acting as secondary stabilizers (Krakenes et al. 2001; Brolin & Halldin 2004; Krakenes & Kaale 2006; Tubbs et al. 2007; Osmotherly et al. 2013a) (Fig. 6.2B).

Key muscle groups acting directly on the CCS and providing dynamic stability and proprioception are the craniocervical flexor (CCF) muscle group

anteriorly (Fig. 6.3A) and the suboccipital muscle (SOM) group posteriorly (Fig. 6.3B) (McPartland & Brodeur 1999; Falla 2004; Schomacher & Falla 2013).

The head, upper cervical spine and neck are innervated by the first 4 cervical spinal nerves. Nerve roots

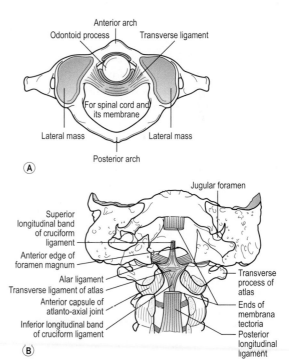

FIG. 6.2 ■ (A) The transverse ligament. (B) The alar ligaments and tectorial membrane. *(From McCarthy 2010, with permission.)*

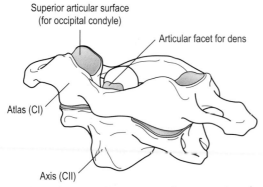

FIG. 6.1 ■ The atlantooccipital and atlantoaxial joints. *(From McCarthy 2010, with permission.)*

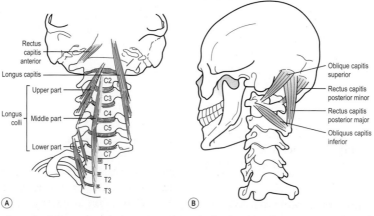

FIG. 6.3 ■ (A) The craniocervical flexor muscle group craniocervical spine muscle group. (B) The suboccipital muscle group. *(From McCarthy 2010, with permission.)*

emerge at each level from C0-C1 downwards and divide into dorsal and ventral branches called rami. The cervical plexus is formed by the anterior rami of C1-C4 and innervates the skin and somatic structures of the anterolateral neck region, occipital, auricular and lateral mastoid regions (see Fig. 6.4). The dorsal rami of the C1-C4 spinal nerves innervate the skin and somatic structures of the posterior cranio-cervical spine (see Figure 6.24).

Upper cervical spinal nerve roots and peripheral nerve trunks can be a source of pain in the head, neck and face. Referral patterns will be dermatomal in the case of nerve root disorders or within the cutaneous field of innervation in the case of peripheral neuropathy (see Fig. 3.16).

Blood is supplied to the brain and brainstem by the internal carotid arteries (ICAs) and vertebral arteries (VAs) communicating via the circle of Willis (Fig. 6.5). The ICAs and the VAs are innervated by the internal carotid plexus and the vertebral nerve respectively. These nerves communicate with the trigeminocervical nucleus and the cervical plexus

(Johnson, 2004). The VAs have a close relationship to the upper cervical vertebrae which means that they are subjected to stretch and deformity on movements of the cervical spine, particularly rotation and extension (Thomas et al. 2015). As a result, the ICAs and the VAs can be a source of pain and symptoms in the upper cervical region due to either damage to the arteries themselves or due to a reduction in blood flow through the arteries to the brain or brainstem. (Taylor & Kerry 2010).

Symptoms Associated with the CCS

The CCS is a common source of symptoms such as head, neck and facial pain, dizziness and nausea. These symptoms may arise due to dysfunction in musculoskeletal structures of the upper three cervical segments; however, due to the close proximity of the UCS to the brainstem, spinal cord and VAs, these structures must also be considered in the differential diagnosis of upper cervical disorders. Symptoms arising from the CCS may have an insidious onset (e.g. primary headache), they may be the result of trauma (e.g. whiplash)

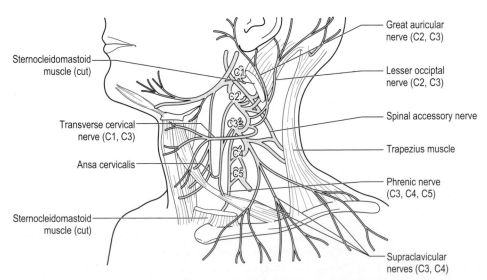

FIG. 6.4 ■ The cervical plexus is composed of the ventral rami of the first four cervical spinal nerves (C1–C4). It innervates the anterolateral upper neck, occipital, auricular and lateral mastoid regions. *(Modified from Netter 2006, with permission.)*

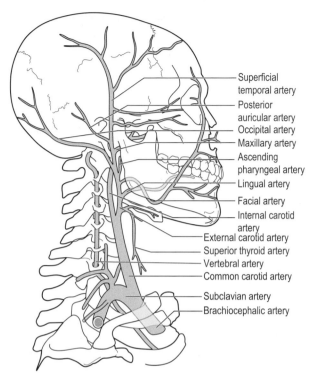

FIG. 6.5 ■ The cervical arterial system. *(From McCance et al., with permission.)*

Labels (from figure):
Superficial temporal artery
Posterior auricular artery
Occipital artery
Maxillary artery
Ascending pharyngeal artery
Lingual artery
Facial artery
Internal carotid artery
External carotid artery
Superior thyroid artery
Vertebral artery
Common carotid artery
Subclavian artery
Brachiocephalic artery

or a specific condition (e.g. rheumatoid arthritis [RA]) or they may be the result of a more serious disorder (e.g. cervical arterial dysfunction [CAD]). Referral of symptoms from the UCS into the head and face is common. The mechanism of referral is thought to be through convergence of afferent fibres from the upper three cervical segments with afferent fibres from the trigeminocervical nerve (cranial nerve V) in the trigeminocervical nucleus (TCN) in the brainstem (Van Griensven 2005; Bogduk & Bartsch 2008; Bogduk & Govind 2009). For further information about referred pain, see Chapter 2.

Headache

Headache is a common disorder, affecting up to 66% of the population (Stovener et al. 2007). The International Headache Society (2013) has identified 14 different headache classifications. Each classification is further subdivided, giving a total of more than 200 different types of headache. Headaches are broadly classified into primary headaches such as migraine and tension-type headache and secondary headaches which are those arising secondary to another disorder, for example, headaches associated with vascular disorders or cervical spine dysfunction. Dysfunction of any innervated somatic structure within the upper three cervical segments, for example the upper cervical facet joints, may refer pain into the head via the proposed convergence theory (see Chapter 2 for more information about referred pain) and this is termed a cervicogenic headache (CGH). There is evidence that physiotherapy can be effective in the management of CGH (Nillson et al. 1997; Jull et al. 2002; Bronfort et al. 2004; Bogduk & Govind 2009). It is important then that the clinician can differentially diagnose between headache types and can also identify headaches that are red flags (Sjaastad et al. 1998; Landtblom et al. 2002; Hall et al. 2008b) (see Table 6.1 and Box 6.1).

For further information regarding the classification of headaches, see the International Headache Society (2013). For further information about differential diagnosis, assessment and management of CGH, see Hall et al. (2008b), Jull et al. (2008b) and Bogduk and Govind (2009).

Cervical Arterial Dysfunction

CAD refers to a range of pathophysiological disorders affecting the cervical arterial system (the VAs and the ICAs), such as arterial stenosis, dissection, thrombus and embolus formation and arterial spasm. These disorders may compromise blood flow to the brain and result in symptomatic ischaemia of the brain and/or brainstem, ranging from minor dysfunctions, due to transient loss of blood flow to specific areas of the brain, to actual ischaemic events, for example, transient ischaemic attack or stroke (Taylor & Kerry 2010, 2015). Intrinsic factors such as atherosclerotic-related changes to the arterial walls, hypertension, vessel hypoplasia and a genetic predisposition along with extrinsic factors, such as trauma, including manipulative therapy or an infection, have been suggested as some of the causative factors in the development of CAD (Thomas 2016). The VA and ICA are most

	Cervicogenic Headache	Migraine	Tension-Type Headache
Onset	Usually starts in the neck or occipital region and radiates forwards	Usually starts in the head and radiates backwards	Starts in the head
Location	Occipital to frontoparietal and orbital	Frontal, periorbital, temporal	Diffuse
Lateralization	Unilateral without side shift	Mostly unilateral with side shift	Diffuse bilateral
Frequency	Chronic, episodic	1–4 per month	Episodic. 1–30 per month
Severity	Moderate to severe	Moderate to severe	Mild to moderate
Duration	1 hour to weeks	4–72 hours	Days to weeks
Pain characteristics	Non-throbbing, non-lancinating	Throbbing, pulsating	Dull, pressing, tightening
Triggers	Neck movement, sustained, awkward head postures	Multiple. Neck movement not typical	Multiple. Neck movement not typical
Associated signs and symptoms	Limited range of neck motion. Tender on palpation over the upper three cervical spinal segments on symptomatic side. Craniocervical flexor weakness. May have nausea, photophobia but milder than migraine	Nausea, vomiting, visual changes, photophobia, phonophobia	No nausea or vomiting. May have photophobia or phonophobia

TABLE 6.1
Differential Diagnosis of Headache (Adapted From Haldeman & Dagenais 2001; Antonaci et al. 2006; Zito et al. 2006; Jull et al. 2008b)

BOX 6.1
HEADACHE RED FLAGS
(HALL et al. 2008b)

- Sudden onset of new severe headache
- A worsening pattern of a pre-existing headache in the absence of obvious predisposing factors
- Headache associated with fever, neck stiffness, skin rash, and with a history of cancer, human immuno-deficiency virus, or other systemic illness
- Headache associated with focal neurological signs other than typical aura
- Moderate or severe headache triggered by cough, exertion or bearing down
- New onset of a headache during or following pregnancy
- N.B.: Patients with one or more red flags should be referred for an immediate medical consultation and further investigation

commonly affected by trauma and/or pathological changes in the UCS (Thomas 2016). For further information see p. 177.

Upper Cervical Instability (UCI)

The close proximity of the CCS to vital structures such as the spinal cord, brainstem and VAs means that excessive movement across the occipitoatlantoaxial complex due to a loss of osseoligamentous integrity caused by pathology or damage to the alar or transverse ligaments, tectorial membrane or odontoid peg can result in spinal cord compression and possible occlusion of the VAs on extreme rotation (Nguyen et al. 2004; Kerry & Taylor 2006; Maak et al. 2006). This can manifest in a wide range of signs and symptoms (see Table 6.4, p. 180) (Osmotherly 2015). UCI is not a common disorder; the populations most affected are those who have sustained major head and neck trauma (e.g. whiplash), patients with RA and patients with congenital disorders such as Down's syndrome (Catrysse et al. 1997; Krakenes et al. 2002, 2003a, b; Nguyen et al. 2004; Dullerud et al. 2010). For further information see p. 178.

SUBJECTIVE EXAMINATION

Details of standard questions asked during the subjective examination can be found in Chapter 2. More specific subjective questioning related to the CCS is described below. The order can be altered as appropriate for the patient being examined and recorded on a subjective examination chart (see Fig. 2.8).

The Patient's Perspective

The therapeutic relationship between the patient and the clinician is important and can impact on treatment outcome (Hall et al. 2010c; Pinto et al. 2012). In order to develop a good rapport with the patient it is helpful to gain an understanding of the patient and his social context at the beginning of the assessment. Asking some of the more straightforward questions from the social history early on, for example, questions about the patient's age, preferred name, whether he is currently working, what he does and if he has any hobbies can help the clinician to build a picture of the patient as an individual and to shift the emphasis away from a problem-focused assessment to a more patient-centred assessment.

Pain is a complex, multidimensional phenomenon (Loeser & Treede 2008). How a person responds to pain largely depends on how that individual's brain interprets it and this will be related to his thoughts, beliefs, emotions and social context (Linton & Shaw 2011). In order to understand fully a patient's disorder and how it affects him as an individual, the clinician needs to explore his psychosocial status. Social history relevant to the onset and progression of the patient's problem, to include information about the patient's employment, home situation and details of any leisure activities, needs to be ascertained. In addition the patient's thoughts, beliefs, emotions and expectations in relation to his disorder need to be explored. The presence of certain psychosocial factors or yellow flags, such as catastrophization, fear avoidance behaviour, stress, anxiety and depression are linked to the transition from acute to chronic pain (Landers et al. 2008; Christensen & Knardahl 2012). These factors are known to increase the pain experienced, affect response to treatment and delay recovery (Linton & Shaw 2011). They are termed yellow flags and are considered to be psychosocial risk factors for chronicity or barriers to recovery. In order to treat the patient appropriately, it is important that yellow flags are identified as early as possible and addressed (Nicholas et al. 2011). This can be done through a series of screening questions and relevant screening questionnaires, e.g. for patients with CGH, the Headache Disability Index Questionnaire and the Headache Disability Questionnaire (Jacobson et al. 1994; Niere & Quin 2009) can provide an indication of the level of disability experienced by the patient and can help identify any personal or environmental factors that may present as a barrier to recovery (see Appendices 6.1 and 6.2). Box 6.2 shows a useful starting point for screening yellow flags in patients with CCS disorders; there are many more yellow-flag questions that can be asked to explore the patient's psychosocial status, and the reader is referred to Waddell (2004).

Body Chart

The following information concerning the area and type of current symptoms can be recorded on a body chart (see Fig. 2.3).

Area of Current Symptoms

The area and type of the patient's symptoms need to be carefully mapped out. Typically, patients with UCS disorders have neck pain high up around the occiput

---

BOX 6.2
YELLOW FLAG SCREENING USING THE MNEMONIC ICE

Using ICE, the clinician may ask the following types of question to establish patients' attitudes and beliefs about their condition

Impression	What do you think is the cause of your pain?
Concerns	Are you worried about anything in relation to your condition?
	Are you worried about anything to do with your home or work life in relation to your condition?
Expectations	What are you expecting will help you?
	Do you think you will return to work? When?
	Do you think physiotherapy will help you?
Additional questions that might be helpful	Have you had time off work in the past with your pain?
	How is your employer/coworkers/family responding to your pain?
	What are you doing to cope with your pain?

and pain over the head and/or face. Patients with CGH usually present with a unilateral, side-consistent headache (Bogduk & Govind 2009).

It is also important to ask about the presence of other symptoms such as disequilibrium, dizziness and altered sensation. Patients with CGH may have associated nausea, photophobia, dizziness and blurred vision but since these are also symptoms of CAD, which can present as a headache in the early stages, careful screening of the risk factors for CAD and the signs and symptoms of brainstem ischemia needs to be carried out (see section on CAD, p. 177). If the patient describes symptoms suggestive of CAD the clinician proceeds with a thorough assessment for potential neurovascular pathology (Kerry & Taylor 2006; Rushton et al. 2014).

If there is more than one area or set of symptoms, the clinician determines which is the worst area or symptom and asks the patient where he feels the symptoms are coming from. Well-localized pain usually suggests a peripheral nociceptive pain mechanism with its origin in upper cervical somatic tissues, e.g. upper cervical joints, muscles, ligaments. Widespread, long-standing pain patterns with no clear anatomical relationship may suggest a more centrally sensitized pain mechanism (Smart & Doody 2010) (see Box 2.2 for the characteristics of pain mechanisms).

Areas Relevant to the Region Being Examined

Check for symptoms in all other related areas, e.g. the lower cervical spine, thoracic spine, head and temporomandibular joint (TMJ), as these may be relevant to the patient's main symptom. Mark unaffected areas with ticks (✓) on the body chart.

Quality of Pain

Establish the quality of the pain. Headaches of cervical origin are often described by the patient as a moderate to severe, non-throbbing pain, which usually starts in the upper neck area and radiates into the head. Migraine headaches are often described as a moderate to severe, throbbing or pulsating pain and tension-type headaches are referred to as a mild, dull, tightening or pressure-type pain (Jull et al. 2008b).

Intensity of Pain

The intensity of pain can be measured using, for example, a visual analogue scale, as shown in Fig. 2.5C. A pain diary may be useful for patients with chronic neck pain or headaches, in order to determine the pain patterns and triggering factors, which may be unusual or complex. Pain intensity, along with other factors such as the presence of night pain, analgesic use, ability to carry out activities of daily living and to continue with work or hobbies, can help to establish the severity of a patient's condition. An understanding of this can help guide the vigour of the physical examination (see Chapter 2 for further information about severity). Pain intensity can also be used as a subjective marker to help judge the effectiveness of treatments for pain.

Abnormal Sensation

Check for any altered sensation locally over the cervical spine and head, as well as the face and upper limbs. Common abnormalities are paraesthesia and numbness. Try to link any areas of altered sensation to upper cervical dermatomes or to the cutaneous field of innervation of upper cervical peripheral nerves (see Fig. 3.15). The presence of altered sensation will also help to determine whether the patient's symptoms are driven by a peripheral neuropathic mechanism (see Box 2.2 for characteristics of pain mechanisms).

The patient may report symptoms of allodynia and secondary hyperalgesia over the face or scalp. These are commonly associated with central sensitization (Smart et al. 2012a) (see Box 2.2).

Constant or Intermittent Symptoms

Ascertain the frequency of the symptoms, and whether they are constant or intermittent. If symptoms are constant, check whether there is variation in the intensity of the symptoms. Constant, unremitting pain may be indicative of malignant disease or other serious pathology. Knowledge of headache frequency may help to diagnose the type of headache differentially (Bogduk & Govind 2009).

Relationship of Symptoms

Determine the relationship between the symptomatic areas – do the symptoms come on together or separately? For example, if the patient has a headache, does he also have neck pain? If so, does one pain start first? Do they both come on together or do they come on independently? Patients with CGH usually complain of a headache that starts in the suboccipital region and radiates forward into the head, face and/or eye (Hall et al. 2008b; Jull et al. 2008b; Bogduk & Govind 2009).

Behaviour of Symptoms

Information about the behaviour of the patient's symptoms allows the clinician to estimate the irritability of the patient's disorder, to determine how easy it will be to reproduce the patient's symptoms during the physical examination and to ascertain whether a full or limited examination needs to be carried out. With an irritable disorder symptoms are brought on quickly after certain positions or movements and take a long time to settle down afterwards. Conversely, patients with a non-irritable condition can tolerate a reasonable amount of movement or sustained positioning before symptoms are reproduced and when they are reproduced they settle down quickly once the movement/position is stopped (Maitland et al. 2005).

- If the patient's symptoms are severe and/or irritable the clinician will aim to limit the content of the physical examination to include only the tests that will help to establish a diagnosis or help with management. The included tests need to be prioritized and examined as far as possible within a symptom-free range or to the point of symptom production/increase of symptoms (P1). Overpressure is not indicated.
- If the patient has constant, severe and/or irritable symptoms, then the clinician will aim to find physical tests that ease the symptoms.
- If the patient's symptoms are non-severe and non-irritable, then the clinician aims to find physical tests that reproduce each of the patient's symptoms. A full examination may be carried out and physical tests and movements can be explored into the painful range.

Symptom behaviour can help to establish the main pain mechanism driving the patient's disorder. Peripheral nociceptive and neuropathic disorders often have clear, consistent, predictable aggravating and easing factors that are related to the involved tissues. Conversely, centrally sensitized conditions usually have unpredictable, inconsistent, unclear aggravating and easing factors that do not relate to a peripheral tissue. Peripheral nociceptive disorders are often less irritable than peripheral neuropathic or centrally sensitized disorders (Smart & Doody 2010; Smart et al. 2012a, b, c) (see Box 2.2 for characteristics of different pain mechanisms).

Symptom behaviour can also give the clinician insight into the possible structure at fault and treatment prognosis; for example, aggravating factors for a peripheral neuropathic disorder may involve movements or positions that load or compress neural tissue. Symptoms that are readily eased may respond more quickly to treatment.

Aggravating Factors

For each symptomatic area, discover what movements and/or positions aggravate the patient's symptoms and how long it takes to bring the symptoms on (or make them worse). Is the patient able to maintain this position or movement? What happens to other symptoms when this symptom is produced (or made worse)? How long does it take for symptoms to ease once the position or movement is stopped? These questions help to confirm the relationship between the symptoms and the irritability of the condition.

The clinician can also ask the patient about theoretically known aggravating factors for structures that could be a source of the symptoms. For example, repeated or sustained neck movements (e.g. rotation) or sustained, awkward head postures (e.g. chin poke position) may be a precipitating factor in CGH (Gadotti et al. 2008). Headaches can also be brought on with eye strain, noise, excessive eating, drinking, smoking, stress or inadequate ventilation.

The clinician may need to ask questions about aggravating factors for other body regions if they are implicated; for example, decreased thoracic mobility has been linked to neck pain (Cleland et al. 2005; Gonzalez-Iglesias et al. 2009; Walser et al. 2009; Lau et al. 2011; Casanova-Méndez et al. 2014).

It is helpful to establish whether the patient is left- or right-handed and which is their dominant eye. Both factors may alter the stresses placed on UCS structures. It is also helpful to ascertain how the symptoms affect the patient's function; for example, what are the symptoms like during static and active postures involving the UCS, e.g. sitting, driving, reading, computer work, watching TV, sport and social activities? The most notable functional restrictions are highlighted with asterisks (*), explored in the physical examination, reassessed at subsequent treatment sessions to evaluate treatment intervention and may be used in the development of treatment goals and advice given.

Easing Factors

For each symptomatic area, the clinician asks what movements and/or positions ease the patient's symptoms, how long it takes to ease them and what happens to other symptoms when this symptom is relieved. These questions help to confirm the relationship between the symptoms and the irritability of the condition.

The clinician can ask the patient about theoretically known easing factors for structures that could be a source of the symptoms. For example, supporting the head or neck may ease symptoms from the UCS. The clinician can analyse the position or movement that eases the symptoms to help determine the structure at fault and to guide treatment selection.

Twenty-Four-Hour Behaviour of Symptoms

The 24-hour pattern of a patient's condition may help to establish whether the patient has a peripheral nociceptive mechanical, inflammatory, ischaemic or degenerative condition. Inflammatory and degenerative disorders commonly have diurnal patterns that are worse in the morning, easier with gentle movement and worsen again in the evening and at night. Ischaemic disorders commonly worsen towards the end of the day or after a prolonged period of sustained activities or posture. Mechanical disorders do not normally have diurnal patterns, they are activity dependent, often related to specific movements or postures.

The clinician determines the pattern of the symptoms first thing in the morning, through the day, at the end of the day and during the night. See Chapter 2 for a full list of questions that can be asked. For the UCS the following questions are of particular interest.

Night Symptoms

- What is your normal sleeping position? Do you sleep on your front?

- What is your present sleeping position?
- How many and what type of pillows do you use? Is your mattress firm or soft?
- Do your symptoms wake you at night? If so, which symptoms?
- How many times in a night/week?
- Can you get back to sleep, how long does it take and what do you have to do?

Morning and Evening Symptoms

- Do you have any stiffness in the morning? How long does it last for? Stiffness in the morning for the first twenty minutes or so might suggest a degenerative disorder such as cervical spondylosis at C2–C3 (this is the only level in the UCS with an intervertebral disc); stiffness and pain for a few hours in the morning may indicate an inflammatory process such as RA, which commonly involves the UCS (Nguyen et al. 2004).

Stage of the Condition

In order to determine the stage of the condition, the clinician asks whether the symptoms are getting better, getting worse or remaining unchanged. This helps the clinician to determine the patient's prognosis. A resolving condition generally has a better prognosis than a worsening one.

Conditions may also be referred to as acute if they are less than 6 weeks in duration, subacute if they are between 6 and 12 weeks in duration and chronic or persistent if they are over 12 weeks in duration.

Special Questions and Red-Flag Screening

The clinician must differentiate between conditions in the UCS that are suitable for conservative management and those that may have a systemic, neoplastic or non-musculoskeletal origin that would require onward referral. Chapter 2 provides full details of general screening questions used to identify any precautions or absolute contraindications to the physical exam and/or treatment. Red flags are physical risk factors indicating the possible presence of serious spinal pathology (Greenhalgh & Selfe 2009). The aim of red-flag screening is to exclude serious or life-threatening pathology in the UCS, such as cranial tumours, spinal metastases, cord compression, spinal infection, inflammatory arthritis and subarachnoid haemorrhage which would require referral to a medical practitioner (Rubio-Ochoa et al. 2016). See Table 6.2 for general red-flag screening relevant to the cervical spine.

For further information about serious spinal conditions that may masquerade as musculoskeletal disorders, see Greenhalgh and Selfe (2009).

In addition to more generalized red-flag screening, specific special questions relevant to the CCS must always be asked. Screening for carotid or VA dysfunction and UCI is routinely carried out (see Tables 6.3 and 6.4, p. 179 & 180).

Cervical Arterial Dysfunction

The close proximity of the cervical arteries to the cervical vertebrae means that movements of the UCS, particularly rotation and extension, can affect blood flow through the cervical arteries and the cervical arteries themselves (Thomas 2016). With an intact circle of Willis and good collateral flow, this is generally not problematic as the body can compensate for changes in flow without incident. However, manual therapy techniques and exercises directed at the UCS could have an adverse effect in patients who have abnormal cervical vessels or in whom collateral flow is inadequate. This could contribute to an 'at-risk' patient having a haemodynamic event as a result of physiotherapy treatment. Early signs and symptoms of CAD can mimic musculoskeletal dysfunction of the UCS (Kerry & Taylor 2006; Bogduk & Govind 2009). In the pre-ischaemic stage CAD can present as pain in the UCS and head (Fig. 6.6).

If the pathology develops, signs and symptoms of brain ischaemia may present (Table 6.3). Although CAD is a rare occurrence, care needs to be taken to differentiate vascular sources of pain from musculoskeletal sources, with the key aim being to avoid any catastrophic neurovascular event (Bogduk & Govind 2009; Thomas 2016).

Current evidence suggests that the most appropriate way to identify the presence of altered

---

TABLE 6.2
General Red-Flag Screening for the Cervical Spine (Greenhalgh & Selfe 2009)

Red Flags

Age of onset 20–55 years	Violent trauma
Constant progressive pain	Systemic steroids
Unremitting night pain	Drug abuse/human immunodeficiency virus
Weight loss	Systemically unwell
Widespread neurology	Past medical history of cancer
Thoracic pain	Structural deformity

Signs and Symptoms of Serious Spinal Pathology in the Cervical Spine

Spinal Cancer	*Cord Compression*	*Spinal Fracture*
■ Age > 50 ■ Previous history of cancer ■ Unexplained weight loss > 5–10% of body weight ■ Failure of > 1 month of conservative treatment	■ Clumsiness of extremities – difficulty with fine motor skills of hands ■ Stumbling gait ■ L'Hermitte's sign ■ Unilateral or bilateral paraesthesias or anaesthesias ■ Bowel or bladder dysfunction	■ Age > 50 ■ History of trauma ■ History of osteoporosis ■ History of systemic steroid use
Cluster of all four red flags provides a very high index of suspicion of spinal cancer with a diagnostic accuracy of sensitivity 1.0 + specificity 0.6		

TABLE 6.3		
Risk Factors, Signs and Symptoms of Cervical Artery Dysfunction (Kerry & Taylor 2010; Rushton et al. 2014; Taylor & Kerry 2015; Thomas 2016)		
	Pre-ischaemic	Ischaemic
Internal carotid artery cervical arterial dysfunction	Neck/temporal/ parietal/frontal pain. Horner's syndrome, pulsatile tinnitus, cranial nerve palsies (CN IX–XII)	Transient ischaemic attack, retinal infarction, stroke
Vertebral artery cervical arterial dysfunction	Acute/recent onset of unusual ipsilateral posterior neck pain or occipital headache	5 Ds: dizziness, diplopia, dysarthria, dysphagia, drop attacks 3 Ns: facial numbness, nystagmus, nausea
Risk factors for cervical arterial dysfunction	■ Recent exposure to minor trauma ■ Recent infection or viral illness ■ Atherosclerosis risk factors ■ Hypertension ■ Hypercholesterolaemia ■ Cardiac disease, vascular disease or history of cerebrovascular accident or transient ischaemic attack ■ Diabetes mellitus ■ Oral contraceptives ■ Long-term use of steroids ■ Smoking ■ Upper cervical instability	

cervical haemodynamics or to predict the risk of a physiotherapy-induced neurovascular event is by careful assessment of the whole vascular system, checking the patient's general cardiovascular health and screening for signs and symptoms associated with CAD (Rushton et al. 2014; Thomas 2016). These are listed in Table 6.3 and can be used by the clinician as a basis for screening questions for CAD.

Many patients present with treatable craniocervical musculoskeletal symptoms, such as neck pain, CGH and cervicogenic dizziness, but also with many of the risk factors identified in Table 6.3. This does not necessarily exclude them from manual therapy treatment. Careful clinical reasoning and monitoring of signs and symptoms are required in the management of these patients (Taylor & Kerry 2010). If frank vascular pathology is identified, however, urgent medical investigation is indicated.

Upper Cervical Instability

UCI can present initially as head and/or neck pain and decreased range of UCS motion due to muscle guarding. With more advanced UCI the patient may present with a myriad of signs and symptoms related to cord compression or cervical artery compromise (Table 6.4) (Forrester & McCarthy 2010; Osmotherly 2015). Identification of UCI, however, is not always easy as symptoms vary so widely and some patients may even be asymptomatic despite marked instability. Currently

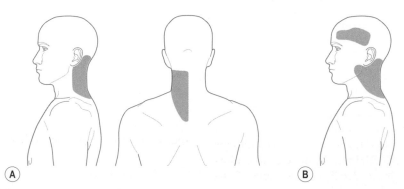

FIG. 6.6 ■ (A) Typical pain presentation for vertebral artery dissection. (B) Typical pain presentation for internal carotid artery dissection. *(From McCarthy 2010, with permission.)*

TABLE 6.4

Risk Factors and Clinical Presentation of Upper Cervical Instability (UCI)
(Forrester & McCarthy 2010; Osmotherly 2015)

Risk Factors for UCI	Early Presentations of UCI	Neurological Signs and Symptoms
▪ History of trauma (e.g. whiplash, rugby neck injury) ▪ Congenital collagenous compromise (e.g. syndromes such as Down's, Ehlers–Danlos, Grisel, Morquio) ▪ Inflammatory arthritis, e.g, rheumatic arthritis, ankylosing spondylitis ▪ Recent neck/head/dental surgery.	▪ Upper cervical or occipital pain ▪ Extreme neck stiffness (muscle guarding) ▪ Anxiety ▪ Poor muscular control ▪ Excessive need for external support for neck (e.g. hands/collar) ▪ Worsening and unpredictability of symptoms ▪ Reports of neck catching/giving way/feeling unstable ▪ Reports of repeated/self-manipulation ▪ Headache ▪ Feeling of lump in throat ▪ Nausea/vomiting ▪ Loss of cervical lordosis	▪ Bilateral or quadrilateral limb paraesthesias ▪ Loss of dexterity ▪ Altered bowel or bladder control ▪ Hyperreflexia ▪ Tinnitus ▪ Occipital numbness/paraesthesia ▪ Paraesthesia of the lips on neck movements ▪ Dizziness ▪ Metallic taste in mouth (CN IX) ▪ Facial pain/paraesthesia ▪ Nystagmus on head or neck moment ▪ Persistent, painfree torticollis ▪ Lingual deviation (CN XII) ▪ Ataxia ▪ L'Hermitte's sign ▪ Clumsy gait

CN, cranial nerve.

there is no set cluster of signs or symptoms predictive of UCI, which means that the clinician will need to be alert and screen for many of the signs and symptoms presented in Table 6.4 in order to establish whether the patient is presenting with UCI. Urgent medical referral is made, if instability is suspected.

Family History

The clinician establishes whether the patient has a family history of RA, atherosclerosis, high blood pressure, myocardial infarction, peripheral vascular disease or cancer, as this may indicate a predisposition to these disorders which may be relevant in the pathogenesis of UCS conditions such as CAD, UCI and headache of malignant origin.

History of the Present Condition

A detailed section on general questions asked in the history of the present condition can be found in Chapter 2. Specific questions related to conditions involving the UCS eg. CGH may be directed to exploring the history in more detail. For example, if the patient complains of a slow, insidious onset of headaches, the clinician determines whether there have

been any factors that precipitated the onset, such as trauma, stress, surgery or occupation. Exploring any changes in the patient's lifestyle, e.g. a new job, hobby or a change in sporting activity, might also help to explain the onset or increase in the patient's symptoms. Detailed questioning about headache history might reveal patterns of presentation that can help to differentially diagnose the type of headache the patient is presenting with, e.g. has the patient had previous headaches? When were they? How many episodes? How often? What was the duration of each episode? Did the patient fully recover between episodes? Similarly, for patients who have had headaches before, establishing if they have received previous treatment, what the treatment was and what the outcomes were can help with differential diagnosis and the development of a management plan.

If there have been no previous attacks, has the patient had any episodes of stiffness in the cervical spine, thoracic spine or any other relevant region?

Past Medical History

The following information is obtained from the patient, past treatment records and/or medical notes:

- any relevant medical history involving the cervical spine and related areas
- a history of trauma or recurrent minor trauma
- the patient's general health status.

Plan of the Physical Examination

When all this information has been collected, the subjective examination is complete. It is useful at this stage to highlight with asterisks (*), for ease of reference, important findings and particularly one or more functional restrictions. These can then be reexamined at subsequent treatment sessions to evaluate treatment intervention.

Information from the subjective examination is used to help the clinician plan an appropriate physical examination (see Fig. 2.9). Clinical reasoning forms can help to guide clinicians through the clinical reasoning process (see Fig. 2.10).

Firstly the clinician needs to decide whether the presenting condition is a musculoskeletal disorder that is suitable for physiotherapy management. Patients with suspected CAD, UCI or headaches that are not believed to be cervicogenic in origin will need to be appropriately referred on for management by other healthcare practitioners.

If the patient presents with a condition that is believed to be musculoskeletal in origin and amenable to physiotherapy management the clinician can use the following questions to organize information collected from the subjective examination to formulate an appropriate physical examination (Gifford & Butler 1997).

- What is the main pain mechanism driving the patient's pain (e.g. peripheral nociceptive, peripheral neuropathic, central sensitization)? This information can help with physical examination planning and the development of management strategies.
- What are the tissue mechanisms in operation in relation to the healing process and the pain mechanisms (e.g. inflammatory, mechanical, ischaemic, degenerative)?
- What are the two or three most likely hypotheses for the source of symptoms? What are the structures or tissues thought to be producing the patient's symptoms? These may include

structures underlying the symptomatic area as well as structures referring into that area. This information can help to plan the physical examination.

- What is the severity and irritability of the patient's condition? This information can help guide the vigour and content of the physical exam.
- Are there any contributing factors to the development and maintenance of the problem? There may be environmental, psychosocial, behavioural, physical or heredity factors. This information can help with physical examination planning, selection of advice provided and the development of management strategies.
- Are there any precautions or contraindications that may affect the physical examination or treatment? This includes the severity and irritability of the patient's symptoms and the nature of the patient's condition – for example, CAD, neurological involvement, recent fracture, trauma, steroid therapy or RA? There may also be certain contraindications to further examination and treatment, e.g. symptoms of cord compression.
- What are the patient's perspectives, preferences and goals? These may be related to their function: abilities and restrictions. Establishing the patients views and priorities can help develop a patient rapport and improve adherence to a management plan.
- What is the patient's prognosis? This can be estimated by considering factors such as the stage and extent of the injury or disorder as well as the patient's expectations, psychological status and lifestyle.

The physical examination plan will include regions and structures that *must* be examined; *should* be examined and *could* be examined in the context of the patient's severity, irritability and any existing precautions or contraindications. For example, some of the tests that *must* be carried out for a patient with a CGH with a potential peripheral nociceptive source of symptoms include examination of upper cervical posture, movements, upper cervical joints and muscle groups. Tests that *should* be carried out include lower cervical posture, movements and cervical muscle strength. Tests that *could* be carried out include scapular position, thoracic spine posture and movements.

Other factors to consider include:

▪ Will it be easy or hard to reproduce the patient's symptoms?
▪ Will additional tests, for example, combined movements and repetitive movements, be necessary to reproduce the patient's symptoms?

Often it is not possible to examine the patient fully at the first attendance and so examination is prioritized over subsequent treatment sessions.

PHYSICAL EXAMINATION

An outline examination chart may be useful for some clinicians and one is suggested in Fig. 2.8. It is important, however, that clinicians do not examine in a rigid manner. Each patient presents differently and this should be reflected in the examination process. The tests and order of testing described below will not be appropriate or relevant to every patient with an UCS disorder. Selected tests need to be matched to the hypotheses generated, severity and irritability. For example, if a peripheral neuropathic pain is suspected a neurological examination will need to be included.

Each significant physical test that either provokes or eases the patient's symptoms is highlighted in the patient's notes by an asterisk (*) for easy reference. The highlighted tests are often referred to as 'asterisks' or 'objective markers'.

Observation

Observation of the patient in dynamic and static situations starts from the moment the clinician begins the subjective examination and continues to the end of the physical examination. Observation can be carried out informally or formally; both are informative. Chapter 3 provides further information about informal observation.

Formal Observation

Observation of Posture. The clinician examines unsupported spinal posture in sitting and standing, particularly noting the head-on-neck posture and observing if the UCS is held in a side-flexed, rotated

or protracted position. The position of the chin in relation to the midline can be used to establish if the head is held in a side-flexed position (Fig. 6.7A). The position of the nose in relation to the midline can be used to establish if the head is held in a rotated position (Fig. 6.7B) and from the side the clinician can establish if the head is held in a forward head position (Fig. 6.7C).

Postural dysfunction rarely influences one region of the body in isolation. It is usually necessary to observe the patient's posture more fully. The position of the lower cervical spine, thoracic spine and scapula should also be examined owing to the close relationship of these regions to the UCS (Ha et al. 2011) (see further information on postural analysis in Chapter 3). A specific abnormal posture relevant to the UCS is the shoulder-crossed syndrome (Janda 2002), which is described in Chapter 3.

Additionally, lumbopelvic posture in unsupported sitting can be observed. A poor lumbopelvic position, which is either too slumped or too extended, can have a direct influence on thoracic and cervical curves as well as on scapular position and cervical muscle function (Jull et al. 2008c). It is useful to assess whether the patient can maintain a neutral spine position in sitting and to determine what affect this has on the patient's symptoms (Fig. 6.8).

There is considerable difference in posture between individuals. It is important for the clinician to establish which postural changes are relevant to the patient's disorder. This can be achieved by passive correction of any observed postural asymmetry and noting any change in the patient's symptoms. See Chapter 3 for further information about postural observation.

Observation of Muscle Form. The clinician observes the muscle bulk and muscle tone of the craniocervical and axioscapular muscles; for example, sternocleidomastoid (SCM), levator scapulae, upper fibres of trapezius and the scalenes, comparing left and right sides. It must be remembered that handedness, level and frequency of physical activity may produce differences in muscle bulk between sides. Some muscles are thought to shorten under stress, e.g. levator scapulae and SCM, whilst other muscles weaken, e.g. CCF, producing muscle imbalance (see Table 3.5). Patterns of muscle imbalance may partly be the cause of postural

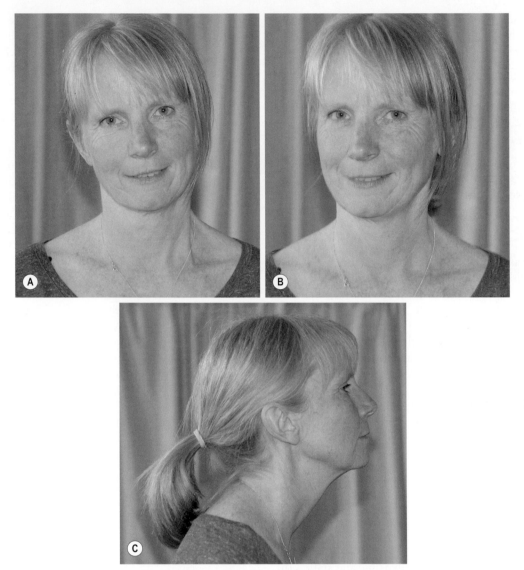

FIG. 6.7 ■ (A) Upper cervical spine held in slight side flexion; note chin swing away from midline. (B) Upper cervical spine held in rotation; note position of nose rotated away from midline. (C) Forward head position, commonly seen in patients with neck pain and headaches. *(From Jull et al. 2008b.)*

changes, for example, the shoulder-crossed syndrome, as well as pain and other symptoms.

Observation of Soft Tissues. The clinician observes the colour of the patient's skin and notes any areas of swelling over the cervical spine or related areas. Skin creases may indicate areas of increased mobility,

whereas soft-tissue thickenings may indicate areas of hypomobility.

Active Physiological Movements

Analysis of upper cervical motion and associated pain response is recognized as an important part of the

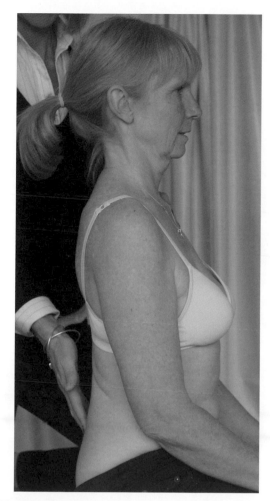

FIG. 6.8 ◼ Neutral spine position. Sacral 'tilt' facilitates normal lumbar lordosis, sternal 'lift' facilitates normal thoracic kyphosis and occipital 'slide' facilitates normal cervical lordosis.

assessment process (Luedtke et al. 2016). Patients with neck pain and headaches often have decreased upper cervical range of motion (Zito et al. 2006; Jull et al. 2007; Ernst et al. 2015). Problematic movements can be identified, which can help to confirm an UCS origin to the disorder. Patterns of movement restriction may indicate the involvement of specific tissues, e.g. articular, muscle and neural, and thus guide subsequent tests used in the physical examination (e.g. selection of passive physiological intervertebral movements [PPIVMs]/passive accessory intervertebral movements [PAIVMs] or muscle length tests). Observation of the

eccentric control offered by the CCF and extensors during sagittal-plane movements can help to identify altered motor control strategies. Reluctance to move in certain directions may indicate fear avoidance behaviour.

Active movements of the UCS are usually tested with the patient in sitting and include upper cervical protraction (extension), retraction (flexion), side flexion and rotation (Fig. 6.9). These movements are commonly performed alongside active movement testing of the cervicothoracic spine (see Chapter 7).

The clinician observes:

- the quality and range of movement
- where the movement is occurring:
  - During full flexion can the patient perform a chin nod prior to lower cervical flexion?
  - During full extension can the patient lift the chin up towards the ceiling prior to lower cervical extension?
  - Does the patient return from full cervical extension in a 'chin poke' position, suggesting reliance on SCM, or can the patient tuck the chin in and curl the spine back from extension?
  - During side flexion does the chin swing laterally, indicating that some side flexion has occurred in the UCS, or does the chin stay more or less in the midline, suggesting lower cervical dominance into side flexion with a potentially hypomobile UCS?
  - During rotation is there a natural head-on-neck 'spinning' motion or does the patient 'carry' the head on the UCS, suggesting a more dominant mid-lower cervical spine movement with potential hypomobility at C1–C2?
- behaviour of pain and resistance through the range of movement and at the end of range of movement
- provocation of any muscle spasm.

The clinician establishes the patient's symptoms at rest and on each movement and corrects any movement deviation to determine its relevance to the patient's symptoms. Overpressure is only added when a movement is full-range and painfree in order to establish if active and passive ranges of motion are similar and if

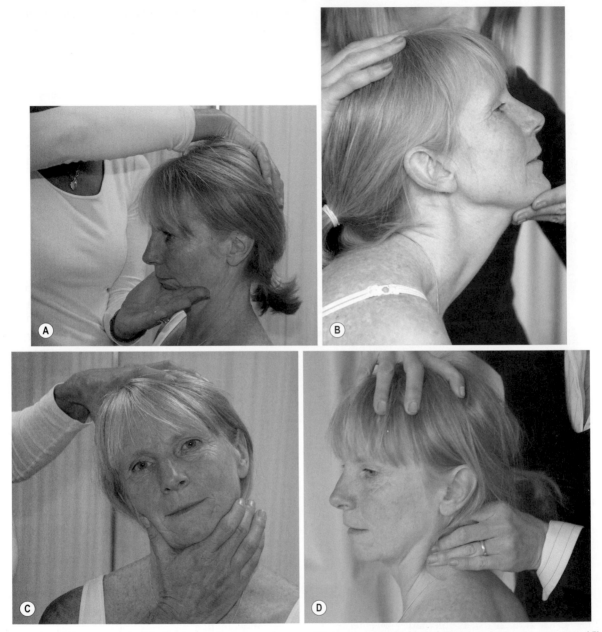

FIG. 6.9 ■ (A) Upper cervical flexion (retraction) + overpressure. (B) Upper cervical extension (protraction) + overpressure. (C) Upper cervical side flexion + overpressure directed towards the opposite shoulder. (D) Upper cervical rotation + overpressure applied through crown of head with C2 stabilized using a pincer grip.

end of range produces pain. Active movement testing can be used as an objective marker.

Additional Testing

If the patient's symptoms are difficult to reproduce on active physiological movement testing or if further movement testing is indicated, many modifications and differentiation tests can be added (see Box 3.4). Movements can be repeated or sustained. Compression or distraction can be added and the UCS quadrant can be tested (Maitland et al. 2005) (Fig. 6.10). Movements can be examined in combination to determine provocative and easing combinations. Table 6.5 and Fig. 6.11 show how upper cervical movements can be combined to apply a stretch to different parts of the joint. This can help confirm structural involvement and guide the selection of the starting position and direction of techniques used for further examination and treatment. For a full account of the combined movement approach see Edwards (1994, 1999) and McCarthy (2010).

Functional movements that reproduce the patient's pain can also be included and differentiated, for example, sitting and working postures, movements of the upper limb and sustained upper cervical rotation.

Differentiation Tests

Numerous differentiation tests can be performed; the choice depends on the patient's signs and symptoms (Maitland et al. 2005) (see Chapter 3). For example, when cervical flexion reproduces the patient's headache in sitting, the addition of slump sitting or knee extension may help to differentiate the structures at fault. Slump sitting or knee extension may increase symptoms if there is a neurodynamic component to the patient's headache. The clinician is constantly aware of the body's attempts to protect hypersensitive neural tissue. For example, a reduction in upper cervical flexion could be due to neural hypersensitivity, not just articular restriction.

Other regions may need to be examined to determine their relevance to the patient's symptoms; they may be the source of the symptoms or a contributing factor. The most likely regions are the TMJ, lower cervical spine and thoracic spine. Studies have demonstrated that movements of upper cervical protraction and retraction involve a 30% contribution from C7–T4 and 10% from T5–T12, suggesting that the thoracic spine and UCS are biomechanically linked (Persson et al. 2007). The joints within these regions can be tested fully (see relevant chapters) or partially with the use of screening tests (see Table 3.4 for further details)

Neurological Testing

A comprehensive neurological examination includes neurological integrity testing, neurodynamic tests and nerve palpation tests. Neurological integrity testing, if

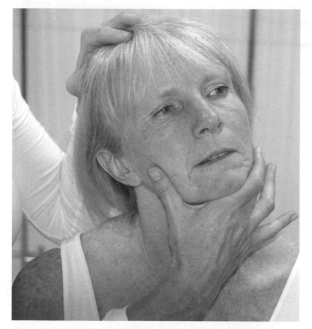

FIG. 6.10 ■ Right upper cervical quadrant. The head is moved into full upper cervical extension, right rotation and right side flexion.

TABLE 6.5		
Combined Physiological Movements in the Craniocervical Spine (Edwards 1994)		
Segmental Level	Anterior Stretch	Posterior Stretch
C0–C1	Extension + contralateral rotation	Flexion + ipsilateral rotation + contralateral side flexion
C1–C2	Rotation + extension + contralateral side flexion	Rotation + flexion + contralateral side flexion

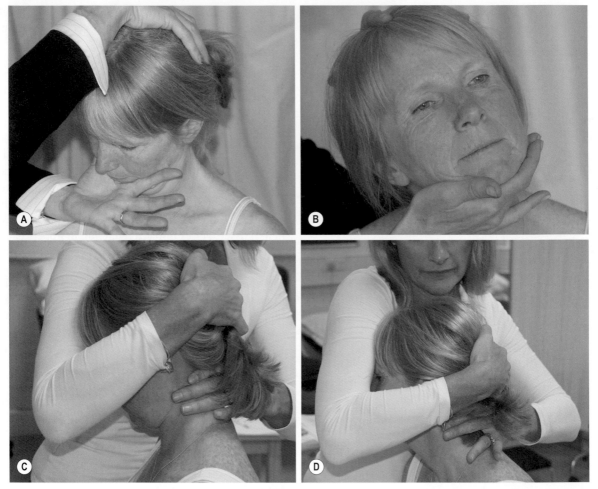

FIG. 6.11 ■ (A) C0–C1 can be examined using a combination of active movements. Upper cervical flexion, a small degree of right rotation and a small degree of left side flexion will increase the stretch on the posterior right C0–C1 capsule. (B) C0–C1 can be examined using a combination of active movements. Upper cervical extension, a small degree of left rotation and a small degree of right side flexion will increase the stretch on the anterior right C0–C1 capsule. (C) C1–C2 can be examined using a combination of active movements. Right rotation and upper cervical flexion will increase the stretch on the posterior right C1–C2 capsule. (D) C1–C2 can be examined using a combination of active movements. Upper cervical right rotation and upper cervical extension will increase the stretch on the posterior right C1–C2 capsule.

indicated, is normally carried out early on in the examination process from a safety perspective. Neurodynamic and nerve palpation testing is usually examined later on.

Integrity of the Nervous System

Generally, if symptoms are localized to the UCS and head, neurological examination can be limited to the cranial nerves and the cervical plexus (C1–C4 nerve roots) (see Table 6.6, p. 187).

Dermatomes/Peripheral Nerves. Light touch and pain sensation of the face, head and neck are tested using cotton wool and pinprick respectively, as described in Chapter 3 and outlined in Table 6.6. Knowledge of dermatomal patterns for the upper

> ## TABLE 6.6
> ### Neurological Conductivity Testing for the Craniocervical Spine

Cranial Nerve Testing

Nerve	Afferent	Efferent	Test
I. Olfactory	Smell		Smell 2–3 familiar items, eyes closed, e,g. coffee/soap/chocolate
II. Optic	Sight		Visual fields: Snellen eye chart
III. Oculomotor		Eye movement: up, down and medial gaze	Patient keeps head still and follows clinician's finger with the eyes. Clinician draws an 'H' shape in front of patient. Then clinician moves finger to patient's nose, to test patient's ability to converge the gaze
IV. Trochlear		Eye movement: down and lateral gaze	
V. Trigeminal	Skin of face	Muscles of mastication	Light touch and pinprick to forehead, cheek and lateral jaw. Clench teeth: clinician palpates masseter and temporalis bilaterally for strength of contraction. Separate jaw: clinician assesses strength of jaw opening against moderate resistance
VI. Abducens		Eye movement: lateral gaze	Tested with H movement test
VII. Facial	Taste anterior aspect of tongue (sweet)	Facial muscles	Patient asked to smile, frown, elevate eyebrows and puff out cheeks
VIII. Vestibulocochlear	Hearing and balance		Hearing: patient's eyes closed, clinician rubs pad of thumb and index finger together next to patient's ear. Determine if the patient can hear it. Test one ear at a time. Hearing should be symmetrical Balance: patient is asked to stand with eyes closed, unsupported for 30 seconds
IX. Glossopharyngeal	Touch and taste posterior tongue (sour)	Gag reflex Ability to swallow	Ask patient to open mouth and say 'ah': watch uvula; it should not deviate laterally. Ability to swallow: ask patient to swallow, watch movement of throat and ask if there are any difficulties
X. Vagus		Muscles of pharynx and larynx	Tested above
XI. Accessory		Sternocleidomastoid and trapezius	Resisted shoulder shrug, check for symmetry and strength and observe for wasting
XII. Hypoglossal		Tongue movement	Patient asked to stick tongue out – should be straight; observe for any side-to-side deviation

Cervical Plexus

Nerve	Afferent (Dermatome)	Efferent (Myotome)
C1		Upper cervical flexion
C2	Skin over posterior aspect of skull	Upper cervical extension
C3	Skin around posterior aspect of neck	Cervical lateral flexion
C4 and CN XI	Skin over shoulder girdle region	Shoulder girdle elevation

CN, cranial nerve.

cervical nerve roots as well as the cutaneous field of innervation of the upper cervical peripheral nerves will enable the clinician to distinguish between any sensory loss due to a nerve root lesion from that due to a peripheral nerve lesion. The UCS cutaneous nerve distribution and dermatomal areas are shown in Fig. 3.16.

Myotomes/Peripheral Nerves. See Table 6.6 and Fig. 3.8 for a description of appropriate myotomal testing in the UCS for the upper cervical and cranial nerves.

Reflex Testing. There are no deep tendon reflexes for C1–C4 nerve roots. The jaw jerk (cranial nerve [CN] V) is elicited by applying a sharp downward tap on the chin with the mouth slightly open. A slight jerk is normal; excessive jerk suggests a bilateral upper motor neuron lesion.

Pathological Reflex Testing for Upper Motor Neuron Lesion

The following reflexes can be tested to check for an upper motor neuron lesion (Fuller 1993). Both of these tests are described in Chapter 3 and are relevant for a CCS neurological examination:

- plantar response
- clonus.

Neurodynamic tests and nerve palpation testing are discussed later in this chapter.

Craniocervical Stability Testing

The tests described below are screening tests designed to identify patients with minor UCI who would be unsuitable for certain manual assessment or treatment techniques in the UCS, such as strong, end-range mobilization or manipulation. However, the diagnostic accuracy of these tests has not been established so it is recommended that they are used in conjunction with findings from the history and physical examination to provide an overall picture of UCS stability and to guide the clinician regarding patient management (Uitvlugt & Indenbaum 1988; Catrysse et al. 1997; Forrester & Barlas 1999; Kaale et al. 2008).

Most of the craniocervical stability tests are provocative and therefore can be potentially harmful. The tests are not indicated for patients with a history of recent head and/or neck trauma; patients with

RA or where subjective indicators of instability are obvious (Table 6.4). Before performing the tests, patients need to be carefully screened for the presence of any gross neurological signs or symptoms indicative of UCI. If any of these are present the clinician should not proceed with the clinical stress tests and the patient should be appropriately referred for a medical opinion (Forrester & McCarthy 2010; Osmotherly 2015).

If there are no cardinal signs and symptoms of UCI on subjective screening, manual testing can proceed; however, care must be taken during the application of the tests. It is recommended that specific further training is undertaken (Pettman 1994).

The following tests are considered positive if excessive movement is evident on testing. It is anticipated that the presence of neurological signs and symptoms will have already been identified in the history and therefore these tests should not provoke any cardinal signs of UCI. If the clinician finds UCI on physical testing or if subjective indicators are suggestive of instability, the patient may require further diagnostic investigations of the UCS (Osmotherly 2015).

Sagittal-Plane Stress Tests

For the following two tests, the forces applied to test the stability across the CCS are directed in an anteroposterior direction (sagittal plane) and are therefore known as sagittal stress tests. They include the Sharp–Purser test and the anterior stress test.

1. **Sharp–Purser test**. (SPT) This test is a relocation test. It assesses the amount of anterior–posterior translation between the atlas and the axis. The transverse ligament and the odontoid peg form an osseoligamentous ring, which provides mechanical stability at this level. If both structures are competent they will prevent the atlas sliding forward on the axis during cervical flexion movements. If there is a loss of integrity in the osseoligamentous ring the atlas will be allowed to slide anteriorly during cervical flexion.
   - For test application, see Fig. 6.12.
   - Test interpretation:
     - A slight posterior gliding movement may be felt when the test is carried out in

cervical flexion due to the natural uptake of the soft tissue; beyond this a hard end feel should be apparent. There should be no posterior gliding movement detected at all when the test is carried out in neutral or upper cervical extension (Forrester & Barlas 1999; Forrester & McCarthy 2010).

◻ The SPT is considered positive, indicating anterior instability of the A-A joint, if there is excessive sliding motion of the head in a posterior direction beyond the normal uptake of the soft tissues when the test is performed in flexion. This will not be the case when the test is repeated in neutral and extension. Excessive movement will be the most common positive finding. Because the SPT is a relocation test, it is suggested that other interpretations of a positive test include symptom modification such as

reduction in the patient's signs and symptoms (pain or central neurological signs and symptoms) brought on by flexion or a 'clunk' sound as the subluxed atlas relocates (Osmotherly 2015).

2. **Anterior shear test**. This is a provocation test that will reproduce any anterior instability at C1–C2 level.
   ■ For test application, see Fig. 6.13.
   ■ Test interpretation:
     ◻ No movement should be detected and no symptoms reproduced if the transverse ligament is competent.
     ◻ A positive test would be indicated by excessive anterior motion of the atlas on the axis, reproduction of cardinal signs of atlanto-axial instability (if the odontoid peg is allowed to migrate into the space occupied by the spinal cord) or a 'lump in the throat' sensation (if the atlas translates anteriorly towards the oesophagus).

Coronal-Plane Stress Tests

For the following tests, the force applied to test the stability of the spine is directed in the coronal plane and they are therefore referred to as coronal stress tests.

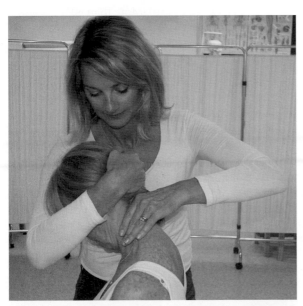

FIG. 6.12 ■ The Sharp–Purser test. Patient in sitting with head and neck flexed. Clinician fixes C2 using a lumbrical grip. The patient's head is cradled by the clinician's opposite arm with the biceps resting on the patient's forehead. A gentle posterior pressure is applied on the patient's forehead through the clinician's biceps and upper arm. This translates the occiput and atlas backwards on a fixed C2. The test is repeated in neutral and extension.

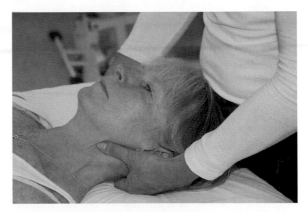

FIG. 6.13 ■ The anterior shear test. Patient supine. Clinician fixes the anterior aspect of C2 transverse processes using the thumbs. Index fingers are placed posteriorly against C1 with remaining fingers supporting the patient's occiput. The clinician applies gentle pressure through the index fingers to the posterior aspect of C1, lifting the head and atlas anteriorly whilst C2 is stabilized.

1. **Side-flexion stress test** for the alar ligaments. The structures limiting lateral flexion are primarily the contralateral alar ligament. This test assesses the integrity of the alar ligaments in side flexion.
   - For test application, see Fig. 6.14.
   - Test interpretation:
     - No movement of the head is possible if the contralateral alar ligament is intact (Forrester & McCarthy 2010).
     - If motion is available in all three positions, the test is considered positive, suggesting an alar tear or arthrotic instability at the C0–C1 joint.

2. **Lateral translation stress test** for the A-A joint. This test assesses the amount of lateral translation of the atlas on the axis. The odontoid peg is the main structure that limits this movement.
   - For test application, see Fig. 6.15.
   - Test interpretation:
     - If the odontoid peg is intact no discernible moment should be detected on application of the test (Forrester & McCarthy 2010).

- Excessive movement or reproduction of the patient's symptoms suggests lateral instability of this joint.

Transverse-Plane Stress Tests

1. **Rotational stress test** for the alar ligament. The key structures that limit rotation are the alar ligaments. This test assesses the integrity of the alar ligaments in rotation. This test is carried out if the previous side-flexion stress test is positive, to determine whether the instability is due to laxity of the alar ligament or to instability at the C0–C1 joint.
   - For test application, see Fig. 6.16.
   - Test interpretation:
     - If the structures limiting craniocervical rotation are intact and C2 is adequately stabilized, rotation of the head will stop between 20 and 40°. A more recent study has suggested that maximum normal range of rotation during this test is 22° (Osmotherly et al. 2013b). More than 40° of rotation indicates a damaged contralateral alar ligament (Krakenes & Kaale 2006).
     - When the excessive rotational motion is in the same direction as the excessive lateral

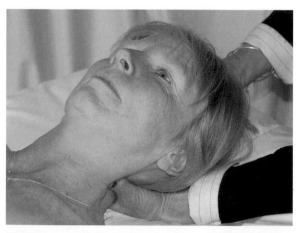

FIG. 6.14 ■ Side-flexion stress test for the alar ligament. Patient supine. Clinician fixes C2 with the left hand using a lumbrical grip; thumb and fingers grip the articular pillars of C2 bilaterally. The right hand grips the crown of the patient's head. Some vertical compression is applied along with a side-flexion movement where the right ear is pushed towards the left side of the neck. The test is repeated in upper cervical flexion and extension.

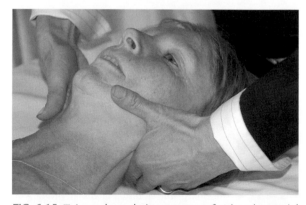

FIG. 6.15 ■ Lateral translation stress test for the atlantoaxial joint. Patient supine. Clinician supports the occiput with fingers 3–5 and using the left index finger makes contact with the left side of C1. The index finger of the right hand is placed over the right side of the C2. A lateral shear from the left to the right of the atlas and occiput on the fixed axis is applied. The test is repeated on the other side.

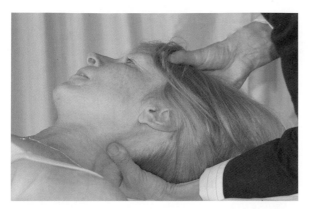

FIG. 6.16 ■ Rotational stress test for the alar ligaments. Patient supine. Clinician fixes C2 with the left hand using a lumbrical grip; thumb and fingers grip the articular pillars of C2 bilaterally. The right hand grips the crown of the patient's head. Some vertical compression is applied along with a right rotation moment. The test is repeated in upper cervical flexion and extension. Hand holds are reversed and the test is performed into left rotation.

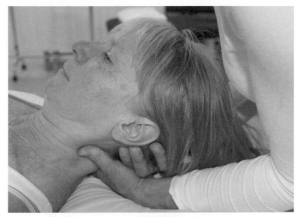

FIG. 6.17 ■ Distraction test for the tectorial membrane. Patient supine. C2 is fixed with the left hand using a lumbrical grip; thumb and fingers grip the articular pillars of C2 bilaterally and apply a slight caudad pressure. The right hand cradles the occiput. The right hand applies a traction and flexion motion to the occiput. The test is repeated in upper cervical flexion and extension.

flexion (from the side-flexion stress test above), this suggests damage to the alar ligament; when the excessive motions are in opposite directions, this suggests arthrotic instability (Pettman 1994).

Distraction Test for the Tectorial Membrane

1. This test assesses the amount of flexion and distraction between the occiput, atlas and axis. The tectorial membrane is the main restraint to this movement.
   ■ For test application, see Fig. 6.17.
   ■ Test interpretation:
     □ Some movement on the application of the distraction movement is normal due to the natural uptake of soft tissues.
     □ The test is considered to be positive in the presence of excessive distraction movement greater than a few millimetres (Pettman 1994; Osmotherly 2015).

Palpation

Palpation of soft tissue, muscle and joint is a useful part of the physical examination as changes in soft tissue and muscle tone can help clinicians to identify the dysfunctional or symptomatic spinal level(s) (see Box 3.5).

With the patient in prone lying the clinician gently palpates the posterior soft tissues in the suboccipital area from the superior nuchal line to the C2–C3 region using the middle three fingers in a circular massage-type motion. This is continued over the articular pillars of C1–C3, from the lateral aspect of the spinous processes to the lateral aspect of the transverse processes (Maitland et al. 2005).

The palpation examination may carry on in the same way into the lower cervical spine, thoracic spine and posterior aspect of the head. The clinician then turns the patient over into supine lying and assesses the anterior soft tissues in a similar manner using the pad of the thumb over the anterior aspect of the mastoid process and the anterolateral aspect of the vertebral bodies from C1–C3 and beyond into the lower cervical spine. Common palpation findings are listed in Box 6.3. It is useful to record palpation findings on a palpation chart (see Fig. 3.35).

Passive Intervertebral Examination

Passive intervertebral examination of the UCS provides information about the amount and quality of physiological or accessory movement available at the individual upper cervical spinal UCS motion segments and any associated pain response. The validity and reliability of passive movements are debatable; however, they continue to be used. It is generally felt that, in conjunction with findings from other physical examination tests, passive movements can assist the clinician in the examination of articular tissue by identifying symptomatic levels, the direction of movement dysfunction and also through mini treatments they can assist with management planning (Luedtke et al. 2016).

Passive Physiological Movements

PPIVMs examine the amount and quality of physiological movement available at each upper cervical spinal level. PPIVMs can be a useful adjunct to PAIVMs to identify segmental hypomobility and hypermobility.

Flexion–Extension PPIVM at C0–C1. For application of technique, see Fig. 6.18A and B.

Side-Flexion PPIVM at C0–C1. For application of technique, see Fig. 6.18C.

Rotation PPIVM at C1–C2. For application of technique, see Fig. 6.18D.

Flexion–Rotation Test. The flexion–rotation test can determine segmental dysfunction at C1–C2 even in the presence of normal active range of movement. Studies have demonstrated that it has very high diagnostic utility (sensitivity = 90% and specificity = 88%) in relation to differentiating CGH of C1–C2 origin from other headache types and it has been shown that therapists can detect these differences reliably (Ogince et al. 2007; Hall et al. 2008a, 2010a, b). Average range of C1–C2 rotation in asymptomatic subjects is between 39° and 42° (Hall & Robinson 2004).

■ For test application, see Fig. 6.19.
■ Test interpretation: the flexion–rotation test is positive if the amount of C1–C2 rotation to the side of pain is less than 32°, although many subjects with CGH often have a range of around 20° towards the symptomatic side (Hall & Robinson 2004).

Accessory Movements

PAIVMs are commonly used in the UCS to gain information about the amount and quality of accessory movement available and the pain response at each upper cervical segmental level (Zito et al. 2006; Jull et al. 2007). PAIVMs can be examined with the patient's UCS in a neutral or combined position and the techniques can be applied with a medial, lateral, cephalad or caudad bias (Maitland et al. 2005). See Box 3.6 for hints on performing accessory movements.

The accessory movements commonly tested at C1–C4 in neutral are:

■ central posteroanterior
■ unilateral posteroanterior
■ unilateral anteroposterior.

On application of the accessory movement being tested, the clinician notes the following during early, mid and late range, taking the patient's severity and irritability into consideration:

■ range and quality of movement
■ resistance through the range and at the end of the range of movement
■ behaviour of pain through the range
■ provocation of any muscle spasm.

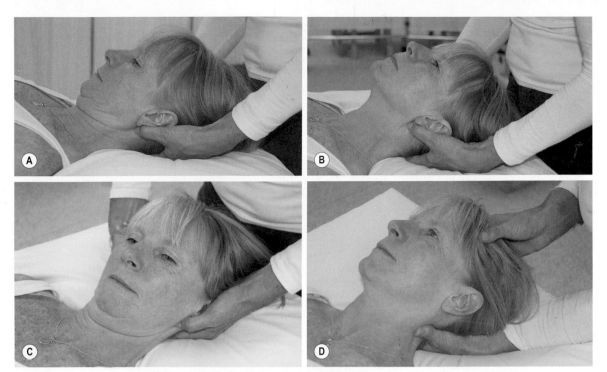

FIG. 6.18 ■ (A, B) Flexion–extension passive physiological intervertebral movement (PPIVM) C0–C1: patient in supine, head on a pillow. Clinician cradles the patient's occiput with fingers 3–5 and palpates between the mastoid process and the lateral aspect of C1 using the tips of the thumbs. Clinician rocks the patient's head forward and backwards in a head-on-neck nodding moment. The small amount of movement between the two bony points on each side is assessed. (C) Side-flexion PPIVM C0–C1: same starting position as for flexion–extension PPIVM. Clinician moves the patient's head into upper cervical side flexion. If the technique is performed correctly, the clinician should see a 'chin swing' to the opposite side of the side flexion being carried out (e.g. left 'chin swing' for right side flexion). The small amount of movement between the two bony points on each side is assessed. (D) Rotation PPIVM C1–C2: patient in supine, head on a pillow. Clinician grips C2 spinous process using a pincer grip with the left hand. The right hand holds the crown of the patient's head. Clinician moves the patient's head into right rotation. The point at which the C2 spinous process is felt to move to the left is assessed. The test is repeated into left rotation. It is usually more accurate to swap hands over. The amount of rotation to both sides is compared.

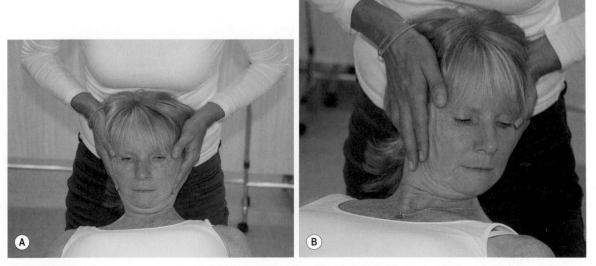

FIG. 6.19 ■ Flexion–rotation test. Patient in supine crook-lying and head extended beyond end of couch. (A) The clinician fully flexes the cervical spine to 'lock up' the subaxial spine and bias rotation to the C1–C2 level. (B) The clinician rotates the patient's head to the right and then to the left. The amount of movement is compared.

See Fig. 6.20. Other cervical levels are shown in Chapter 7.

It is useful to record findings on a palpation chart and/or movement diagrams (see Figs 3.38–3.45). These are explained in detail in Chapter 3.

Accessory Movements as a Combined Technique. Accessory movements can be applied in combined positions in order to increase or decrease the stretch on upper cervical facet joints, joint capsules or surrounding paravertebral muscles. The different combinations can be quite confusing. Table 6.7 shows some possible combinations of starting positions and accessory movements that will increase the stretch on different aspects of the A-O and A-A joints. For a full description of upper cervical accessory movements in combined positions, see Edwards (1994, 1999).

Following accessory movements to the UCS the clinician reassesses all the physical asterisks (movements or tests that have been found to reproduce the patient's symptoms) in order to establish the effect of the accessory movements on the patient's signs and symptoms.

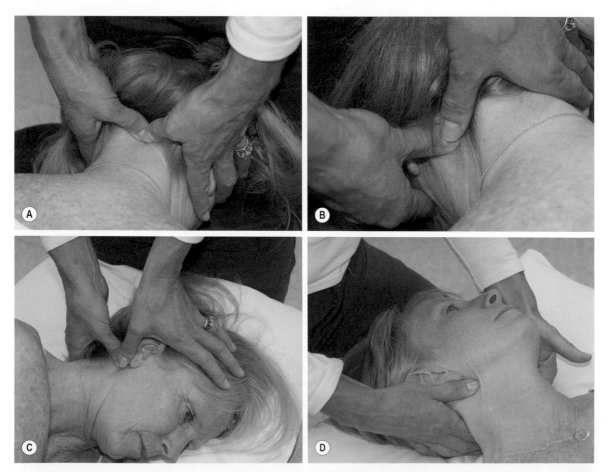

FIG. 6.20 ▪ Accessory movement to C1 (A) Central posterior–anterior accessory movement. Pressure is applied through the thumbs on to the posterior arch of C1, directed cephalady towards the patient's eyes. (B) Unilateral posterior-anterior accessory movement. Thumb pressure is applied laterally over the posterior arch of C1. (C) Transverse pressure. Thumb pressure is applied to the transverse process of C1. (D) Unilateral anteroposterior accessory movement. Thumb pressure is applied over the anterior aspect of C1 transverse process.

<table>
<tr><td colspan="4" align="center">TABLE 6.7</td></tr>
<tr><td colspan="4" align="center">Passive Accessory Intervertebral Movements as a Combined Technique</td></tr>
</table>

Level	Combined Starting Position	Accessory	Effect
Atlantooccipital joint	In prone: flexion + right rotation (nose stays within head hole)	Unilateral posteroanterior right C1	Increase stretch posterior aspect C0–C1
	In supine: extension + left rotation	Unilateral anteroposterior on right C1	Increase stretch anterior aspect C0–C1
Atlantoaxial joint	In prone: right rotation to 30° (nose rotated out of head hole) + flexion	Unilateral posteroanterior on right C2	Increase stretch posterior aspect C1–C2
	In prone: right rotation to 30° (nose rotated out of head hole) + extension	Unilateral posteroanterior on right C2	Increase stretch anterior aspect C1–C2

Passive physiological and accessory movements can then be tested in other regions suspected to be a source of, or contributing to, the symptoms. Regions likely to be examined are the TMJ, lower cervical spine and upper thoracic spine.

Sustained Natural Apophyseal Glides (SNAGs). SNAGs are indicated for peripheral nociceptive, arthrogenic, mechanical disorders. When correctly selected and applied SNAGs should:

- Decrease or relieve the patient's pain immediately
- increase the range of movement
- increase function.

For patients complaining of headaches, Mulligan (2010) describes four examination techniques:

1. headache SNAGs (Fig. 6.21A)
2. reverse headache SNAGs Fig. 6.21B
3. upper cervical traction (Fig. 6.21C)
4. SNAGs for restricted cervical rotation at C1–C2.

For patients with upper cervical neck pain and loss of movement, suggested techniques include:

- SNAG to spinous process of C2–C4 + dysfunctional movement, e.g. rotation
- SNAG to transverse process of C2–C4 + dysfunctional movement.

For a full description of each technique, see Chapter 3 and Mulligan (2010).

Symptom Modification and Mini Treatments

In addition to gathering information throughout the physical examination about pain reproduction, resistance profiles and movement dysfunction, the clinician may decide to perform 'mini treatments' on the symptomatic or dysfunctional spinal segment using carefully reasoned and selected techniques, for example PPIVMs, PAIVMs, natural apophyseal glides (NAGs) and SNAGs, trigger points or hold–relax muscle techniques. Assessing the effect of the mini treatments using selected objective markers can help the clinician to confirm a working hypothesis for the patient's disorder and can also help to determine which treatment may have the biggest impact.

Muscle Testing

Normal muscle function in the CCS requires normal muscle strength, length, control and coordination. In order to 'rule in' or 'rule out' myogenic involvement in a patient's disorder a comprehensive examination of muscle tissue will assess all these functions.

Muscle Strength

Changes in muscle strength, endurance and fatigability have been identified in the cervical flexors, extensors and axioscapular muscles in patients with neck pain and CGH of both insidious and traumatic onset (Jull et al. 1999, 2004, 2008a; Jull, 2000; Falla 2004a; Falla et al. 2004b; O'Leary et al. 2007).

Isotonic Testing. The clinician may want to test the general strength of the cervical muscles isotonically

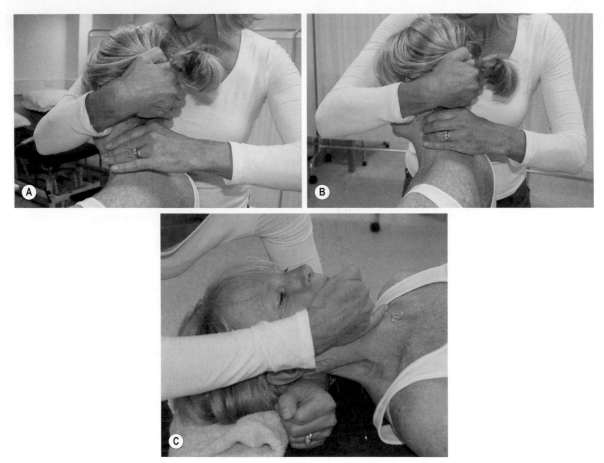

FIG. 6.21 ■ (A) Headache sustained natural apophyseal glide (SNAG). (B) Reverse Headache SNAG. (C) Cervical traction at C1–C2.

whilst observing the quality of muscle contraction and motor recruitment patterns. This can be done in supine or prone with the head in a neutral or rotated position by asking the patient simply to lift the head off the bed. Different starting positions will bias strength testing to different muscle groups. Pillows can be used to make the test easier.

Isometric Testing. This can help to differentiate symptoms from inert structures and contractile structures. The CCS is positioned in neutral and the patient is asked to hold this position against the resistance of the clinician. The clinician can provide resistance to any direction of movement and also in different parts of the range. If symptoms are reproduced on contraction this may suggest a contractile tissue disorder.

For details of these general tests, see Jull et al. (2008c). Testing the strength of these muscles is also described in Chapter 3.

Sensorimotor Control

Sensorimotor control is the integration and coordination of sensory and motor information by the central nervous system in order to regulate joint stability, movement acuity, coordination and balance (Roijezon et al. 2015). Afferent information from the periphery (visual, vestibular and proprioceptive systems) is combined and used to elicit an appropriate motor response from the postural muscles before and during movement (Treleaven 2008).

Clinically, alterations in sensorimotor function in the CCS are associated with lasting pain, loss of movement, dizziness, nausea, visual disturbance, hearing disturbances and loss of postural stability (Jull et al. 2008e; Treleaven 2008).

A growing body of evidence suggests that proprioception and motor control in the cervical spine are altered in response to pain, effusion, trauma and fatigue (Jull 2000; Falla 2004a; Falla et al. 2004a; Jull et al. 2004; Treleaven 2011; de Vries et al. 2015; Roijezone et al. 2015). Changes include:

- increased cervical joint position sense error
- poor oculomotor function
- inhibition of the deep CCF and semispinalis
- increased activation of superficial neck muscles (scalenes, SCM, splenius capitis)
- delayed onset of CCF activation
- decreased strength and endurance capacity of the CCF and deep cervical extensors
- poor balance.

These poor muscle recruitment strategies between groups of muscles and between deep and superficial muscles along with proprioceptive deficits in the cervical region have been shown to be associated with UCS symptoms (O'Leary et al. 2007; Falla et al. 2011; Lindstrom et al. 2011; Schomacher & Falla 2013; Schomacher et al. 2013; de Vries et al. 2015).

Sensorimotor Testing

Sensorimotor deficits can be tested by assessment of the proprioceptive system and motor control. A range of tests can be used, including cervical joint position sense tests, postural stability tests, oculomotor function tests and motor control tests. Assessment of the proprioceptive system is described in Chapter 7. Motor control assessment is described below. For further information, see Jull et al. (2008c), Treleaven (2008), Clark et al. (2015) and Roijezon et al. (2015).

Motor control can be assessed indirectly by:

- observing posture (for example, patients with forward head position are likely to have long, weak CCF)
- noting any changes in muscle recruitment patterns during active movements
- observing the quality of movement and where the movement is occurring
- palpating muscle activity in various positions.

In addition to this, specific muscle testing can be undertaken in the UCS.

Deep Cervical Muscle Testing. The deep cervical muscles (CCF and SOM groups) have been shown to have a high density of muscle spindles, particularly the SOMs. This suggests that, in addition to their role in controlling head-on-neck movements, they play a significant role in craniocervical proprioception (Boyd-Clark et al. 2001, 2002; O'Leary et al. 2009).

Deep Craniocervical Flexors. Assessment of the recruitment and endurance of the deep CCFs (longus colli, longus capitis, rectus capitis anterior and lateralis) is made using the low-load craniocervical flexion test (Jull et al. 2008c, d). A pressure biofeedback unit (PBU: Chattanooga, Australia) is used to measure the function of the deep neck flexors.

- For starting position, see Fig. 6.22.
- The patient is then taught the correct nodding action of upper cervical flexion, as if indicating 'yes'.
    - The patient is instructed to put the tongue on the roof of the mouth, to close the lips but not to clench the jaw. This helps to prevent substitution strategies by other muscle groups.
    - It is important that the head is not lifted or retracted. When the CCFs are weak, the SCM initiates the movement, causing the jaw to lead the movement, and the UCS hyperextends.
- Testing is then undertaken in two stages: because pain inhibits CCF activity, testing should never induce symptoms (Arendt-Nielsen & Falla 2009).
    - Stage 1 – analysis of movement patterning. This is a five-level test whereby the patient attempts to increase the pressure progressively on the PBU in a correct motor strategy. Using visual feedback from the PBU, the patient attempts to hold a nod at 22, 24, 26, 28 and 30 mmHg with a few seconds' rest between each stage. Ideally, subjects are able to progress through all five levels. Observation and palpation for overuse of superficial muscles (SCM, plus the scalene and hyoid groups) are made; these muscles may be active, but not

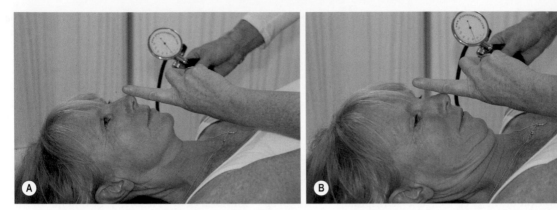

FIG. 6.22 ■ (A, B) Craniocervical flexion test: Patient in supine crook-lying. Folded towel under occiput to ensure the head and neck are in a neutral position. A pressure biofeedback unit is placed under the cervical spine, against the occiput and inflated to 20 mmHg. Patient is asked to perform a head 'nod'. To facilitate the correct movement the patient is asked to slide her nose down her finger.

dominant. A positive test is recorded when a patient is unable to achieve a level without either initiating a retraction movement and/or recruiting superficial flexors as the dominant group. A recording is made of both the level achieved and the quality of movement (Jull et al. 2008c).

■ Stage 2 – holding capacity of deep neck flexors. This stage is only undertaken when training in stage 1 has resulted in normal patterning at all five levels. Beginning at 22 mmHg (2 mmHg above a baseline of 20 mmHg), the patient attempts to hold the test position (nod) for 10 seconds. Ten 10-second repetitions are aimed for at each level. The number of 10-second repetitions is recorded and used as the patient's baseline score. As in stage 1, a positive finding is when there is superficial muscle dominance or retraction of the neck. The clinician also observes the quality of movement, looking for jerky, poor control of the head (Jull et al. 2008c).

Deep Cervical Extensors. Although most clinical and research attention has been focused towards the CCF, the deep extensors also contribute towards sensorimotor control of the head on the neck. Assessment of these muscle groups is therefore justified particularly

for those patients who present with forward head position and neck pain or headaches (Schomacher et al. 2015).

For the first two tests below, the inability to perform a smooth, coordinated movement along with excessive movement in the lower cervical spine is suggestive of poor extension motor control (Jull et al. 2008c):

■ craniocervical extension test (rectus capitis posterior group):
  ■ With the patient in four-point kneeling or prone sitting, the patient performs craniocervical flexion and extension (a head-on-neck 'nodding' movement) whilst maintaining the lower cervical spine in a neutral position. The clinician can palpate this muscle group to assess for activation strategies.
■ craniocervical rotation test (obliquus capitis group):
  ■ With the patient in the same position as above, the patient performs craniocervical rotation (to less than 40°), as if saying 'no' whilst maintaining the lower cervical spine in a neutral position. This muscle group is palpable, allowing the clinician to assess muscle recruitment strategies.
■ deep cervical extensor test (semispinalis cervicis and multifidus muscle groups)

- For test application, see Fig. 6.23.
- This position will bias muscle activity towards semispinalis cervicis, and discourage activity in the superficial semispinalis capitis and splenius capitis.
- If there is good control between the CCF (holding the CCS in neutral) and the deep cervical extensors (producing the movement), the movement should be seen to occur around the cervicothoracic junction rather than at the craniovertebral junction or as a shearing extension movement around C5.

Axioscapular Muscles. Owing to their attachments in the UCS and the occiput, activity of the upper fibres of trapezius, levator scapulae, scalenae group and SCM will influence movement patterns in the UCS. Additionally, scapular positioning and control are associated with cervical dysfunction, specifically following whiplash trauma (Jull et al. 2008c). Therefore assessment of control and patterning of these muscle groups together with scapular control via the middle and

lower fibres of trapezius and serratus muscles should be considered (see Chapter 9 for further details).

Muscle Length

The clinician tests the length of muscles, in particular those thought prone to shortening (Janda 2002); that is, levator scapulae, upper trapezius, SCM, pectoralis major and minor, scalenes and the deep occipital muscles. Testing the length of these muscles is described in Chapter 3 (see Table 3.9 and Fig. 3.13).

Neurodynamic Tests

The following neurodynamic tests may be carried out in order to ascertain the degree to which neural tissue is responsible for the production of the patient's symptom(s) in the UCS:

- passive neck flexion
- upper-limb neurodynamic tests
- straight-leg raise
- slump.

These tests are described in detail in Chapter 3.

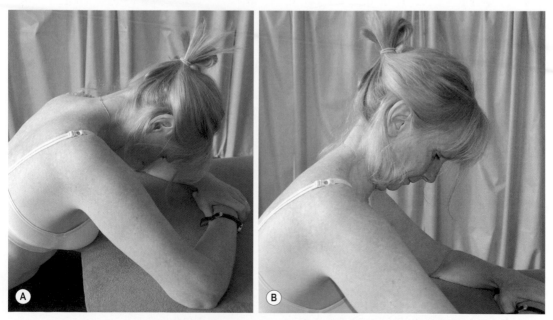

FIG. 6.23 ■ (A, B) Deep cervical extensor test. Patient in prone propped on elbows with craniocervical spine in neutral and lower cervical spine in full flexion. Patient performs extension of the cervical spine, around cervicothoracic junction, returning to a head neutral position whilst maintaining the upper cervical spine in neutral.

Nerve Palpation

Table 6.8 and Fig. 6.24 show the peripheral nerves that can be palpated in the UCS. If the peripheral nerves are involved in the patient's disorder they will be tender to touch and may reproduce the patient's symptoms (see Chapter 3 for further information).

TABLE 6.8		
Nerves That Can Be Palpated in the Craniocervical Spine		
Nerve	**Level**	**Area of Palpation**
Greater occipital nerve	Dorsal ramus of C2	2 cm lateral to midline – a thumb's width out and down from occipital protuberance
Lesser occipital nerve	Ventral ramus of C2	2 cm medial from mastoid process, located in a dip
Third occipital nerve	Dorsal ramus of C3	Over the posterior aspect of C2–C3 facet joint

Cervical Arterial Dysfunction Testing

If vascular dysfunction is suspected following the subjective examination, further information regarding the integrity of the cervical arterial system can be gained from the following examination procedures. Further reading is recommended to support understanding of the following procedures (Kerry & Taylor 2010).

1. Blood pressure. In the event of acute arterial dysfunction, it is likely that there will be a systemic cardiovascular response manifesting in dramatic change in blood pressure (usually increasing). Blood pressure can be taken using appropriate, validated procedures and equipment, in either sitting or lying.
2. Functional positional testing. In recent years there has been a shift of emphasis away from physical testing of the cervical arterial system owing to the poor reported diagnostic accuracy of these tests in detecting incompetent VA or ICA vessels (Rushton et al. 2014). Whilst positional testing is not able to screen for all different types of CAD pathology, current research

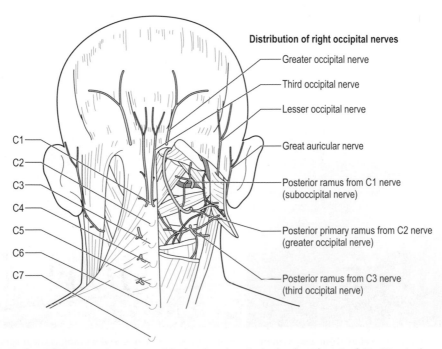

Distribution of right occipital nerves
- Greater occipital nerve
- Third occipital nerve
- Lesser occipital nerve
- Great auricular nerve
- Posterior ramus from C1 nerve (suboccipital nerve)
- Posterior primary ramus from C2 nerve (greater occipital nerve)
- Posterior ramus from C3 nerve (third occipital nerve)

C1
C2
C3
C4
C5
C6
C7

FIG. 6.24 ■ Innervation of the posterior aspect of the head and neck via the dorsal rami of C1–C4 spinal nerves showing location of craniocervical peripheral nerves for palpation. *(Modified from Rubin & Safdieh 2007, with permission.)*

suggests that these tests may still have a role in assessing the compensatory capacity of the cervical arterial system as a whole rather than testing the structure or function of individual arteries (Thomas 2016). The tests may therefore still be used to assess the integrity of the collateral cervical arterial system and brain perfusion during end-range cervical movements with the aim of detecting those patients with insufficient compensatory blood flow who may then go on to suffer from cerebral ischaemic events (Thomas et al. 2015). Findings from positional testing, however, should not be used in isolation to arrive at a diagnosis but considered in conjunction with findings from other aspects of the subjective and physical examination. Classically the positional tests have a minimum requirement of a passive 10-second hold into end-range cervical rotation (Magarey et al. 2004). A positive test is considered if reproduction of symptoms suggestive of hindbrain ischaemia is found (e.g. dizziness, nystagmus). The tests can be repeated in cervical extension or a combination of cervical extension plus rotation.

3. Pulse palpation. The VA pulses are difficult to palpate due to their size and depth. The ICA is easily accessible at the midcervical level, medial to the SCM. Gross pathologies, such as aneurysm formation, are characteristic in the nature of their pulse, that is, a pulsatile, expandable mass. Pain and exaggerated pulse on palpation of the temporal artery may support a hypothesis of temporal arteritis.

4. Cranial-nerve examination. Cranial nerves are peripheral nerves, which mostly arise from the brainstem. Cranial-nerve dysfunction can be a result of cervical arterial compromise; although this is rare, it tends to affect the lower cranial nerves, in particular the hypoglossal nerve (swallowing) (Thomas 2016). Careful screening for gross asymmetries and variations from the norm in cranial nerve function is indicated if CAD is suspected (Kerry & Taylor 2010). Table 6.6 shows a method of cranial nerve assessment.

5. Proprioception tests. Hindbrain ischaemia associated with vertebrobasilar insufficiency can result in gross loss of proprioceptive function. Simple proprioception testing such as tandem gait, heel-to-knee, Romberg's test and Hautant's test is undertaken to assess proprioception dysfunction.

6. Differentiation test. Differentiation between dizziness produced from the vestibular apparatus of the inner ear and that from neck movements due to either cervical vertigo or compromised cervical arteries may be required (Maitland et al. 2005, p. 246).

■ For test application, see Fig. 6.25.
■ Test interpretation:
   ■ The test is considered positive and stopped immediately if dizziness, nausea or any

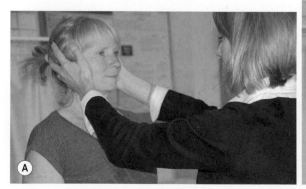 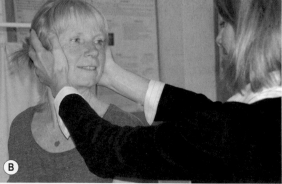

FIG. 6.25 ■ Differential diagnosis of dizziness. (A) In standing, the clinician maintains the patient's head in neutral; this prevents movement within the vestibular system. (B) The patient moves the trunk to the left then to the right in order to produce cervical rotation. Each position is held for 10 seconds, with a 10-second rest period between directions. *(From Magarey et al. 2004.)*

other symptom associated with cervical artery insufficiency is provoked.

■ This test may help to differentiate between vestibular causes of dizziness and cervicogenic or vascular causes; however, it cannot differentiate between vascular (CAD) and cervicogenic causes of dizziness.

■ Test findings therefore need to be considered in conjunction with a number of other tests in order to rule in or rule out CAD. The presence of CAD contraindicates certain treatment techniques to the cervical spine (see Table 2.4).

COMPLETION OF THE EXAMINATION

Having carried out the above tests, the examination of the UCS is now complete. The subjective and physical examinations produce a large amount of information, which needs to be recorded accurately and quickly. It is vital at this stage to highlight with an asterisk (*) important findings from the examination. These findings are reassessed at, and within, subsequent treatment sessions to evaluate the effects of treatment on the patient's condition.

The physical testing procedures that specifically indicate joint, nerve or muscle tissues, as a source of the patient's symptoms, are summarized in Table 3.9.

On completion of the physical examination, the clinician will review and refine hypotheses developed at the end of the subjective examination (see Box 2.1). Following this the clinician will:

1. Evaluate the examination findings, formulate a clinical diagnosis and write up a problem list.
2. Determine the objectives of treatment in collaboration with the patient and devise an initial treatment plan and ongoing management strategy.
3. Explain the findings of the examination to the patient, explore any misconceptions the patient may have regarding the injury or disorder and discuss the prognosis.
4. Warn the patient of possible exacerbation up to 24–48 hours following the examination.
5. Request the patient to report details on the behaviour of the symptoms following examination at the next attendance.

For guidance on treatment and management principles, the reader is directed to the companion textbook (Petty & Barnard 2017).

APPENDIX 6.1 HEADACHE DISABILITY INDEX QUESTIONNAIRE

Patient name: _____   Date _____

INSTRUCTIONS: Please CIRCLE the correct response:

1. I have headache: (1) 1 per month   (2) more than 1 but less than 4 per month   (3) more than 1 per week
2. My headache is: (1) mild   (2) moderate   (3) severe

Please read carefully: the purpose of the scale is to identify difficulties that you may be experiencing because of your headache. Please check off 'YES', 'SOMETIMES', or 'NO' to each item. Answer each question as it pertains to your headache only.

YES	SOMETIMES	NO	
____	____	____	Because of my headaches I feel disabled.
____	____	____	Because of my headaches I feel restricted in performing my routine daily activities.
____	____	____	No one understands the effect my headaches have on my life.
____	____	____	I restrict my recreational activities (e.g. sports, hobbies) because of my headaches.
____	____	____	My headaches make me angry.
____	____	____	Sometimes I feel that I am going to lose control because of my headaches.
____	____	____	Because of my headaches I am less likely to socialize.
____	____	____	My spouse (significant other), or family and friends have no idea what I am going through because of my headaches.
____	____	____	My headaches are so bad that I feel that I am going to go insane.
____	____	____	My outlook on the world is affected by my headaches.
____	____	____	I am afraid to go outside when I feel that a headache is starting.
____	____	____	I feel desperate because of my headaches.
____	____	____	I am concerned that I am paying penalties at work or at home because of my headaches.
____	____	____	My headaches place stress on my relationships with family or friends.
____	____	____	I avoid being around people when I have a headache.
____	____	____	I believe my headaches are making it difficult for me to achieve my goals in life.
____	____	____	I am unable to think clearly because of my headaches.
____	____	____	I get tense (e.g. muscle tension) because of my headaches.
____	____	____	I do not enjoy social gatherings because of my headaches.
____	____	____	I feel irritable because of my headaches.
____	____	____	I avoid travelling because of my headaches.
____	____	____	My headaches make me feel confused.
____	____	____	My headaches make me feel frustrated.
____	____	____	I find it difficult to read because of my headaches.
____	____	____	I find it difficult to focus my attention away from my headaches and on other things.

Instructions: 1. Using this system, if 'YES' is checked on any given line, that answer is given 4 points ... a 'SOMETIMES' answer is given 2 points and a 'NO' answer is given zero. 2. Using this system, a score of 10–28% is considered to constitute mild disability; 30–48% is moderate; 50–68% is severe; 72% or more is complete.

Patient's signature: _____   Date: _____

From Jacobson et al. (1994).

APPENDIX 6.2 HEADACHE DISABILITY QUESTIONNAIRE

Name: _____   Date: _____   Score: _____ /90

Please read each question and circle the response that best applies to you

1. How would you rate the usual pain of your headache on a scale from 0 to 10?

0	1	2	3	4	5	6	7	8	9	10
No pain										Worst pain

2. When you have headaches, how often is the pain severe?

Never	1–9%	10–19%	20–29%	30–39%	40–49%	50–59%	60–69%	70–79%	80–89%	90–100% Always
0	1	2	3	4	5	6	7	8	9	10

1. On how many days in the last month did you actually lie down for an hour or more because of your headaches?

None	1–3	4–6	7–9	10–12	13–15	16–18	19–21	22–24	25–27	28–31 Every day
0	1	2	3	4	5	6	7	8	9	10

2. When you have a headache, how often do you miss work or school for all or part of the day?

Never	1–9%	10–19%	20–29%	30–39%	40–49%	50–59%	60–69%	70–79%	80–89%	90–100% Always
0	1	2	3	4	5	6	7	8	9	10

5. When you have a headache while you work (or are at school), how much is your ability to work reduced?

Not reduced	1–9%	10–19%	20–29%	30–39%	40–49%	50–59%	60–69%	70–79%	80–89%	90–100% Unable to work
0	1	2	3	4	5	6	7	8	9	10

6. How many days in the last month have you been kept from performing housework or chores for at least half of the day because of your headaches?

None	1–3	4–6	7–9	10–12	13–15	16–18	19–21	22–24	25–27	28–31 Every day
0	1	2	3	4	5	6	7	8	9	10

7. When you have a headache, how much is your ability to perform housework or chores reduced?

Not reduced	1–9%	10–19%	20–29%	30–39%	40–49%	50–59%	60–69%	70–79%	80–89%	90–100% Always
0	1	2	3	4	5	6	7	8	9	10

8. How many days in the last month have you been kept from non-work activities (family, social or recreational) because of your headaches?

None	1–3	4–6	7–9	10–12	13–15	16–18	19–21	22–24	25–27	28–31 Every day
0	1	2	3	4	5	6	7	8	9	10

9. When you have a headache, how much is your ability to engage in non-work activities (family, social or recreational) reduced?

Not reduced	1–9%	10–19%	20–29%	30–39%	40–49%	50–59%	60–69%	70–79%	80–89%	90–100% Always
0	1	2	3	4	5	6	7	8	9	10

From Niere and Quin (2009).

REFERENCES

Amiri, M., et al., 2003. Measurement of upper cervical flexion and extension with the 3-space fastrak measurement system: a repeatability study. J. Man. Manip. Ther. 11, 198–203.

Antonaci, F., et al., 2006. Diagnosing cervicogenic headache. J. Headache Pain 7, 145.

Arendt-Nielsen, L., Falla, D., 2009. Motor control adjustments in musculoskeletal pain and the implications for pain recurrence. Pain 142, 171–172.

Bogduk, N., 2002. Biomechanics of the cervical spine. In: Grant, R. (Ed.), Physical therapy of the cervical and thoracic spine, third ed. Churchill Livingstone, New York.

Bogduk, N., Bartsch, T., 2008. Cervicogenic headache. In: Silberstein, S.D., et al. (Eds.), Wolff's headache, eighth ed. Oxford University Press, New York, pp. 551–570.

Bogduk, N., Govind, J., 2009. Cervicogenic headache: an assessment of the evidence on clinical diagnosis, invasive tests, and treatment. Lancet Neurol. 8, 959–968.

Bogduk, N., Mercer, S., 2000. Biomechanics of the cervical spine. I: Normal kinematics. Clin. Biomech. (Bristol, Avon) 15, 633–648.

Boyd Clark, L., et al., 2001. Comparative histochemical composition of muscle fibres in a pre and post-vertebral muscle of the cervical spine. J. Anat. 199, 709–716.

Boyd Clark, L., et al., 2002. Muscle spindle distribution, morphology and density in longus colli and multifidus muscles of the cervical spine. Spine 27, 694–701.

Brolin, K., Halldin, P., 2004. Development of a finite model of the upper cervical spine in a parameter study of ligament characteristics. Spine 29, 376–385.

Bronfort, G., et al., 2004. Non-invasive physical treatments for chronic/recurrent headache. Cochrane Database Syst. Rev. (3), CD001878.

Casanova-Méndez, A., et al., 2014. Comparative short-term effects of two thoracic spinal manipulation techniques in subjects with chronic mechanical neck pain: a randomized controlled trial. Man. Ther. 19, 331–337.

Catrysse, E., et al., 1997. Upper cervical instability: are clinical tests reliable? Man. Ther. 2, 91–97.

Chancey, V., et al., 2007. A kinematic and anthropometric study of the upper cervical spine and the occipital condyles. J. Biomech. 40, 1953–1959.

Christensen, J., Knardahl, S., 2012. Work and headache: a prospective study of psychological, social, and mechanical predictors of headache severity. Pain 153, 2119–2132.

Clark, N., et al., 2015. Proprioception in musculoskeletal rehabilitation. Part 2: clinical assessment and intervention. Man. Ther. 20, 378–387.

Cleland, J., et al., 2005. Immediate effects of thoracic manipulation in patients with neck pain: a randomized clinical trial. Man. Ther. 10, 127–135.

de Vries, J., et al., 2015. Joint position sense error in people with neck pain: A systematic review. Man. Ther. 20, 736e–744.

Dullerud, R., et al., 2010. MRI of ligaments and membranes in the craniovertebral junction in whiplash associated injury and healthy control subjects. Acta Radiol. 51, 207–212.

Edwards, B., 1994. Examination of the high cervical spine (occiput–C2) using combined movements. In: Boyling, J.D., Palastanga, N. (Eds.), Grieve's modern manual therapy, second ed. Churchill Livingstone, Edinburgh.

Edwards, B., 1999. Manual of combined movements: their use in the examination and treatment of mechanical vertebral column disorders, second ed. Butterworth-Heinemann, Oxford.

Ernst, M., et al., 2015. Extension and flexion in the upper cervical spine in neck pain patients. Man. Ther. 20, 547–552.

Falla, D., 2004a. Unravelling the complexity of muscle impairment in chronic neck pain. Man. Ther. 9, 125–133.

Falla, D., et al., 2004b. Feedforward activity of the cervical flexor muscles during voluntary arm movements is delayed in chronic neck pain. Exp. Brain Res. 157, 43–48.

Falla, D., et al., 2011. Association between intensity of pain and impairment in onset and activation of deep cervical flexors in patients with persistent neck pain. Clin. J. Pain 27, 309–314.

Forrester, G., Barlas, P., 1999. Reliability and validity of the Sharp–Purser test in the assessment of atlantoaxial instability in patients with rheumatoid arthritis. Physiotherapy 85, 376.

Forrester, G., McCarthy, C., 2010. Upper cervical spine. In: McCarthy, C. (Ed.), Combined movement theory. Elsevier, London (Chapter 8).

Fuller, G., 1993. Neurological examination made easy. Churchill Livingstone, Edinburgh.

Gadotti, I., et al., 2008. Cervical musculoskeletal impairments in cervicogenic headache: a systematic review and a meta-analysis. Phys. Ther. Rev. 13, 149–166.

Gifford, L., Butler, D., 1997. The integration of pain sciences into clinical practice. J. Hand Ther. 10, 86–95.

Gonzalez-Iglesias, J., et al., 2009. Thoracic spine manipulation on the management of patients with neck pain: a randomized clinical trial. J. Orthop. Sports Phys. Ther. 39, 20–27.

Greenhalgh, S., Selfe, J., 2009. Red flags II: a guide to identifying serious pathology of the spine. Elsevier, Edinburgh.

Haldeman, S., Dagenais, S., 2001. Cervicogenic headaches: a critical review. Spine J. 1, 31–46.

Hall, T., et al., 2008b. Clinical evaluation of cervicogenic headache: a clinical perspective. J. Man. Manip. Ther. 16, 73–80.

Hall, T., et al., 2010a. Reliability of manual examination and frequency of symptomatic cervical motion segment dysfunction in cervicogenic headache. Man. Ther. 15, 542–546.

Hall, T., et al., 2010b. Comparative analysis and diagnostic accuracy of the cervical flexion rotation test. J. Headache Pain 11, 391–397.

Hall, A.M., et al., 2010c. The influence of the therapist–patient relationship on treatment outcome in physical rehabilitation: a systematic review. Phys. Ther. 90, 1099–1110.

Ha, S., et al., 2011. Effects of passive correction of scapular position on pain, proprioception, and range of motion in neck-pain patients with bilateral scapular downward-rotation syndrome. Man. Ther. 16, 585–589.

Hall, T., Robinson, K., 2004. The flexion-rotation test and active cervical mobility: a comparative measurement study in cervicogenic headache. Man. Ther. 9, 197–202.

Hall, T., et al., 2008a. Inter-tester reliability and diagnostic validity of the cervical flexion-rotation test in cervicogenic headache. J. Manipulative Physiol. Ther. 31, 293–300.

International Headache Society, 2013. The international classification of headache disorders, 3rd edn. Cephalalgia 33, 629–808.

Ishii, T., et al., 2004. Kinematics of the cervical spine in rotation in vivo three-dimensional analysis. Spine 29, E139–E144.

Jacobson, G.P., et al., 1994. The Henry Ford Hospital Headache Disability Inventory (HDI). Neurology 44, 837–842.

Janda, V., 2002. Muscles and motor control in cervicogenic disorders. In: Grant, R. (Ed.), Physical therapy of the cervical and thoracic spine, third ed. Churchill Livingstone, New York.

Jull, G., 2000. Deep cervical flexor dysfunction in whiplash. J. Musculoskelet. Pain 8, 143–154.

Jull, G., et al., 2007. Cervical musculoskeletal impairment in frequent intermittent headache. Part 1: subjects with single headaches. Cephalalgia 27, 793–802.

Jull, G., et al., 1999. Further clinical clarification of the muscle dysfunction in cervical headache. Cephalalgia 19, 179–185.

Jull, G., et al., 2004. Impairment in the cervical flexors: a comparison of whiplash and insidious onset neck pain patients. Man. Ther. 9, 89–94.

Jull, G., et al., 2008d. Clinical assessment of the deep cervical muscles: the craniocervical; flexion test. J. Manipulative Physiol. Ther. 31, 525–533.

Jull, G., et al., 2008a. Alterations in cervical muscle function in neck pain. In: Whiplash, headache and neck pain. Research based directions for physical therapists. Churchill Livingstone, Elsevier, Edinburgh (Chapter 4).

Jull, G., et al., 2008b. Cervicogenic headache: differential diagnosis. In: Whiplash, headache and neck pain. Research based directions for physical therapists. Churchill Livingstone, Elsevier, Edinburgh (Chapter 9).

Jull, G., et al., 2008c. Clinical assessment: physical examination of the cervical region. In: Whiplash, headache and neck pain. Research based directions for physical therapists. Churchill Livingstone, Elsevier, Edinburgh (Chapter 12).

Jull, G., et al., 2008e. Disturbances in postural stability, head and eye movement control in cervical disorders. In: Whiplash, headache and neck pain. Research based directions for physical therapists. Churchill Livingstone, Elsevier, Edinburgh (Chapter 6).

Jull, G., et al., 2002. A randomized controlled trial of exercise and manipulative therapy for cervicogenic headache. Spine 27, 1835–1843.

Kaale, B., et al., 2008. Clinical assessment techniques for detecting ligament and membrane injuries in the upper cervical spine region – a comparison with MRI results. Man. Ther. 13, 397–403.

Kerry, R., Taylor, A., 2006. Cervical arterial dysfunction assessment and manual therapy. Man. Ther. 11, 243–253.

Kerry, R., Taylor, A., 2010. Haemodynamics. In: McCarthy, C. (Ed.), Combined movement theory. Elsevier, London (Chapter 6).

Krakenes, J., Kaale, B., 2006. Magnetic resonance imaging assessment of craniovertebral ligaments and membranes after whiplash trauma. Spine 31, 2820–2826.

Krakenes, J., et al., 2002. MRI assessment of the alar ligaments in the late stage of whiplash injury: a study of structural abnormalities and observer agreement. Neuroradiology 38, 44–50.

Krakenes, J., et al., 2003b. MR analysis of the tectorial and posterior antlanto-occipital membranes in the late stage of whiplash injury. Neuroradiology 45, 585–591.

Krakenes, J., et al., 2003a. MR analysis of the transverse ligament in the late stage of whiplash injury. Acta Radiol. 44, 637–644.

Krakenes, J., et al., 2001. MRI assessment of normal ligamentous structures in the craniovertebral junction. Neuroradiology 43, 1089–1097.

Landers, M., et al., 2008. The use of fear-avoidance beliefs and nonorganic signs in predicting prolonged disability in patients with neck pain. Man. Ther. 13, 239–248.

Landtblom, A., et al., 2002. Sudden onset headache: a prospective study of features, incidence and causes. Cephalalgia 22, 354–360.

Lau, H., et al., 2011. The effectiveness of thoracic manipulation on patients with chronic mechanical neck pain – a randomized controlled trial. Man. Ther. 16, 141–147.

Lindstrom, R., et al., 2011. Association between neck muscle coactivation, pain and strength in women with neck pain. Man. Ther. 16, 80–86.

Linton, S., Shaw, W., 2011. Impact of psychological factors in the experience of pain. Phys. Ther. 91, 700–711.

Loeser, J., Treede, R., 2008. The Kyoto protocol of IASP basic pain terminology. Pain 137, 473–477.

Luedtke, K., et al., 2016. International consensus on the most useful physical examination tests used by physiotherapists for patients with headache: a Delphi study. Man. Ther. 23, 17–24.

Maak, T., et al., 2006. Alar, transverse and apical ligament strain due to head-turned rear impact. Spine 31, 632–638.

Magarey, M., et al., 2004. Pre-manipulative testing of the cervical spine review, revision and new clinical guidelines. Man. Ther. 9, 95–108.

Maitland, G., et al., 2005. Maitland's vertebral manipulation, seventh ed. Butterworth-Heinemann, Oxford.

McCarthy, C., 2010. Combined movement theory: rational mobilization and manipulation of the vertebral column. Elsevier, Edinburgh.

McPartland, J., Brodeur, R., 1999. Rectus capitus posterior minor: a small but important suboccipital muscle. J. Bodyw. Mov. Ther. 3, 30–35.

Mulligan, B., 2010. Manual therapy 'Nags', 'Snags', 'MWMs' etc., sixth ed. Orthopaedic Physical Therapy Products, New Zealand.

Netter, F.H., 2006. Atlas of human anatomy, fourth ed. Elsevier, Philadelphia.

Nguyen, H., et al., 2004. Rheumatoid arthritis of the cervical spine. Spine J. 4, 329–334.

Nicholas, M., et al., 2011. Early identification and management of psychological risk factors ('yellow flags') in patients with low back pain: a reappraisal. Phys. Ther. 91, 737–753.

Niere, K., Quin, A., 2009. Development of a headache-specific disability questionnaire for patients attending physiotherapy. Man. Ther. 14, 45–51.

Nillson, N., et al., 1997. The effect of spinal manipulation in the treatment of cervicogenic headache. J. Manipulative Physiol. Ther. 2, 326–330.

Ogince, M., et al., 2007. The diagnostic validity of the cervical flexion-rotation test in C1/2-related cervicogenic headache. Man. Ther. 12, 256–262.

O'Leary, S., et al., 2009. Muscle dysfunction in cervical spine pain: implications for assessment and management. J. Orthop. Sports Phys. Ther. 39, 324–333.

O'Leary, S., et al., 2007. Cranio-cervical flexor muscle impairment at maximal, moderate, and low loads is a feature of neck pain. Man. Ther. 12, 34–39.

Osmotherly, P., 2015. Pre-manipulative screening for craniocervical ligament integrity. In: Jull, G., et al. (Eds.), Grieve's modern musculoskeletal physiotherapy, fourth ed. Elsevier, Edinburgh (Chapter 35.3).

Osmotherly, P., et al., 2013a. Revisiting the clinical anatomy of the alar ligaments. Eur. Spine J. 22, 6–64.

Osmotherly, P., et al., 2013b. Towards understanding normal craniocervical rotation occurring during the rotation stress test for the alar ligaments. Phys. Ther. 93, 986–992.

Persson, P., et al., 2007. Associated sagittal spinal movements in performance of head pro- and retraction in healthy women: a kinematic analysis. Man. Ther. 12, 119–125.

Pettman, E., 1994. Stress tests of the craniovertebral joints. In: Boyling Palastanga, N. (Ed.), Grieve's modern manual therapy, second ed. Churchill Livingstone, Edinburgh.

Petty, N.J., Barnard, K., 2017. Principles of musculoskeletal treatment and management: a handbook for therapists, third ed. Elsevier, Edinburgh.

Pinto, R., et al., 2012. Patient-centred communication is associated with positive therapeutic alliance: a systematic review. J. Physiother. 58, 77–87.

Roijezon, U., et al., 2015. Proprioception in musculoskeletal rehabilitation. Part 1: Basic science and principles of assessment and clinical interventions. Man. Ther. 20, 368–377.

Rubin, M., Safdieh, J.E., 2007. Netter's concise neuroanatomy. Saunders, Philadelphia.

Rubio-Ochoa, J., et al., 2016. Physical examination tests for screening and diagnosis of cervicogenic headache: a systematic review. Man. Ther. 21, 35–40.

Rushton, A., et al., 2014. International framework for examination of the cervical region for potential of cervical arterial dysfunction prior to orthopaedic manual therapy intervention. Man. Ther. 19, 222–228.

Salem, W., et al., 2013. In vivo three-dimensional kinematics of the cervical spine during maximal axial rotation. Man. Ther. 18, 339–344.

Schomacher, J., et al., 2013. Localized pressure pain sensitivity is associated with lower activation of the semispinalis cervicis muscle group in patients with chronic neck pain. Clin. J. Pain 29, 898–906.

Schomacher, J., et al., 2015. Can neck exercises enhance the activation of semispinalis cervicis relative to splenius capitis at specific spinal levels? Man. Ther. 20, 694–702.

Schomacher, J., Falla, D., 2013. Function and structure of the deep cervical extensor muscles in patients with neck pain. Man. Ther. 18, 360–366.

Sjaastad, O., et al., 1998. Cervicogenic headache: diagnostic criteria. The CGHA International Study Group. Headache 38, 442–445.

Smart, K., et al., 2012a. Mechanisms-based classification of musculoskeletal pain: part 1 of 3: Symptoms and signs of central sensitisation in patients with LBP +/– leg pain. Man. Ther. 17, 336–344.

Smart, K., et al., 2012b. Mechanisms-based classification of musculoskeletal pain: part 2 of 3: Symptoms and signs of peripheral neuropathic pain in patients with LBP +/– leg pain. Man. Ther. 17, 345–351.

Smart, K., et al., 2012c. Mechanisms-based classification of musculoskeletal pain: part 3 of 3: Symptoms and signs of nociceptive pain in patients with LBP +/– leg pain. Man. Ther. 17, 352–357.

Smart, K., Doody, C., 2010. Clinical indicators of nociceptive, peripheral neuropathic and central mechanisms of MSK pain. A Delphi survey of expert clinicians. Man. Ther. 15, 80.

Stovener, L., et al., 2007. The global burden of headache: a documentation of headache of prevalence and disability worldwide. Cephalagia 27, 193–210.

Taylor, A., Kerry, R., 2010. A 'system based' approach to risk assessment of the cervical spine prior to manual therapy. Int. J. Osteopath. Med. 13, 85–93.

Taylor, A., Kerry, R., 2015. Haemodynamics and clinical practice. In: Jull, G., et al. (Eds.), Grieve's modern musculoskeletal physiotherapy, fourth ed. Elsevier, Edinburgh (Chapter 35.2).

Thomas, L., 2016. Cervical arterial dissection: an overview and implications for manipulative therapy practice. Man. Ther. 21, 2–9.

Thomas, L., et al., 2015. The effect of end-range cervical rotation on vertebral and internal carotid artery blood flow and cerebral inflow: a sub analysis of an MRI study. Man. Ther. 20, 475–480.

Treleaven, J., 2008. Sensorimotor disturbances in neck disorders affecting postural stability, head and eye movement control. Man. Ther. 13, 2–11.

Treleaven, J., 2011. Dizziness, unsteadiness, visual disturbances and postural control implications for the transition to chronic symptoms after a whiplash trauma. Spine 36, S211–S217.

Tubbs, S., et al., 2007. The tectorial membrane: anatomical, biomechanical and histological analysis. Clin. Anat. 20, 382–386.

Uitvlugt, G., Indenbaum, S., 1988. Clinical assessment of atlantoaxial instability using the Sharp-Purser test. Arthritis Rheumatol. 31, 918–922.

Van Griensven, H., 2005. Pain in practice theory and treatment strategies for manual therapists. Elsevier, Edinburgh.

Waddell, G., 2004. The back pain revolution, second ed. Elsevier, Edinburgh.

Walser, R., et al., 2009. The effectiveness of thoracic spine manipulation for the management of musculoskeletal conditions: a systematic review and meta-analysis of randomised clinical trials. J. Man. Manip. Ther. 17, 237–246.

Zito, G., et al., 2006. Clinical tests of musculoskeletal dysfunction in the diagnosis of cervicogenic headache. Man. Ther. 11, 118–129.

7

EXAMINATION OF THE CERVICOTHORACIC REGION

CHRIS WORSFOLD

CHAPTER CONTENTS

INTRODUCTION

The cervical spine is the most complex articular system in the body, comprising 37 separate joints and moving over 600 times per hour (Giles & Singer 1998), with a total sagittal plane excursion in excess of 1 000 000° per day (Sterling et al. 2008); no other part of the articular system is in such a state of constant motion. Common conditions relevant to this region include nerve root, intervertebral disc and facet joint disorders and whiplash injury. Narrowing of the spinal foramen and canal may occur (stenosis) and osseous anomalies (e.g. cervical rib) can be present (Giles & Singer 1998). Structural changes are not strongly associated with pain, however, and are commonly found in asymptomatic subjects (Nakashima et al. 2015). The cervicothoracic region is defined here as the region between C3 and T4, and includes the joints and their surrounding soft tissues. Note that the order of subjective questioning

and the physical tests described below can be altered as appropriate for the patient being examined.

SUBJECTIVE EXAMINATION

Patients' Perspective on Their Experience

This includes the patient's perspectives, experience and expectations, age, employment, home situation and details of any leisure activities. In order to treat the patient appropriately, it is important that the condition is managed within the context of the patient's social and work environment.

Psychosocial factors need to be assessed, as they will strongly influence recovery and treatment response. Screening for psychosocial risk factors such as a posttraumatic stress reaction is important in whiplash injury. Posttraumatic stress reactions are characterized by intrusive thoughts and flashbacks regarding the trauma (i.e. motor vehicle collision) and a state of hyperarousal that can involve feelings of irritability, and difficulty concentrating and falling asleep at night (Worsfold 2014).

The clinician may ask the following types of questions to elucidate psychosocial factors:

- Have you had time off work in the past with your pain?
- How is your employer/coworkers/family responding to your pain?
- Do you think you will return to work? When?
- What do you understand to be the cause of your pain?
- What are you expecting will help you?
- Do you expect to recover?
- Do you feel you can control your pain?
- What are you doing to cope with your pain?
- Do you feel overwhelmed by the pain?

Body Chart

The following information concerning the area and type of current symptoms can be recorded on a body chart (see Fig. 2.3).

Area of Current Symptoms

Be exact when mapping out the area of the symptoms. Patients may have symptoms over a large area. As well as symptoms over the cervical spine, they may have symptoms over the head and face, thoracic spine and upper limbs. Ascertain which is the worst symptom and record where the patient feels the symptoms are coming from.

Areas Relevant to the Region Being Examined

All other relevant areas are checked for symptoms; it is important to ask about pain or even stiffness, as this may be relevant to the patient's main symptom. Mark unaffected areas with ticks on the body chart. Check for symptoms in the head, temporomandibular joint, thoracic spine, shoulder, elbow, wrist and hand and ascertain whether the patient has ever experienced any disequilibrium or dizziness. Dizziness and unsteadiness are commonly associated with whiplash injury and, less frequently, atraumatic neck pain and may indicate sensorimotor disturbance (Treleaven 2008). A high index of suspicion is warranted in any symptoms

arising from the cervical spine. Such an approach serves to minimize the risk that potentially fatal but rare pathologies, such as cervical arterial dysfunction (CAD), are not overlooked or provoked by physical examination and subsequent treatment. If symptoms suggestive of CAD are described by the patient, the clinician proceeds with a thorough assessment for potential neurovascular pathology (Barker et al. 2000; Kerry & Taylor 2006; Kerry et al. 2008). The clinician's aim during the patient history is to make the best judgement on the probability of serious pathology and contraindications to treatment based on available evidence; furthermore, a 'risk factors' versus 'benefit of intervention' model is advocated (Rushton et al. 2012).

Quality of Pain

Establish the quality of the pain. Complaints of burning and electric shock-like pains and pains that 'have a mind of their own' are suggestive of neuropathic pain, a risk factor for poor recovery in whiplash injury (Sterling & Pedler 2009). If the patient suffers from associated headaches, consider carrying out a full upper cervical spine examination (see Chapter 6).

Intensity of Pain

The intensity of pain can be measured using, for example, a visual analogue scale, as shown in Fig. 2.5. A pain diary may be useful for patients with chronic neck pain with or without headaches to determine the pain patterns and triggering factors.

Abnormal Sensation

Check for any altered sensation locally in the cervical spine and in other relevant areas such as the upper limbs or face.

Constant or Intermittent Symptoms

Ascertain the frequency of the symptoms, whether they are constant or intermittent. If symptoms are constant, check whether there is variation in the intensity of the symptoms, as constant unremitting pain may be indicative of neoplastic disease.

Relationship of Symptoms

Determine the relationship between the symptomatic areas – do they come together or separately? For example, the patient could have shoulder pain without cervical pain, or the pains may always be present together.

Behaviour of Symptoms

Aggravating Factors

For each symptomatic area, discover what movements and/or positions aggravate the patient's symptoms, i.e. what brings them on (or makes them worse)? Is the patient able to maintain this position or movement (severity)? What happens to other symptoms when this symptom is produced (or is made worse)? How long does it take for symptoms to ease once the position or movement is stopped (irritability)? These questions help to confirm the relationship between the symptoms.

The clinician also asks the patient about theoretically known aggravating factors for structures that could be a source of the symptoms. The clinician ascertains how the symptoms affect function, such as static and active postures, e.g. sitting, standing, lying, washing, ironing, dusting, driving, reading, writing, work, sport and social activities. Note details of the training regimen for any sports activities.

Common aggravating movements and positions for the cervical spine involve looking up, e.g. attending a fireworks display or painting a ceiling (cervical extension), reversing the car (cervical rotation), reading (sustained flexion) and sleeping postures (cervical rotation and side flexion). Hair washing, shaving, applying make-up, tying shoe laces and crossing the road are all potential aggravating factors, requiring a relatively large excursion of cervical range of motion (Bible et al. 2010). Aggravating factors for other regions, which may need to be queried if they are suspected to be a source of the symptoms, are shown in Table 2.2. The clinician finds out if the patient is left- or right-handed.

Detailed information on each of the above activities is useful in order to help determine the structure(s) at fault and identify functional restrictions. This information can be used to determine the aims of treatment and any advice that may be required. The most notable functional restrictions are highlighted with asterisks (*), explored in the physical examination and reassessed at subsequent treatment sessions to evaluate treatment intervention.

Easing Factors

For each symptomatic area, the clinician asks what movements and/or positions ease the patient's symptoms, how long it takes to ease them and what happens to other symptoms when this symptom is relieved. These questions help to confirm the relationship between the symptoms.

The clinician asks the patient about theoretically known easing factors for structures that could be a source of the symptoms. For example, symptoms from the cervical spine may be eased by supporting the head or neck, whereas symptoms arising from a cervical rib may be eased by shoulder girdle elevation and/or depression. The clinician can analyse the position or movement that eases the symptoms, to help determine the structure at fault. For example, the patient may obtain relief from nerve root inflammation by placing her arm/hand on top of her head, thus reducing strain on sensitized neural structures (Malanga et al. 2003).

Twenty-Four-Hour Behaviour of Symptoms

The clinician determines the 24-hour behaviour of symptoms by asking questions about night, morning and evening symptoms.

Night Symptoms. The following questions may be asked:

- Do you have any difficulty getting to sleep?
- What position is most comfortable/uncomfortable?
- What is your normal sleeping position?
- What is your present sleeping position?
- Do your symptoms wake you at night? If so,
  - Which symptoms?
  - How many times in the past week?
  - How many times in a night?
  - How long does it take to get back to sleep?
- How many and what type of pillows are used?

Morning and Evening Symptoms. The clinician determines the pattern of the symptoms first thing in the morning, through the day and at the end of the day. Stiffness lasting no longer than 20–30 minutes in the morning might suggest cervical spondylosis; stiffness and pain for a few hours are suggestive of an inflammatory process such as rheumatoid arthritis.

Neck pain that tends to occur towards the end of the day can indicate muscle weakness and/or lack of endurance.

Stage of the Condition

In order to determine the stage of the condition, the clinician asks whether the symptoms are getting better, getting worse or remaining unchanged.

Special Questions

Additional to the routine special questions identified in Chapter 3 are the following areas.

Cervical Spine Fracture

Although cervical spine fracture is rare in physiotherapy practice, a high index of suspicion is indicated in patients who have sustained trauma involving dangerous mechanisms of injury, e.g. fall > 1 metre/5 steps, high-speed motor vehicle collisions, axial loading to the head (e.g. diving) and > 65 years of age, presenting with bilateral < 45° cervical rotation and paraesthesia in the extremities. This screening method is termed the 'Canadian C-spine rule' (Stiell et al. 2001). Any suspicion of cervical spine fracture requires urgent referral for medical investigation.

Cervical Arterial Dysfunction

Although rare, cervical arterial dissection has been associated with manipulation, whiplash injury and sports injuries (Hauser et al. 2010; Willett & Wachholtz 2011). In the initial stages CAD could present as stiffness and pain in the neck. Thus the clinician needs to maintain a high index of suspicion. The clinician needs to ask about symptoms that may be related to pathologies of the arterial vessels, which course through the neck, namely, the vertebral arteries and the internal carotid arteries. Pathologies of these vessels can result in neurovascular insult to the brain (stroke). These pathologies are known to produce signs and symptoms similar to musculoskeletal dysfunction of the upper cervical spine (Bogduk 1994; Kerry & Taylor 2006). Care must be taken to differentiate vascular sources of pain from musculoskeletal sources. Urgent medical investigation is indicated if frank vascular pathology is identified.

CAD can present initially with pain in the upper cervical spine and head. This is referred to as the

---

BOX 7.1
RISK FACTORS FOR CERVICAL ARTERIAL DYSFUNCTION (BARKER ET AL. 2000; KERRY & TAYLOR 2006; KERRY ET AL. 2008)

- Past history of trauma to cervical spine/cervical vessels
- History of migraine-type headache
- Hypertension
- Hypercholesterolaemia/hyperlipidaemia
- Cardiac disease, vascular disease, previous cerebrovascular accident or transient ischaemic attacks
- Diabetes mellitus
- Blood-clotting disorders/alterations in blood properties (e.g. hyperhomocysteinaemia)
- Anticoagulant therapy
- Oral contraceptives
- Long-term use of steroids
- A history of smoking
- Infection
- Immediately postpartum

---

preischaemic stage. If the pathology develops, signs and symptoms of brain ischaemia may develop. Risk factors associated with CAD are given in Box 7.1. The clinician uses further screening questions to help establish the nature and possible causes and sources of the patient's complaints.

Many patients present with treatable musculoskeletal causes of symptoms, but also with many of the risk factors identified in Box 7.1. This does not necessarily exclude them from manual therapy treatment, and careful clinical reasoning and monitoring of signs and symptoms are required in the management of these patients (Kerry & Taylor 2009).

Family History

Family history relevant to the onset and progression of the patient's problem is recorded.

History of the Present Condition

For each symptomatic area, the clinician needs to know how long the symptom has been present, whether there was a sudden or slow onset and whether there was a known cause that provoked the onset of the symptom. If the onset was slow, the clinician should find out if there has been any change in the patient's lifestyle, e.g. a new job or hobby or a change in sporting activity, which may have affected the stresses on the cervical spine and related areas. To confirm the relationship between the symptoms, the clinician asks what happened to other symptoms when each symptom began.

Past Medical History

The following information is obtained from the patient and/or the medical notes:

- The details of any relevant medical history, particularly related to the cervical spine, cranium and face.
- The history of any previous attacks: how many episodes? When were they? What was the cause? What was the duration of each episode? Did the patient recover fully between episodes? If there have been no previous attacks, has the patient had any episodes of stiffness in the cervical or thoracic spine? Check for a history of trauma or recurrent minor trauma.
- Ascertain the results of any past treatment for the same or similar problem. Past treatment records may be obtained for further information.

Plan of the Physical Examination

When all this information has been collected, the subjective examination is complete. It is useful at this stage to highlight with asterisks (*), for ease of reference, important findings and particularly one or more functional restrictions. These can then be reexamined at subsequent treatment sessions to evaluate treatment intervention.

In order to plan the physical examination, the following hypotheses need to be developed from the subjective examination:

- The regions and structures that need to be examined as a possible cause of the symptoms, e.g. temporomandibular region, upper cervical spine, cervical spine, thoracic spine, acromioclavicular joint, sternoclavicular joint, glenohumeral joint, elbow, wrist and hand, muscles and nerves. Often, it is not possible to examine fully at the first attendance and so examination of the structures needs to be prioritized over the subsequent treatment sessions. Using clinical reasoning

skills, the clinician needs to prioritize and justify what 'must' be examined in the initial session and what 'should' or 'could' be followed up at subsequent sessions.

- Other factors that need to be examined, e.g. working and everyday postures, vertebral artery, sensorimotor impairment, muscle weakness.
- In what way should the physical tests be carried out? Will it be easy or hard to reproduce each symptom? Will it be necessary to use combined movements or repetitive movements to reproduce the patient's symptoms? Are symptoms severe and/or irritable? If symptoms are severe, physical tests may be carried out to just before the onset of symptom production or just to the onset of symptom production; no overpressures will be carried out, as the patient would be unable to tolerate this. If symptoms are irritable, physical tests may be examined to just before symptom production or just to the onset of provocation, with fewer physical tests being examined to allow for a rest period between tests.
- Are there any precautions and/or contraindications to elements of the physical examination that need to be explored further, such as CAD, neurological involvement, recent fracture, trauma, steroid therapy or rheumatoid arthritis? There may also be certain contraindications to further examination and treatment, e.g. symptoms of spinal cord compression.

A physical examination planning form can be useful for clinicians to help guide them through the clinical reasoning process (see Fig. 2.9).

PHYSICAL EXAMINATION

The information from the subjective examination helps the clinician to plan an appropriate physical examination. The severity, irritability and nature of the condition are the major factors that will influence the choice and priority of physical testing procedures. The first and overarching question the clinician might ask is: 'Is this patient's condition suitable for me to manage as a therapist?' For example, a patient presenting with symptoms suggestive of cervical myelopathy (i.e. neurological deficit due to spinal cord pathology) may only need neurological integrity testing, prior to an urgent medical referral. The nature of the patient's condition has had a major impact on the physical examination. The second question the clinician might ask is: 'Does this patient have a musculoskeletal dysfunction that I may be able to help?' To answer that, the clinician needs to carry out a full physical examination; however, this may not be possible if the symptoms are severe and/or irritable. If the patient's symptoms are severe and/or irritable, the clinician aims to explore movements as much as possible, within a symptom-free range. If the patient has constant and severe and/or irritable symptoms, then the clinician aims to find physical tests that ease the symptoms. If the patient's symptoms are non-severe and non-irritable, then the clinician aims to find physical tests that reproduce each of the patient's symptoms.

Each significant physical test that either provokes or eases the patient's symptoms is highlighted in the patient's notes by an asterisk (*) for easy reference. The highlighted tests are often referred to as 'asterisks' or 'markers'.

The order and detail of the physical tests described below need to be appropriate to the patient being examined; some tests will be irrelevant, some tests will be carried out briefly, while it will be necessary to investigate others fully. It is important that readers understand that the techniques shown in this chapter are some of many; the choice depends mainly on the relative size of the clinician and patient, as well as the clinician's preference. For this reason, novice clinicians may initially want to copy what is shown, but then quickly adapt to what is best for them.

Observation

Informal Observation

The clinician needs to observe the patient in dynamic and static situations; the quality of movement is noted, as are the postural characteristics and facial expression. Informal observation will have begun from the moment the clinician begins the subjective examination and will continue to the end of the physical examination.

Formal Observation

Observation of Posture. The clinician examines the patient's spinal posture in sitting and standing, noting the posture of the head and neck, thoracic spine and upper limbs. It should be noted that, in the cervicothoracic region, associations between forward head 'chin poke' posture and neck pain are poor (Richards et al. 2016), despite there being a strong tradition within physiotherapy of 'correcting posture' (Kendall et al. 1993). The clinician is encouraged however to correct the patient's posture actively or passively to determine its relevance to the patient's problem whilst keeping in mind that any changes in posture will rarely influence one region of the body in isolation.

Observation of Muscle Form. The clinician observes the muscle bulk and tone of the patient, comparing left and right sides. It must be remembered that handedness and level and frequency of physical activity may well produce differences in muscle bulk between sides.

Observation of Soft Tissues. The clinician observes the quality and colour of the patient's skin and any area of swelling or presence of scarring, and takes cues for further examination.

Observation of the Patient's Attitudes and Feelings. The age, gender and ethnicity of patients and their cultural, occupational and social backgrounds will all affect their attitudes and feelings towards themselves, their condition and the clinician. The clinician needs to be aware of and sensitive to these attitudes, and to empathize and communicate appropriately so as to develop a rapport with the patient and thereby enhance the patient's compliance with the treatment.

Active Physiological Movements

For active physiological movements, the clinician notes the:

■ quality of movement
■ range of movement
■ behaviour of pain through the range of movement
■ resistance through the range of movement and at the end of the range of movement
■ provocation of any muscle spasm.

The active movements with overpressure listed below and shown in Fig. 7.1 are tested with the patient in sitting. Assessment can be enhanced with the use of

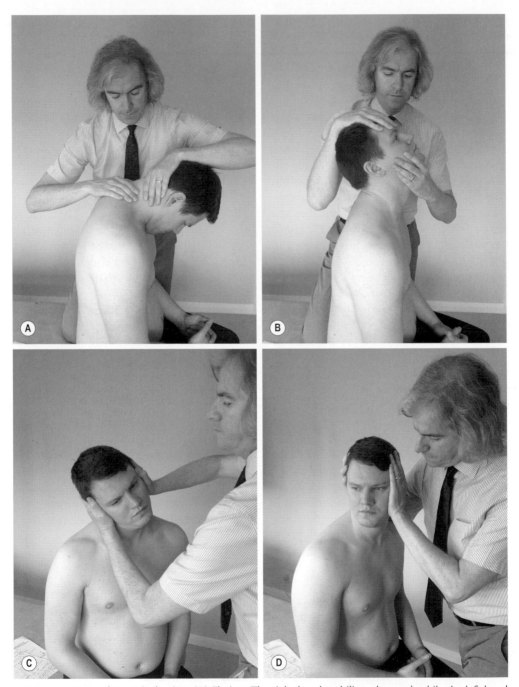

FIG. 7.1 ■ Overpressures to the cervical spine. (A) Flexion. The right hand stabilizes the trunk while the left hand moves the head down so that the chin moves towards the chest. (B) Extension. The right hand rests over the head to the forehead while the left hand holds over the mandible. Both hands then apply a force to cause the head and neck to extend backwards. (C) Lateral flexion. Both hands rest over the patient's head around the ears and apply a force to cause the head and neck to tilt laterally. (D) Rotation. The left hand lies over the zygomatic arch while the right hand rests over the occiput. Both hands then apply pressure to cause the head and neck to rotate.

Continued

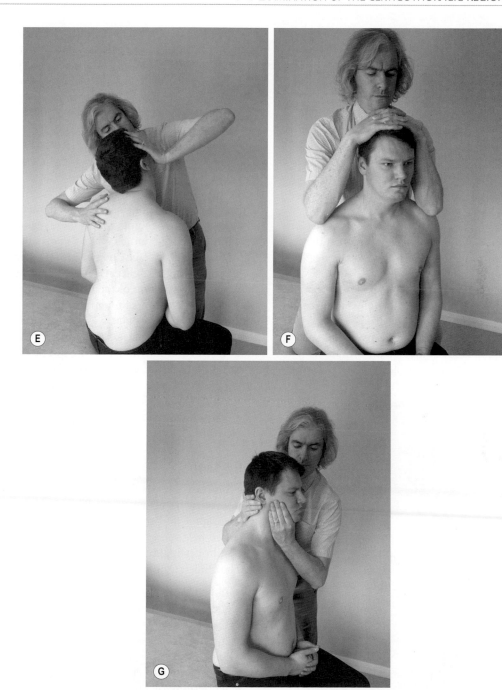

FIG. 7.1, cont'd ▪ (E) Left extension quadrant. This is a combination of extension, left rotation and left lateral flexion. The patient actively extends and, as soon as the movement is complete, the clinician passively moves the head into left rotation and then lateral flexion by applying gentle pressure over the forehead with the left hand. (F) Compression. The hands rest over the top of the patient's head and apply a downward force. (G) Distraction. The left hand holds underneath the mandible while the right hand grasps underneath the occiput. Both hands then apply a force to lift the head upwards.

combined movements (Edwards 1980, 1985, 1999) (Fig. 7.2). The clinician establishes the patient's symptoms at rest and prior to each movement, and corrects any movement deviation to determine its relevance to the patient's symptoms.

For the cervical spine the active movements and possible modifications are shown in Table 7.1. Numerous differentiation tests (Hengeveld & Banks 2001) can be performed; the choice depends on the patient's signs and symptoms. For example, when turning the head around to the left reproduces the patient's left-sided infrascapular pain, differentiation between the cervical and thoracic spine may be required. The clinician can increase and decrease the rotation at the cervical and thoracic regions to find out what effect this has on the infrascapular pain. The patient turns the head and trunk around to the left; the clinician maintains the position of the cervical spine and derotates the thoracic spine, noting the pain response. If symptoms remain the same or increase, this might suggest the cervical spine is the source of the symptoms. The position of cervical and thoracic rotation is then resumed and this time the clinician maintains the position of the thoracic spine and derotates the cervical spine, noting the pain response. If the symptoms remain the same or increase, this implicates the thoracic spine, and this may be further tested by increasing overpressure to the thoracic spine, which would be expected to increase the symptoms.

It may be necessary to examine other regions to determine their relevance to the patient's symptoms; they may be the source of the symptoms, or they may be contributing to the symptoms. The most likely regions are the temporomandibular, shoulder, elbow, wrist and hand. The joints within these regions can be tested fully (see relevant chapter) or partially with the use of screening tests (see Chapter 3 for further details).

Some functional ability has already been tested by the general observation of the patient during the subjective and physical examinations, e.g. the postures adopted during the subjective examination and the ease or difficulty of undressing prior to the examination. Any further functional testing can be carried out at this point in the examination and may include sitting postures and aggravating movements of the upper limb. Clues for appropriate tests can be obtained from the subjective examination findings, particularly aggravating factors.

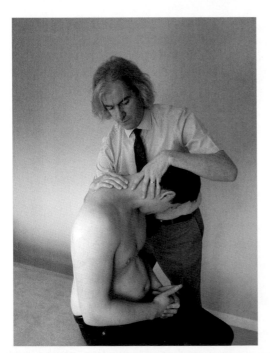

FIG. 7.2 ■ Combined movement to the cervical spine. The right hand supports the trunk while the left hand moves the head into flexion, then lateral flexion then rotation.

Palpation

The clinician palpates the cervicothoracic spine and, if appropriate, the patient's upper cervical spine, lower thoracic spine and any other relevant areas. It is useful to record palpation findings on a body chart (see Fig. 2.3) and/or palpation chart (see Fig. 3.35).

The clinician notes the following:

- the temperature of the area
- increased skin moisture
- the presence of oedema or effusion
- mobility and feel of superficial tissues, e.g. ganglions, nodules
- the presence or elicitation of any muscle spasm
- tenderness of bone, ligaments, muscle, tendon, tendon sheath and nerve; nerves in the upper limb can be palpated at the following points:
  - the suprascapular nerve along the superior border of the scapula in the suprascapular notch

TABLE 7.1
Active Physiological Movements With Possible Modifications

Active Movements	Modifications
Cervical spine	Repeated movements
Flexion	Speed altered
Extension	Movements combined (Edwards 1980, 1985, 1999), e.g.
Left lateral flexion	▪ Extension quadrant: extension, ipsilateral rotation and lateral flexion
Right lateral flexion	
Left rotation	▪ Flexion then rotation
Right rotation	▪ Extension then rotation
Compression	▪ Flexion then lateral flexion then rotation (Fig. 7.2)
Distraction	▪ Extension then lateral flexion
Upper cervical extension/protraction (pro)	Compression or distraction sustained
Repetitive protraction (rep pro)	Injuring movement
Repetitive flexion (rep flex)	Differentiation tests
Upper cervical flexion/retraction (ret)	Function
Repetitive retraction (rep ret)	
Repetitive retraction and extension (rep ext)	
Left repetitive lateral flexion (rep lat flex)	
Right repetitive lateral flexion (rep lat flex)	
Left repetitive rotation (rep rot)	
Right repetitive rotation (rep rot)	
Retraction and extension lying supine	
Repetitive retraction and extension lying supine	
Static (maximum of 3 minutes) retraction and extension lying supine or prone	
?Temporomandibular	
?Shoulder	
?Elbow	
?Wrist and hand	

- the brachial plexus in the posterior triangle of the neck, at the lower third of sternocleidomastoid
- the suprascapular nerve along the superior border of the scapula in the suprascapular notch
- the dorsal scapular nerve medial to the medial border of the scapula
- the median nerve over the anterior elbow joint crease, medial to the biceps tendon; also at the wrist between palmaris longus and flexor carpi radialis
- the radial nerve around the spiral groove of the humerus, between brachioradialis and flexor carpi radialis; also in the forearm and at the wrist in the snuffbox
- increased sensitivity to light palpation (hyperalgesia/allodynia) suggests neuropathic or 'central sensitization' pain states
- increased or decreased prominence of bones
- symptoms (often pain) provoked or reduced on palpation. Posterior midline tenderness can indicate vertebral fracture (Stiell et al. 2001).

Passive Intervertebral Examination

Passive intervertebral examination of the cervical spine is intended to produce information regarding the quantity (range) and quality (through range and end-feel) of specific motion segments and additionally to identify the source of the patient's symptoms. The validity and reliability of this concept have been challenged in recent years, demonstrating varying results (Pool et al. 2004; Piva et al. 2006). Despite this variance, there is continuing use of these techniques, with a belief that findings from passive examination contribute towards valid diagnosis, clinical decision making and management planning (van Trijffel et al. 2005, 2009; Abbott et al. 2009). It appears that when passive intervertebral examination techniques are utilized within a cluster of tests they are useful both for diagnosing the facet joint as the source of pain and for clinical decision making (De Hertogh et al. 2007; Schneider et al. 2014). The sensitivity and specificity of these tests are shown in Table 7.2.

Passive Physiological Movements

This can take the form of passive physiological intervertebral movements (PPIVMs), which examine the movement at each segmental level. PPIVMs can be a useful adjunct to passive accessory intervertebral movements to identify segmental hypomobility and hypermobility. With the patient supine, the clinician palpates the gap between adjacent spinous processes and articular pillars to feel the range of intervertebral movement during flexion, extension, lateral flexion and rotation. Fig. 7.3 demonstrates a rotation PPIVM at the C4–C5 segmental level. It may be necessary to examine other regions to determine their relevance to the patient's symptoms; they may be the source of the symptoms, or they may be contributing to the

symptoms. The most likely regions are the temporomandibular region, shoulder, elbow, wrist and hand.

Passive Accessory Intervertebral Movements

It is useful to use the palpation chart and movement diagrams (or joint pictures) to record findings. These are explained in detail in Chapter 3.

The clinician notes the following:

- quality of movement
- range of movement
- resistance through the range and at the end of the range of movement
- behaviour of pain through the range
- provocation of any muscle spasm.

The cervical and upper thoracic spine (C2–T4) accessory movements are shown in Fig. 7.4 and listed in Table 7.3.

Following accessory movements to the cervicothoracic region, the clinician reassesses all the physical

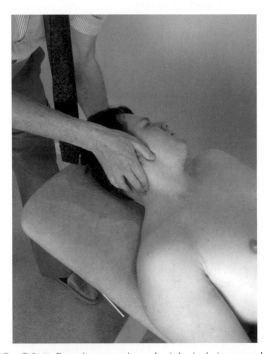

FIG. 7.3 ■ Rotation passive physiological intervertebral movement at the C4–C5 segmental level. The clinician places the index finger over the right C4–C5 zygapophyseal joint region, feeling for tissue texture changes as the head is passively rotated to the left.

TABLE 7.2		
Diagnosing Facet Joint Pain: Sensitivity and Specificity of Passive Intervertebral Examination (Schneider et al. 2014)		
Diagnostic Test	Sensitivity (%)	Specificity (%)
Passive intervertebral examination (PIE)	92	71
Palpation for segmental tenderness (PST)	94	73
Combined extension-rotation (ER)	83	59
PIE, PST and ER	79	84

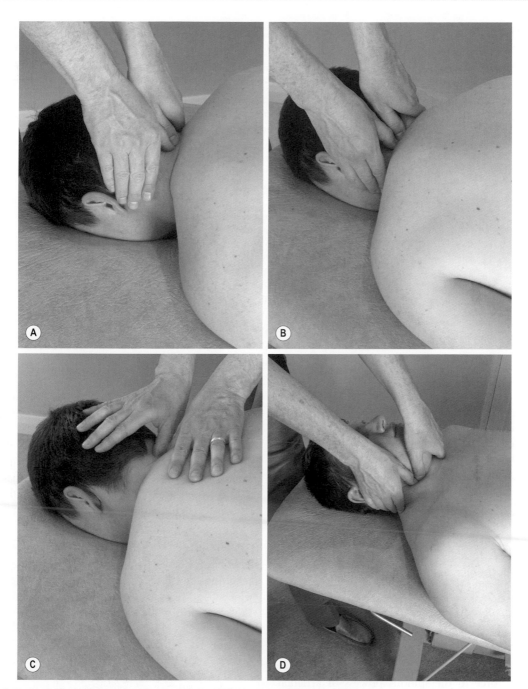

FIG. 7.4 ■ Cervical accessory movements. (A) Central posteroanterior. Thumb pressure is applied to the spinous process. (B) Unilateral posteroanterior. Thumb pressure is applied to the articular pillar. (C) Transverse. Thumb pressure is applied to the lateral aspect of spinous process. (D) Unilateral anteroposterior. In the supine position, thumb pressure is applied to the anterior aspect of the transverse process. Care is needed to avoid pressure over the carotid artery

TABLE 7.3

Accessory Movements, Choice of Application and Reassessment of the Patient's Asterisks

Accessory Movements		Choice of Application	Identify Any Effect of Accessory Movements on Patient's Signs and Symptoms
C2–T4		Alter speed of force application	Reassess all asterisks
	Central posteroanterior	Start position, e.g.	
	Unilateral posteroanterior	■ In flexion	
	Transverse	■ In extension	
	Unilateral anteroposterior (C2–T1 only)	■ In lateral flexion	
Ribs 1–4			■ In flexion and rotation
Caud	Longitudinal caudad first rib	■ In flexion and lateral flexion	
	Anteroposterior	■ In extension and rotation	
	Posteroanterior	■ In extension and lateral flexion	
Med	Medial glide	Direction of the applied force	
		Point of application of applied force	
Upper cervical spine		As above	Reassess all asterisks
Lower thoracic spine		As above	Reassess all asterisks
Shoulder region		As above	Reassess all asterisks
Elbow region		As above	Reassess all asterisks
Wrist and hand		As above	Reassess all asterisks

asterisks (movements or tests that have been found to reproduce the patient's symptoms) in order to establish the effect of the accessory movements on the patient's signs and symptoms. Accessory movements can then be tested for other regions suspected to be a source of, or contributing to, the patient's symptoms (Fig. 7.5). Again, following accessory movements to any one region, the clinician reassesses all the asterisks. Regions likely to be examined are the upper cervical spine, lower thoracic spine, shoulder, elbow, wrist and hand (Table 7.3).

Natural Apophyseal Glides (NAGs)

These can be applied to the apophyseal joints between C2 and T3. The patient sits and the clinician supports the patient's head and neck and applies a static or oscillatory force to the spinous process or articular pillar in the direction of the facet joint plane of each vertebra (Mulligan 1999). Fig. 7.6 demonstrates a unilateral NAG on C5. This is repeated 6–10 times. The patient should feel no pain, but may feel slight discomfort.

Reversed Natural Apophyseal Glides

The patient sits and the clinician supports the head and neck and applies a force to the articular pillars of a vertebra using the index and thumb of the hand (Fig. 7.7). A force is then applied to the pillars in the direction of the facet plane.

Sustained Natural Apophyseal Glides (SNAGs)

The painful cervical spine movements are examined in sitting. The clinician applies a force to the spinous process and/or transverse process in the direction of the facet joint plane of each cervical vertebra as the patient moves slowly towards the pain. All cervical movements can be tested in this way. Fig. 7.8 demonstrates a C5 extension SNAG. For further details on these techniques, see Chapter 3 and Mulligan (1999).

Muscle Tests

Muscle tests include those examining muscle strength, control, length and isometric muscle contraction.

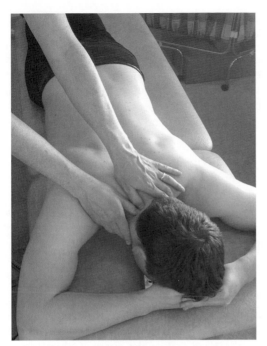

FIG. 7.5 ■ Palpation of accessory movements using a combined movement. Thumb pressure over the right articular pillar of C5 is carried out with the cervical spine positioned in left lateral flexion.

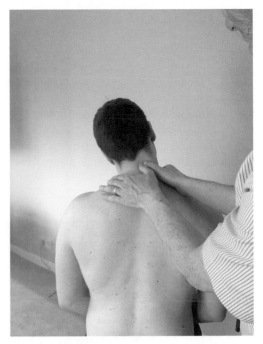

FIG. 7.6 ■ Unilateral natural apophyseal glide on C6. Thumb pressure is applied to the right articular pillar of C5 as the patient laterally flexes to the left.

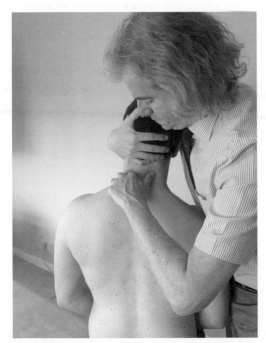

FIG. 7.7 ■ Reversed flexion natural apophyseal glide to C5. The right hand supports the head and neck. The index and thumb of the left hand apply an anterior force to the articular pillars of C5.

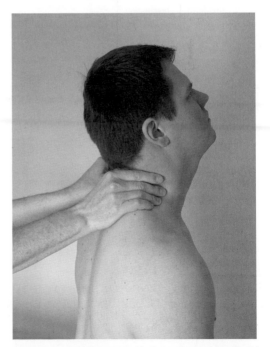

FIG. 7.8 ■ Extension sustained natural apophyseal glide to C5. Thumb pressure is applied to the spinous process of C5 as the patient slowly extends.

Movement Control

A battery of tests can be used to examine movement control formally (Table 7.4). These tests have been shown to have 'substantial to excellent' intrarater and interrater reliability ($k = 0.86$ and $k = 0.69$, respectively) (Segarra et al. 2015). The tests have been shown to discriminate between normal healthy controls and patients with neck pain (Elsig et al. 2014). The battery of tests includes cervicothoracic extension, sitting cervical retraction and protraction and quadruped cervical rotation (Fig. 7.9).

TABLE 7.4
Movement Control (MC) Tests (Elsig et al. 2014)

MC test 1: extension cervicothoracic junction	**Instruction** Make a double chin. Then, try to look at the ceiling without losing the double-chin position and without making a hollow back **Compensatory movements** Protraction of the head Loss of the flexion in the upper cervical spine Elevation or protraction of the shoulders
MC test 2: pro- and retraction of head	**Instruction** Push the chin horizontally forward and backward. **Compensatory movements** Elevation or protraction of the shoulder Excessive flexion or extension in the lower cervical spine Flexion of the thoracic spine The line between the ear and the nose cannot be held horizontally
MC test 3: quadruped cervical rotation	**Instruction** Make a straight back. Turn your head and neck slowly to the right and back to the starting position. Try to make the rotation around an axis that runs longitudinally through your head, neck and spine. Then you do the same movement to the left **Compensatory movements** Lateral flexion of the cervical spine Flexion or extension in the cervical spine Flexion, extension or lateral flexion in the thoracic spine Elevation of the shoulders

Specific muscle testing can be undertaken as follows.

Deep Cervical Muscle Testing. Deep muscles in the cervical spine are important in the support and control of the head and neck. See Chapter 6 for testing of the deep cervical flexors and extensors.

Scapular Strength. To assess gross muscle function, specific functional tests can be carried out. For example, the clinician can observe the patient performing a slow push-up from the prone position to assess function of the serratus anterior muscle. Weakness will cause the scapula to wing (the medial border moves away from the thorax).

Isometric Muscle Testing

The cervical flexor endurance test records the length of time the supine patient can maintain her head 2 cm above the plinth before the onset of 'chin thrust', i.e. fatigue (Fig. 7.10). The clinician places his index finger on the patient's chin to identify the first onset of fatigue or 'chin thrust' (Grimmer 1994). Normal values are 14 seconds for females and 18 seconds for males (Grimmer 1994). Good intratester and intertester reliability of the cervical endurance test has been reported (Grimmer 1994; Olson et al. 2006; Domenech et al. 2011). The clinician can also test isometric resisted tests of neck flexor and extensor strength in the neutral head position and, if indicated, in different parts of the physiological range; testing flexion or extension in combination with rotation allows useful comparison of left- and right-side differences (Fig. 7.11). The clinician also observes the quality of the muscle activity, e.g. does there appear to be excessive effort or muscle activity? These would suggest lack of muscular endurance or patient fear of performing the movement.

Muscle Length

The clinician tests the length of muscles, e.g. levator scapulae, upper trapezius, sternocleidomastoid, pectoralis major and minor, scalenes and the deep occipital muscles. Testing the length of these muscles is described in Chapter 3.

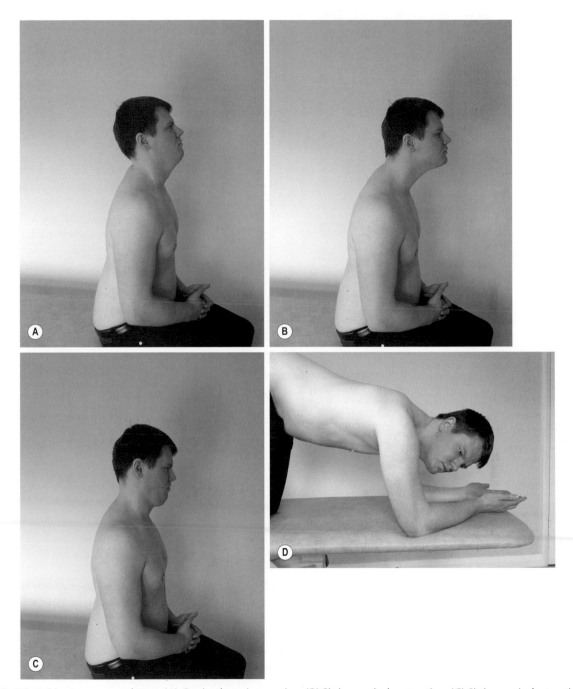

FIG. 7.9 ■ Movement control tests. (A) Cervicothoracic extension. (B) Sitting cervical protraction. (C) Sitting cervical retraction. (D) Quadruped cervical rotation.

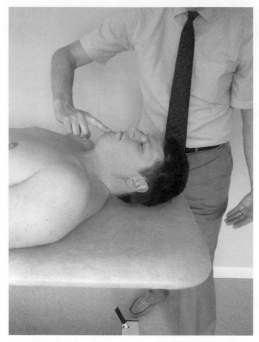

FIG. 7.10 ■ Cervical flexor endurance test. Record the length of time the supine patient can maintain the head 2 cm above the plinth, prior to the first onset of fatigue. The clinician's index finger is placed on the patient's chin to identify the onset of 'chin thrust'.

Neurological Tests

The neurological examination includes neurological integrity testing, tests for neural sensitization and other nerve tests.

Integrity of Nervous System

As a general guide, a neurological examination is indicated if symptoms are felt below the acromion.

Dermatomes/Peripheral Nerves. Light touch and pain sensation of the upper limb are tested using cotton wool and pinprick, respectively, as described in Chapter 3. Knowledge of the cutaneous distribution of nerve roots (dermatomes) and peripheral nerves enables the clinician to distinguish the sensory loss due to a root lesion from that due to a peripheral nerve lesion. The cutaneous nerve distribution and dermatome areas are shown in Chapter 3.

Myotomes/Peripheral Nerves. The following myotomes are tested and are shown in Chapter 3:

- C4: shoulder girdle elevation
- C5: shoulder abduction
- C6: elbow flexion
- C7: elbow extension
- C8: thumb extension
- T1: finger adduction.

A working knowledge of the muscular distribution of nerve roots (myotomes) and peripheral nerves enables the clinician to distinguish motor loss due to a root lesion from that due to a peripheral nerve lesion. Peripheral nerve distributions are shown in Chapter 3.

Reflex Testing. The following deep tendon reflexes are tested (see Chapter 3):

- C5–C6: biceps
- C7: triceps and brachioradialis.

Neurodynamic Tests

The following neurodynamic tests may be carried out in order to ascertain the degree to which neural tissue is responsible for the production of the patient's symptom(s):

- passive neck flexion
- upper-limb neurodynamic tests
- straight-leg raise
- long-sitting slump
- slump.

These tests are described in detail in Chapter 3.

Other Nerve Tests

Plantar Response to Test for an Upper Motor Neuron Lesion (Walton 1989). Pressure applied from the heel along the lateral border of the plantar aspect of the foot produces flexion of the toes in the normal individual. Extension of the big toe with downward fanning of the other toes occurs with an upper motor neuron lesion.

Tinel's Sign. The clinician taps the skin overlying the brachial plexus. Reproduction of distal pain/paraesthesia denotes a positive test indicating regeneration of an injured sensory nerve (Walton 1989).

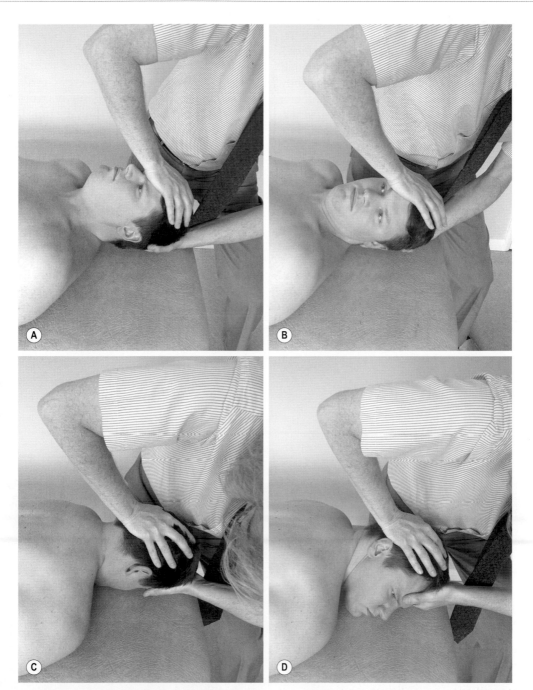

FIG. 7.11 ■ Isometric muscle tests. The clinician tests isometric contractions of the neck flexors and extensors. The clinician must ensure that: (1) no movement takes place during the test; (2) the patient's head is supported firmly throughout the test; and (3) the pain response is monitored closely. (A) Flexion neutral head position. The right hand is resisting the patient's efforts to flex the neck. (B) Flexion and left cervical rotation test. The right hand is resisting the patient's efforts to flex the neck in the sagittal plane. (C) Extension neutral head position. The right hand is resisting the patient's efforts to extend the neck. (D) Extension and right cervical rotation test. The right hand is resisting the patient's efforts to extend the neck in the sagittal plane.

Sensorimotor Tests

Sensorimotor control has been discussed in Chapter 3. Clinically, dizziness and unsteadiness are commonly associated with whiplash injury and, less frequently, atraumatic neck pain and may indicate sensorimotor disturbance (Treleaven 2008). It is hypothesized that afferent output from the cervical spine (e.g. from muscle spindles and/or mechanoreceptors) is impaired in neck pain and injury, and this in turn can lead to disruption of the reflexive balance mechanisms involving the eyes and the vestibular system, manifesting in unsteadiness and dizziness. Thus cervical proprioception, eye movement control and postural stability can all be impaired to a lesser or greater degree (Treleaven et al. 2003, 2008, 2011).

Sensorimotor impairment testing therefore involves assessing proprioception (joint position error), oculomotor control and postural stability (Fig. 7.12).

Proprioception

Cervical joint position error tests measure an individual's ability to relocate her head accurately to the same point in space with the eyes closed. Evidence suggests that cervical joint position error measured with a laser and target in the clinical setting has acceptable validity (compared with laboratory-based electromagnetic tracking, e.g. Fastrak system) and reliability (intraclass correlation coefficient > 0.75) and can discriminate between healthy controls and subjects with neck pain (Heikkila & Astrom 1996; Heikkila & Wenngren 1998; Chen & Treleaven 2013; Jørgensen et al. 2014).

Oculomotor Tests

The smooth-pursuit test involves the patient sitting and following a moving object with her eyes whilst keeping the head still. The object – usually the

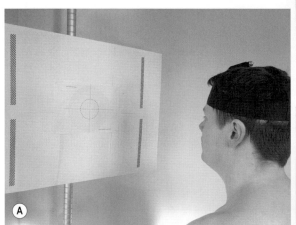
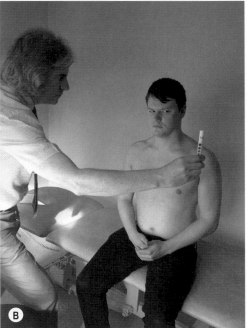

FIG. 7.12 ■ Sensorimotor tests. (A) Proprioception/joint position error (JPE). The patient sits 90 cm from a wall with eyes closed in a neutral head position. He moves the head in the direction being tested as far as is comfortable. He attempts to return to the precise starting position, keeping the eyes closed. The JPE between the starting point and the return point is measured in centimetres. JPE > 5 cm suggests impairment. (B) Oculomotor control smooth-pursuit test. The patient follows an object with his eyes moving 30° either side of the midline whilst maintaining neutral head position.

clinician's finger – is panned slowly, taking 5 seconds to cross an arc 30° either side of the patient's midline. Onset of pain, dizziness or increased effort suggests sensorimotor impairment. The smooth-pursuit test has good interrater reliability and has been shown to discriminate between healthy controls and subjects with chronic neck pain (Della Casa et al. 2014).

Postural Stability

Tests of postural stability include comfortable, narrow and tandem standing, tested with both eyes open and eyes closed. The test is timed to 30 seconds maximum. Patients 'fail' the test if they step or require support during the test (Field et al. 2008).

Miscellaneous Tests

Spurling's Neck Compression Test

The test is performed by extending, laterally flexing and rotating the neck to the same side and then applying downward axial pressure through the head (Fig. 7.13). The test is considered positive if radicular symptoms radiate into the limb ipsilateral to the side to which the head is laterally flexed and rotated (Malanga et al. 2003). The test appears to have high specificity and sensitivity (95% and 92%, respectively) and good to fair interrater reliability (Malanga et al. 2003; Shah & Rajshekhar 2004).

Shoulder Abduction Test

The test is performed by actively or passively abducting the symptomatic arm and placing the patient's arm on top of her head. The test is considered positive with reduction or relief of ipsilateral cervical radicular symptoms (Malanga et al. 2003).

Cervical Arterial Dysfunction Testing

If vascular dysfunction is suspected following the subjective examination (see above), further information regarding the integrity of the cervical arterial system can be gained from the following examination procedures. Further reading (Kerry & Taylor 2006) is recommended to support understanding of these procedures.

Blood Pressure

In the event of acute arterial dysfunction, it is likely that there will be a systematic cardiovascular response

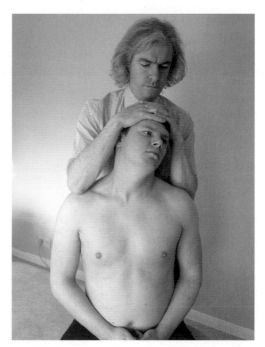

FIG. 7.13 ■ Spurling's neck compression test. Performed by extending, laterally flexing and rotating the neck to the same side and then applying downward axial pressure through the head. The test is considered positive if radicular symptoms radiate into the limb ipsilateral to the side to which the head is laterally flexed and rotated.

manifesting in a dramatic change in blood pressure (usually increasing). Blood pressure is taken using appropriate, validated procedures and equipment, in either sitting or lying.

Functional Positional Testing

Passive repositioning of the head has been classically considered a test for vertebrobasilar insufficiency. A minimum requirement of a passive 10-second hold into cervical rotation has been proposed (Magarey et al. 2004). A positive test is considered if reproduction of symptoms suggestive of hindbrain ischaemia is found. The diagnostic utility of this procedure is, however, not certain (Thiel & Rix 2005; Kerry 2006) and, like any of the individual parts of CAD testing, reliance on one result alone is not indicative of pathology.

Cranial Nerve Examination

Cranial nerve dysfunction can be a component part of arterial compromise in the neck and head, and this may be an indication of vascular dysfunction. Careful screening for gross asymmetries and variations from the norm in cranial nerve function are indicated if CAD is suspected (Kerry & Taylor 2008).

Test for Thoracic Outlet Syndrome

There are several tests for this syndrome, which are described in Chapter 9.

COMPLETION OF THE EXAMINATION

Having carried out the above tests, the examination of the cervical spine is now complete. The subjective and physical examinations produce a large amount of information, which needs to be recorded accurately and quickly. It is important, however, that the clinician does not examine in a rigid manner, simply following the suggested sequence outlined in the chart. Each patient presents differently and this needs to be reflected in the examination process. It is vital at this stage to highlight with an asterisk (*) important findings from the examination. These findings are reassessed at, and within, subsequent treatment sessions to evaluate the effects of treatment on the patient's condition.

The physical testing procedures which specifically indicate joint, nerve or muscle tissues, as a source of the patient's symptoms, are summarized in Table 3.9. The strongest evidence that a joint is the source of the patient's symptoms is that active and passive physiological movements, passive accessory movements and joint palpation all reproduce the patient's symptoms, and that, following a treatment dose, reassessment identifies an improvement in the patient's signs and symptoms. Weaker evidence includes an alteration in range, resistance or quality of physiological and/or accessory movements and tenderness over the joint, with no alteration in signs and symptoms after treatment. One or more of these findings may indicate a dysfunction of a joint which may or may not be contributing to the patient's condition.

The strongest evidence that a muscle is the source of a patient's symptoms is if active movements, an isometric contraction, passive lengthening and palpation of a muscle all reproduce the patient's symptoms, and that, following a treatment dose, reassessment identifies an improvement in the patient's signs and symptoms. Further evidence of muscle dysfunction may be suggested by reduced strength or poor quality during the active physiological movement and the isometric contraction, reduced range and/or increased/decreased resistance, during the passive lengthening of the muscle, and tenderness on palpation, with no alteration in signs and symptoms after treatment. One or more of these findings may indicate a dysfunction of a muscle which may or may not be contributing to the patient's condition.

The strongest evidence that a nerve is the source of the patient's symptoms is when active and/or passive physiological movements reproduce the patient's symptoms, which are then increased or decreased with an additional sensitizing movement, at a distance from the patient's symptoms. In addition, there is reproduction of the patient's symptoms on palpation of the nerve and neurodynamic testing, sufficient to be considered a treatment dose, resulting in an improvement in the above signs and symptoms. Further evidence of nerve dysfunction may be suggested by reduced range (compared with the asymptomatic side) and/or increased resistance to the various arm movements, and tenderness on nerve palpation.

On completion of the physical examination the clinician will:

- explain the findings of the physical examination and how these findings relate to the subjective assessment. An attempt should be made to clear up any misconceptions patients may have regarding their illness or injury
- collaborate with the patient and via problem solving together devise a treatment plan and discuss the prognosis
- warn the patient of possible exacerbation up to 24–48 hours following the examination
- request the patient to report details on the behaviour of the symptoms following examination at the next attendance
- evaluate the findings, formulate a clinical diagnosis and write up a problem list
- determine the objectives of treatment
- devise an initial treatment plan.

In this way, the clinician develops the following hypotheses categories (adapted from Jones & Rivett 2004):

- function: abilities and restrictions
- patient's perspective on his/her experience
- source of symptoms. This includes the structure or tissue that is thought to be producing the patient's symptoms, the nature of the structure or tissues in relation to the healing process and the pain mechanisms involved
- contributing factors to the development and maintenance of the problem. There may be environmental, psychosocial, behavioural, physical or heredity factors
- precautions/contraindications to treatment and management. This includes the severity and irritability of the patient's symptoms and the nature of the patient's condition
- management strategy and treatment plan
- prognosis – this can be affected by factors such as the stage and extent of the injury as well as the patient's expectation, personality and lifestyle.

For guidance on treatment and management principles, the reader is directed to the companion textbook (Petty & Barnard 2017).

REFERENCES

Abbott, J.H., et al., 2009. Manual physical assessment of spinal segmental motion: intent and validity. Man. Ther. 14, 36–44.

Barker, S., et al., 2000. Guidance for pre-manipulative testing of the cervical spine. Man. Ther. 5, 37–40.

Bible, J.E., et al., 2010. Normal functional range of motion of the cervical spine during 15 activities of daily living. J. Spinal Disord. Tech. 23, 15–21.

Bogduk, N., 1994. Cervical causes of headache and dizziness. In: Boyling, J.D., Palastanga, N. (Eds.), Grieve's modern manual therapy, second ed. Churchill Livingstone, Edinburgh, p. 317.

Chen, X., Treleaven, J., 2013. The effect of neck torsion on joint position error in subjects with chronic neck pain. Man. Ther. 18, 562–567.

De Hertogh, W., et al., 2007. The validity of the manual examination in the assessment of patients with neck pain. Spine 7, 628–629.

Della Casa, E., et al., 2014. Head-eye movement control tests in patients with chronic neck pain; inter-observer reliability and discriminative validity. BMC Musculoskelet. Disord. 15, 16.

Domenech, M.A., et al., 2011. The deep neck flexor endurance test: normative data scores in healthy adults. PM R 3, 105–110.

Edwards, B.C., 1980. Combined movements in the cervical spine (C2–7): their value in examination and technique choice. Aust J Physiother 26, 165–169.

Edwards, B.C., 1985. Combined movements in the cervical spine (their use in establishing movement patterns). In: Glasgow, E.F., Twomey, L.T., et al. (Eds.), Aspects of manipulative therapy. Churchill Livingstone, Melbourne (Chapter 19).

Edwards, B.C., 1999. Manual of combined movements: their use in the examination and treatment of mechanical vertebral column disorders, second ed. Butterworth-Heinemann, Oxford.

Elsig, S., et al., 2014. Sensorimotor tests, such as movement control and laterality judgment accuracy, in persons with recurrent neck pain and controls. A case-control study. Man. Ther. 19, 555–561.

Field, S., et al., 2008. Standing balance: a comparison between idiopathic and whiplash-induced neck pain. Man. Ther. 13, 183–191.

Giles, L., Singer, K., 1998. Clinical anatomy and management of cervical spine pain. Clinical anatomy and management of back pain series. Elsevier, Oxford.

Grimmer, K., 1994. Measuring the endurance capacity of the cervical short flexor muscle group. Australian Journal of Physiotherapy 40, 251–254.

Hauser, V., et al., 2010. Late sequelae of whiplash injury with dissection of cervical arteries. Eur. Neurol. 64, 214–218.

Heikkila, H., Astrom, P.G., 1996. Cervicocephalic kinesthetic sensibility in patients with whiplash injury. Scand. J. Rehabil. Med. 28, 133–138.

Heikkila, H.V., Wenngren, B.I., 1998. Cervicocephalic kinesthetic sensibility, active range of cervical motion, and oculomotor function in patients with whiplash injury. Arch. Phys. Med. Rehabil. 79, 1089–1094.

Hengeveld, E., Banks, K. (Eds.), 2001. Maitland's vertebral manipulation, sixth ed. Butterworth-Heinemann, Oxford.

Jones, M.A., Rivett, D.A., 2004. Clinical reasoning for manual therapists. Butterworth-Heinemann, Edinburgh.

Jørgensen, R., et al., 2014. Reliability, construct and discriminative validity of clinical testing in subjects with and without chronic neck pain. BMC Musculoskelet. Disord. 15, 408.

Kendall, F.P., et al., 1993. Muscles testing and function, fourth ed. Williams & Wilkins, Baltimore, MD.

Kerry, R. 2006 Vertebral artery testing: how certain are you that your pre-cervical manipulation and mobilisation tests are safe and specific? HES 2nd International Evidence Based Practice Conference, London.

Kerry, R., Taylor, A.J., 2006. Masterclass: cervical arterial dysfunction assessment and manual therapy. Man. Ther. 11, 243–253.

Kerry, R., Taylor, A.J., 2008. Arterial pathology and cervicocranial pain – differential diagnosis for manual therapists and medical practitioners. Int. Musculoskelet. Med. 30, 70–77.

Kerry, R., Taylor, A.J., 2009. Cervical arterial dysfunction: knowledge and reasoning for manual physical therapists. J Orthop Sports Phys Ther 39, 378–387.

Kerry, R., et al., 2008. Cervical arterial dysfunction and manual therapy: a critical literature review to inform professional practice. Man. Ther. 13, 278–288.

Magarey, M.E., et al., 2004. Pre-manipulative testing of the cervical spine review, revision and new clinical guidelines. Man. Ther. 9, 95–108.

Malanga, G.A., et al., 2003. Provocative tests in cervical spine examination: historical basis and scientific analyses. Pain Physician 6, 199–205.

Mulligan, B.R., 1999. Manual therapy 'NAGs', 'SNAGs', 'MWMs' etc., fourth ed. Plane View Services, New Zealand.

Nakashima, H., et al., 2015. Abnormal findings on magnetic resonance images of the cervical spines in 1211 asymptomatic subjects. Spine 40, 392–398.

Olson, L.E., et al., 2006. Reliability of a clinical test for deep cervical flexor endurance. J. Manipulative Physiol. Ther. 29, 134–138.

Petty, N.J., Barnard, K., 2017. Principles of musculoskeletal treatment and management: a handbook for therapists, third ed. Elsevier, Edinburgh.

Piva, S.R., et al., 2006. Inter-tester reliability of passive intervertebral and active movements of the cervical spine. Man. Ther. 11, 321–330.

Pool, J.J., et al., 2004. The interexaminer reproducibility of physical examination of the cervical spine. J. Manipulative Physiol. Ther. 27, 84–90.

Richards, K.V., et al., 2016. Neck posture clusters and their association with biopsychosocial factors and neck pain in Australian adolescents. Phys. Ther. 96, 1576–1587.

Rushton, A., et al., 2012. International framework of the cervical region for potential of cervical arterial dysfunction prior to orthopaedic manual therapy intervention. Man. Ther. 2012, 1–37.

Schneider, G.M., et al., 2014. Derivation of a clinical decision guide in the diagnosis of cervical facet joint pain. Arch. Phys. Med. Rehabil. 95, 1695–1701.

Segarra, V., et al., 2015. Inter- and intra-tester reliability of a battery of cervical movement control dysfunction tests. Man. Ther. 20, 570–579.

Shah, K.C., Rajshekhar, V., 2004. Reliability of diagnosis of soft cervical disc prolapse using Spurling's test. Br. J. Neurosurg. 18, 480–483.

Sterling, M., Pedler, A., 2009. A neuropathic pain component is common in acute whiplash and associated with a more complex clinical presentation. Man. Ther. 14, 173–179.

Sterling, A.C., et al., 2008. Annual frequency and magnitude of neck motion in healthy individuals. Spine 33, 1882–1888.

Stiell, I.G., et al., 2001. The Canadian C-spine rule for radiography in alert and stable trauma patients. JAMA 286, 1841–1848.

Thiel, H., Rix, G., 2005. Is it time to stop functional pre-manipulative testing of the cervical spine? Man. Ther. 10, 154–158.

Treleaven, J., 2008. Sensorimotor disturbances in neck disorders affecting postural stability, head and eye movement control. Part 2: Case studies. Man. Ther. 13, 266–275.

Treleaven, J., et al., 2003. Dizziness and unsteadiness following whiplash injury: characteristic features and relationship with cervical joint position error. J. Rehabil. Med. 35, 36–43.

Treleaven, J., et al., 2008. Comparison of sensorimotor disturbance between subjects with persistent whiplash-associated disorder and subjects with vestibular pathology associated with acoustic neuroma. Arch. Phys. Med. Rehabil. 89, 522–530.

Treleaven, J., et al., 2011. Head eye co-ordination and gaze stability in subjects with persistent whiplash associated disorders. Man. Ther. 16, 252–257.

van Trijffel, E., et al., 2005. Inter-examiner reliability of passive assessment of intervertebral motion in the cervical and lumbar spine: a systematic review. Man. Ther. 10, 256–269.

van Trijffel, E., et al., 2009. Perceptions and use of passive intervertebral motion assessment of the spine: a survey among physiotherapists specializing in manual therapy. Man. Ther. 14, 243–251.

Walton, J.H., 1989. Essentials of neurology, sixth ed. Churchill Livingstone, Edinburgh.

Willett, G.M., Wachholtz, N.A., 2011. A patient with internal carotid artery dissection. Phys. Ther. 91, 1266–1274.

Worsfold, C., 2014. When range of motion is not enough: towards an evidence-based approach to medico-legal reporting in whiplash injury. J. Forensic Leg. Med. 25, 95–99.

8

EXAMINATION OF THE THORACIC REGION

LINDA A. EXELBY

CHAPTER CONTENTS

POSSIBLE CAUSES OF PAIN AND/OR LIMITATION OF MOVEMENT

The curvature of the thoracic spine normally exhibits a mild kyphosis (posterior curvature) and mobility of the thoracic spine plays an important role in determining overall posture and optimal movement patterns in the rest of the spine and shoulder girdle (Edmondston & Singer 1997). An intact ribcage with its complex ligamentous attachments to the thoracic spine has been shown to play a significant role in thoracic spine stability (Oda et al. 2002). The multiple articulations of the thoracic spine, ribs and sternum should not be considered in isolation and it is proposed that where there are anterior attachments the true functional spinal unit of the thorax should be considered as a 'ring' (Lee 2013). For example, the sixth thoracic ring would comprise left and right sixth ribs,

the sternum, the T5–T6 vertebrae and T5–T6 disc. The ribcage also serves as a site for the attachment of a large number of cervical, lumbar and shoulder girdle muscles.

The thoracic spine and ribcage provide protection for the heart and lungs and are essential for respiration. The multiple somatic structures that make up this region can be the cause of local pain; however, consideration should also be given to the fact that symptoms from pathological conditions of the viscera within the ribcage and abdomen may be referred to this region (Magee 2014). Common musculoskeletal pathologies that can affect this region include symptoms from arthogenic structures such as facet joints, discs and costal joints. Myofascial strain may also cause symptoms. Symptoms from disc herniation have been reported as extremely rare in the upper thoracic spine but may occur more frequently from T6–T7

231

down; 72% of these herniations are central (Mellion & Ladeiro 2001). Facet and costal joint degeneration are also common by the fourth decade (Edmondston & Singer 1997). However, degenerative changes do not necessarily correlate with symptoms (Brinjikjia et al. 2014).

Age may provide a clue about the nature of the underlying pathology; for example, Scheuermann's disease is found mostly in teenagers and is aggravated by physical activities. Idiopathic scoliosis is most commonly found in adolescent females. Osteoporotic-related injuries are found more commonly in the older population.

The thoracic spine examination is appropriate for patients with symptoms in the spine or thorax between T3 and T10. This region includes the intervertebral joints between T3 and T10 as well as the costovertebral, costotransverse, sternocostal, costochondral and interchondral joints with their surrounding soft tissues. To test the upper thoracic spine above T4, it is more appropriate to carry out an adapted cervical spine examination (see Chapter 7). Similarly, to test the lower thoracic spine below T10, an adapted lumbar spine examination can be performed (see Chapter 12).

The order of the subjective questioning and the physical tests described below can be altered as appropriate for the patient.

SUBJECTIVE EXAMINATION

Further details of questions asked during the subjective examination and tests carried out in the physical examination can be found in Chapters 2 and 3, respectively.

Patients' Perspective on Their Experience

The structure of the session needs to be explained to the patient and consent gained. Social and family history relevant to the onset and progression of the patient's problem is recorded. This includes patients' perspectives, experience and expectations, their age, employment, home situation and details of any leisure activities. The age, gender and ethnicity of patients and their cultural, occupational and social backgrounds will all affect their attitudes and feelings towards themselves, their condition and the clinician. The clinician needs to be aware of, and sensitive to, these attitudes

to empathize and communicate appropriately so as to develop a rapport with the patient.

In order to treat the patient appropriately, it is important that the condition is managed within the context of the patient's social and work environment.

The clinician may ask the following types of question to elucidate psychosocial factors:

- Have you had time off work in the past with your pain?
- What do you understand to be the cause of your pain?
- What are you expecting will help you?
- How is your employer/coworkers/family responding to your pain?
- What are you doing to cope with your pain?
- Do you think you will return to work? When?

Validated, reliable questionnaires may be used to identify various psychosocial risk factors and may be useful in patients with more persistent pain.

Body Chart

The information concerning the type and area of current symptoms can be recorded on a body chart (see Fig. 2.3).

Area of Current Symptoms

Be exact when mapping out the area of the symptoms. Symptoms may be felt in the following areas: posteriorly over the thoracic spine, laterally around the chest wall and anteriorly over the sternum. They may follow the course of a rib, run horizontally or be a deep 'through the chest' sensation. Facet joint syndromes usually present as local pain (Dreyfuss et al. 1994) and thoracic nerve root pain is usually referred as a band following the intercostal space. Band-like chest pain or abdominal pain has been reported as a common initial symptom of disc herniation (Mellion & Ladeiro 2001). The central nature of lower thoracic disc herniation would lead the clinician to question about spinal cord compromise and symptoms in the lower extremity The clinician needs to be aware that cervical spine structures (between C3 and C7) can refer pain to the scapula and upper arm (Cloward 1959; Bogduk & Marsland 1988). The upper thoracic spine can refer symptoms to the upper limbs, and the lower thoracic spine to the lower lumbar spine and groin region.

Areas Relevant to the Region Being Examined

All other relevant areas are checked for symptoms; it is important to ask about pain or even stiffness, as this may be relevant to the patient's main symptom. Mark unaffected areas with ticks (✓) on the body chart. Check for symptoms in the cervical spine and upper limbs if it is an upper thoracic problem, or in the lumbar spine and lower limbs if it is a lower thoracic problem. If the patient has symptoms that may emanate from these areas it may be appropriate to assess them more fully. See relevant chapters in this book.

Quality of Pain

Establish the quality of the pain (see Chapter 2).

Intensity of Pain

The intensity of pain can be measured using, for example, a visual analogue scale, as shown in Fig. 2.5. The intensity of pain informs clinical reasoning severity, may provide guidance to the structures producing the symptoms and guides the extent and vigour of the examination.

Abnormal Sensation

Check for any altered sensation or paraesthesia over the thoracic spine, ribcage and other relevant areas.

Constant or Intermittent Symptoms

Ascertain the frequency of all the symptoms, whether they are constant or intermittent. If symptoms are constant, check whether there is variation in the intensity of the symptoms, as constant unremitting pain may be indicative of serious pathology. Special questions relating to visceral function may be appropriate. If there is a relationship, a referral from viscera may need to be considered.

Relationship of Symptoms

Determine the relationship between the symptomatic areas – do they come together or separately? For example, the patient could have shoulder pain without thoracic spine pain, or the pains may always be present together. If one symptomatic area becomes more severe, what happens to the other symptomatic areas?

Behaviour of Symptoms

Aggravating Factors

For each symptomatic area, discover what movements and/or positions aggravate the patient's symptoms. Is the patient able to maintain this position or movement (severity)? What happens to other symptoms when this symptom is produced (or is made worse)? And how long does it take for symptoms to ease once the position or movement is stopped (irritability)? Irritability and severity are explained in Chapter 2.

The clinician ascertains how the symptoms affect function, such as static and active postures, e.g. sitting, standing, lying, performing domestic chores, driving (and reversing the car, which requires trunk rotation), work, sport and social activities. Common aggravating factors for the thoracic spine are rotation of the thorax and deep breathing. Sustained positioning or repetitive movements may often affect the thoracic spine. Examples of these would be working at a desk or check-out counter or where work requires a semirotated position or repetitive rotation (racket sports). Note details of ergonomics at work and the training regimen for any sports activities. Check whether the patient is avoiding activities that exacerbate the symptoms as this may influence the severity and irritability rating.

Detailed information on each of the above activities is useful in order to help determine the structure(s) at fault and identify potential functional restrictions and movement impairments. This information can be used to determine the aims of treatment and any advice that may be required.

Easing Factors

For each symptomatic area, the clinician asks what movements and/or positions ease the patient's symptoms, how long it takes to ease them and what happens to other symptoms when this symptom is relieved. These questions help to confirm the relationship between the symptoms and determine their irritability. Collating the information between aggravating and easing factors helps formulate a hypothesis, plan the physical examination and inform initial advice on the modification of functional tasks. If the patient's symptoms do not fit a musculoskeletal presentation then the clinician needs to be alert to other possible serious causes.

Twenty-Four-Hour Behaviour of Symptoms

The clinician determines the 24-hour behaviour of each symptomatic area by asking questions about night, morning and evening symptoms.

Night Symptoms. (See Chapter 2 for details of questions that must be asked.) In addition, questions specific to the positioning of the spine would be:

- What position is most comfortable/uncomfortable?
- What is your normal sleeping position?
- What is your present sleeping position?
- How many and what type of pillows are used?
- Is your mattress firm or soft and has it been changed recently?

Morning and Evening Symptoms. The clinician determines the pattern of the symptoms in the morning (on waking and on rising), through the day and at the end of the day. The status of symptoms on first waking establishes whether the patient is better with rest. Pain/stiffness on waking would suggest an inflammatory component whereas no pain on waking but pain on rising would suggest a more mechanical origin. Stiffness in the morning for the first few minutes might suggest spondylosis; stiffness and pain for a few hours may be suggestive of an inflammatory process such as ankylosing spondylitis. If symptoms are worse after work compared with when off work, it is important to explore work activities that may be aggravating the symptoms.

Stage of the Condition

In order to determine the stage of the condition, the clinician asks whether the symptoms are getting better, getting worse or remaining unchanged.

Special Questions

As detailed in Chapter 2, the clinician must differentiate between conditions that are suitable for conservative treatment and other systemic, neoplastic and non-musculoskeletal conditions.

General Health

The clinician ascertains the state of the patient's general health to find out if the patient suffers from any osteoporosis, respiratory disorders, cardiovascular disease, breathlessness, chest pain, malaise, fatigue, fever, abdominal cramps, nausea or vomiting, stress, anxiety or depression. Questions relating to change in visceral function may be appropriate owing to the referral pain patterns of these structures.

For full details of all special questions see Chapter 2. Questions relevant to this region include the following.

Serious Pathology

Cancer. Does the patient have a history of cancer? Is there a familial history of cancer? The vertebral column is a common site of skeletal metastasis.

Tuberculosis. Most extrapulmonary tuberculosis presents in the spine at T10–L1 and patients in the early stages may well present with backache.

Osteoporosis. Osteoporosis is the most prevalent of the metabolic bone diseases; incidence increases with age, so it is especially common in postmenopausal women and there can be a familial history. Compression vertebral fractures most commonly occur in the lumbar or midthoracic spine. There are a number of potential causes, some of which can include early menopause, major gynaecological surgery (hysterectomy), endocrinal and metabolic diseases (diabetes and hypothyroidism) and diet (low calcium and vitamin D intake).

Inflammatory Conditions. Has the patient (or a member of the family) been diagnosed as having rheumatoid arthritis or ankylosing spondylitis? Costochondritis and Tietze syndrome are forms of inflammation of the cartilage where ribs attach to the sternum; in Tietze syndrome localized swelling is the distinguishing finding.

Drug Therapy

If medication is taken specifically for the thoracic spine condition, is the patient taking the medication regularly? What effect does it have? How long before this appointment was the medication taken? Has the patient been prescribed long-term (6 months or more) steroids or anticonvulsants, as this may have an impact on bone density.

Radiograph and Medical Imaging

Has the patient been radiographed or had any other investigative scans recently? Has the patient had a dual-energy X-ray absorptiometry (DEXA) scan? This will measure bone density. Other tests may include blood tests if systematic inflammatory conditions or infection are suspected.

Neurological Symptoms

Has the patient experienced symptoms of spinal cord compression, for example, numbness, tingling and/or electric shocks in the hands and feet either bilaterally or unilaterally, depending on the site of the compression? Also, has the patient experienced weakness or difficulty using the arms or legs? Sympathetic function is difficult to measure but questions about changes in swelling, sweating, skin changes (pitting oedema, shiny and inelastic skin) and circulation need to be included. Reporting of a painful red, skin rash with vesicles in a band of skin would implicate herpes zoster.

Vascular Symptoms

The vascular supply to the upper limb passes through the thoracic outlet. Questions should include how good the patient's circulation is and whether the patient has any swelling, coldness, cyanosis, fatigability or cramping in the upper extremities.

History of the Present Condition

- For each symptomatic area, the clinician needs to know how long the symptom has been present, whether there was a sudden or slow onset and whether there was a known cause that provoked the onset of the symptom. The mechanism of injury gives some important clues as to the injured structure. If the onset was slow, the clinician finds out if there has been any change in the patient's lifestyle, e.g. a new job or hobby or a change in sporting activity, which may have affected the stresses on the thoracic spine and related areas. Was there a sudden onset of pain as a result of a traumatic episode or repetitive minor trauma? Rib injuries are commonly caused by trauma. Sudden onset of pain as a result of minor trauma in someone with osteoporosis may be the result of a vertebral compression fracture. Further questioning regarding loss of

height, increased deformity, pain on standing, walking, coughing and sneezing, which is eased with lying down, may make the clinician suspicious. To confirm the relationship between symptoms, the clinician asks what happened to other symptoms and when each symptom began. Clarify the progression and impact of the symptoms on the patient's normal function from the initial onset of this episode to the present time. Find out details about any treatment interventions and advice given: what was it and what was the effect? How do the interventions align with patients' understanding and beliefs of their condition?

Past Medical History

The following information is obtained from the patient and/or the medical notes:

- The history of any previous attacks: symptom distribution, behaviour and cause of initial symptoms. Since then, how many episodes? When were they? What was the cause? What was the duration of each episode? And did the patient fully recover between episodes? If there have been no previous attacks, has the patient had any episodes of stiffness in the cervical, thoracic or lumbar spine or any other relevant region? Check for a history of trauma or recurrent minor trauma. Ascertain the results of any past treatment for the same or similar problem.

Plan of the Physical Examination

After allowing the patient an opportunity to add anything that may not have been mentioned so far, the purpose and plan for the physical examination will need to be explained and consent obtained.

Highlighting with asterisks (*) the important subjective examination findings and particularly one or more functional restrictions will inform your physical examination. A planning form can help guide clinicians through the clinical reasoning process and ensure the development of a working hypothesis of the most likely cause of the patient's symptoms (see Fig. 2.9). A 'must, should, could' list will help prioritize your examination procedures to ensure that your hypothesis is supported (see Chapter 2).

The hypothesis is developed from the subjective examination by identifying:

- The regions and structures that need to be examined as a possible cause of the symptoms. Often, it is not possible to examine fully at the first attendance and so examination of the structures must be prioritized (must, should, could) over subsequent treatment sessions.
- Other factors that need to be examined, e.g. working and everyday postures, breathing patterns and muscle weakness.
- The predominant pain mechanisms that might be driving the patient's symptoms. Pain has been classified into nociceptive (mechanical, inflammatory or ischaemic), peripheral, neurogenic, central, autonomic and affective (Gifford 1996). For the clinical features of pain mechanisms, see Box 2.2.
- In what way should the physical tests be carried out? Will it be easy or hard to reproduce each symptom? Will it be necessary to use combined movements or repetitive movements to reproduce the patient's symptoms? Are symptoms severe and/or irritable? If symptoms are severe, physical tests may be carried out to just before or to the initial onset of symptom production. No overpressures will be carried out. If symptoms are irritable, physical tests may be examined to just before or to initial symptom production, with fewer physical tests being examined.
- Are there any precautions and/or contraindications to elements of the physical examination that need to be explored further, such as neurological involvement, recent fracture, trauma, osteoporosis, steroid or anticoagulant therapy and inflammatory conditions? There may also be certain contraindications to further examination and treatment, e.g. symptoms of cord compression.

PHYSICAL EXAMINATION

The information from the subjective examination helps the clinician to plan an appropriate physical examination. The severity, irritability, nature and pain mechanisms of the condition are the major factors that will influence the choice and priority of physical testing procedures. The first and overarching question the clinician might ask is: 'Is this patient's condition suitable for me to manage as a therapist?' For example, a patient presenting with spinal cord compression symptoms may only need neurological integrity testing, prior to an urgent medical referral. The nature of the patient's condition has a major impact on the physical examination. The second question the clinician might ask is: 'Does this patient have a musculoskeletal dysfunction that I may be able to help?' To answer that, the clinician needs to carry out a full physical examination; however, this may not be possible if the symptoms are severe and/or irritable. The clinician would then aim to explore movements as much as possible, within a symptom-free range, or find physical tests that ease the symptoms. If the patient's symptoms are non-severe and non-irritable, then the clinician aims to find physical tests that reproduce each of the patient's symptoms.

Each significant physical test that either provokes or eases the patient's symptoms is highlighted in the patient's notes by an asterisk (*) for easy reference.

The order and detail of the physical tests described below need to be appropriate to the patient being examined and to the hypotheses (primary or alternatives) developed. It is important that readers understand that the techniques shown in this chapter are only some of many.

Observation

Informal Observation

The clinician observes the patient in dynamic and static situations; the quality of movement is noted, as are the postural characteristics and facial expression. Informal observation occurs throughout the consultation.

Formal Observation

Observation of Posture. The clinician examines the spinal posture of the patient in sitting and standing, noting the level of the pelvis, scoliosis, kyphosis or lordosis and the posture of the upper and lower limbs. Common postural types are described in Chapter 3.

The clinician passively corrects any asymmetry to determine its relevance to the patient's problem. In addition, the clinician observes for any chest deformity, such as pigeon chest, where the sternum lies forward and downwards; funnel chest, where the sternum lies posteriorly (which may be associated with an increased thoracic kyphosis); or barrel chest, where the sternum lies forward and upwards (associated with emphysema) (Magee 2014). The clinician notes the patient's quiet breathing pattern – this includes quality of movement of the ribcage and which part of the ribcage is being used primarily – respiratory rate (normal quiet breathing is 8–14 breaths per minute), rhythm and the effort required to inhale and exhale. Observing the muscles used by the patient will indicate the ease of breathing; for example, excessive use of the accessory muscles of respiration, which can include sternocleidomastoid, pectoralis minor, trapezius, serrati and erector spinae (Innocenti & Troup 2008).

Observation of Muscle Form. The clinician observes the muscle bulk and tone of the patient, comparing the left and right sides. It must be remembered that handedness and level and frequency of physical activity may well produce differences in muscle bulk between sides. Some muscles are thought to shorten under stress, while other muscles weaken, producing movement or postural impairments (see Table 3.7).

Observation of Soft Tissues. The clinician observes the quality and colour of the patient's skin and any area of swelling, or presence of scarring, and takes cues for further examination.

Observation of Gait. The clinician observes the gait pattern if it is applicable to the patient's presenting symptoms.

Active Physiological Movements

The anatomical design of the thoracic spine offers little mobility in the sagittal plane (flexion 32°, extension 25°) and frontal planes (side flexion 26°). The largest range of motion is that of axial rotation with a mean (standard deviation) total range (left and right rotation) of 85 ± 15° (Heneghan & Rushton 2016). The amount of rotation possible depends on the ability of the ribs to undergo distortion. With age the costal cartilages ossify, less distortion occurs and rotation is reduced. Rotation range is significantly decreased in flexion when compared with neutral or extended

postures (Edmondston et al. 2007). Rotation in the thoracic spine is essential for optimal functional movement; a stiff painfree thoracic spine may create excessive loading and mobility demands in adjacent regions which may ultimately become symptomatic. Being the longest and most anatomically complex region there has not been the development of reliable and valid measurement tools and most measurements rely on gross measures of the thoracic and lumbar spine combined (Heneghan & Rushton 2016).

For active physiological movements the spine will normally curve segmentally evenly and smoothly without areas of excessive or reduced movement. The clinician notes the:

- quality of the movement
- range of the movement
- behaviour of the pain through the range of movement
- provocation of any muscle spasm.

A movement diagram can be used to depict this information. The active movements with overpressure shown in Fig. 8.1 are tested with the patient in sitting. The clinician establishes the patient's symptoms at rest prior to each movement and corrects any movement deviation to determine its relevance to the patient's symptoms. If these movements do not reproduce symptoms and the clinician is searching for the patient's pain, then movements may be combined (Edwards 1992). The order in which movements are combined depends on the aggravating activities and the patient's response to primary movement. The patient actively performs the first (primary movement), the clinician maintains this position and passively adds the second movement. The patient reports any changes in symptoms (Fig. 8.1E and F).

Active movements of the thoracic spine and possible modifications are shown in Table 8.1. It is worth mentioning the work of Robin McKenzie. If all movements are full and symptom-free on overpressure, but symptoms are aggravated by certain postures and eased with postural correction, the condition is categorized as a postural syndrome (McKenzie & May 2006). If there are local, intermittent spinal symptoms with at least one movement and the restricted movement consistently produces concordant pain at end range with no reduction, abolition or peripheralization of

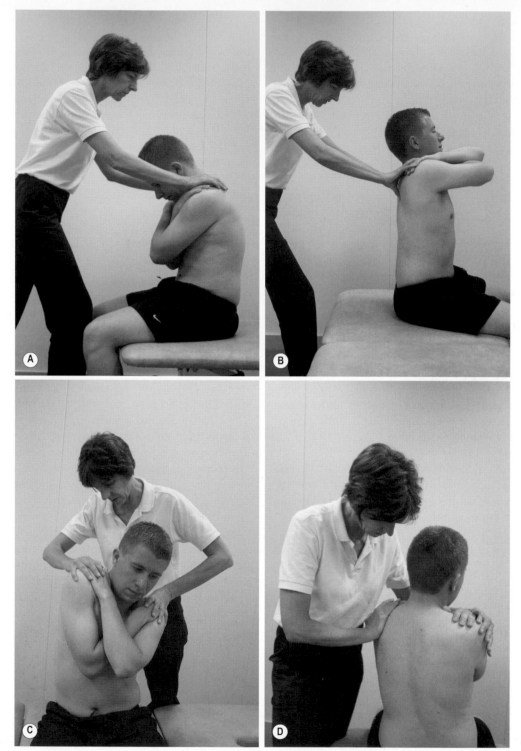

FIG. 8.1 ■ Overpressures to the thoracic spine. These movements are all carried out with the patient's arms crossed. (A) Flexion. Both hands on top of the shoulders, angle pressure down and posteriorly through the midthoracic spine to increase thoracic flexion. (B) Extension. Both hands on top of shoulders, angle pressure down and anteriorly through the sternum. The pelvis may be positioned into a posterior rotation to isolate extension to the thoracic spine. (C) Lateral flexion. Both hands on top of the shoulders, apply a force to increase thoracic lateral flexion. (D) Rotation. The right hand rests behind the patient's left shoulder and the left hand lies on the front of the right shoulder. Both hands then apply a force to increase right thoracic rotation.

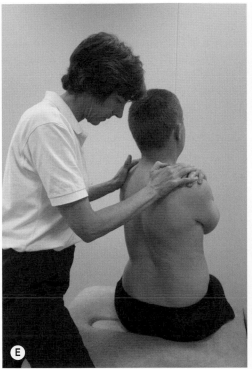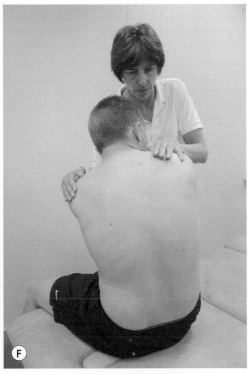

FIG. 8.1, cont'd ■ (E) Combined right rotation/extension. This movement is a combination of right rotation and extension. Both hands are placed on top of the shoulders; the patient then actively rotates – note the symptoms produced – the clinician then passively extends the thoracic spine as for extension overpressure and notes any change in symptoms. (F) Combined flexion/right rotation. Both hands are placed on top of the shoulders and a flexion force is localized to the thoracic spine. Note the symptoms produced. Maintaining flexion, both hands apply a right rotation. Note change in symptoms.

TABLE 8.1	
Active Movements and Possible Modifications	
Active Physiological Movements	**Modifications**
Thoracic spine	Repeated
Flexion	Speed altered
Extension	Combined (Edwards 1999)
Left lateral flexion	e.g.
Right lateral flexion	■ Flexion then rotation
Left rotation	■ Extension then rotation
Right rotation	Compression or distraction
Repetitive flexion (rep flex)	Sustained
Repetitive extension (rep ext)	Injuring movement
Repetitive rotation left (rep rot)	Differentiation tests
Repetitive rotation right (rep rot)	Function
?Cervical spine	
?Upper limb	
?Lumbar spine	
?Lower limbs	

symptoms, the condition is categorized as a dysfunction syndrome (McKenzie & May 2006). If on repeated movement, centralization or abolition of symptoms occurs and is maintained over time, this is characterized as a reducible derangement syndrome. Two types of derangement are described (Table 8.2).

Numerous differentiation tests can be performed; the choice depends on the patient's signs and symptoms. For example, when turning the head around to the left reproduces the patient's left-sided infrascapular pain, differentiation between the cervical and thoracic spine may be required. The clinician can increase and decrease the rotation at the cervical and thoracic regions to find out what effect this has on the infrascapular pain. The patient turns the head and trunk around to the left; the clinician maintains the position of the cervical spine and derotates the thoracic spine, noting

TABLE 8.2
Derangement Syndromes of the Thoracic Spine (McKenzie & May 2006)

Reducible Derangement

Centralization: in response to therapeutic loading strategies, pain is progressively abolished in a distal to proximal direction, and each progressive abolition is retained over time, until all symptoms are abolished

If back pain only is present this moves from a widespread to a more central location and then is abolished

Pain is decreased and then abolished during the application of therapeutic loading strategies

The change in pain location, or decrease or abolition of pain, remains better, and should be accompanied or preceded by improvements in the mechanical presentation (range of movement and/or deformity)

Irreducible Derangement

Peripheralization of symptoms: increase or worsening of distal symptoms in response to therapeutic loading strategies, and/or no decrease, abolition, or centralization of pain

---

the pain response. If symptoms remain the same or increase, this might suggest the cervical spine is the source of the symptoms. The position of cervical and thoracic rotation is then resumed and this time the clinician maintains the position of the thoracic spine and derotates the cervical spine to neutral, noting the pain response (Fig. 8.2A). If the symptoms remain the same or increase, this implicates the thoracic spine. It may be necessary to examine other regions to determine their relevance to the patient's symptoms as they may be the source of the symptoms, or they may be contributing to the symptoms (see relevant chapter).

Observation of Aggravating Functional Activities or Positions

Depending on the irritability, severity and nature of the symptoms it is important to observe at least one key functional restriction of the patient as this may be contributing to ongoing symptoms; it also ensures that

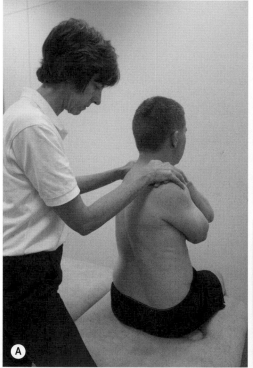
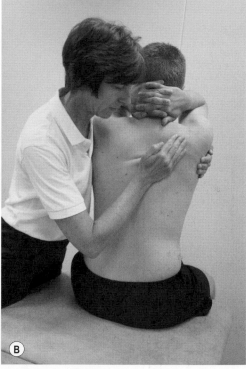

FIG. 8.2 ▪ Differentiation testing. (A) The clinician maintains right rotation of the thoracic spine while the patient returns the head to neutral. (B) Using a sustained natural apophyseal glide on T6 with left rotation, the clinician applies a cephalad posteroanterior glide to the T6 right transverse process while the patient moves into left rotation. Any changes in symptoms are noted.

you maintain a patient-focused perspective. Altering any impairments and noting the symptom response on retesting will guide further relevant testing. For example, a patient may have symptoms with rotation to the left; the clinician observes that this movement is performed in flexion. Placing the patient in a more neutral posture and repeating left rotation may reduce symptoms.

Symptom Modification

Symptom modifications are applied to the thoracic vertebrae or ribs whilst the patient performs a painful active movement. For example, a glide can be performed either centrally or unilaterally on a thoracic vertebra in the direction of the facet joint plane. If there is a reduction in pain, this segment is implicated as a source of the pain. Fig. 8.2B demonstrates a left rotation modification procedure on the T6 transverse process. In this example, the technique aims to facilitate the glide of the right inferior facet of T6 upwards on T7. This can then be used as a treatment technique (Mulligan 2010).

Passive Physiological Movements

These can take the form of passive physiological intervertebral movements (PPIVMs), which examine the movement at each segmental level. PPIVMs can be a useful adjunct to passive accessory intervertebral movements to identify segmental hypomobility and hypermobility. PPIVMs are usually performed in sitting for the midthoracic region. The clinician palpates between adjacent spinous processes or transverse processes to feel the range of intervertebral movement during thoracic flexion, extension, rotation and lateral flexion. Fig. 8.3 demonstrates PPIVMs for flexion of the thoracic spine. For a full description of PPIVMs, see Hengeveld and Banks (2013).

Muscle Tests

The muscles that need to be tested will depend on the area of symptoms and the functional aggravating movements. Because of the interdependence of this area this may include other regions.

Muscle Strength

The clinician may test the trunk flexors, extensors, lateral flexors and rotators and other relevant muscle

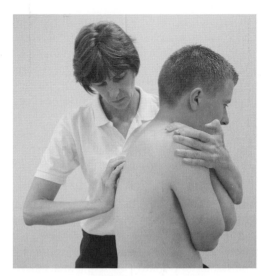

FIG. 8.3 ■ Passive physiological intervertebral movements for flexion of the thoracic spine. The clinician's right middle or index finger is placed in the gap between adjacent spinous processes and the patient is passively flexed by grasping around the thorax with the left hand.

groups as necessary. For details of these general tests readers are directed to Hislop et al. (2013), and Kendall et al. (2010). Details of strength testing are given in Chapter 3.

Muscle Control

The functional recruitment of muscles is considered to be more important than the overall strength of a muscle group (Sahrmann 2010). This is assessed initially by observing posture and the quality of movement, noting any changes in muscle recruitment patterns and by palpating the relevant muscles.

Movement impairment around the scapula has been described by a number of workers and may cause thoracic spine symptoms (Sahrmann 2010); these can be assessed by observation and modification of upper-limb movement impairments, noting the effect on symptoms.

The abdominal and thoracolumbar erector spinae which attach to the ribcage are the superficial muscles and are responsible for movement of this region. During trunk rotation it has been demonstrated via electromyogram (needle and surface electrodes) that the deeper muscles (i.e. laminar fibres of multifidus) are differentially active to the superficial muscles and have been shown to be less direction-specific and to be more variable in their activation, suggesting that they may have a role in segmental control. This differential activation between deep and superficial muscles has not been demonstrated with sagittal loading (Lee et al. 2005, 2011).

Observation and palpation can help identify changes in the balance of recruitment patterns which may result in thoracic spine and ribcage dysfunction.

These recruitment patterns can vary from:

- overactivity of superficial muscles, resulting in increased compression and reduced mobility of passive structures, to
- underactivity of deeper muscles, resulting in lack of stability or control of segmental movement (Lee et al. 2005, 2011).

Muscle Length

The clinician tests the length of muscles, in particular those thought prone to shorten (Janda 2002). Details of testing of the length of these muscles are given in Chapter 3.

Neurological Testing

This includes neurological integrity testing, neurodynamic tests and some other nerve tests.

Neurological Integrity

The distribution of symptoms will determine the appropriate neurological examination to be carried out. Symptoms confined to the midthoracic region require dermatome/cutaneous nerve testing only, since there is no myotome or reflex that can be tested. If symptoms spread proximally or distally, a neurological examination of the upper or lower limbs, respectively, is indicated (see Chapter 3).

Dermatomes/Peripheral Nerves. In the thoracic spine there is a great deal of overlap of the dermatomes and absence of one dermatome is unlikely to lead to a loss of sensation. Light touch and pain sensation are tested using cotton wool and pinprick, respectively (see Chapter 3). Knowledge of the cutaneous distribution of nerve roots (dermatomes) and peripheral nerves enables the clinician to distinguish sensory loss due to

a root lesion from that due to a peripheral nerve lesion. The cutaneous nerve distribution and dermatome areas are shown in Fig. 3.16.

Neurodynamic Tests

The following tests may be carried out in order to ascertain the degree to which neural tissue is responsible for the production of the patient's symptom(s):

- passive neck flexion
- upper-limb neural sensitization tests (in particular upper-limb neurodynamic test [ULNT] 3, which biases the ulnar nerve C8, T1)
- straight-leg raise
- slump (if symptoms are reproduced or increased when adding unilateral or bilateral knee extension and ankle dorsiflexion to an active thoracic spine movement, a neural component to the symptoms may be implicated).

These tests are described in detail in Chapter 3.

Central Nervous System Testing – Upper Motor Nerve Lesions

Plantar Response – Babinski's Sign (Fuller 2013). Pressure applied from the heel along the lateral border of the plantar aspect of the foot produces flexion of the toes in the normal individual. Extension of the big toe with downward fanning of the other toes occurs with an upper motor neuron lesion.

Clonus. Dorsiflex the ankle briskly, maintain the foot in that position and a rhythmic contraction may be found. More than three beats is considered abnormal.

Miscellaneous Tests

Respiration

There is a close relationship between the respiratory and musculoskeletal systems. Dysfunction in one can lead to dysfunction in the other (Hodges et al. 2001; Wirth et al. 2014). The importance of breathing retraining is becoming more widely recognized. Normal breathing function relies on correct postural alignment, thoracic and ribcage mobility and the absence of overdominance of accessory muscles (Innocenti & Troup 2008; Lee et al. 2010). Observation is key but costovertebral joint movement can be determined by measuring chest expansion. This may be particularly useful for conditions that include severe scoliosis and ankylosing spondylitis. A tape measure is placed around the chest at the fourth intercostal space. The patient is asked to exhale fully and pause and a measurement is taken; the patient is then asked to inhale fully and hold the breath while the second measurement is taken. The normal difference between exhalation and inhalation is 3–7.5 cm. Also ask the patient to take a deep breath and then to cough to determine if these actions reproduce the symptoms.

Vascular Tests

Tests for thoracic outlet syndrome are described in Chapter 9.

Palpation

The clinician palpates the thoracic spine and, if appropriate, the cervical/lumbar spine and upper/lower limbs. It is useful to record palpation findings on a body chart and/or palpation chart (see Fig. 3.35).

The clinician notes the following:

- the temperature of the area
- bony anomalies: increased or decreased prominence of bones; deviation of the spinous process from the centre; vertebral rotation – assessed by palpating the position of the transverse processes
- mobility and feel of superficial tissues, e.g. scarring
- muscle tone
- tenderness of bone and muscle trigger points (shown in Fig. 3.36)
- symptom reproduction (usually pain).

Passive Accessory Intervertebral Movements

It is useful to use the palpation chart and movement diagrams (or joint pictures) to record findings. These are explained in detail in Chapter 3.

The clinician notes the following:

- quality of movement
- range of movement
- resistance through the range and at the end of the range of movement
- behaviour of pain through the range
- any provocation of muscle spasm.

The thoracic spine (T1–T12) accessory movements and rib accessory movements are shown in Figs 8.4–8.6 and listed in Table 8.3. Accessory movements can then be tested in other regions suspected to be a source of, or contributing to, the patient's symptoms. Following accessory movements to the thoracic region, the clinician reassesses all the physical asterisks (movements or tests that have been found to reproduce the patient's symptoms) in order to establish the effect of the accessory movements on the patient's signs and symptoms.

EXAMINATION OF THE RIBCAGE

The ribs are strongly attached to the thoracic spine via the costovertebral and costotransverse joints and their associated ligaments. It may therefore be necessary to test these joints for mobility and pain provocation. Very few studies have been done on the biomechanics of the intact thoracic spine and ribcage. However, a model proposed by Lee (2003) is useful for clinical assessment. Lee proposes that movements of the rib joints are influenced by the mechanics of the thoracic spine. For example, flexion results in the inferior facet joint of the upper vertebra and its same-numbered rib gliding/rolling in a superior, anterior direction – a rib's mobility into flexion could therefore be palpated by applying a cephalad glide to it near the costotransverse joint (Fig. 8.5A). The reverse occurs with extension and the glide direction applied to the rib would be caudad. This is particularly applicable to the ribs that attach to the sternum (ribs 2–7). The lower ribs are less strongly attached to the thoracic spine and are therefore less influenced by thoracic spine movements.

A posteroanterior glide applied to the rib angle will test the anatomical structures that resist anterior translation of the rib. First, fix the contralateral transverse processes of the two vertebrae to which the rib is attached. For example, when applying a posteroanterior glide to the fourth rib on the right, fix T3 and T4 on the left (Fig. 8.5B). If no movement is allowed to occur at the thoracic spine and symptoms are reproduced the costal joints and ligaments are implicated.

Rib Mechanics During Respiration

During inspiration the first rib elevates, moving the manubrium into an anterior superior direction. A

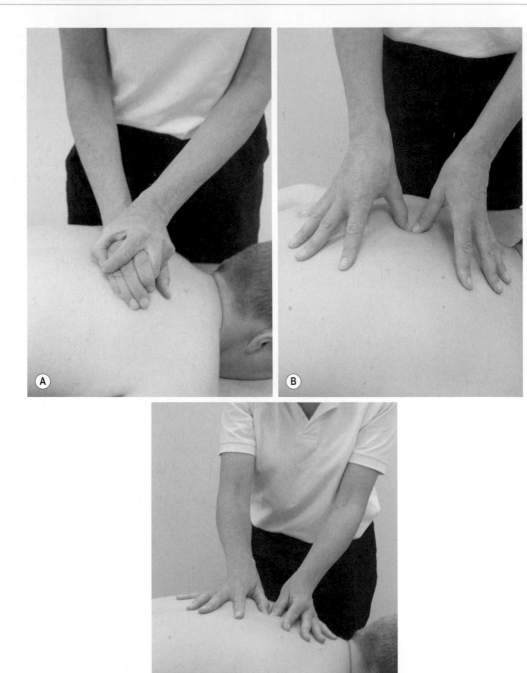

FIG. 8.4 ■ Thoracic spine (T1–T12) accessory movements. (A) Central posteroanterior. A pisiform grip is used to apply pressure to the spinous process. (B) Unilateral posteroanterior. Thumb pressure is applied to the transverse process. (C) Transverse. Thumb pressure is applied to the lateral aspect of the spinous process.

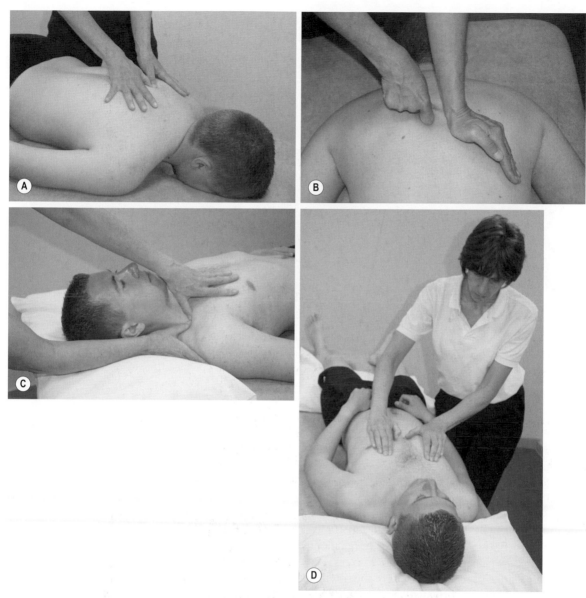

FIG. 8.5 ■ Accessory movements to ribs. (A) Unilateral posteroanterior cephalad glide. Thumb pressure is applied to the rib lateral to the costotransverse joint. (B) Posteroanterior glide. Thumb pressure is applied to the posterior aspect of the rib whilst the contralateral transverse processes of the vertebrae to which the rib is attached are fixed. (C) Longitudinal caudad glide first rib. Thumb pressure is applied to the superior aspect of the first rib and pressure is applied downwards towards the feet. Pressure can be applied anywhere along the superior aspect of the rib. The rib can also be motion-tested with respiration. (D) Motion testing of the sternal ribs (2–7) with respiration. Anteroposterior pressure can also be applied to the anterior aspect of the rib, testing for symptom reproduction and stiffness.

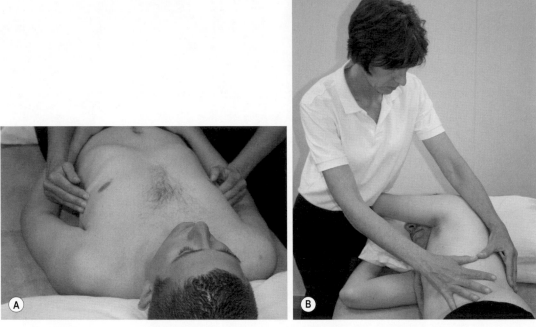

FIG. 8.6 ■ Rib lateral motion testing and accessory movement. (A) Motion testing to the lower ribs with lateral costal breathing. (B) A caudad glide is applied to the lateral part of the rib with the patient in side-lying. The thumb is placed along the line of the rib.

common dysfunction of the first and second ribs is when they remain in elevation. This can be caused by joint stiffness or scaleni overactivity. These ribs can be motion-tested by palpation with breathing and/or longitudinal caudad glides (Fig. 8.5C).

The biomechanics of ribs and thoracic spine during inspiration are largely the same as extension, whilst expiration and flexion are similar. Rib dysfunctions can be assessed by palpating rib mobility with respiration. The mechanics of the costal joints of the ribs that attach to the sternum are oriented largely to facilitate upward and superior movement of the sternum during inspiration – pump-handle motion (Levangie & Norkin 2011). The reverse occurs during expiration. The mobility of individual ribs can be palpated over the anterior ribcage whilst the patient is asked to breathe (Fig. 8.5D); this is best done in supine lying but can be assessed in functional positions. An anteroposterior glide will assess for pain provocation and mobility. Sternocostal and costochondral can be palpated anteriorly for tenderness.

The lower ribs have a more upward and lateral motion and increase the transverse diameter of the lower thorax during inspiration – bucket-handle motion (Levangie & Norkin 2011). Individual rib movement can be motion-tested by the clinician palpating laterally whilst asking the patient to do lateral costal breathing (Fig. 8.6A). A cephalad or caudad glide applied laterally along the rib will assess for mobility and pain provocation. This can be done with the patient in supine lying where both sides can be compared, or a more detailed assessment of the ribs laterally can be done with the patient in side-lying (Fig. 8.6B). Further details on a proposed model of rib dysfunction can be found in Magee (2014, Chapter 8).

COMPLETION OF THE EXAMINATION

■ At this stage the clinician highlights with an asterisk (*) important findings from the examination. These findings need to be reassessed at,

TABLE 8.3

Accessory Movements, Choice of Application and Reassessment of the Patient's Asterisks

Accessory Movements	Choice of Application	Identify any Effect of Accessory Movements on Patient's Signs and Symptoms
Thoracic Spine	*Start Position, e.g.*	*Reassess all Asterisks*
↕	Central posteroanterior	■ In flexion (with various cephalad/caudad angles)
⌐ ⌐	Unilateral posteroanterior	■ In extension (with various cephalad/caudad angles)
⇄	Transverse	■ In lateral flexion
Accessory Movements to Ribs 1–12	■ In flexion and rotation	
↔ Caud/ceph		■ In extension and rotation
↕	Anteroposterior	Speed of force application
↕	Posteroanterior	Direction of the applied force
Costochondral, Interchondral and Sternocostal Joints		
↕ Anteroposterior		
?Cervical spine	As above	Reassess all asterisks
?Upper-limb joints	As above	Reassess all asterisks
?Lumbar spine	As above	Reassess all asterisks
?Lower-limb joints	As above	Reassess all asterisks

and within, subsequent treatment sessions to evaluate the effects of treatment on the patient's condition. For full details, see Chapter 3.

■ The clinician should collate the information collected, reflect on the findings and compare them with the expected clinical presentation based on the initial primary hypothesis and alternative hypotheses. Aspects of the hypotheses categories may need reviewing or refining (Jones & Rivett 2004).

■ What can the patient do and what is the patient unable to do? How are the symptoms impacting on the patient's life?

■ What are the patient's beliefs? Are they helpful or unhelpful in terms of driving behaviours?

■ What is the source of symptoms? This includes the structure or tissue that is thought to be producing the patient's symptoms (e.g. arthrogenic, myogenic, neurogenic), the mechanism of the injury, the stage of the tissue-healing process and the pain mechanisms.

■ What are the contributing factors that have resulted in the development and maintenance of the problem? There may be environmental, psychosocial, behavioural, local or distant physical movement impairments or heredity factors.

■ Are there any precautions/contraindications to treatment and management? This includes the severity and irritability of the patient's symptoms and the nature of the patient's condition.

■ Where will initial management and treatment be focused?

■ Assessing the prognosis – this can be affected by factors such as the stage and extent of the injury as well as the patient's expectation, personality and lifestyle. Included in the prognosis should be an initial estimate of percentage improvement, the number of treatments required to achieve this and the time period for this to occur.

Before leaving the clinician needs to:

■ Explain the findings of the physical examination and how these findings relate to the subjective assessment. An attempt should be made to clear up any misconceptions patients may have regarding their illness or injury.

■ Allow patients sufficient opportunity to discuss their thoughts and beliefs after the examination and your explanation.

■ Collaborate with the patient and via problem solving together devise a treatment plan and discuss the prognosis, initially offering some advice if appropriate.

■ Warn the patient of possible exacerbation up to 24–48 hours following the examination.

■ Request the patient to report details on the behaviour of the symptoms following examination at the next attendance.

For guidance on treatment and management principles, the reader is directed to the companion textbook (Petty & Barnard 2017).

REFERENCES

Bogduk, N., Marsland, A., 1988. The cervical zygapophyseal joints as a source of neck pain. Spine 13, 610–617.

Brinjikjia, W., et al., 2014. Systematic literature review of imaging features of spinal degeneration in asymptomatic populations. AJNR Am. J. Neuroradiol. 36, 811–816.

Cloward, R.B., 1959. Cervical discography: a contribution to the etiology and mechanism of neck, shoulder and arm pain. Ann. Surg. 150, 1052–1064.

Dreyfuss, P., et al., 1994. Thoracic zygapophyseal joint pain patterns: a study in normal volunteers. Spine 19, 807–811.

Edmondston, S.J., et al., 2007. Influence of posture on the range of axial rotation and coupled lateral flexion of the thoracic spine. J. Manipulative Physiol. Ther. 30, 193–199.

Edmondston, S.J., Singer, K.P., 1997. Thoracic spine: anatomical and biomechanical considerations for manual therapy. Man. Ther. 2, 132–143.

Edwards, B.C., 1992. Manual of combined movements: their use in the examination and treatment of mechanical vertebral column disorders, second ed. Butterworth-Heinemann, Oxford.

Edwards, B.C., 1999. Manual of combined movements: their use in the examination and treatment of mechanical vertebral column disorders, second ed. Butterworth-Heinemann, Oxford.

Fuller, G., 2013. Neurological examination made easy, fifth ed. Churchill Livingstone, Edinburgh.

Gifford, L., 1996. The clinical biology of aches and pains (course manual), fifth ed. Neuro-Orthopaedic Institute UK, Falmouth.

Heneghan, N.R., Rushton, A., 2016. Understanding why the thoracic region is the 'Cinderella' region of the spine. Man. Ther. 21, 274–276.

Hengeveld, E., Banks, K., 2013. Maitland's vertebral manipulation: management of neuromusculoskeletal disorders, vol. 1, eighth ed. Churchill Livingstone, Edinburgh (Chapter 5).

Hislop, H., et al., 2013. Daniels and Worthingham's muscle testing: techniques of manual examination and performance testing, nineth ed. W.B. Saunders, Philadelphia.

Hodges, P.W., et al., 2001. Postural activity in the diaphragm is reduced in humans when respiratory demand increases. J. Physiol. (Lond.) 537, 999–1008.

Innocenti, D.M., Troup, F., 2008. Dysfunctional breathing. In: Pryor, J.A., Prasad, A.S. (Eds.), Physiotherapy for respiratory and cardiac problems: adults and paediatrics, fourth ed. Churchill Livingstone, Edinburgh.

Janda, V., 2002. Muscles and motor control in cervicogenic disorders. In: Grant, R. (Ed.), Physical therapy of the cervical and thoracic spine, third ed. Churchill Livingstone, New York, p. 182.

Jones, M.A., Rivett, D.A., 2004. Clinical reasoning for manual therapists. Butterworth-Heinemann, Edinburgh.

Kendall, F.P., et al., 2010. Muscles testing and function, fifth ed. Lippincott Williams and Wilkins, Baltimore.

Lee, D., 2003. The thorax: an integrated approach, second ed. Orthopedic Physical Therapy, White Rock, BC, Canada.

Lee, L.J., 2013. Thoracic ring control: a missing link? MPA In Touch 4: 13–16.

Lee, L.J., et al., 2010. Changes in sitting induce multiplanar changes in chest wall shape and motion in breathing. Respir. Physiol. Neurobiol. 170, 236–245.

Lee, L.J., et al., 2005. Differential activation of the thoracic multifidus and longissimus thoracis during trunk rotation. Spine 30, 870–876.

Lee, L.J., et al., 2011. En bloc control of deep and superficial thoracic muscles in sagittal loading and unloading of the trunk. Gait Posture 33, 588–593.

Levangie, P.K., Norkin, C.C., 2011. Joint structure and function. A comprehensive analysis, fifth ed. F.A. Davis, Philadelphia (Chapter 5).

Magee, D.J., 2014. Orthopedic physical assessment, sixth ed. W.B. Saunders, Philadelphia (Chapter 8).

McKenzie, R.A., May, S.J., 2006. The cervical and thoracic spine: mechanical diagnosis and therapy, second ed. Spinal Publications New Zealand, Waikanae, New Zealand.

Mellion, L.R., Ladeiro, C., 2001. The herniated thoracic disc: a review of the literature. J. Man. Manip. Ther. 9, 154–163.

Mulligan, B.R., 2010. Manual therapy 'NAGs', 'SNAGs', 'MWMs' etc., sixth ed. Plane View Services, New Zealand.

Oda, I., et al., 2002. An in vitro human cadaveric study investigating the biomechanical properties of the thoracic spine. Spine 27, E64–E70.

Petty, N.J., Barnard, K., 2017. Principles of musculoskeletal treatment and management: a handbook for therapists, third ed. Elsevier, Edinburgh.

Sahrmann, S.A., 2010. Movement system impairment syndromes of the extremities, cervical and thoracic spines. Mosby, St Louis.

Wirth, B., et al., 2014. Respiratory dysfunction in patients with chronic neck pain – influence of thoracic spine and chest mobility. Man. Ther. 19, 440–444.

9

EXAMINATION OF THE SHOULDER REGION

COLETTE RIDEHALGH ■ KEVIN HALL

CHAPTER CONTENTS

INTRODUCTION

Pain in the shoulder region can be due to local structures, spinally referred pain or from referral from non-musculoskeletal conditions – masqueraders (Grieve 1994). Some of these masqueraders may be red flags which will require urgent medical attention (e.g. neoplasm). The differentiation process is therefore of great importance and needs to be considered from the outset.

Local structures potentially responsible for symptoms include: the sternoclavicular, acromioclavicular and glenohumeral joints and their surrounding soft tissues. Particular conditions include:

- trauma which may result in a number of soft-tissue and bony injuries, including:
  - fracture of the clavicle, humerus or scapula
  - dislocation of one of the above joints
  - ligamentous sprain
  - muscular strain
  - rotator cuff tear
- tendinopathy, particularly of the rotator cuff or long head of biceps
- spontaneous conditions, e.g. adhesive capsulitis and rupture of the long head of biceps
- bursitis
- instability
- impingement
- osteoarthritis
- inflammatory disorders, e.g. rheumatoid arthritis:
  - referred pain
  - referral of pain from the cervical spine or thoracic spine
- thoracic outlet syndrome
- red flags and masqueraders

- infection, e.g. tuberculosis
- neoplasm
- referral from the viscera, e.g. lungs, heart, diaphragm, gallbladder and spleen (Brown 1983).

Further details of the questions asked during the subjective examination and the tests carried out in the physical examination can be found in Chapters 2 and 3, respectively.

The order of the subjective questioning and the physical tests described below can be altered as appropriate for the patient being examined.

SUBJECTIVE EXAMINATION

Patients' Perspectives on Their Experience

It is essential that the patients' narrative is considered. Their experience of the events that have occurred and are still occurring will have a significant impact on their outcome to treatment. It will also enable the clinician to understand better patients' perspectives on not only what they think is the problem, but also on their expectations of the clinician.

Any social history that is relevant to the onset and progression of the patient's problem will be recorded. This includes the patient's employment status, home situation and details of any leisure/sporting activities. The age, gender and ethnicity of patients and their cultural, occupational and social backgrounds may all affect their attitudes and feelings towards themselves, their condition and the clinician. The clinician needs to be aware of, and sensitive to, these attitudes, and to empathize and communicate appropriately so as to develop a rapport with the patient and thereby enhance the patient's compliance with the treatment.

Factors from this information may indicate direct or indirect mechanical influences on the management of the patient and the prognosis. In order to treat the patient appropriately, it is important that the condition is managed within the context of the patient's social and work environment.

The clinician may ask the following types of questions to elucidate psychosocial factors:

- Have you had time off work in the past with your pain?
- What do you understand to be the cause of your pain?
- What are you expecting will help you?
- How is your employer/co-workers/family responding to your pain?
- What are you doing to cope with your pain?
- Do you think you will return to work? When?

Although these questions are described in relation to psychosocial risk factors for poor outcomes for patients with low-back pain (Waddell 2004), they may be relevant to patients with shoulder pain. Research on prognostic indicators suggests that recovery from shoulder conditions can be affected by high levels of disability and pain at onset, educational background and the number of comorbidities present (Chester et al. 2013; Dunn et al. 2014).

Body Chart

The following information concerning the type and area of current symptoms can be recorded on a body chart (see Fig. 2.3).

Area of Current Symptoms

Be exact when mapping out the area of the symptoms. Symptoms from the glenohumeral joint are commonly felt commonly felt over the anterior deltoid, often extending into the region of the distal deltoid and into the biceps. Acromioclavicular and sternoclavicular joint lesions are often felt locally around the joint, although it is not uncommon for the acromioclavicular joint to refer pain proximally over the area of the upper trapezius. Ascertain which is the worst symptom and record where the patient feels the symptoms are coming from.

Areas Relevant to the Region Being Examined

All other relevant areas are checked for symptoms; it is important to ask about pain or even stiffness, as this may be relevant to the patient's main symptom. Mark unaffected areas with ticks (✓) on the body chart. Check for symptoms in the cervical spine, thoracic spine, elbow, wrist and hand.

Quality of Pain

Establish the quality of the pain. Catching pain or arcs of pain are typical of impingement-related problems around the shoulder. Clunking felt within the shoulder joint may indicate labral pathology or instability.

Intensity of Pain

The intensity of pain can be measured using, for example, a visual analogue scale, as shown in Fig. 2.5.

Abnormal Sensation

Check for any altered sensation locally around the shoulder region as well as over the spine and distally in the arm.

Constant or Intermittent Symptoms

Ascertain the frequency of the symptoms, whether they are constant or intermittent. If symptoms are constant, check whether there is variation in the intensity of the symptoms, as constant unremitting pain may be indicative of more serious pathology.

Relationship of Symptoms

Determine the relationship between symptomatic areas – do they come together or separately? For example, the patient may have shoulder pain without neck pain, or the pains may always be present together. This is a critical element of the examination as there is such a close relationship between the spine and shoulder region.

Behaviour of Symptoms

Aggravating Factors

For each symptomatic area a series of questions can be asked:

- What movements, activities or positions bring on or make the patient's symptoms worse?
- How long does it take before symptoms are aggravated?
- Is the patient able to maintain this position or movement?
- What happens to other symptoms when this symptom is produced or made worse?
- How do the symptoms affect function, e.g. reaching, dressing, overhead activities, sport and social activities?
- Does the patient have a feeling of instability in the shoulder?

The clinician also asks the patient about theoretically known aggravating factors for structures that could be a source of the symptoms. Common aggravating factors for the shoulder are hand behind back, above-head activities, lifting and lying on the shoulder. Aggravating factors for other regions, which may need to be queried if they are suspected to be a source of the symptoms, are shown in Table 2.2.

Detailed information on each of the aggravating activities is useful in order to help determine the structures at fault and identify functional restrictions. This information can be used to determine the aims of treatment and any advice that may be required. The most notable functional restrictions are highlighted with asterisks (*), explored in the physical examination and reassessed at subsequent treatment sessions to evaluate treatment intervention.

Easing Factors

For each symptomatic area a series of questions can be asked to help determine what eases the symptoms:

- What movements and/or positions ease the patient's symptoms?
- How long does it take before symptoms are eased? If symptoms are constant but variable it is important to know what the baseline is and how long it takes for the symptoms to reduce to that level.
- What happens to other symptoms when this symptom is eased?

Twenty-Four-Hour Behaviour of Symptoms

The clinician determines the 24-hour behaviour of symptoms by asking questions about night, morning and evening symptoms.

Night Symptoms. The following questions may be asked:

- Do you have any difficulty getting to sleep?
- What position is most comfortable/uncomfortable?
- What is your normal sleeping position?
- What is your present sleeping position?
- Can you lie on the affected shoulder?
- Do your symptoms wake you at night? If so, which symptom(s)?
- How many times in the past week?
- How many times in a night?
- How long does it take to get back to sleep?
- How many and what type of pillows are used?

Morning and Evening Symptoms. The clinician determines the pattern of the symptoms first thing in the morning, through the day and at the end of the day. Morning stiffness that lasts more than 2 hours is suggestive of an inflammatory condition such as rheumatoid arthritis. Stiffness lasting only 30 minutes or less is likely to be mechanical or degenerative in nature.

Stage of the Condition

In order to determine the stage of the condition, the clinician asks whether the symptoms are getting better, getting worse or remaining unchanged.

Special Questions

Special questions must always be asked, as they may identify certain precautions or contraindications to the physical examination and/or treatment (Table 2.4). As mentioned in Chapter 2, the clinician must differentiate between conditions that are suitable for conservative management and systemic, neoplastic and other non-musculoskeletal conditions, which require referral to a medical practitioner. The reader is referred to Chapter 2 for details of serious pathological processes that can mimic musculoskeletal conditions.

Previous Shoulder Dislocation

If the patient has a history of previous dislocation, care must be taken during the physical examination, e.g. for anterior dislocation the clinician should take care when positioning the shoulder in lateral rotation and abduction.

Neurological Symptoms

Has the patient experienced symptoms of spinal cord compression, which are bilateral tingling in the hands or feet and/or disturbance of gait? Does the patient complain of gross weakness or altered sensation in the arm? This may indicate more than one level of nerve root compression at the cervical spine. Does the patient complain of altered sensation in the arm during abduction and lateral rotation, e.g. throwing activities? This may indicate anterior shoulder instability (Hill et al. 2008).

Vascular Symptoms

Does the patient complain of coldness, change in colour or loss of sensation in the arm or hands? Does the patient get symptoms when the arms are raised or if working with the arms overhead? This may indicate a vascular problem and will need further testing (e.g. thoracic outlet syndrome).

Cervical Artery Dysfunction (CAD)

This is relevant where there are symptoms of pain, discomfort and/or altered sensation emanating from the cervical spine, where CAD may be the source of symptoms. Further questions and testing for CAD are described more fully in Chapter 6.

History of the Present Condition

For each symptomatic area the clinician needs to know how long the symptom has been present, whether there was a sudden or slow onset and whether there was a known cause that provoked the onset of the symptom. If the onset was slow, the clinician finds out if there has been any change in the patient's lifestyle, e.g. a new job or hobby or a change in sporting activity; this may have contributed to the patient's condition. To confirm the relationship of the symptoms, the clinician asks what happened to other symptoms when each symptom began.

The clinician should ask whether the patient has a history of spontaneous dislocation/subluxation or a history of voluntary dislocation/subluxation (party trick movements).

Has the patient taken any medication for the pain, and if so what was its effect?

Past Medical History

The following information is obtained from the patient and/or the medical notes:

- The details of any relevant medical history.
- The history of any previous shoulder pain: how many episodes? When were they? What was the cause? What was the duration of each episode? And did the patient fully recover between episodes? If there has been no previous history of shoulder pain, has the patient had any episodes of stiffness in the cervical spine, thoracic spine, shoulder or any other relevant region? Check for a history of trauma or recurrent minor trauma.
- Ascertain the results of any past treatment for the same or a similar problem. Past treatment records may be obtained for further information

General Health

The clinician ascertains the state of the patient's general health, and finds out if the patient suffers from any cough, breathlessness, chest pain, malaise, fatigue, fever, nausea or vomiting, stress, anxiety or depression. Symptoms in the shoulder may be referred from the lungs, pleura, heart, diaphragm, gallbladder and spleen (Brown 1983).

Weight Loss

Has the patient noticed any recent unexplained weight loss?

Rheumatoid Arthritis

Has the patient (or a member of the family) been diagnosed as having rheumatoid arthritis?

Drug Therapy

What drugs are being taken by the patient? Has the patient been prescribed long-term (6 months or more) medication/steroids? Has the patient been taking anticoagulants?

Further Investigations

Has the patient been X-rayed or had any other medical tests recently? The medical tests may include blood tests, magnetic resonance imaging (MRI), diagnostic ultrasound, arthroscopy and arthrogram.

Plan of the Physical Examination

When all this information has been collected, the subjective examination is complete. It is useful at this stage to highlight with asterisks (*), for ease of reference, important findings and particularly one or more functional restrictions. These can then be reexamined at subsequent treatment sessions to evaluate treatment intervention.

In order to plan the physical examination, the following hypotheses need to be developed from the subjective examination:

- The regions and structures that should be examined as a possible source of the symptoms, e.g. rotator cuff, glenohumeral joint, cervical spine. Often it is not possible to examine fully at the first attendance and so examination of the

structures must be prioritized over subsequent treatment sessions.
- Other contributing factors that should be examined, e.g. instability, posture, muscle control and sporting technique, such as service and strokes for tennis.
- In what way should the physical tests be carried out? Will it be easy or hard to reproduce each symptom? Will it be necessary to use combined movements or repetitive movements to reproduce the patient's symptoms?
- Are symptoms severe and/or irritable? If symptoms are severe, physical tests may be carried out to just before the onset of symptom production or just to the onset of symptom production; no overpressures will be carried out, as the patient would be unable to tolerate this. If symptoms are irritable, physical tests may be examined to just before symptom production or just to the onset of provocation, with fewer physical tests being examined to allow for a rest period between tests.
- Are there any precautions or contraindications to elements of the physical examination that need to be explored further, e.g. cervical artery dysfunction, neurological involvement, cardiac problems?

A physical examination planning form can be useful for clinicians to help guide them through the clinical reasoning process (see Fig. 2.9).

Physical Examination

The information from the subjective examination helps the clinician to plan an appropriate physical examination. The severity, irritability and nature of the condition are the major factors that will influence the choice and priority of physical testing procedures. The first and overarching question the clinician might ask is: 'Is this patient's condition suitable for me to manage as a therapist?' The second question the clinician might ask is: 'Does this patient have a musculoskeletal dysfunction that I may be able to help?' To answer that, the clinician needs to carry out a full physical examination; however, this may not be possible if the symptoms are severe and/or irritable. If the patient's symptoms are severe and/or irritable, the clinician aims to explore movements as much as possible, within a symptom-free range. If the patient has constant and severe and/or irritable symptoms, then the clinician aims to find physical tests that ease the symptoms. If the patient's symptoms are non-severe and non-irritable, then the clinician aims to find physical tests that reproduce each of the patient's symptoms.

Each significant physical test that either provokes or eases the patient's symptoms is highlighted in the patient's notes by an asterisk (*) for easy reference. The highlighted tests are often referred to as 'asterisks' or 'markers'.

The order and detail of the physical tests described below need to be appropriate to the patient being examined. It is important that readers understand that the techniques shown in this chapter are only some of many examination techniques available. They represent some of the most commonly used techniques. The clinician is encouraged to consider the validity and reliability of all tests used. A brief mention of these issues follows the description of each test in the following text.

Observation

Informal Observation

The clinician needs to observe the patient in dynamic and static situations; the quality of movement is noted, as are the postural characteristics and facial expression. Informal observation will have begun from the moment the clinician begins the subjective examination and will continue to the end of the physical examination.

Formal Observation

Observation. The clinician examines the posture of the patient in sitting and standing, noting the posture of the shoulders, head and neck, thoracic spine and upper limbs. The clinician also notes bony and soft-tissue contours around the region. The clinician examines the muscle bulk and muscle tone of the patient, comparing left and right sides. It must be remembered that handedness and level and frequency of physical activity may well produce differences in muscle bulk between sides. The clinician may check the alignment of the head of the humerus with the acromion as this can give clues about possible mechanical insufficiencies. The clinician pinch-grips the anterior and posterior edges of the acromion with one hand and with the other hand pinch-grips the anterior and posterior aspects of the humerus. It is generally thought that, normally, no more than one-third of the humeral head lies anterior to the acromion. The clinician passively corrects any asymmetry to determine its relevance to the patient's problem.

It is worth noting that pure postural dysfunction rarely influences one region of the body in isolation and it may be necessary to observe the patient more fully for a full postural examination.

Active Physiological Movements

For active physiological movements (Table 9.1), the clinician notes:

- quality of movement
- range of movement
- behaviour of pain through the range of movement
- resistance through the range of movement and at the end of the range of movement
- provocation of any muscle spasm.

A movement diagram can be used to depict this information. The active movements with overpressure are shown in Fig. 9.1 and can be tested with the patient in standing and/or sitting. Movements are carried out on the left and right sides. The clinician establishes the patient's symptoms at rest, prior to each movement and corrects any movement deviation to determine its relevance to the patient's symptoms. Physiological movements can be examined in isolation or combined to provoke symptoms in presentations that are non-severe and non-irritable. The physiological movements that the clinician chooses to combine should be guided by the aggravating factors from the subjective examination.

Once a symptomatic movement has been identified the clinician can apply shoulder symptom modification procedures (SSMPs) (Lewis 2009, 2016) in an attempt to restore painfree movement. The symptomatic movement can be a planar physiological movement, a combined movement or any functional activity described by the patient in the subjective examination (aggravating factors). Once the pain-provoking movement has been established the clinician can investigate the effect of applying an SSMP to that movement and

TABLE 9.1	
Active Physiological Movements and Possible Modifications	
Active Physiological Movements	Modifications
Shoulder girdle	Repeated
Elevation	Speed altered
Depression	Combined, e.g.
Protraction	■ Abduction with medial or lateral rotation
Retraction	■ Medial/lateral rotation with flexion
Glenohumeral joint	
Flexion	Compression or distraction to scapulothoracic, glenohumeral or acromioclavicular joints
Extension	
Abduction	
Adduction	
Medial rotation	Sustained
Lateral rotation	Injuring movement
Hand behind neck (HBN)	Differentiation tests
Hand behind back (HBB)	Functional ability
Horizontal flexion	
Horizontal extension	
?Cervical spine	
?Thoracic spine	
?Elbow	
?Wrist and hand	

notes how symptoms are affected. SSMPs include thoracic posture, scapular position and humeral head position. The clinician applies an SSMP and asks the patient to repeat the pain-provoking movement. If the pain is lessened by the application of the SSMP then the clinician notes the extent of pain relief and moves on to the next SSMP in a systematic way. For example, if active abduction reproduces 5/10 pain at 90° and this is reduced to 2/10 by reducing the patient's thoracic kyphosis, then this is noted by the clinician and may be incorporated into the exercise and treatment regime. The clinician will then go on to repeat abduction with scapular facilitation, and modification of the head of humerus position to see if symptoms can be reduced further or eliminated completely (Fig. 9.2). If the symptoms improve with the addition of these assessment techniques then the technique becomes part of the treatment programme. Multiple techniques can be used for a patient if indicated by the pain response. For a fuller description of SSMPs, see Lewis (2009, 2016).

It may be necessary to examine other regions to determine their relevance to the patient's symptoms; they may be the source of the symptoms, or they may be contributing to the symptoms. The most likely regions are the shoulder, sternoclavicular joint, cervical spine, thoracic spine, elbow, wrist and hand. The joints within these regions can be tested fully (see Chapter 7) or partially with the use of screening tests (see Chapter 3 for further details).

Some functional ability has already been tested by general observation of the patient during the subjective and physical examinations, e.g. the postures adopted during the subjective examination and the ease or difficulty of undressing prior to the examination. Any further functional testing can be carried out at this point in the examination and may include various sitting postures or aggravating movements of the upper limb. Clues for appropriate tests can be obtained from the subjective examination findings, particularly aggravating factors.

Capsular Pattern

Cyriax (1982) described the capsular pattern of the glenohumeral joint as a limitation of lateral rotation, abduction and medial rotation. Historically a capsular pattern has been used to describe conditions relating to pathology of the capsule (frozen shoulder), stiffness following immobilization and osteoarthritis of the glenohumeral joint. However, this creates some confusion as osteoarthritis is a multitissue pathology involving bony and soft tissue structures. For this reason a better term to describe conditions which result in multidirectional stiffness of the glenohumeral joint would be a 'stiff shoulder'. Conditions that present with multidirectional stiffness include frozen shoulder contracture syndrome (FSCS), osteoarthritis of the glenohumeral joint, osteochondromatosis and, on very rare occasions, neoplasm. FSCS is a common condition which presents as shoulder pain and stiffness in patients around the age of 50 years. Bunker (2009) and Lewis (2015) describe a simple diagnostic process whereby FSCS is suspected if there is a restriction of active and passive external rotation in equal amounts and a normal X-ray. A thorough description of the aetiology, diagnosis and management can be found in Lewis (2015).

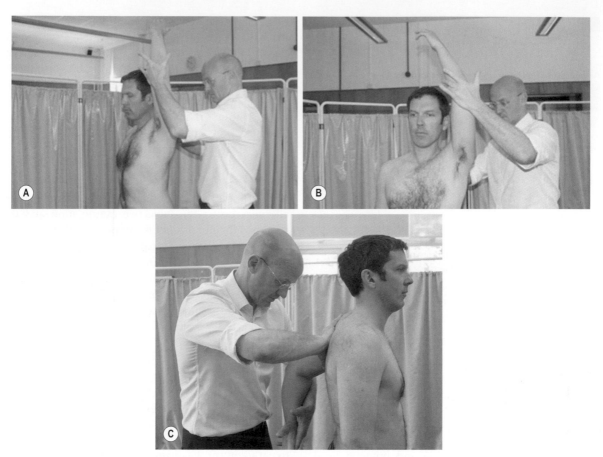

FIG. 9.1 ▪ Active movements with overpressure. (A) Flexion: apply pressure on the humerus into flexion whilst stabilizing the scapula. (B) Overpressure into a functional position of abduction and lateral rotation: with the patient's arm in HBH position, apply further pressure into combined flexion, abduction and lateral rotation individually to test each component of the movement. (C) Hand behind back (HBB): with the patient's arm in HBB position, apply further pressure into medial rotation, adduction and extension individually to test each component of the movement.

Passive Physiological Movements

All the active movements described above can usually be examined passively with the patient in the supine position, comparing left and right sides. In addition, medial and lateral rotation of the scapula can be examined. A comparison of the response of symptoms to the active and passive movements can help to determine whether the structure at fault is non-contractile (articular) or contractile (extraarticular) (Cyriax 1982). If the lesion is non-contractile, such as ligament, then active and passive movements will be

painful and/or restricted in the same direction. If the lesion is in a contractile tissue (i.e. muscle), active and passive movements are painful and/or restricted in opposite directions.

Posterior Shoulder Tightness

Posterior shoulder tightness has been linked to several pathologies of the shoulder, including tendinopathy, labral pathology and subacromial pain syndrome (SAPS) (Dashottar & Borstad 2012). Supporting evidence has emerged from cadaveric studies that have

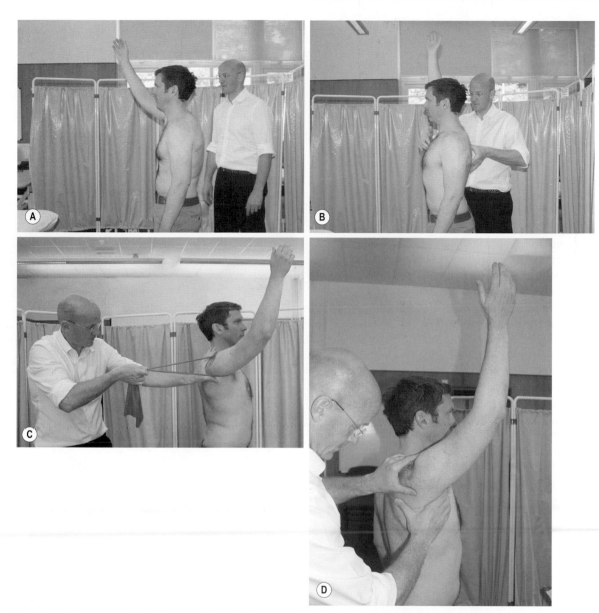

FIG. 9.2 ■ Symptom modification procedure. (A) Note restriction in shoulder flexion with thoracic spine in kyphosed position. (B) Increased shoulder flexion with change in posture. (C) Applying an anteroposterior glide to the humeral head using Thera-Band. (D) Scapular facilitation.

experimentally shortened the posterior capsule and observed a translation of the humeral head with glenohumeral joint movement. This translation is thought to cause irritation of local soft-tissue structures.

Posterior shoulder tightness can be assessed using three clinical tests. Validity of these tests is supported by cadaveric research that has measured strain in the posterior capsule with different movements of the shoulder (Borstad & Dashottar 2011). The three tests are:

1. Supine internal rotation in 90° abduction (Fig. 9.3). The scapula is stabilized through the coracoid process and the angle of internal rotation is measured (maintaining 90° shoulder abduction). Reliability values of intratester intraclass correlation coefficient (ICC) of 0.81 have been reported (Wilk et al. 2011).
2. Horizontal adduction (Fig. 9.4). The lateral border of the scapula is stabilized with the clinician's caudad hand and the glenohumeral joint is moved into horizontal adduction, maintaining neutral rotation. The clinician records the angle the humerus makes with the vertical. Reliability values of intratester ICC of 0.91 have been reported (Laudner et al. 2006).
3. Low flexion (Fig. 9.5). With the patient supine and with 90° of elbow flexion, the arm is elevated to 60° flexion and then internally rotated to end of range. The angle the arm makes with the horizontal is measured. Reliability values of

intertester ICC of 0.90–0.96 have been reported (Borstad et al. 2015).

For all three tests the range in the symptomatic arm is compared with the range in the asymptomatic arm. The greater the difference between the contralateral shoulder and the symptomatic shoulder, the more significant the findings.

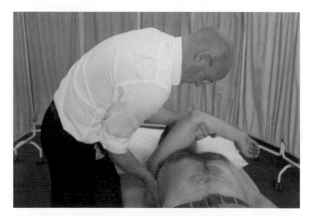

FIG. 9.4 ▪ Horizontal adduction.

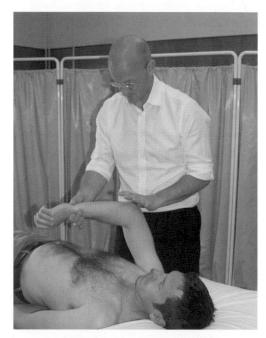

FIG. 9.5 ▪ Low flexion test.

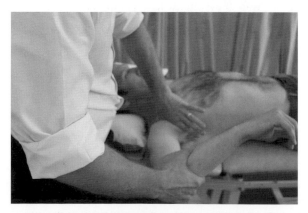

FIG. 9.3 ▪ Supine internal rotation in 90° abduction.

In the next few sections there will be discussion regarding the clinical diagnosis of different shoulder conditions. These conditions are based on a pathoanatomical diagnosis, that is, the presence of structural pathology within the shoulder. We will describe tests that can be performed in the examination to aid in the diagnosis of each condition, e.g. rotator cuff pathology, and we will comment on the ability of these tests to identify the condition when it is present (specificity) or to exclude it when absent (sensitivity). The diagnostic accuracy of clinical tests in identifying anatomical structures responsible for symptoms, however, is fraught with difficulty. The result of a test (positive or negative) must be compared to a gold-standard investigation, usually ultrasound, MRI or surgical observation, that visualizes the structure in question to determine if the structural pathology is present. A comparison is then made with the results of the orthopaedic test to determine its accuracy. One of the problems is that these investigations/procedures are not 100% accurate at identifying the pathology in question. Further complicating the issue of the structural diagnosis is the high incidence of pathology in asymptomatic shoulders, so lots of people without pain have changes that will be identified through imaging or at surgery. So, if the structure is asymptomatic in so many cases, how do we know it is the cause of symptoms in this patient? This lack of certainty means that the results of these tests should be interpreted with caution and careful consideration of the subjective history of the patient.

Joint Integrity Tests

Instability is a common but complex area. The definitions and classifications of shoulder instability are varied and have historically been related to being traumatic or atraumatic, but this has not allowed for the complexities of understanding the many factors responsible for the continuation of symptoms relating to instability that many people face. Gerber and Ganz (1984) described a continuum of instability from translation ('some pain or discomfort when I lift') to subluxation ('it feels like it's going to come out') to dislocation ('shoulder comes out'). More recently a classification system has been developed which incorporates the complex presentation and causes of continuing instability (Fig. 9.6) (Lewis et al. 2004). The

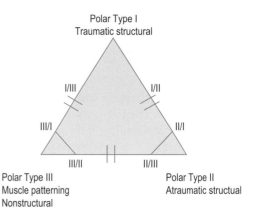

FIG. 9.6 ■ Stanmore triangle. *(Modified from Lewis et al. 2004.)*

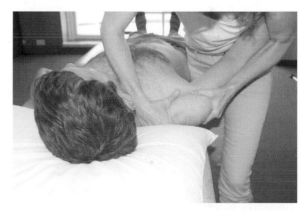

FIG. 9.7 ■ Anterior shoulder drawer test.

system allows for individuals to be considered in relation to the most predominant features of the condition, e.g. they may have had a traumatic dislocation (polar type I) but also have a muscle patterning dysfunction (polar type III). The following tests predominantly move the glenohumeral joint towards the direction of the instability and therefore should be used with caution and common sense. They are not suitable when a patient has recently had a dislocation.

Anterior Shoulder Instability

Anterior Shoulder Drawer Test (Gerber & Ganz 1984) *(Fig. 9.7).* With the patient supine and the shoulder in abduction (80–120°), forward flexion (0–20°) and lateral rotation (0–30°), the clinician stabilizes the scapula and glides the humerus anteriorly. Excessive movement, a click and/or patient apprehension suggest that there is anterior shoulder instability.

Apprehension Test (Fig. 9.8). With the patient supine, the clinician takes the shoulder into 90° abduction and adds lateral rotation. The test is considered positive – indicating anterior instability – if the patient becomes apprehensive. Further confirmation can be achieved by using the relocation test (Jobe et al. 1989), where an anteroposterior force is applied to the head of the humerus (using the heel of the hand); apprehension is lessened and the clinician is able to take the shoulder further into lateral rotation. It has been proposed by Lo et al. (2004) that an additional component can be added to the test – a quick release of the posteriorly directed force. This so-called surprise test, taken with the findings of the apprehension and relocation test, has been shown to have a positive predictive value of 93.6% and negative predictive value of 71.9% (Lo et al. 2004), but will only be safe to use in a very limited numbers of cases. All three tests have been shown to have strong specificity. Overall the apprehension test has the strongest diagnostic odds ratio (53.6), suggesting a good strength of association between the test and the condition (Hegedus et al. 2012)

Load and Shift Test (Fig. 9.9). With the patient in sitting or supine the clinician stabilizes the scapula and applies a posteroanterior force to the humeral head whilst palpating the joint line to assess the amount of movement. This test can be graded from 0 to 3, with 0 being no movement and 3 being full dislocation. This can also be used as a test for posterior instability with the direction of force applied in a posterior direction. The test has been found to have a specificity of 100% and a sensitivity of 50% (Tzannes & Murrell 2002).

Posterior Shoulder Instability

There are relatively few studies which describe tests for posterior instability. Gerber and Ganz (1984) described the load and shift test (as described above) and posterior drawer tests.

Posterior Drawer Test (Fig. 9.10). With the patient lying supine, the arm is flexed between 80 and 120°,

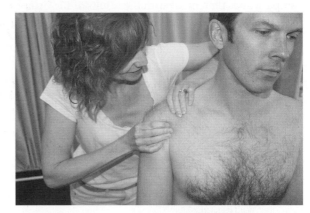

FIG. 9.9 ■ Load and shift test.

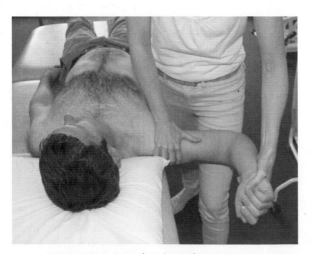

FIG. 9.8 ■ Apprehension/relocation test.

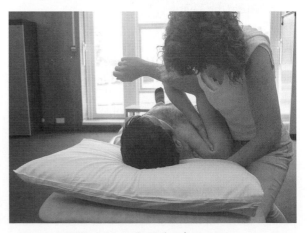

FIG. 9.10 ■ Posterior drawer test.

and horizontally flexed 20–30°. Fixing the scapula, the humeral head is translated posteriorly whilst simultaneously medially rotating slightly and flexing the glenohumeral joint.

Inferior Shoulder Instability

Sulcus Sign (Matsen et al. 1990) (Fig. 9.11). The clinician applies a longitudinal caudad force to the humerus with the patient sitting and the arm relaxed in the lap to ensure the biceps muscle is not contracted. A positive test is indicated if a sulcus appears distal to the acromion, suggesting inferior instability of the shoulder. The glenohumeral joint can then be externally rotated and the test repeated. This maneuver causes a tightening of the middle glenohumeral ligament (Terry et al. 1991), and therefore may limit translation of the humeral head. Therefore if the test remains positive, a suspected greater amount of instability may be apparent, whereas a negative test upon application of the external rotation suggests a localized superior glenohumeral ligament or coracohumeral ligament dysfunction. The specificity of this test has been found to be 72% and the sensitivity 85% for positive tests >1 cm (Tzannes & Murrell 2002).

Rotator Cuff Pathology Tests

Rotator cuff pathology has been described as a very common cause of shoulder pain (Lewis 2010, 2016).

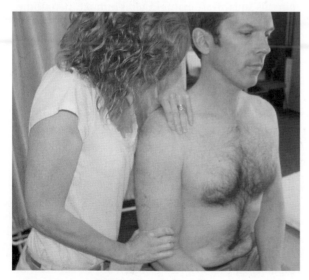

FIG. 9.11 ▪ Sulcus sign.

There appears to be a continuum of pathology of the rotator cuff, with minor tendinopathy at one end of the continuum and massive full-thickness tears at the other end. A normal tendon is thought to develop tendinopathy, partial tears then full-thickness tears of increasing size as pathology progresses. Many studies have demonstrated that partial and full-thickness tears of the rotator cuff are common in asymptomatic shoulders, resulting in controversy relating to the clinical relevance of rotator cuff tears (Milgrom et al. 1995). Tears occur most commonly in supraspinatus. Isolated infraspinatus tears are very uncommon, but do occur commonly with supraspinatus tears. Broadly there are two types of tests used in the physical examination of the rotator cuff: cuff integrity tests and lag signs. The cuff integrity tests (e.g. resisted lateral rotation, full/empty can) determine the force of contraction generated and monitor pain provocation and the lag signs (external rotation/drop sign/Gerber lift-off) determine if a position can be maintained and are used to identify full-thickness tears of the rotator cuff.

Empty- and Full-Can Tests for Supraspinatus Tear or Tendinopathy (Jobe & Moynes 1982) (Fig. 9.12)

The patient abducts the arm to 90° in the scapular plane with the arm internally rotated so the thumb points downwards. The clinician applies a downward force to the distal forearm. Pain or weakness is a positive finding (Itoi et al. 1999). Three studies of low to moderate bias have reported sensitivity of 75–90% and specificity of 32–68% (Hegedus et al. 2012). The test can also be performed in external rotation with the thumb pointing up (full-can test). It was previously thought that this test can isolate activity in the supraspinatus muscle; however, electromyogram studies have demonstrated that this movement generates high levels of activity in the majority of muscles in the shoulder and therefore cannot isolate supraspinatus activity (Boettcher et al. 2009).

Gerber 'Lift-Off' for Subscapularis Tendinopathy (Fig. 9.13)

For patients with full internal rotation this test can be performed by placing the hand behind the back in the area of the midlumbar spine so that the dorsum of the hand is resting against the lumbar spine. The patient is asked to lift the hand away from the body. The

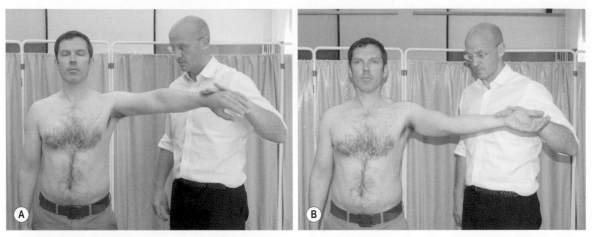

FIG. 9.12 ■ (A) Empty-can test. (B) Full-can test.

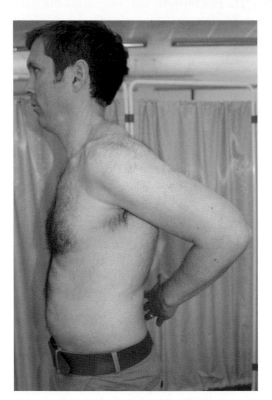

FIG. 9.13 ■ Gerber lift-off test.

External Rotation Lag Sign for Full-Thickness Tears of the Supraspinatus and Infraspinatus (Hertel et al. 1996; Castoldi et al. 2009) (Fig. 9.14)

With the elbow flexed to 90°, the arm is placed in 20° abduction in the scapular plane and the shoulder is externally rotated to end range (−5° to reduce the effect of elastic recoil of the glenohumeral joint). The patient is asked to resist external rotation in this position. If no resistance can be provided the patient is asked to hold the arm in this position and the clinician releases the arm. If the arm drops towards the body the test is considered positive for a full-thickness tear of supraspinatus and infraspinatus (± teres minor). Two studies of low to moderate bias have reported sensitivity of 46–100% and excellent specificity of 93–98% (Hegedus et al. 2012).

Biceps Tests

Speed's Test for Bicipital Tendinopathy (Fig. 9.15)

Tenderness in the bicipital groove when shoulder forward flexion is resisted (with forearm supination and elbow joint extension) suggests bicipital tendinopathy.

Yergason's Test (Fig. 9.16)

The patient has the elbow flexed to 90° and forearm in full pronation. The clinician resists supination whilst palpating in the bicipital groove. Pain or subluxation of the tendon in the groove constitutes a positive test.

inability to lift the hand away from the body is considered a positive test and is thought to indicate pathology of the subscapularis tendon. Four studies of low to moderate bias have reported sensitivity of 6–50% and specificity of 23–79% (Hegedus et al. 2012).

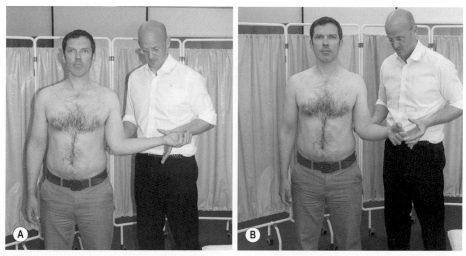

FIG. 9.14 ■ (A, B) External rotation lag sign.

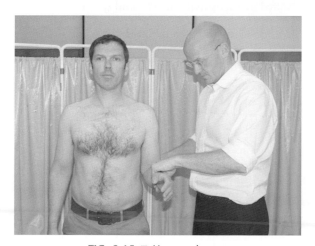

FIG. 9.15 ■ Yergason's test.

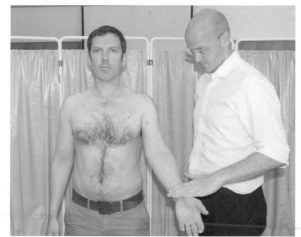

FIG. 9.16 ■ Speed's test.

Holtby and Razmjou (2004) found specificity of 79% and sensitivity of 43%.

Superior Labral Anterior–Posterior (SLAP) Tests

A SLAP lesion occurs predominantly either due to trauma, such as a fall on an outstretched arm, or repeated overload of the long head of biceps, for example, in overhead athletes. Symptoms include clunking within the shoulder joint, with associated pain and loss of function, particularly in overhead positions (Powell et al. 2004). There is a seemingly endless number of tests described for SLAP lesions, and dependent on the study they have varied results in terms of validity. The tests described therefore are ones which are used commonly in practice with some evidence of validity. There is controversy in the literature regarding the clinical relevance of labral tears as there is a high incidence of superior labral tears in asymptomatic individuals (Schwartzberg et al. 2016).

Biceps Load Tests I and II (Fig. 9.17)

■ Biceps load test I: in 90° of abduction, with the patient's elbow in 90° flexion and the forearm supinated, the clinician resists elbow flexion. Pain reproduction indicates a positive test for a SLAP lesion. Improvement in pain or apprehension indicates the absence of a SLAP lesion.

■ Biceps load test II is the same as test I, performed at 120° of abduction. The choice of test should be guided by the range of abduction that is most provocative. Kim et al. (2001) found specificity to be 96.9% and sensitivity to be 89.7%.

Passive Distraction Test (Schlechter et al. 2009) (Fig. 9.18)

With patient in supine and the glenohumeral joint in 150° abduction with the elbow extended, forearm supinated and humerus maintained in neutral rotation, the examiner applies passive pronation of the forearm. Pain within the shoulder joint is indicative of a positive test.

Active Compression Test (O'Brien et al. 1998) (Fig. 9.19)

With the patient in standing, the shoulder flexed to 90°, adduction 10–15°, medial rotation so thumb is pointing down and elbow in full extension, the examiner applies a downward force which the patients resists. The forearm is then supinated and the force reapplied. A positive test is confirmed with pain and/or clicking inside the shoulder on the first part of the test, which diminishes or is relieved after the supination is applied.

Schlechter et al. (2009) found that a combination of passive distraction and active compression tests resulted in a sensitivity of 70% and specificity of 90%.

Shoulder Impingement Syndrome

Shoulder impingement is a condition first described by Neer in 1983. The initial description suggested that the bursa and tendons of the shoulder become compressed in positions of shoulder elevation by the undersurface of the acromion. This model has been challenged over the last decade, as many anatomical observations do not fit the proposed mechanisms of compression. A more appropriate term to describe this condition might be Rotator Cuff Related Shoulder Pain (RCRSP) (Lewis 2016). Two tests commonly used to assess for RCRSP are:

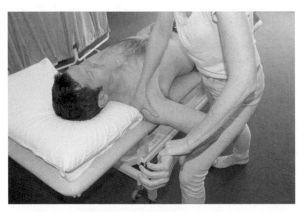

FIG. 9.17 ■ Biceps load test.

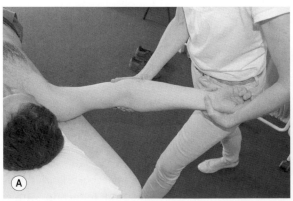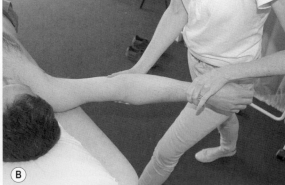

FIG. 9.18 ■ (A, B) Passive distraction test.

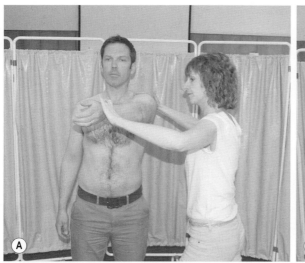
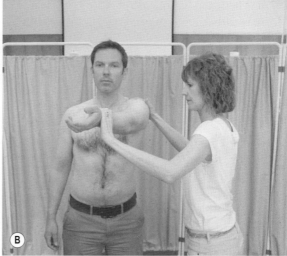

FIG. 9.19 ■ (A, B) Active compression test.

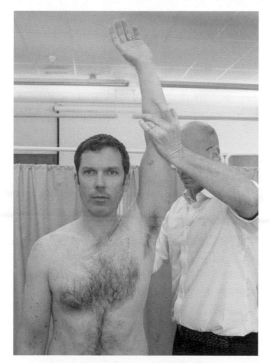

FIG. 9.20 ■ Neer test.

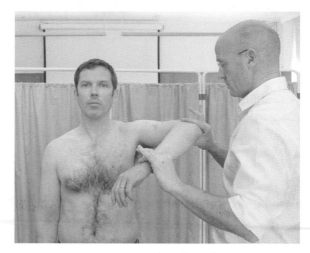

FIG. 9.21 ■ Hawkins–Kennedy test.

studies of low to moderate bias have reported sensitivity of 54–81% and specificity of 10–95% (Hegedus et al. 2012).

1. Neer test (1983) (Fig. 9.20) This can be performed with the patient in standing or sitting. The clinician elevates the internally rotated shoulder whilst stabilizing the scapula. Reproduction of pain is positive for this test. Four

2. Hawkins–Kennedy (Hawkins & Bokor 1990) (Fig. 9.21) The patient is examined with 90° of shoulder flexion and 90° of elbow flexion. The shoulder is then internally rotated to end range; further abduction/adduction of the shoulder can be added if the test is negative. Reproduction of pain is positive for this test. Five studies of low to moderate bias have reported sensitivity of

63–74% and specificity of 40–89% (Hegedus et al. 2012).

Cluster Signs for Impingement

Due to the inherent inaccuracies of individual tests, combining tests can improve the diagnostic accuracy of the examination. Park et al. (2005) described a cluster of signs for the diagnosis of shoulder impingement. When the following three tests were positive for pain the likelihood ratios (LRs) were: +LR 10.56 and –LR 0.17:

1. Hawkins–Kennedy
2. painful arc
3. infraspinatus isometric test.

Muscle Tests

Muscle Strength

The clinician may choose to test the shoulder girdle elevators, depressors, protractors and retractors as well as the shoulder joint flexors, extensors, abductors, adductors, medial rotators and lateral rotators. For details of these general tests readers are directed to Hislop et al. (2013) and Kendall et al. (2005). Greater detail may be required to test the strength of muscles, in particular those thought prone to become weak (see Table 3.7); that is, serratus anterior, middle and lower fibres of trapezius and the deep neck flexors (Janda 2002). Testing the strength of these muscles is described in Chapter 3.

Isometric Muscle Testing for Assessing Muscle as a Source of Symptoms

The therapist may choose to test the shoulder girdle elevators, depressors, protractors and retractors, as well as the shoulder joint flexors, extensors, abductors, adductors, medial rotators and lateral rotators in the resting position and, if indicated, in different parts of the physiological range. In addition, the clinician observes the quality of the muscle contraction to hold this position (this can be done with the patient's eyes shut). The patient may, for example, be unable to prevent the joint from moving or may hold with excessive muscle activity; either of these circumstances may suggest a neuromuscular dysfunction.

Muscle Control

Muscle control is of particular interest in the shoulder in relation to scapular function. The role of the scapula is to provide a stable base for the glenohumeral joint and to orientate the glenoid in the optimal position for glenohumeral joint function. The lack of bony articulation in the scapulothoracic region means the scapula is very mobile and reliant on well-coordinated muscle activity to control its position and function. The coordinated motion between the scapula and humerus is called scapulohumeral rhythm (McClure et al. 2009).

Scapular motion that deviates from what is considered normal is called scapular dyskinesis (Kibler et al. 2013), where 'dys' means 'alteration of' and 'kinesis' means 'motion'. It is a general term and does not identify the cause of abnormal movement.

Scapular dyskinesis has been linked with many types of shoulder pathology (McClure et al. 2006), although it is unclear if dyskinesis is the cause or the result of pain in the shoulder. The dyskinesis may result from pathology, as in the case of acromioclavicular joint strain or long thoracic nerve injury, or the presence of dyskinesis may be a causative factor in the development of pain. The picture is further complicated by the high incidence of scapular dyskinesis in the asymptomatic population, making it difficult to determine the clinical relevance (McClure et al. 2006).

Many methods of measuring scapular dyskinesis have developed which have not always demonstrated good reliability or validity. The scapula is very mobile and its movement is in complex three-dimensional planes, making reliable evaluation of the nature of its movement difficult. McClure et al. (2009) developed a method of identifying scapular dyskinesis that appears to demonstrate good reliability and validity. This method involves the observation and identification of:

■ winging of the inferior scapular border
■ winging of the medial scapular border
■ lack of smooth scapular movement during arm elevation (specifically early elevation of the scapula during arm elevation or a sudden downward rotation during arm lowering).

If any of these is observed then dyskinesis is considered to be present. However, how relevant this is for specific shoulder conditions is not clear. Ratcliffe et al. (2014), following systematic review, have not been able to identify a typical pattern of scapular dyskinesis in patients with RCRSP and suggested this may be due to the complex multifactorial nature of the condition; with further research, subgroups may emerge.

The current recommendation is to observe and identify scapular dyskinesis and then evaluate the effect of manual correction on symptoms. If correction reduces symptoms then this correction can be incorporated into the treatment strategy.

Muscle Length

The clinician may choose to test the length of muscles, in particular those thought prone to shorten (Janda 2002); that is, latissimus dorsi, pectoralis major and minor, upper trapezius, levator scapulae and sternocleidomastoid. Testing the length of these muscles is described in Chapter 3.

Neurological Tests

Neurological examination includes neurological integrity testing and neurodynamic tests. These are not routinely examined, and are only indicated if the patient complains of neurological symptoms, or has pain in a distribution that may indicate neurological involvement. Readers are referred to Chapter 3 for neural integrity testing of the upper limb.

Neurodynamic Tests

The upper-limb neurodynamic tests (ULNTs) may be carried out in order to ascertain the degree to which neural tissue is responsible for producing the patient's symptoms. The choice of tests should be influenced by the distribution of the patient's symptoms, e.g. if the patient has posterior upper-arm and lateral elbow pain, then ULNTs with a radial nerve bias may be indicated. These tests are described in detail in Chapter 3.

Nerves may also be palpated to ascertain the presence of mechanosensitivity. Palpable nerves in the upper limb are as follows:

- The suprascapular nerve can be palpated along the superior border of the scapula in the suprascapular notch.

- The dorsal scapular nerve can be palpated medial to the medial border of the scapula.
- The brachial plexus can be palpated in the posterior triangle of the neck; it emerges at the lower third of sternocleidomastoid.
- The median nerve can be palpated over the anterior elbow joint crease, medial to the biceps tendon, also at the wrist between palmaris longus and flexor carpi radialis.
- The radial nerve can be palpated around the spiral groove of the humerus, between brachioradialis and flexor carpi radialis, in the forearm and also at the wrist in the snuffbox.

Vascular Tests

Allen Test

With the patient sitting and the arm abducted to 90°, the clinician horizontally extends and laterally rotates the arm (Magee 2014). Disappearance of the radial pulse on contralateral cervical rotation is indicative of thoracic outlet syndrome.

Adson's Manoeuvre

In sitting, the patient's head is rotated towards the tested arm (Magee 2014). The patient then extends the head while the clinician extends and laterally rotates the shoulder. The patient then takes a deep breath and disappearance of the radial pulse indicates a positive test. It should be noted that disappearance of the pulse has been found to occur in a large percentage of asymptomatic subjects (Young & Hardy 1983; Swift & Nichols 1984).

Palpation of Pulses

If it is suspected that the circulation is compromised, the brachial pulse is palpated on the medial aspect of the humerus in the axilla.

Palpation

The shoulder region is palpated, as well as the cervical spine and thoracic spine and upper limbs as appropriate. It is useful to record palpation findings on a body chart (see Fig. 2.3) and/or palpation chart (see Fig. 3.35).

The clinician notes the following:

- the temperature of the area
- localized increased skin moisture
- the presence of oedema or effusion
- mobility and feel of superficial tissues, e.g. ganglions, nodules and scar tissue
- the presence or elicitation of any muscle spasm
- tenderness of bone, bursae (subacromial and subdeltoid), ligaments, muscle, tendon (long head of biceps, subscapularis, infraspinatus, teres minor, supraspinatus, pectoralis major and long head of triceps), tendon sheath, trigger points (shown in Fig. 3.36) and nerve.

Accessory Movements

It is useful to use the palpation chart and movement diagrams (or joint pictures) to record findings. These are explained in detail in Chapter 3.

The clinician notes the:

- quality of movement
- range of movement
- resistance through the range and at the end of the range of movement
- behaviour of pain through the range
- provocation of any muscle spasm.

Glenohumeral, acromioclavicular and sternoclavicular joint accessory movements should be tested in provocative positions/ranges when the patient is non-severe and non-irritable, as this is most likely to reproduce symptoms and guide treatment. Some accessory movements to the glenohumeral joint are shown in Fig. 9.22. A list of accessory movements with possible modifications is provided in Table 9.2. The neutral position can be useful in severe and irritable patients, or as an initial testing procedure to familiarize the patient with handling techniques. Following accessory movements to the shoulder region, the clinician reassesses all the physical asterisks in order to establish the effect of the accessory movements on the patient's signs and symptoms. Accessory movements can then be tested for other regions suspected to be a source of, or contributing to, the patient's symptoms. Again, following accessory movements to any one region, the clinician reassesses all the asterisks. Regions that may be examined are the cervical spine, thoracic spine, elbow, wrist and hand.

COMPLETION OF THE EXAMINATION

Having carried out the above tests, the examination of the shoulder region is now complete. The subjective and physical examinations produce a large amount of information, which must be recorded accurately and quickly. It is vital at this stage to highlight with an asterisk (*) important findings from the examination. These findings must be reassessed at, and within, subsequent treatment sessions to evaluate the effects of treatment on the patient's condition.

The physical testing procedures which specifically indicate joint, nerve or muscle tissues as a source of the patient's symptoms are summarized in Table 3.9. It must be remembered that no one physical test for shoulder dysfunction provides a perfect diagnosis. It is the full exploration of both the subjective and physical findings which enables the clinician to prioritize certain tissues or contributing factors as those which are most pertinent to the patient's condition. These include physical, but importantly also psychological and social, factors (Chester et al. 2016) in the overall picture.

On completion of the physical examination the clinician will:

- Explain the findings of the physical examination and how these findings relate to the subjective assessment. An attempt should be made to clear up any misconceptions patients may have regarding their illness or injury.
- Collaborate with the patient and via problem solving together devise a treatment plan and discuss the prognosis.
- Warn the patient of possible exacerbation up to 24–48 hours following the examination.
- Request the patient to report details on the behaviour of the symptoms following examination at the next attendance.
- Explain the findings of the physical examination and how these findings relate to the subjective assessment. It is helpful to clear up any misconceptions patients may have regarding their illness or injury.
- Evaluate the findings, formulate a clinical hypothesis and write up a problem list.
- Determine the objectives of treatment alongside the patient.

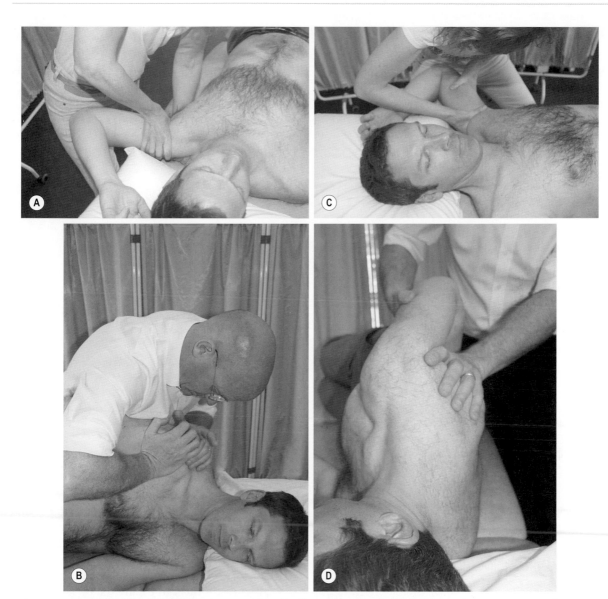

FIG. 9.22 ■ Accessory movement. (A) Anteroposterior glenohumeral joint in abduction/external rotation: support the patient's scapula with one hand and apply an anteroposterior force through the head of humerus with the other hand. (B) Anteroposterior glenohumeral joint in side-lying, hand behind back position. (C) Longitudinal caudad in abduction/external rotation: support the patient's scapula with one hand and apply a force towards the patient's feet, pushing through the humeral head. (D) Longitudinal cephalad scapula with hand behind back. These techniques can be applied in different ranges of movement depending on the patient presentation.

TABLE 9.2		
Accessory Movements, Choice of Application and Reassessment of the Patient's Asterisks		
Accessory Movements	Choice of Application	Identify Any Effect of Accessory Movements on Patient's Signs and Symptoms
Glenohumeral joint	Start position, e.g.	Reassess all asterisks
↕ Anteroposterior	■ Glenohumeral joint in flexion, abduction	
Posteroanterior	■ Acromioclavicular joint accessory movements	
←·· Caud Longitudinal caudad	■ Carried out with glenohumeral joint in horizontal flexion	
←·· Ceph Longitudinal cephalad	Speed of force application	
·· Lat Lateral	Direction of the applied force	
·· Med Medial	Point of application of applied force	
Acromioclavicular joint		
↕ Anteroposterior		
Posteroanterior		
←·· Caud Longitudinal caudad		
Sternoclavicular joint		
↕ Anteroposterior		
Posteroanterior		
←·· Caud Longitudinal caudad		
←·· Ceph Longitudinal cephalad		
Cervical spine	As above	Reassess all asterisks
Thoracic spine	As above	Reassess all asterisks
Elbow	As above	Reassess all asterisks
Wrist and hand	As above	Reassess all asterisks

■ Devise an initial treatment plan alongside the patient.

In this way, the clinician will have developed the following hypotheses categories (adapted from Jones & Rivett 2004):

■ function: abilities and restrictions
■ patients' perspective on their experience
■ source of symptoms, including the structure or tissue that is thought to be producing the patient's symptoms, the nature of the structure or tissues in relation to the healing process and the pain mechanisms
■ contributing factors to the development and maintenance of the problem. There may be environmental, psychosocial, behavioural, physical or heredity factors

■ precautions/contraindications to treatment and management. This includes the severity and irritability of the patient's symptoms and the nature of the patient's condition
■ management strategy and treatment plan
■ prognosis – this can be affected by factors such as the stage and extent of the injury as well as the patient's expectations, personality and lifestyle.

For guidance on treatment and management principles, the reader is directed to the companion textbook (Petty & Barnard 2017).

REFERENCES

Boettcher, C.A., et al., 2009. The 'empty can' and 'full can' tests do not selectively activate supraspinatus. J. Sci. Med. Sport 12, 435–439.

Borstad, J.D., Dashottar, A.B., 2011. Quantifying strain on posterior shoulder tissues during 5 simulated clinical tests: a cadaver study. J. Orthop. Sports Phys. Ther. 41, 90–99.

Borstad, J.D., et al., 2015. Validity and reliability of the low flexion measurement for posterior glenohumeral joint capsule tightness. Man. Ther. 20, 875–878.

Brown, C., 1983. Compressive, invasive referred pain to the shoulder. Clin. Orthop. Relat. Res. 173, 55–62.

Bunker, T., 2009. Time for a new name for frozen shoulder – contracture of the shoulder. Shoulder Elbow 1, 4–9.

Castoldi, F., et al., 2009. External rotation lag sign revisited: accuracy for diagnosis of full thickness supraspinatus tear. J. Shoulder Elbow Surg. 18, 529–534.

Chester, R., et al., 2013. Predicting response to physiotherapy treatment for musculoskeletal shoulder pain: a systematic review. BMC Musculoskelet. Disord. 14, 203.

Chester, R., et al., 2016. Psychological factors are associated with the outcome of physiotherapy for people with shoulder pain: a multicentre longitudinal cohort study. Br. J. Sports Med. 0, 1–8.

Cyriax, J., 1982. Textbook of orthopaedic medicine – diagnosis of soft tissue lesions, eighth ed. Baillière Tindall, London.

Dashottar, A., Borstad, J.D., 2012. Posterior glenohumeral joint capsule contracture. Shoulder Elbow 4, 230–236.

Dunn, W.R., et al., 2014. Symptoms of pain do not correlate with rotator cuff tear severity: a cross-sectional study of 393 patients with a symptomatic atraumatic full-thickness rotator cuff tear. J. Bone Joint Surg. 96, 793–800.

Gerber, C., Ganz, R., 1984. Clinical assessment of instability of the shoulder. J. Bone Joint Surg. 66B, 551–556.

Grieve, G.P., 1994. Thoracic musculoskeletal problems. In: Grieve, G.P. (Ed.), Modern manual therapy of the vertebral column. Churchill Livingstone, Edinburgh, pp. 401–428.

Hawkins, R.J., Bokor, D.J., 1990. Clinical evaluation of shoulder problems. In: Rockwood, C.A., Matsen, F.A. (Eds.), The shoulder. W.B. Saunders, Philadelphia, p. 149.

Hegedus, E.J., et al., 2012. Which physical examination tests provide clinicians with the most value when examining the shoulder? Update of a systematic review with meta-analysis of individual tests. Br. J. Sports Med. 46, 964–978.

Hertel, R., et al., 1996. Lag signs in the diagnosis of rotator cuff rupture. J. Shoulder Elbow Surg. 5, 307–313.

Hill, A.M., et al., 2008. The clinical assessment and classification of shoulder instability. Curr. Orthop. 22, 208–225.

Hislop, H., et al., 2013. Daniels and Worthingham's muscle testing, techniques of manual examination, ninth ed. Elsevier Saunders, St Louis.

Holtby, R., Razmjou, H., 2004. Accuracy of the Speeds and Yergasons tests in detecting biceps pathology and SLAP lesions; comparison with arthroscopic findings. Arthroscopy 20, 231–236.

Itoi, E., et al., 1999. Which test is more useful, the full can test or the empty can test, in detecting a torn supraspinatus tendon? Am. J. Sports Med. 27, 65–68.

Janda, V., 2002. Muscles and motor control in cervicogenic disorders. In: Grant, R. (Ed.), Physical therapy of the cervical and thoracic spine, third ed. Churchill Livingstone, New York, p. 195.

Jobe, F.W., Moynes, D.R., 1982. Delineation of diagnostic criteria and a rehabilitation program for rotator cuff injuries. Am. J. Sports Med. 10, 336–339.

Jobe, F.W., et al., 1989. Shoulder pain in the overhand or throwing athlete: the relationship of anterior instability and rotator cuff impingement. Orthop. Rev. 18, 963–975.

Jones, M.A., Rivett, D.A., 2004. Clinical reasoning for manual therapists. Butterworth-Heinemann, Edinburgh.

Kendall, F.P., et al., 2005. Muscles testing and function, fifth ed. Williams & Wilkins, Baltimore.

Kibler, W.B., et al., 2013. Clinical implications of scapular dyskinesis in shoulder injury: the 2013 consensus statement from the 'scapular summit'. Br. J. Sports Med. 47, 877–885.

Kim, S.H., et al., 2001. Biceps load test II: a clinical test for SLAP lesions of the shoulder. Arthroscopy 17, 160–164.

Laudner, K.G., et al., 2006. Assessing posterior shoulder contracture: the reliability and validity of measuring glenohumeral joint horizontal adduction. J. Athl. Train. 41, 375–380.

Lewis, J., 2009. Rotator cuff tendinopathy/subacromial impingement syndrome: is it time for a new method of assessment? Br. J. Sports Med. 43, 259–264.

Lewis, J., 2010. Rotator cuff tendinopathy: a model for the continuum of pathology and related management. Br. J. Sports Med. 44, 918–923.

Lewis, J.S., 2011. Subacromial impingement syndrome: a musculoskeletal condition or clinical illusion? Phys. Ther. Rev. 16, 388–398.

Lewis, J., 2015. Frozen shoulder contracture syndrome – aetiology, diagnosis and management. Man. Ther. 20, 2–9.

Lewis, J., 2016. Rotator cuff related shoulder pain: assessment, management and uncertainties. Man. Ther. 23, 57–68.

Lewis, A., et al., 2004. The classification of shoulder instability: new light through old windows. Orthop. Trauma 18, 97–108.

Lo, I.K., et al., 2004. An evaluation of the apprehension, relocation and surprise tests for anterior shoulder instability. Am. J. Sports Med. 32, 301–307.

Magee, D.J., 2014. Orthopedic physical assessment, sixth ed. Elsevier Saunders, St Louis.

Matsen, F.A., et al., 1990. Anterior glenohumeral instability. In: Rockwood, C.A., Matsen, F.A. (Eds.), The shoulder. W.B. Saunders, Philadelphia, p. 526.

McClure, P., et al., 2006. Shoulder function and 3-dimensional scapular kinematics in people with and without shoulder impingement syndrome. Phys. Ther. 86, 1075–1090.

McClure, P., et al., 2009. A clinical method for identifying scapular dyskinesis: part 1: reliability. J. Athl. Train. 44, 160–164.

Milgrom, C., et al., 1995. Rotator-cuff changes in asymptomatic adults: the effect of age, hand dominance and gender. Bone Joint Surg. Br. 77-B, 296–298.

Neer, C.S., 1983. Impingement lesions. Clin. Orthop. Relat. Res. 173, 70–77.

O'Brien, S.J., et al., 1998. The active compression test: a new and effective test for diagnosing labral tears and acromioclavicular joint abnormality. Am. J. Sports Med. 26, 610–613.

Park, H.B., et al., 2005. Diagnostic accuracy of clinical tests for the different degrees of subacromial impingement syndrome. Bone Joint Surg. Am. 87, 1446–1455.

Petty, J.N., Barnard, K., 2017. Principles of musculoskeletal treatment and management: a handbook for therapists, third ed. Elsevier, Edinburgh.

Powell, S.E., et al., 2004. The diagnosis, classification, and treatment of SLAP lesions. Oper. Tech. Sports Med. 12, 99–110.

Ratcliffe, E., et al., 2014. Is there a relationship between subacromial impingement syndrome and scapular orientation? A systematic review. Br. J. Sports Med. 48, 1251–1256.

Schlechter, J.A., et al., 2009. The passive distraction test: a new diagnostic aid for clinically significant superior labral pathology. Arthroscopy 25, 1374–1379.

Schwartzberg, R., et al., 2016. High prevalence of superior labral tears diagnosed by MRI in middle-aged patients with asymptomatic shoulders. Orthop. J. Sports Med. 5, 1.

Swift, T.R., Nichols, F.T., 1984. The droopy shoulder syndrome. Neurology 34, 212–215.

Terry, G.C., et al., 1991. The stabilizing function of passive shoulder restraints. Am. J. Sports Med. 19, 26–34.

Tzannes, A., Murrell, G.A.C., 2002. Clinical examination of the unstable shoulder. Sports Med. 32, 447–457.

Waddell, G., 2004. The back pain revolution, second ed. Churchill Livingstone, Edinburgh.

Wilk, K.E., et al., 2011. Correlation of glenohumeral internal rotation deficit and total rotational motion to shoulder injuries in professional baseball pitchers. Am. J. Sports Med. 39, 329–335.

Young, H.A., Hardy, D.G., 1983. Thoracic outlet syndrome. Br. J. Hosp. Med. 29, 459–461.

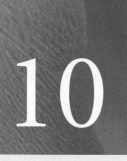

10

EXAMINATION OF THE ELBOW REGION

COLLEEN BALSTON ■ DIONNE RYDER

CHAPTER CONTENTS

INTRODUCTION TO THE ELBOW REGION

The elbow complex is composed of three bones, the humerus, ulna and radius, which together form three separate articulations or joints; the humeroulnar joint, the humeroradial joint and the superior radioulnar joint. The joint capsule is thin and continuous for all three joints. The capsule is reinforced anteriorly by the collateral ligaments, which contribute to elbow stability. The humeroulnar joint provides most of the elbow structural stability due to the tight fit between the trochlea and the trochlear notch. It is primarily involved in flexion and extension. The humeroradial joint allows flexion and extension movements as well as pronation and supination (Hengeveld et al. 2014). The elbow is not considered a typical weight-bearing joint; however, pushing activities and press-ups do subject the humeroradial joint to compression forces and should be considered in patients with lateral elbow pain. The superior and inferior radioulnar joints are usually considered one joint; however, in this text the inferior radioulnar joint is discussed in Chapter 11. They are primarily involved in supination and pronation movements and therefore are essential in fine-tuning wrist and hand spatial positioning.

The muscles associated primarily with the elbow include three flexors (brachialis, biceps brachii and brachioradialis) and two extensors (triceps and anconeus). The role these muscles have in elbow movement depends on many factors; including functional anatomy, elbow and forearm positions, type of muscle contraction and associated load. These factors are important to consider during manual muscle testing. In

273

addition, the humerus provides a stable base of attachment for many of the wrist and hand muscles (common flexor and extensor muscles of wrist and hand), which are susceptible to overload and degenerative changes.

Anatomically the elbow forms part of the kinetic chain for the upper limb, sitting between the mobile shoulder, wrist and hand joints. The elbow's primary role is to optimize hand function by enabling an individual to place the hand in a variety of positions to perform functional activities. Normal elbow physiological ranges for flexion and extension range between −5° hypertension and 145° flexion, although most functional activities usually occur between 30° and 130° of flexion.

The superior radioulnar joint has on average 75° of forearm pronation and 85° of supination (Neumann 2010). These physiological ranges enable a wide variety of activities. For example, elbow flexion and supination are used to bring the hand to the face and body in activities of daily living, such as eating, dressing and carrying objects. Similarly, elbow extension and pronation together enable the hand to be used in reaching, pushing, throwing and weight bearing, e.g. through a walking stick. The elbow joints therefore allow transmission of forces to or from the hand such as traction/distraction (e.g. pulling or carrying activities), torque as a result of twisting (e.g. using a screwdriver) or compression (e.g. pushing a heavy door). Any gross loss of flexion or extension range may significantly limit the level of functional independence for an individual (Lockard 2006). In contrast, compensations at the elbow may arise when there are dysfunctions at the wrist or shoulder, reminding us of the importance of screening these regions too.

Elbow injuries affect people of all ages and activity levels and often result in significant pain and disability (Aviles et al. 2008). Elbow pain potentially may be described as arthrogenic, myogenic, neurogenic or a combination of these 'genics', depending on the structures involved. Knowledge of the epidemiology of potential diagnoses and the aetiology of suspected conditions is critical for recognition of common patterns. For example, sports involving overhead throwing, repeated use of power grips (golf and tennis) and compression (divers, gymnasts and weightlifters) are particularly associated with acute, chronic and repetitive elbow pathologies.

In trauma-related elbow injuries, identifying the mechanism of injury is essential when establishing a diagnosis (Aviles et al. 2008). In atraumatic disorders, particular symptoms may be indicative of certain conditions or joint dysfunctions. For example, numbness and tingling in the little finger while talking on the phone (and at night) may suggest ulnar neuropathy, twinges of pain on turning a key may be related to the superior radioulnar joint and an inability to extend the elbow fully may suggest synovitis or osteoarthritis (MacDermid & Michlovitz 2006). See Table 10.1 for possible causes of pain and/or limitation of

TABLE 10.1	
Possible Causes of Pain and/or Limitation of Movement	
Trauma/defined mechanism of injury	▪ Fracture of humerus, radius or ulna – fall on outstretched hand ▪ Dislocation of the head of the radius (most commonly seen in young children) ▪ Ligamentous sprain – 'pop' may suggest collateral ligament injury ▪ Muscular strain
Inflammatory	▪ Inflammatory disorders: rheumatoid arthritis ▪ Bursitis (of subcutaneous olecranon, subtendinous olecranon, radioulnar or bicipitoradial bursa)
Degenerative/repetitive conditions	▪ Common extensor origin dysfunction/lateral epicondylalgia/tennis elbow ▪ Common flexor origin dysfunction/medial epicondylalgia/golfer's elbow ▪ Degenerative conditions: osteoarthritis and loose bodies ▪ Calcification of tendons or muscles, e.g. myositis ossificans
Peripheral nerve sensitization/neuropathy entrapment	▪ Compression of, or injury to, the median, radial and ulnar nerve
Sinister pathologies	▪ Infection, e.g. tuberculosis ▪ Primary bone tumours
Other	▪ Hypermobility syndrome ▪ Haemophilia ▪ Referral of symptoms from the cervical spine, thoracic spine, shoulder, wrist or hand ▪ Volkmann's ischaemic contracture e.g. supracondylar fracture of humerus

movement. Poor posture of cervical, thoracic spine and upper limbs has been noted in patients with elbow pain and should always be considered during the examination (Wilke et al. 2002).

SUBJECTIVE EXAMINATION

Further details of the questions asked during the subjective examination and the tests carried out in the physical examination can be found in Chapters 2 and 3, respectively. The order of the subjective questioning and the physical tests described below should be justified through sound clinical reasoning and may depend on the type of presenting symptoms as well as the patient's expectations.

Patients' Perspective on Their Experience

In order to treat the patient appropriately, it is important that the condition is managed within the context of the patient's social and work environment. Social history that is relevant to the onset and progression of the patient's problem is recorded. This includes age, employment, home situation, including sleep postures, and details of any leisure and sporting activities (MacDermid & Michlovitz 2006). It is essential to gain an understanding of the functional demands on the elbow. For example, does the patient's job involve sustained positions of wrist flexion or extension, so implicating the common flexor/extensor origins at the elbow? Alternatively does the patient undertake repetitive activities, e.g. sustained computer or production line work? This information may indicate direct and/ or indirect mechanical influences on the elbow. In cases of athletes, trauma or work-related injuries, ask specifically about details of work status and any potential compensation claims.

Identifying the patient's expectations and possible presence of unhelpful thoughts/beliefs and psychosocial factors will help effectively plan both the subjective and physical examinations. For example, by examining the expectations of the patient, the suitability of using manual therapy can be established and modified if the patient is expecting a 'hands off approach' such as exercise and advice. Being mindful of patient groups at risk of psychosocial factors will also alert the perceptive clinician to investigate further. Examples of elbow patient groups at higher risk of psychosocial factors

such as depression, anxiety and fear avoidance include those associated with feelings of low job control and support as well as those with lateral epicondylalgia (Alizadehkhaiyat et al. 2007; van Rijn et al. 2009). Helpful psychosocial screening questions are as follows:

- What is your main problem?
- What do you think physiotherapy can do for you?
- How do you feel about physical activity?

Early identification of known psychosocial risk factors such as depression and low mood is important as their presence is linked to the development of chronic musculoskeletal pain and poorer clinical outcomes (Linton et al. 2011).

Patient-reported outcome measures or questionnaires are also recommended in order to measure the impact of the dysfunction on the patient's perceptions and functional limitations. Useful outcome measures include the Oxford Elbow Score (Joint-specific), Patient-Rated Tennis Elbow Evaluation (Condition-specific), Disabilities of the Arm, Shoulder and Hand (DASH) and Patient Specific Functional Scale (PSFS) (The et al. 2013).

Body Chart

The following information concerning the type and area of current symptoms can be recorded on a body chart (see Fig. 2.3). It is useful to document the patient's hand preference (left- or right-handed) on the body chart. This helps to determine the impact that symptoms in the upper limb may have on normal function. Handedness and frequency of physical activity may well produce differences in muscle bulk between sides.

Area of Current Symptoms

Be precise when mapping out the area of the symptoms. Elbow symptoms can be felt locally or may refer symptoms distally to the forearm and hand. Localized pain may be felt over the joint lines, especially the humeroradial joint, the olecranon process, ulnar notch and medial and lateral epicondyles. Elbow symptoms which refer distally to the forearm and hand may have their source in the cervical spine (C5–C6 with lateral elbow pain and C7–C8 with medial elbow pain) or thoracic spine (Neumann 2010). Ascertain which is the worst symptom and record where the patient feels the symptoms are coming from.

Areas Relevant to the Region Being Examined

Symptoms around the elbow complex may be referred from more proximal and distal structures, including arthrogenic, myogenic or neurogenic structures in the region of the cervical and thoracic spine, shoulder, wrist and hand. For example, lateral elbow pain radiating symptoms distally to the forearm may arise from the common extensor tendon or more proximally from the cervical spine. Be sure to negate all possible areas that might refer or contribute to the area of pain. Mark unaffected areas with ticks (✓) on the body chart.

Quality of Pain

Establish the quality of the pain in order to assist in determining possible pain mechanisms, e.g. sharp, catching pain may indicate an intraarticular dysfunction, whereas a deep ache localized to the lateral epicondyle with or without distal referral may be indicative of tennis elbow/lateral epincondylalgia.

Intensity of Pain

The intensity of pain can be measured as shown in Chapter 2 (see Fig. 2.5) and informs clinical reasoning of symptom severity, which may help guide the extent and vigour of the physical examination.

Abnormal Sensation

Check for any altered sensation locally around the elbow region and any other relevant areas, such as the wrist and hand. Sensory and motor loss in the peripheral nerve distribution of the median, radial and ulnar nerves can occur either through compression or traction injuries. Symptoms of paraesthesia, burning pain and sensitivity to touch (allodynia or hyperalgesia) may indicate nerve entrapment.

Constant or Intermittent Symptoms

Ascertain the frequency of the symptoms, whether they are constant or intermittent. If symptoms are constant, check whether there is variation in the intensity of the symptoms, as constant unremitting pain may be indicative of a serious pathology.

Relationship of Symptoms

The relationship between the symptomatic areas can be explored by careful questioning, e.g. do the symptoms come together or separately? Can the patient experience elbow pain without shoulder or neck pain or are the pains always present together? Which symptom comes on first? Understanding the relationship between symptomatic areas is invaluable in identifying order and selection of assessment and management techniques.

Behaviour of Symptoms

Aggravating Factors

For each symptomatic area, identify what movements and/or positions aggravate the patient's symptoms, i.e. what brings them on (or makes them worse)? Is the patient able to maintain this position or movement (severity)? What happens to other symptoms when this symptom is produced (or is made worse)? How long does it take for symptoms to ease once the position or movement is stopped (irritability)? These questions help to confirm the relationship between the symptoms. The concepts of severity and irritability are discussed in Chapter 2.

The clinician also asks the patient about theoretically known aggravating factors for structures that could be a source of the symptoms. Common aggravating factors such as pain and stiffness on eating or reaching for an object may implicate the humeroulnar and humeroradial joints (joint dysfunction) whereas pain with gripping, turning a key in a lock and opening a bottle may implicate the common extensor tendon or the superior radioulnar joint. Other known aggravating factors include leaning on the forearm or hand, writing, typing, lifting, carrying, sport and leisure activities. Identify past and current training regimen for sporting populations and ensure careful examination of throwing actions where applicable. It is important for the clinician to be as specific as possible when investigating aggravating factors. Where possible, break the movement or activity down into individual components as this may provide clues for what to expect during the physical examination.

Aggravating factors for other regions may need to be considered if they are suspected to be a proximal or contributing source of the symptoms (see Table 2.2).

Easing Factors

For each symptomatic area, the clinician needs to explore the easing factors (positions/movements and timing) to confirm the relationship between the symptoms and determine their irritability.

The clinician asks the patient about theoretically known easing factors for structures that could be a source of the symptoms. For example, symptoms from the elbow joint may be relieved by pulling the forearm away from the upper arm, thereby creating some joint distraction. Painful and swollen elbows may be eased when held in the resting position with the hand supported. The resting position of approximately 70° flexion is typically adopted in painful and swollen elbows, as in this position the elbow has maximum joint volume. It is also important to explore and confirm the relationship of symptoms when altering the position or moving proximal or distal joints. For example, symptoms from neural tissues may be relieved by shoulder girdle elevation, which reduces tension on the brachial plexus and nerve roots. Establishing what happens to symptoms during these easing positions or movements is important as it will help the clinician to clinically reason the source of symptoms and confirm the relationship of more than one symptom if present.

Using clinical reasoning skills the clinician can then analyse the positions or movements that aggravate or ease the symptoms to help determine the structure(s) at fault. This information can be used to determine the irritability of the condition, the appropriate vigour/extent of the physical examination, the aims of treatment and any advice that may be required.

The most notable functional restrictions are highlighted with asterisks (*), then explored in the physical examination and reassessed at subsequent treatment sessions to evaluate treatment intervention.

Twenty-Four-Hour Behaviour of Symptoms

The clinician determines the 24-hour behaviour of symptoms by asking questions about night, morning and evening symptoms.

Night Symptoms. Suggested questions to establish the behaviour of symptoms at night are detailed in Chapter 2. Night pain may arise from sleep positions such as sustained elbow flexion (e.g. ulnar neuropathy) or

from compression, if the patient is unable to lie on the affected side.

Morning and Evening Symptoms. The clinician determines the pattern of the symptoms first thing in the morning, through the day and at the end of the day. The status of symptoms on first waking establishes whether the patient is better with rest. Pain/stiffness on waking would suggest an inflammatory component whereas no pain on waking but pain on activity would suggest a more mechanical origin.

Stage of the Condition

In order to determine the stage of the condition the clinician asks whether the symptoms are getting better, getting worse or remaining unchanged.

Special Questions

Special questions as highlighted in Chapter 2 are routinely asked, as these identify certain precautions or contraindications to the physical examination and/or treatment, as well as screen for the presence of serious pathologies. Routine special questions include the patient's recent general health, unexplained weight loss, medications, including over-the-counter medications, medical imaging and the presence or absence of neurological symptoms. The clinician must differentiate between musculoskeletal conditions that are suitable for treatment and management and systemic, neoplastic and other non-musculoskeletal conditions which require referral to a medical practitioner.

In relation to the elbow, the following conditions and findings are particularly relevant and should be noted during the subjective assessment to determine their contribution to the elbow dysfunction and symptoms.

Comorbidities and Serious Illness

Thyroid dysfunction is associated with a higher incidence of musculoskeletal conditions such as adhesive capsulitis and Dupuytren's contracture (Cakir et al. 2003). Similarly, diabetes mellitus is linked with delayed tissue healing and peripheral neuropathy (Boissonnault 2011). The presence of specific comorbid conditions may have an effect on the patient's prognosis with delayed or suboptimal healing and should be taken into account during treatment planning.

Primary bone tumours around the elbow are generally rare. The suspicion of a tumour however, should be raised in the patient with unremitting, unexplained, non-mechanical bony elbow pain (Goodman 2010a, b).

Past Medical and Family History

The following information is obtained from the patient and/or medical notes and should include details of any medical history such as major or long-standing illnesses, accidents or surgery that are relevant to the patient's condition. Family history that is relevant to the onset and progression of the patient's problem is also recorded. Check for a history of trauma or recurrent minor trauma. Patients with a history of elbow dislocation or fractures may be at risk of developing elbow instability secondary to the original injury (Bell 2008). Ascertain the results of any past treatment for the same or a similar problem. Past treatment records may be obtained for further information.

Elbow Stiffness or Arthritic Conditions

Elbow arthritis can be classified into degenerative (osteoarthritis), inflammatory, including rheumatoid arthritis and ankylosing spondylitis, and posttraumatic arthritis (Lim et al. 2008). The patient's family history of inflammatory arthritis should be explored, as rheumatoid arthritis commonly affects the elbow, either unilaterally or bilaterally. Primary degenerative arthritis is less common. Posttraumatic arthritis should be considered in patients with a history of trauma. Comorbid conditions with known predisposition to elbow stiffness such as haemophilia should be investigated (Nandi et al. 2009). In haemophiliacs, the elbow is prone to haemarthrosis and is cited as the second most commonly affected joint after the knee (Utukuri & Goddard 2005).

Osteoporosis

Patients, especially females who present with a combination of factors such as long-term corticosteroid use, early menopause, history of fractures and family history of osteoporosis, should be considered at risk and investigated (Greenhalgh & Selfe 2010).

Sudden Swelling

Sudden swelling in the absence of trauma suggests infection or inflammation of the joint. Septic arthritis is uncommon in the elbow, but it may be seen in patients with a suppressed immune system or diabetes, those taking cortisone medications or intravenous drug abusers.

Neurological Symptoms

Patients may report neural tissue symptoms such as tingling, paraesthesia, pain or hypersensitivity in the upper limb and/or hand. Consider whether symptoms are likely to be peripheral or spinal nerve in origin. Are these symptoms unilateral or bilateral? Has the patient noticed any weakness in the hand? Or has the patient experienced symptoms of spinal cord compression, which are bilateral tingling in the hands or feet and/or disturbance of gait? Progressive or deteriorating neurological symptoms of nerve root compression or symptoms of cord compression would require immediate onward referral.

Radiography and Medical Imaging

X-rays are the first choice following a traumatic elbow injury as this helps to establish initial injury and any associated fractures or dislocations. These results will also provide information on postreduction alignment that will help guide rehabilitation and indicate the likely prognosis. Other medical tests may include blood tests, magnetic resonance imaging or a bone scan.

History of the Present Condition

For each symptomatic area, the clinician needs to know how long the symptoms have been present. Did these symptoms develop suddenly or gradually? Was there a known cause that provoked the onset of the symptoms? If the onset of symptoms was associated with trauma, e.g. a fall, the clinician establishes how the patient fell. Did the patient fall on the outstretched hand, possibly fracturing the radial head, or on the tip of the elbow, injuring the olecranon? If associated with a throwing action, did the patient feel a 'pop', which may indicate an acute ligamentous injury? (Cain et al. 2003)?

Elbow ligamentous injuries can result from acute injuries such as a dislocation or fracture, or chronic from repetitive overloading, possibly leading to chronic recurrent instability. Three elbow instabilities occur: posterolateral rotatory instability is the most common and usually occurs as a consequence of previous dislocation or fracture. Medial collateral instability is more common than an isolated lateral elbow instability due to its vulnerability in overhead throwing positions. Patients with ligament instability may report a diffuse ache and other symptoms, such as clicking, snapping, clunking and apprehension in certain positions. If these are noted then part of the examination should include judicious use of joint integrity and ligament tests (Aviles et al. 2008).

If the onset was gradual, consider if the development of symptoms is associated with a change in the patient's lifestyle, e.g. a new job or leisure activity or a change in sporting activity. To confirm the relationship of symptoms, the clinician asks what happened when symptoms first began and how over time symptoms have developed or changed. In addition the clinician needs to identify what treatment, if any, the patient has sought so far and its outcome. Is this the first episode or is there a history of elbow problems? If so, how many episodes? When were they? Was there a cause? What was the duration of each episode? Did the patient fully recover between episodes? If there have been no previous episodes, has the patient had any episodes of stiffness in the cervical spine, thoracic spine, shoulder, elbow, wrist, hand or any other relevant region?

When all this information has been collected, the subjective examination is complete. For ease of reference highlight with asterisks (*) important subjective findings and one or more functional restrictions. These can be reexamined at subsequent treatment sessions to evaluate treatment intervention.

Plan of the Physical Examination

During the subjective examination the clinician will begin to form hypotheses based on verbal and non-verbal communication. This information enables the clinician to plan the physical examination whilst addressing the following key questions.

Precautions and Contraindications

The clinician must first establish whether the patient has a musculoskeletal dysfunction and then identify whether this musculoskeletal dysfunction is suitable for manual and exercise therapy. Within the elbow, specific contraindications and precautions may include recent fracture, trauma, suspicion of myositis ossificans, long-term steroid therapy or rheumatoid arthritis. Beyond the elbow, contraindications such as neurological nerve root compression with deteriorating symptoms or symptoms of cord compression will also need consideration. Identifying and reviewing any precautions or contraindications will indicate if caution is needed and help the clinician decide on the sequencing, extent and suitability of clinical examination tests. It will also identify if onward referral is required (e.g. high suspicion of an undiagnosed fracture). The elbow extension test can be used as a screening test for suspected fractures, confirming the need for onward referral/radiological evaluation (Appleboam et al. 2008).

Developing Working and Alternative Hypotheses

Based on the subjective information the clinician's clinical reasoning will help to identify a prioritized list of working hypotheses and possible sources/structures (arthrogenic, myogenic and neurogenic) that could be the cause of the patient's symptoms. The possible sources may include the structures underneath the symptomatic area, e.g. joints, muscles, nerves and fascia, as well as the regions referring into the area. Proximal and distal regions which refer to the area may need to be examined as a possible cause of symptoms, e.g. cervical spine, thoracic spine, shoulder and wrist and hand. In complex cases it is not always possible to examine fully at the first attendance and so, using clinical reasoning skills, the clinician will need to prioritize and justify what 'must' be examined in the first assessment session and what 'should' or 'could' be followed up at subsequent sessions. Table 10.2 shows a suggested planning sheet for use in clinical reasoning of the 'must', 'should' and 'could'.

What Is the Predominant Pain Mechanism?

Pain has been classified into nociceptive (mechanical, inflammatory or ischaemic), peripheral neuropathic pain, central sensitization and autonomic (van Griensven 2014). The subjective examination should enable the clinician to reason clinically the symptoms' predominant pain mechanism. For example, localized intraarticular pain at the end range of elbow extension is likely to be due to a mechanical nociceptive pain mechanism. A patient who thinks that pain is harmful may demonstrate fear avoidance behaviours.

TABLE 10.2		
Must, Should and Could List of Planning[a]		
Must	**Should**	**Could**

■ Observation (informal and formal)
■ Posture: cervical and thoracic spine, shoulder/shoulder girdle, elbow, wrist and hand.
■ Body chart and relationship of symptoms
■ Brief appraisal of cervical and thoracic spine active range
■ Brief appraisal of shoulder/shoulder girdle position and relationship to elbow
■ Functional demonstration
■ Active range of movements, noting range, quality and symptom response
■ Flexion
■ Extension
■ Supination
■ Pronation
■ Passive range of movements, noting range, quality and symptom response
■ Flexion, flexion abduction and flexion adduction
■ Extension, extension abduction and extension adduction
■ Palpate elbow structures:
  ■ Olecranon and fossa, humeroulnar, humeroradial and superior radioulnar joint
  ■ Anterior capsule, collateral ligaments, annular ligament
  ■ Relevant nerve palpation points for ulnar, radial and median nerves
  ■ Flexor and extensor muscle insertions
  ■ Common flexor and extensor tendons
■ Accessory movements
■ Muscle testing, including grip assessment, length and strength tests
■ Ligamentous testing
	■ Brief appraisal of shoulder, wrist and hand active movements
	■ Neural and neurodynamic tests
		■ Differentiation testing – neural, arthrogenic and myogenic
		■ Brief appraisal of the thoracic spine active movements
		■ Passive physiological and accessory intervertebral movements of cervical/thoracic spine.

[a]Tests would be selected depending on the type of dysfunction/condition and therefore would be prioritized according to the presenting patient's symptoms.

Psychosocial factors may enhance the patient's pain experience and therefore understanding what patients think about their pain and how it makes them feel is important. Clearly establishing which pain mechanisms may be causing and/or maintaining the condition will help the clinician manage both the condition and the patient appropriately.

Sequence and Extent of Physical Tests

The severity, irritability and nature of the condition are the key factors that will influence the choice and priority of physical testing procedures. If symptoms are severe, physical tests may be carried out to just before or to the initial onset of symptom production.

No overpressures will be carried out. If symptoms are irritable, physical tests may be examined to just before or to initial symptom production with fewer physical tests being examined. If the patient has constant and severe and/or irritable symptoms, then the clinician aims to find physical tests that ease the symptoms. If the patient's symptoms are non-severe and non-irritable, then the clinician aims to find physical tests that reproduce each of the patient's symptoms and these may include the use of combined, sustained or repetitive movements.

The planning of the physical examination should provide the clinician with a clear outline of examination which is safe and purposeful.

PHYSICAL EXAMINATION

The clinician should have a preferred primary clinical hypothesis after the subjective examination and the purpose of the physical examination is to confirm or refute this hypothesis. The physical planning sheet should clearly outline what needs to be examined. The order and detail of the physical tests described below will need to be modified for the patient being examined; some tests will be irrelevant, some tests will be carried out briefly, while it will be necessary to investigate others more fully. It is important to recognize that the techniques shown in this chapter are not exhaustive and that there are many modifications and variations which can be used. It is also important to understand that the reliability, sensitivity and specificity will vary between all physical tests (see Chapter 3). The diagnostic accuracy of the elbow tests which have good evidence to support their use has been presented and this may be helpful for the clinician in appraising the usefulness of the clinical test. Each significant physical test that either provokes or eases the patient's symptoms is highlighted in the patient's notes by an asterisk (*) for easy reference.

Observation

Informal Observation

Informal observation occurs throughout the consultation. The clinician should observe the patient in dynamic and static situations, and assess the patient's ability and willingness to move the upper limb, the quality of movement and any associated facial expressions.

Formal Observation

This is particularly useful in helping to determine the presence of predisposing factors such as abnormal bony alignments, preferred patterns of muscle use and observation of resting muscle lengths.

Observation of Posture. The clinician assesses the bony landmarks and soft-tissue contours of the elbow region, as well as the patient's neck and head posture and alignment of the shoulder girdle in both sitting and standing. Careful examination of the neck and shoulder should be performed in elbow pain of insidious onset so as to exclude possible referral of symptoms. Poor posture of the neck, trunk and upper limbs, e.g. tight pectoralis minor and weak lower trapezius, has been identified in sports people with elbow pathology (Wilke et al. 2002). The clinician should attempt to modify the patient's posture and note any change in the patient's symptoms. Similarly, the clinician should always correct any faulty shoulder alignments first and note the effect on the elbow and forearm alignment and or pain. This will help determine if the elbow alignment is a result of a proximal dysfunction/impairment, e.g. a winging or anteriorly tilted scapula (Caldwell & Khoo-Summers 2010).

Observation of Bony Alignment. The clinician may initially observe the relative position of the olecranon and the medial and lateral epicondyles. They should form a straight line with the elbow in extension and an isosceles triangle with the elbow in 90° flexion (Fig. 10.1) (Magee 2014). Anatomical and gender variations of the distal humerus do exist which may alter this alignment; however, gross alterations in this positioning may indicate a fracture or dislocation.

In standing normal alignment of the elbow and forearm includes slight elbow flexion, neutral forearm rotation with thumb facing anteriorly with the palm oriented towards the body. The clinician can assess

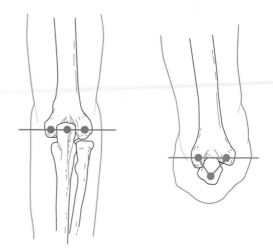

FIG. 10.1 The position of the olecranon and medial and lateral epicondyles should form a straight line with the elbow in extension and an isosceles triangle with the elbow flexed to 90°. *(From Magee 2014, with permission.)*

the carrying angle of the elbow by placing the patient's arm in the anatomical position. The normal carrying angle is 5–10° in males and 10–15° in females; >15° is cubital valgus and <5–10° is cubital varus (Magee 2014). The carrying angle should be symmetrical on each side. A fracture of the distal humerus may result in a cubital varus and is sometimes known as a gun stock deformity. Cubital varus and valgus may also result from collateral ligament instability.

The patient should be able to achieve the functional positon of the elbow, which is 90° of flexion with forearm in midway of supination and pronation. Habitual flexion and extension elbow postures are also noted. Hyperextension of up to −5/−10° in the elbow, especially in females, can be normal. Increased resting elbow extension may be a result of hyperextension/lax anterior capsule, small olecranon, weakness or decreased stiffness of elbow flexors. If the patient demonstrates increased elbow hyperextension then screening for generalized hypermobility should be considered (Simmonds & Keer 2007). Decreased resting elbow flexion may suggest short or overactive elbow flexors.

Observation of Swelling. Swelling at the elbow can occur within the joint or be discrete. Since the elbow joints share a capsule, joint swelling will affect all three joints and the elbow may be held in a semiflexed position (approximately 70°). On the lateral aspect of the elbow intraarticular swelling may be noted in the triangular space between the lateral epicondyle, head of the radius and tip of the olecranon. Posteriorly discrete swelling of the olecranon bursa may be observed (Magee 2014). An infected olecranon bursa may be associated with fever and erythema.

Observation of Muscle Form. The clinician examines the muscle bulk and muscle tone of the patient, comparing left and right sides. It must be remembered that handedness and level and frequency of physical activity may well produce differences in muscle bulk between sides.

Functional Testing

Informal and formal observation would already include some assessment of functional ability. Normal functional elbow position is often described as 90° flexion with the forearm in midposition between pronation and supination. However, many functional activities will involve elbow flexion or extension in combination with pronation and supination. Clues for assessment of suitable functional movements can be obtained from the subjective examination findings or patient-reported outcome measures or questionnaires such as the Patient Rated Elbow Evaluation (PREE), the American Shoulder and Elbow Surgeons Elbow Index (ASES-e) (King et al. 1999) and DASH (The et al. 2013). Asking the patient to demonstrate a simple functional task such as eating will help provide invaluable clues as to the potential structures involved. For example, eating involves elbow flexion (up to 120°), supination (for positioning a spoon or fork) and shoulder flexion. Any elbow flexion or extension deficits will quickly become apparent. Other examples of functional activities may include using the arm to rise out of a chair, throwing an object, gripping and carrying a briefcase.

Active Physiological Movements

Flexion and extension are the primary movements that occur at the humeroulnar and humeroradial joints. Pronation and supination are predominantly centred around the superior/inferior radioulnar joints, although there will be some contribution from the humeroradial joint (Magee 2014). Active physiological movements of the elbow complex should be performed first, comparing right and left sides, and be sequenced so that the most painful movements are performed last. The clinician establishes symptoms at rest prior to each movement, and corrects any compensatory movement to determine its relevance to the patient's symptoms. Active physiological movements of the elbow and forearm and possible modifications are shown in Table 10.3. The clinician notes the following:

- range of movement
- quality of movement – can the patient perform the movement without compensations? For example, compensatory shoulder adduction and abduction can occur during supination and pronation respectively, giving the appearance of a normal range

TABLE 10.3
Active Physiological Movements and Possible Modifications

Active physiological movements
Elbow flexion
Elbow extension
Forearm pronation
Forearm supination
Possible modifications to physiological movements
Repeated
Speed altered
Combined movements and sequencing, e.g.

■ Elbow flexion with pronation or supination
■ Elbow pronation with elbow flexion or extension
Added compression or distraction, e.g.

■ Compression to humeroulnar joint in / during flexion
Sustained
Injuring movement
Differentiation tests
Functional movements
Identify any effect of the modifications of physiological movements on patient's signs and symptoms
Reassess all *asterisks
If necessary screen any proximal and distal regions that may refer to the area
Cervical spine
Thoracic spine
Shoulder
Wrist and hand

■ behaviour of pain through the range of movement
■ resistance through the range of movement and at the end of the range of movement
■ provocation of any muscle spasm or apprehension which may be indicative of ligament instability.

Where appropriate, active movements can be tested with overpressure with the patient lying supine or sitting (Fig. 10.2).

Symptom Modification or Differentiation Testing

Various differentiation tests (Hengeveld et al. 2014) can be performed and selection will depend on the patient's signs and symptoms. For example, when elbow flexion reproduces the patient's elbow pain, differentiation between the humeroradial and humeroulnar joint may be required. In this case, the clinician takes the elbow into flexion to produce the symptoms and then in turn adds a compression force through the radius and then through the ulna by radial and ulnar deviation of the wrist and compares the pain response in each case (Fig. 10.3). If symptoms are from the radioulnar joint, for example, then the patient may feel an increase in pain when compression is applied to the humeroradial joint but not when compression is applied to the humeroulnar joint. The converse would occur for the humeroulnar joint.

It may be necessary to examine other regions to determine their relevance to the patient's symptoms; they may be the source of the symptoms, or they may be contributing to the symptoms. The most likely regions are the shoulder, cervical spine, thoracic spine, wrist and hand. The joints within these regions can be tested fully (see relevant chapter) or partially with the use of screening tests provided in Chapter 3.

Passive Physiological Movements

All active movements described above can be examined passively with the patient usually in supine, comparing left and right sides. In addition to these movements, passive ranges of flexion and extension can be combined with adduction and abduction, to explore the joint fully. The few degrees of abduction and adduction occur as a result of the incongruent joint surfaces of the humeroulnar and humeroradial joint. Loss of these subtle degrees of movement has been found in patients with lateral epicondylalgia and extension-related pain (Hyland et al. 1990; Lockard 2006). The clinician feels through range for restriction and/or reproduction of symptoms and assesses end-feel of the joint in the following movements (Fig. 10.4):

■ abduction
■ adduction
■ flexion/abduction
■ flexion/adduction
■ extension/abduction
■ extension/adduction.

Joint Integrity Tests

Joint integrity tests are included in the assessment when the subjective history suggests an instability

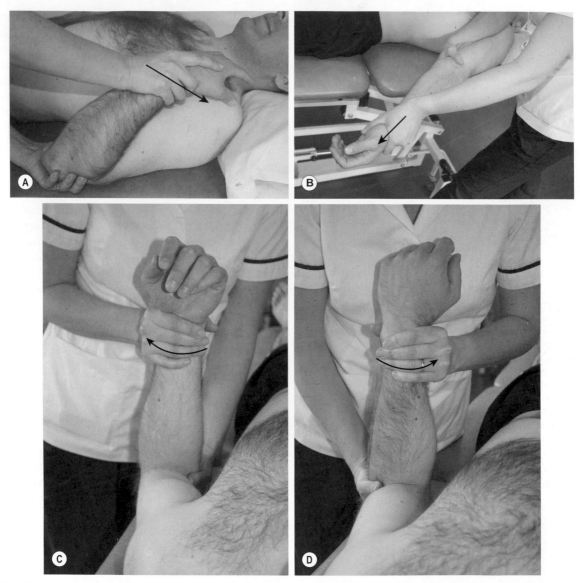

FIG. 10.2 Overpressures to the elbow complex. (A) Flexion. The left hand supports underneath the elbow while the right hand flexes the elbow. (B) Extension. The right hand supports underneath the elbow while the left hand extends the elbow. (C) Supination. (D) Pronation. The arrows represent the direction of the clinician's force.

(clicking, loss of control or performance). Medial, lateral and posterolateral rotatory instabilities exist. For all of the joint integrity tests below, a positive test is traditionally indicated by excessive movement relative to the unaffected side. However in the presence of laxity, 'patient apprehension' should also be considered positive and the patient referred for further testing, e.g.

magnetic resonance imaging and passive examination under anaesthesia.

Medial Collateral Ligament Testing

THE VALGUS TEST. The integrity of the medial (ulnar) collateral ligament (MCL) is tested by applying an abduction force to the forearm with the elbow in

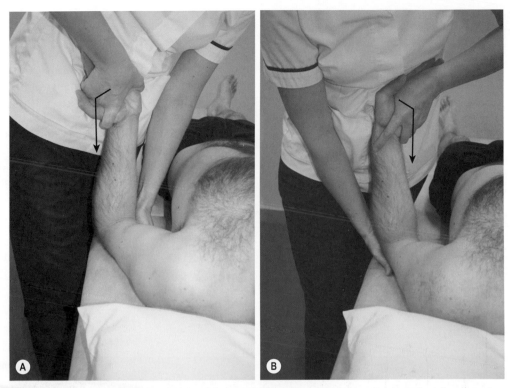

FIG. 10.3 Differentiation test between the humeroradial and humeroulnar joint. The clinician takes the elbow into flexion to produce the symptoms and then in turn adds a compression force through the radius (A) and then the ulna (B) by taking the wrist into radial and ulnar deviation respectively. The arrows represent the direction of the clinician's force.

20–30° flexion, to unlock olecranon from the fossa and the forearm in supination. The clinician should use one hand to stabilize the humerus in external rotation, thereby ensuring that the tension is directed at the MCL. No diagnostic accuracy studies of this test have been performed to determine the sensitivity and specificity values (Fig. 10.4E).

The moving valgus stress test examines the MCL through range (Fig. 10.5). In the seated position, the clinician externally rotates and abducts the shoulder to 90° and then passively extends the elbow whilst simultaneously applying a constant valgus force. Medial elbow pain between an arc of 120° and 70° of elbow flexion is considered a positive test (O'Driscoll et al. 2005). The moving valgus stress test for MCL tears of the elbow has been found to be sensitive (100%) and specific (75%), with likelihood ratios (LRs) of LR+ 4 and LR– 0 in a small population study by O'Driscoll et al. (2005). This suggests that the test is highly

sensitive within a similar population group of predominantly males with a sporting background.

Lateral Collateral Ligament Testing

The lateral (radial) collateral ligament is tested by applying an adduction force to the forearm with the elbow in 20–30° flexion, to unlock the olecranon from the fossa. The clinician should use one hand to stabilize the humerus in internal rotation. Quality of end-feel, excessive movement or reproduction of the patient's symptoms is a positive test and suggests instability of the elbow joint (Volz & Morrey 1993). No diagnostic accuracy studies of this test have been performed to determine the sensitivity and specificity values.

POSTEROLATERAL PIVOT SHIFT APPREHENSION TEST (O'DRISCOLL ET AL. 1991). Recurrent posterolateral instability of the elbow can be difficult to diagnose and requires a careful history and physical examination. A provocative test is used to investigate the presence of instability and therefore care should always be taken. There is much debate as to the structures responsible for posterolateral instability; however, the lateral portion of the ulnar collateral ligament is often cited as a primary culprit. For the test, the patient lies supine with the arm raised above the head whilst the clinician grasps the patient's wrist and elbow (Fig. 10.6). A supination and axial compression force is applied through the wrist. The elbow is then flexed to 20° whilst a valgus stress is applied to the forearm. Patient apprehension with increasing flexion (usually between 40° and 70°) indicates a positive test. Posterolateral rotatory instability results from a rotatory subluxation of the radius and ulna relative to the humerus. No diagnostic accuracy studies of this test have been performed to determine the sensitivity and specificity values.

Muscle Tests

Muscle tests include examining muscle strength, length and isometric muscle testing. The muscles that need to be tested will depend on the area of symptoms, the functional aggravating movements and observed postures. The common diagnostic muscle tests used in the clinical practice of the elbow, such as the Mills test or passive tennis elbow test, medial and lateral epicondylalgia tests, have not been studied for diagnostic accuracy. The tests suggested are commonly advocated by consensus and expert opinion. See Chapter 3 for details of muscle testing.

Muscle Strength

A complete assessment of a muscle's strength would include the clinician testing the muscle isotonically through the available range. During the physical

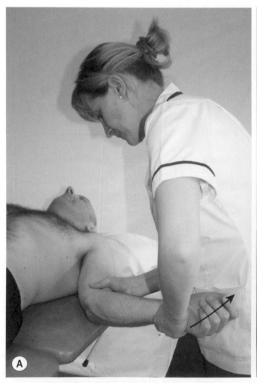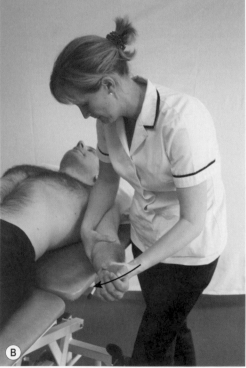

FIG. 10.4 Passive physiological movements to the elbow complex. (A) Abduction. The right hand stabilizes the humerus while the left hand abducts the forearm. (B) Adduction. The right hand stabilizes the humerus while the left hand adducts the forearm.

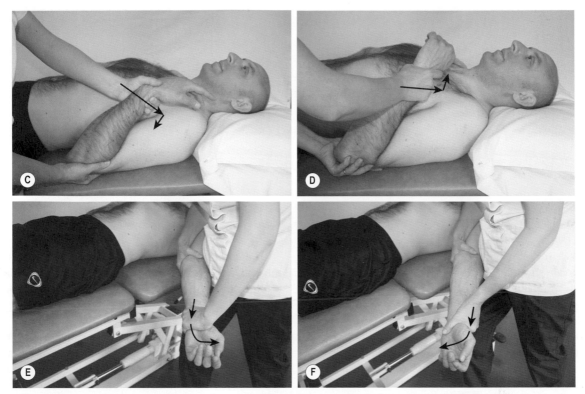

FIG. 10.4, cont'd ■ (C) Flexion/abduction. The right hand supports underneath the upper arm while the left hand takes the arm into flexion and abduction. (D) Flexion/adduction. The left hand supports underneath the upper arm while the right hand takes the arm into flexion and adduction. (E) Extension/abduction. The right hand supports underneath the upper arm while the left hand takes the arm into extension and abduction. (F) Extension/adduction. The right hand supports underneath the upper arm while the left hand takes the forearm into extension and adduction. The arrows represent the direction of the clinician's force.

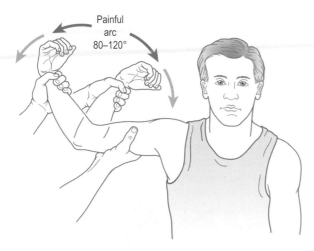

FIG. 10.5 Moving valgus stress test. *(From Magee et al. 2009, with permission.)*

examination of the elbow, it may be appropriate to test the elbow flexors/extensors, pronators and supinators, wrist flexors, extensors, radial deviators and ulnar deviators and any other relevant muscle groups of relevant regions.

For further details of these tests readers are directed to Kendall et al. (2010) and Hislop et al. (2013). Details of strength testing are also given in Chapter 3.

Muscle Length

To determine if the muscles of the elbow, wrist and hand are tight, passive muscle length tests are performed. The outcome of the length test may be affected by factors such as starting position of shoulder, elbow and forearm and whether the muscles are two-joint muscles. For example, passive tension in the triceps

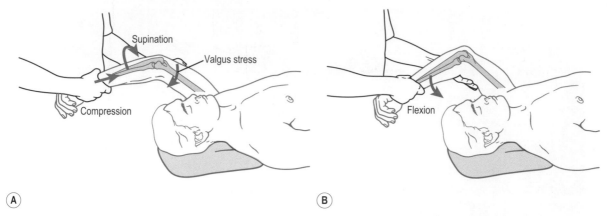

FIG. 10.6 (A, B) Posterolateral instability test. *(From Magee et al. 2008, with permission.)*

muscle may limit elbow flexion if the test starting position is in shoulder flexion or if the shoulder simultaneously moves into flexion during the test. To test triceps, the patient should be tested in sitting with the arm passively taken into full shoulder elevation while the elbow is extended. The elbow is then passively flexed and range and end-feel of elbow flexion noted.

The clinician tests for lateral epicondylalgia by stretching the extensor muscles of the wrist and hand. This is done by extending the elbow, pronating the forearm and then flexing the wrist and fingers (Mills test or passive elbow tennis elbow test). A positive test (i.e. muscle shortening) is indicated if the patient's symptoms are reproduced or if range of movement is limited compared with the other side. This position will, however, also load the radial nerve and so if positive a neural component may be suspected and the addition of neural sensitizers, such as shoulder girdle depression, may be added to confirm or negate (Butler 2000).

The length of the flexor muscles of the wrist and hand should be tested, especially if medial epicondylalgia is suspected. In supine with the elbow extended, the clinician passively supinates the forearm and then extends the wrist and fingers. A positive test is indicated if the patient's symptoms are reproduced or if the range of movement is limited compared with the other side. This position will also load the median nerve and, if positive, the clinician will need to consider a neural component and look at the addition of neural sensitizers such as cervical lateral flexion (Butler 2000).

The clinician may need to test the length of other muscles in the upper quadrant and further descriptions of the tests for muscle length are given in Chapter 3.

Isometric Muscle Testing

The clinician tests the elbow flexors, extensors, forearm pronators, supinators, wrist flexors, extensors, radial deviators and ulnar deviators (and any other relevant muscle group) in resting position, in different parts of the physiological range and, if indicated, in sustained positions with or without load. In the elbow, the greatest amount of isometric elbow flexion is found in the position of 90–100° with the forearm supinated. Elbow flexion ranges above or below this position significantly reduce the available isometric power (Magee 2014). The clinician notes the strength and quality of the contraction, as well as any reproduction of the patient's symptoms. Fig. 10.7 demonstrates basic isometric elbow and wrist muscle strength tests.

Special Tests

Repeated microtrauma to the common flexor and extensor origins produces degenerative changes within the tendon, resulting in persistent symptoms. Common provocative tests are commonly used; however, no diagnostic accuracy studies are available to determine the values of sensitivity and specificity for these tests (Cook & Hegedus 2013).

Common provocative tests are as follows.

Lateral Epicondylalgia (Tennis Elbow Tests). Pain over the lateral epicondyle accompanying gripping and

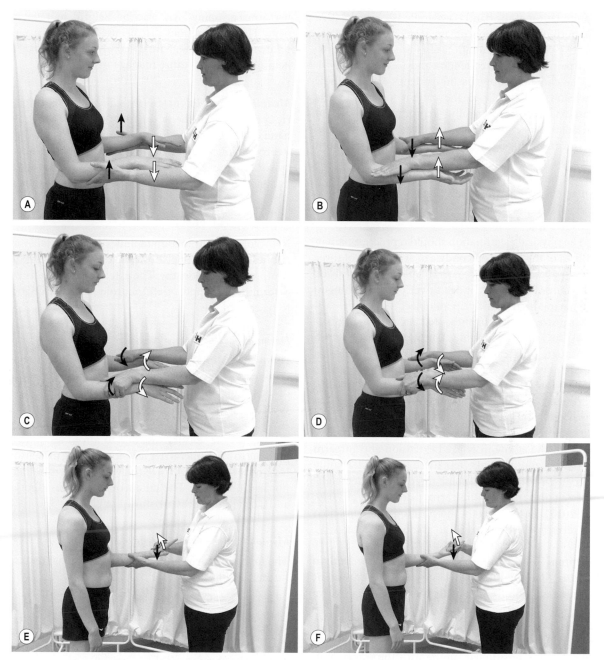

FIG. 10.7 Positioning for isometric resisted movements. Black arrows indicate clinician's direction of resistance and white arrows represent the patient's action. (A) Elbow extension. (B) Elbow flexion. (C) Elbow/forearm supination. (D) Elbow/forearm pronation. (E) Wrist extension. (F) Wrist flexion.

manipulation of the hand is generally associated with a diagnosis of tennis elbow or lateral epicondylalgia. Provocative clinical examination tests are used to reproduce pain in the affected tendon and are as follows.

The clinician supports the patient's arm in elbow extension and then asks the patient to contract the wrist extensors isometrically – reproduction of pain at the lateral aspect of the elbow indicates a positive test. Variations of this test exist. For example, the basic test can be sensitized by an isometric contraction or extension of the third proximal interphalangeal joint activating extensor carpi radialis brevis – reproduction of pain or weakness over the lateral epicondyle indicates a positive test.

The physical examination should reproduce pain in the area of the lateral epicondyle in at least one of three ways: palpation of the lateral epicondyle; resisted extension of the wrist, index finger or middle finger; and having the patient grip an object.

Grip strength can be measured using a dynamometer to provide some baseline quantitative data on which to evaluate progress. Left and right sides can be compared but variance due to hand dominance will need to be accounted for. The painfree grip test is a reliable, valid and sensitive measure of the physical or functional impairment of lateral epicondylalgia (Coombes et al. 2009). Most protocols recommend performing the test with the elbow in relaxed extension and forearm pronation, repeating the test three times at 1-minute intervals. The average of these three tests is then compared against the uninjured arm (Coombes et al. 2009; Lim 2013). Ensure that the test position is documented as alternative test positions can also be used.

Symptom Modification for Lateral Epicondylalgia (Tennis Elbow). Although largely seen as treatment techniques, mobilization with movements can serve as a useful differentiation tool. In the elbow, accessory glides to the humeroulnar joint and the radial head may reduce pain during gripping activities. To test, the patient is positioned supine with the upper limb fully supported and holding a grip dynamometer. The clinician applies a lateral glide to the humeroulnar joint as the patient actively grips (Fig. 10.8). For patients with suspected tennis elbow, pain relief is a positive finding. Similarly, applying a posteroanterior glide to the radial head while the patient performs gripping may also be helpful in relieving pain. These techniques can be used to confirm and refute hypotheses of lateral epicondylalgia and may be helpful in guiding future management.

Medial Epicondylalgia (Golfer's Elbow Test). Isometric contraction of the flexor muscles of the wrist and hand can be examined for common flexor origin pain. Reproduction of pain or weakness over the medial epicondyle indicates a positive test. Tenderness on palpation of the area will also help confirm a diagnosis.

Neurological Tests

Neurological examination includes neurological integrity testing, neural sensitization tests and testing for compression neuropathy. The extent of symptoms will determine the appropriate neurological examination to be carried out.

Dermatomes/Peripheral Nerves

Following trauma or compression to peripheral nerves, it is vital to assess the cutaneous sensation. Knowledge of the cutaneous distribution of nerve roots (dermatomes) and peripheral nerves – radial (C5–T1), median (C5–T1) and ulnar (C7–T1) – enables the clinician to distinguish the sensory loss due to a root lesion from that due to a peripheral nerve lesion. Testing for sensory loss must therefore involve the whole upper limb and not just the elbow. The cutaneous nerve distribution and dermatome areas are shown in Chapter 3.

Myotomes/Peripheral Nerves

The following myotomes are tested (see Chapter 3 for further details):

- C4: shoulder girdle elevation
- C5: shoulder abduction
- C6: elbow flexion
- C7: elbow extension
- C8: thumb extension
- T1: finger adduction.

A working knowledge of the muscular distribution of nerve roots (myotomes) and peripheral nerves enables the clinician to distinguish motor loss due to a root lesion from that due to a peripheral nerve lesion.

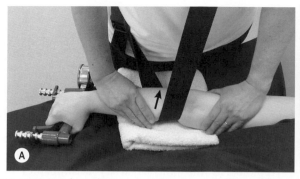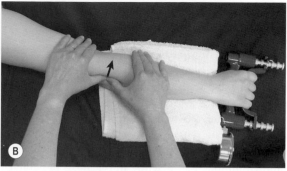

FIG. 10.8 (A) Lateral elbow mobilization with movement. The clinician applies a sustained lateral humeroulnar accessory glide while the patient grips and relaxes the dynamometer or performs the painful action. If there is significant improvement in the painfree grip then the clinician repeats the technique for 6–10 repetitions. A belt as in the example may be used to assist the accessory glide. (B) Radial head posteroanterior mobilization with movement. The clinician applies a sustained posterior–anterior accessory glide over the radial head whilst the patient grips and relaxes the dynamometer or performs the painful action. If there is significant improvement in the painfree grip then the clinician repeats the technique for 6–10 repetitions. The arrows represent the direction of the clinician's force.

The peripheral nerve distributions are shown in Chapter 3.

Reflex Testing

The following deep tendon reflexes are tested (see Chapter 3 for further details):

- C5–C6: biceps
- C6: brachioradialis
- C7: triceps.

Neurodynamic Tests

The upper-limb neurodynamic tests (1, 2a, 2b and 3) may be carried out in order to ascertain the degree to which neural tissue is responsible for the production of the patient's elbow symptom(s). These tests are described in detail in Chapter 3.

Testing for Compression Neuropathy

Compression neuropathies are common in the elbow. Ulnar neuropathy of the elbow is the second most common entrapment neuropathy in the upper extremity.

Ulnar Nerve Compression Neuropathy Tests. Ulnar neuropathy can be caused by habitual and repetitive activities (such as leaning on the elbows), trauma,

including fractures and dislocations, rheumatic and degenerative joint disease and immobilization during surgery.

TINEL'S TEST. At the elbow Tinel's test is most useful during the middle stages of the condition where a positive test will indicate the presence of sensory nerve regeneration distal to the site of compression. Using a reflex hammer, the clinician taps the cord-like ulnar nerve where it lies in the groove between the olecranon and the medial epicondyle and repeats four to six times. A positive sign is indicated by paraesthesia in the distribution of the ulnar nerve (Hattam & Smeatham 2010; Magee 2014). Novak et al. (1994) investigated the diagnostic accuracy of this test and found values of 70% for sensitivity and 98% for specificity in a small population group. This suggests that it may be a useful test in helping to diagnose cubital tunnel syndrome when included in the clinical examination and combined with the patient history.

ELBOW FLEXION TEST FOR CUBITAL TUNNEL SYNDROME. The cubital tunnel is formed by a tendinous arch connecting humeral and ulnar heads of flexor carpi ulnaris approximately 1–2 cm distal to the medial epicondyle. During elbow flexion, the cubital tunnel narrows, causing an increase in pressure on the nerve. To test for cubital tunnel syndrome the patient sits with elbow fully flexed with the forearm in supination and wrist in neutral for at least 1 minute.

Variations in both the test position and the length of hold recommended do exist; however, sustained elbow flexion is common to all. A positive sign is indicated by paraesthesia or numbness in the distribution of the ulnar nerve (Buehler & Thayer 1988). The sensitivity of elbow flexion with a hold of 30 seconds has been demonstrated by Novak et al. (1994) at just 32% and this increases to 75% with a hold of 60 seconds. This low to moderate sensitivity suggests that the clinical examination needs to be combined with the subjective examination to aid sufficiently in diagnosis of cubital tunnel syndrome. The most sensitive provocative test in the diagnosis of cubital tunnel syndrome was elbow flexion with a hold of 60 seconds when combined with pressure on the ulnar nerve (sensitivity 98% and specificity 95%; Novak et al. 1994).

Median Nerve Compression Neuropathy Tests.
Median nerve entrapment is less common in the elbow; however, proximal injury is well described, particularly around the origin of the anterior interosseous nerve (anterior interosseous syndrome), around pronator teres (pronator syndrome) or at the ligament of Struthers (supracondylar process syndrome). Common provocative tests are commonly used; however, no diagnostic accuracy studies are available to determine the sensitivity and specificity for these particular tests (Cook & Hegedus 2013).

PINCH-GRIP TEST. This tests for anterior interosseous nerve entrapment (anterior interosseous syndrome) between the two heads of pronator teres muscle (Magee 2014). The test is considered positive if the patient is unable actively to pinch the tips of the distal interphalangeal joints of the index finger and thumb together. Symptoms and findings are mainly motor and sensory loss should not be observed. The test is also known as the OK sign.

TEST FOR PRONATOR SYNDROME. With the elbow flexed to 90°, the clinician resists pronation as the elbow is extended. Tingling in the distribution of the median nerve is a positive test. This involves compression of the median nerve just proximal to the formation of the anterior interosseous nerve (Magee 2014). In addition to the anterior interosseous syndrome, described previously, the flexor carpi radialis, palmaris longus and flexor digitorum muscles are affected, thus weakening grip strength; there is also sensory loss in the distribution of the median nerve.

TEST FOR SUPRACONDYLAR PROCESS SYNDROME. This test involves compression or entrapment of the median nerve as it passes under the ligament of Struthers which connects the medial epicondyle to the distal humerus. This ligament is rare and found in less than 3% of individuals and typically will only be problematic following trauma. Pain is reproduced on elbow, wrist or finger extension or forearm supination. In addition pinch and grip weakness may be present (Ay et al. 2002). There may also be associated vascular symptoms as the brachial artery accompanies the nerve.

Radial Nerve Compression Neuropathy Test. The posterior interosseous nerve which is a branch of the radial nerve may be injured at the elbow as it passes through the supinator (arcade of Frohse), causing posterior interosseous nerve syndrome. Posterior interosseous nerve syndrome may occur secondary to fracture or subluxation of proximal radius and repetitive pronation and supination activities.

TEST FOR RADIAL TUNNEL SYNDROME. This involves compression of the posterior interosseous nerve between the two supinator heads in the arcade of Frohse (found in 30% of the population) (Magee 2014). Forearm extensor muscles may be affected, resulting in a functional wrist drop. Weakness may also occur, during finger extension; there are usually no sensory symptoms. This syndrome can mimic lateral epicondylalgia.

Vascular Considerations in Examination and Assessment

Palpation of Pulses

The incidence of elbow neurovascular injury is rare but may occur following elbow dislocation and reduction. Cyanosis, pallor, lack of pulses and marked pain may suggest vascular injury or possible compartment syndrome. If compromised circulation is suspected then palpate the brachial artery pulse on the medial aspect of the humerus in the axilla and in the cubital fossa and check the radial artery pulse at the wrist (Carter et al. 2010).

Palpation

The structures in the elbow region are relatively superficial and hence readily accessible to palpation. Sound knowledge of anatomy and structural relations will help the clinician to conduct a systematic and informative examination, whilst noting the following:

- the temperature of the area
- the presence of oedema or effusion; this can be measured using a tape measure and comparing left and right sides
- mobility and feel of superficial tissues, e.g. ganglions, nodules and scar tissue
- the presence or elicitation of any muscle spasm and local trigger points in supinator/ brachioradialis/pronator teres
- pain provoked or reduced on palpation; positive Tinel's sign on nerve palpation
- crepitus or clicking.

Suggested Approach to Systematic Palpation

- Anteriorly: palpate the cubital fossa, biceps tendon, median nerve medial to the biceps tendon and brachial artery, coronoid process of ulna and head of the radius – the radial head is confirmed by pronation and supination of the forearm.
- Medially: palpate wrist flexor pronator muscles, fan-shaped MCL and the ulnar nerve posterior to medial epicondyle.
- Laterally: palpate wrist extensors, brachioradialis and supinator, cord-like lateral collateral ligament and annular ligament.
- Posteriorly – palpate the olecranon process in 90° flexion: triceps and anconeus tendon insertions.

Common palpation findings:

- On the medial aspect of the elbow, a thickened ulnar nerve may be palpable in cases of ulnar nerve neuropathy.
- On the lateral aspect of the elbow, fullness in the infracondylar fold may indicate synovial proliferation or an increase in synovial fluid and tenderness of the lateral epicondyle/common extensor tendon is typical of lateral epicondylalgia
- On the posterior aspect, the olecranon bursa, if inflamed, may be palpable and visible. Rheumatoid nodules may be present on the posteromedial aspect of the elbow.

The cervical spine and thoracic spine, shoulder, wrist and hand should also be palpated as appropriate. It is useful to record palpation findings on a body chart (see Fig. 2.3) and/or palpation chart (see Fig. 3.35).

Accessory Movements

It is useful to use the palpation chart and movement diagrams (or joint pictures) to record findings. These are explained in detail in Chapter 3.

The clinician notes the:

- quality of movement
- range of movement
- resistance through the range and at the end of the range of movement
- behaviour of pain through the range
- provocation of any muscle spasm.

Humeroulnar joint (Fig. 10.9), humeroradial joint (Fig. 10.10), superior radioulnar joint (Fig. 10.11) and inferior radioulnar (Fig. 10.12) joint accessory movements are listed in Table 10.4. Note that each of these accessory movements will move more than one of the joints in the elbow complex – a medial glide on the olecranon, for example, will cause movement at the superior radioulnar joint as well as the humeroulnar joint.

Following accessory movements to the elbow region, the clinician reassesses all the physical asterisks (movements or tests that have been found to reproduce the patient's symptoms) in order to establish the effect of the accessory movements on the patient's signs and symptoms. Accessory movements can then be tested for other regions suspected to be a source of or contributing to the patient's symptoms. Again, following accessory movements to any one region the clinician reassesses all the asterisks. Regions likely to be examined are the cervical spine, thoracic spine, shoulder, wrist and hand (Table 10.4).

Completion of the Examination

On completion of the physical examination, the clinician will need to collate the information to evaluate and revisit how findings compare with expected findings, based on the initial primary working hypothesis and alternative hypotheses. Throughout the physical examination the clinician will have been revisiting

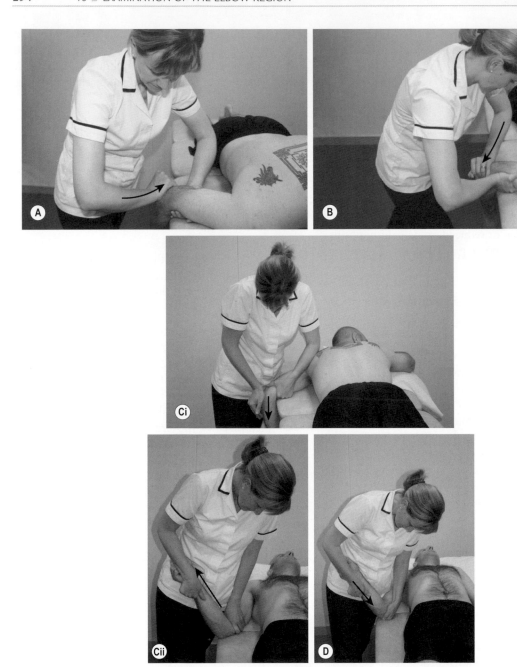

FIG. 10.9 Humeroulnar accessory movements. (A) Medial glide on the olecranon. The left hand supports underneath the upper arm and the right heel of the hand applies a medial glide to the olecranon. (B) Lateral glide on the olecranon. The right hand supports the forearm while the left hand applies a lateral glide to the olecranon. (C) Longitudinal caudad. Longitudinal caudad can be applied directly on the olecranon; (Ci) the left hand supports underneath the upper arm and the right heel of the hand applies a longitudinal caudad glide to the olecranon or (Cii) the left hand stabilizes the upper arm and the right hand grips the shaft of the ulna and pulls the ulna upwards to produce a longitudinal caudad movement at the humeroulnar joint. (D) Compression. The left hand supports underneath the elbow while the right hand pushes down through the shaft of the ulna. The arrows represent the direction of the clinician's force.

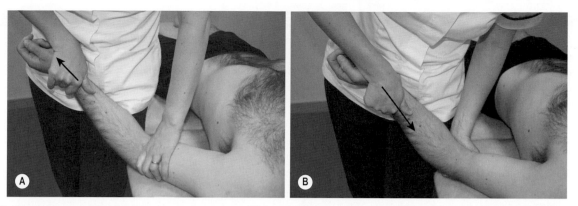

FIG. 10.10 Humeroradial joint accessory movements. (A) Longitudinal caudad. The left hand blocks the upper arm movement and the right hand pulls the radial side of the forearm. (B) Longitudinal cephalad. The left hand supports underneath the elbow and the right hand pushes down through the radial side of the forearm. The arrows represent the direction of the clinician's force.

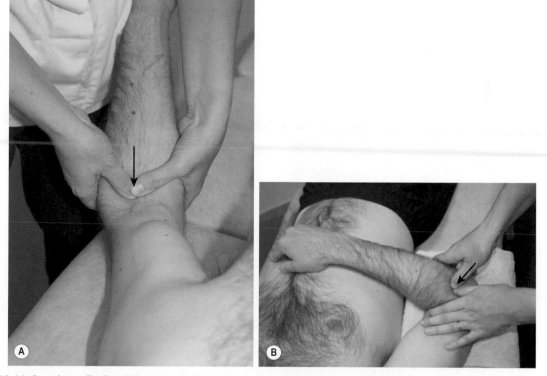

FIG. 10.11 Superior radioulnar joint accessory movements. (A) Anteroposterior. Thumb pressure is applied slowly through the soft tissue to the anterior aspect of the head of the radius. (B) Posteroanterior. Thumb pressure is applied to the posterior aspect of the head of the radius. The arrows represent the direction of the clinician's force.

TABLE 10.4
Accessory Movement, Choice of Application and Reassessment of the Patient's Asterisks

Accessory Movements of Elbow Joints

Humero-ulnar joint	Humero-radial joint	Superior radioulnar joint	Inferior radioulnar joint
Med Medial glide on olecranon or coronoid	Caud Longitudinal caudad	Anteroposterior	Anteroposterior
Lat Lateral glide on olecranon or coronoid	Ceph Longitudinal cephalad	Posteroanterior	Posteroanterior
Caud Longitudinal caudad			
Comp Compression			

Choice of Application and Modifications to the Above Joints or Regions

Start position of the joint:

- in flexion
- in extension
- in pronation
- in supination
- in flexion and supination
- in flexion and pronation
- in extension and supination
- in extension and pronation

Speed of force application

Direction of the applied force

Point of application of applied force

Identify Any Effect of Accessory Movements on Patient's Signs and Symptoms

Reassess all *asterisks

If Necessary Screen Any Proximal and Distal Regions That May Refer to the Area

Cervical spine
Thoracic spine
Shoulder
Wrist and hand

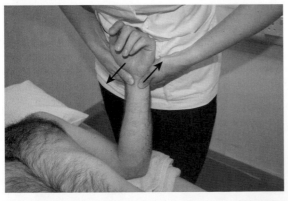

FIG. 10.12 Inferior radioulnar joint accessory movements: anteroposterior/posteroanterior glide. The left and right hands each grasp the anterior and posterior aspects of the radius and ulna. The hands then apply a force in opposite directions to produce an anteroposterior/posteroanterior glide. The arrows represent the direction of the clinician's force.

and refining the hypotheses categories (adapted from Jones & Rivett 2004):

- What can the patient do and what is the patient unable to do? How are these symptoms impacting on the patient's life?
- What are the patient's beliefs and are they helpful or unhelpful in terms of driving behaviours?
- What are the mechanisms of symptoms (include anatomy, biomechanics, mechanism of injury, pain mechanism, stages of tissue healing, tissues at fault). Are they arthrogenic/myogenic/neurogenic?
- What are the physical impairments and associated structures/tissue sources driving the patient's symptoms?
- Does this patient's problem have any other contributing factors that may be influencing the

onset or maintenance of symptoms? For example, environmental, psychosocial, behavioural, physical or heredity factors.

- Are there any precautions/contraindications to treatment and management? This includes the severity and irritability of the patient's symptoms and the underlying cause(s) of the patient's symptoms.
- Where will initial management/treatment be focused?
- Assessing prognosis – this can be affected by factors such as the stage and cause of symptoms, the patient's expectations, personality and lifestyle. Included in the prognosis should be an initial estimate of the percentage improvement for the patient, the number of treatments required to achieve this and the time period over which it will occur.

Before the patient leaves the clinician:

- explains the findings of the physical examination and how these findings relate to the subjective assessment, offering some initial advice if appropriate
- allows the patient sufficient opportunity to discuss thoughts and beliefs which may well have changed over the course of the examination
- revisits the patient's initial expectations and through collaboration with the patient identifies an agreed treatment strategy in order to achieve agreed goals
- warns the patient of possible exacerbation up to 24–48 hours following the examination
- requests the patient to report details on the behaviour of the symptoms following examination at the next attendance.

For guidance on treatment and management principles, the reader is directed to the companion textbook (Petty & Barnard 2017).

REFERENCES

Alizadehkhaiyat, O., et al., 2007. Pain, functional disability, and psychologic status in tennis elbow. Clin. J. Pain 23, 482–489.

Appleboam, A., et al., 2008. Elbow extension test to rule out elbow fracture: multicentre, prospective validation and observational study of diagnostic accuracy in adults and children. Br. Med. J. 337, a2428.

Aviles, A., et al., 2008. Elbow. In: Magee, D.J., Zachazewski, J.E., et al. (Eds.), Pathology and intervention in musculoskeletal rehabilitation. Saunders, St Louis, MO.

Ay, S., et al., 2002. An unusual supracondylar process syndrome. J. Hand Surg. Am. 27, 913–915.

Bell, S., 2008. Elbow instability, mechanisms and management. Curr. Orthop. 22, 90–103.

Boissonnault, W.G., 2011. Primary care for the physical therapist: examination and triage, 2nd ed. Elsevier Saunders, St Louis, MO.

Buehler, M.J., Thayer, D.T., 1988. The elbow flexion test; a clinical test for cubital tunnel syndrome. Clin. Orthop. 233, 213–216.

Butler, D., 2000. The sensitive nervous system. Neuro Orthopaedic Institute, Adelaide.

Cain, L., et al., 2003. Elbow injuries in throwing athletes: a current concept review. Am. J. Sports Med. 31, 621–635.

Cakir, M., et al., 2003. Musculoskeletal manifestations in patients with thyroid disease. Clin. Endocrinol. (Oxf) 59, 162–167.

Caldwell, C., Khoo-Summers, L., 2010. Movement system impairment syndromes of the wrist and hand. In: Sahrmann, S.A. (Ed.), Movement system impairment syndromes of the extremities, cervical and thoracic spines. Mosby, St Louis, pp. 165–236.

Carter, S.J., et al., 2010. Orthopaedic pitfalls in the ED: neurovascular injury associated with posterior elbow dislocations. Am. J. Emerg. Med. 28, 960–965.

Cook, C.E., Hegedus, E., 2013. Orthopedic physical examination tests: an evidence-based approach, 2nd ed. Prentice Hall, Upper Saddle River, NJ.

Coombes, B.K., et al., 2009. A new integrative model of lateral epicondylalgia. Br. J. Sports Med. 43, 252–258.

Goodman, C.C., 2010a. Screening for medical problems in patients with upper extremity signs and symptoms. J. Hand Ther. 23, 105–125.

Goodman, C.C., 2010b. Screening for gastrointestinal, hepatic/biliary, and renal/urologic disease. J. Hand Ther. 23, 140–156.

Greenhalgh, S., Selfe, J., 2010. Red flags II. A guide to solving serious pathology of the spine. Churchill Livingstone, London.

Hattam, P., Smeatham, A., 2010. Special tests in musculoskeletal examination. An evidence-based guide for clinicians. Churchill Livingstone Elsevier, Edinburgh (Chapter 3).

Hengeveld, E., Banks, K., 2014. Maitland's peripheral manipulation: management of neuromusculoskeletal disorders, vol. 2, 5th ed. Butterworth-Heinemann Elsevier, London.

Hislop, H., et al., 2013. Daniels and Worthingham's muscle testing: techniques of manual examination and performance testing, 9th ed. W.B. Saunders, Philadelphia.

Hyland, S., et al., 1990. The extension-adduction test in chronic tennis elbow: soft tissue components and joint biomechanics. Aust. J. Physiother. 36, 147–153.

Jones, M.A., Rivett, D.A., 2004. Clinical reasoning for manual therapists. Butterworth-Heinemann, Edinburgh.

Kendall, F.P., et al., 2010. Muscles testing and function in posture and pain, 5th ed. Williams & Wilkins, Baltimore.

King, G., et al., 1999. A standardized method for assessment of elbow function. J. Shoulder Elbow Surg. 8, 351–354.

Lim, E.C., 2013. Pain free grip strength test. J. Physiother. 59, 59.

Lim, Y.W., et al., 2008. Pattern of osteophyte distribution in primary osteoarthritis of the elbow. J. Shoulder Elbow Surg. 17, 963–966.

Linton, S.J., et al., 2011. The role of depression and catastrophizing in musculoskeletal pain. Eur. J. Pain 15, 416–422.

Lockard, M., 2006. Clinical biomechanics of the elbow. J. Hand Ther. 19, 72–81.

MacDermid, J.C., Michlovitz, S.L., 2006. Examination of the elbow: linking diagnosis, prognosis, and outcomes as a framework for maximizing therapy interventions. J. Hand Ther. 19, 82–97.

Magee, D.J., 2014. Orthopedic physical assessment, 6th ed. Saunders Elsevier, Philadelphia (Chapter 6).

Magee, D.J., et al., 2009. Pathology and intervention in musculoskeletal rehabilitation. Saunders, St Louis, MO.

Nandi, S.L., et al., 2009. The stiff elbow. Hand (NY) 4, 368–379.

Novak, C.B., et al., 1994. Provocative testing for the cubital tunnel syndrome. J. Bone Joint Surg. Am. 19, 817–820.

Neumann, D.A., 2010. Kinesiology of the musculoskeletal system. Foundations for rehabilitation, 2nd ed. Mosby Elsevier, St Louis (Chapter 7).

O'Driscoll, S.W., et al., 1991. Posterolateral rotary instability of the elbow. J. Bone Joint Surg. Am. 73, 441.

O'Driscoll, S.W., et al., 2005. The "moving valgus stress test" for medial collateral ligament tears of the elbow. Am. J. Sports Med. 33, 231–239.

Petty, N.J., Barnard, K., 2017. Principles of neuromusculoskeletal treatment and management: a handbook for therapists, 3rd ed. Elsevier, Edinburgh.

Simmonds, J., Keer, R., 2007. Hypermobility and the hypermobility syndrome. Man. Ther. 12, 298–309.

The, B., et al., 2013. Elbow-specific clinical rating systems: extent of established validity, reliability, and responsiveness. J. Shoulder Elbow Surg. 22, 1380–1394.

Utukuri, M., Goddard, N.J., 2005. Haemophilic arthropathy of the elbow. Haemophilia 11, 565–570.

van Griensven, H., 2014. Neurophysiology of pain. In: van Griensven, H., Strong, J., Unruh, A. (Eds.), Pain. A textbook for health professionals, 2nd edn, Churchill Livingstone, Edinburgh, pp. 77–90.

van Rijn, R.M., et al., 2009. Associations between work-related factors and specific disorders at the elbow: a systematic literature review. Rheumatology 48, 528–536.

Volz, R.C., Morrey, B.F., 1993. The physical examination of the elbow. In: Morrey, B.F. (Ed.), The elbow and its disorders, 2nd ed. W.B. Saunders, Philadelphia.

Wilke, K.E., et al., 2002. Current concepts in the rehabilitation of the overhead throwing athlete. Am. J. Sports Med. 30, 136–151.

11

EXAMINATION OF THE WRIST AND HAND

DIONNE RYDER

CHAPTER CONTENTS

WRIST AND HAND: AN OVERVIEW

The wrist and hand are a complex of 28 bones, a series of joints – the superior and inferior radioulnar, radiocarpal, midcarpal, intercarpal, carpometacarpal (CMC), intermetacarpal, metacarpophalangeal (MCP) and interphalangeal joints, 19 intrinsic and 20 extrinsic muscles plus supporting soft tissues, all supplied by three peripheral nerves. The wrist and hand are part of a kinetic chain, encompassing the cervical spine, shoulder and elbow, all allowing for optimal positioning of the hand for function.

The main functional requirement of the hand is prehension, which can be defined as the application of a functionally effective force, by the hand, to an object for a specific task. Prehension is fundamental to a patient's independence, especially if the patient's dominant hand is affected. The action of gripping will be dependent on normal movement and control throughout the whole kinetic chain. The role of the hand as a

sensory organ providing information on temperature and texture, known as stereognosis, is also fundamental to normal function. Due to its anatomical structure and functional requirements, the hand has significant representation on both the sensory and primary motor cortex (homunculi). Effective prehension will depend on sufficient stability, flexibility, strength, dexterity and proprioception of the whole upper quadrant.

Additionally, the hand is an important tool for communication, for example, through gesturing or sign language. Second to the face, the hand is the most visible part of the body, so deformity or dysfunction can have a significant psychological impact on an individual.

There are many musculoskeletal pathologies that impact on normal function of the wrist and hand. Trauma is relatively common; for example, following a fall on the outstretched hand, accounting for fractures of the distal radius, ulna or scaphoid, as well as tears of the triangular fibrocartilaginous complex

(TFCC) and ligamentous injuries resulting in carpal instabilities. Patients can also present with tendinopathies or neural tissue sensitization associated with overuse/overload (Baker et al. 2007). Alternatively, systemic inflammatory conditions such as rheumatoid arthritis (RA) and degenerative joint conditions such as osteoarthritis (OA) can mean pain and associated deformities impact significantly on normal function.

In light of the functional significance of the hand, patients with hand conditions may be managed by a dedicated hand therapy team which will include physiotherapists and occupational therapists with additional skills, including the provision of static and dynamic splints.

A thorough working knowledge of anatomy and biomechanics, in addition to an appreciation of the functional role, of the wrist and hand will help inform clinical reasoning, ensuring that the initial examination is informed and management strategies seek to optimize all aspects of functional restoration.

SUBJECTIVE EXAMINATION

Further details of the questions asked during the subjective examination and the tests carried out in the physical examination can be found in Chapters 2 and 3, respectively.

The order of the subjective questioning and the physical tests described below should be justified through sound clinical reasoning and altered as appropriate for the patient being examined.

Patients' Perspectives on Their Experience

Most patients will seek treatment because they have symptoms and/or functional limitations which are impacting on their activities of daily living, such as self-care or work-related/sport or social activities. An understanding of the patient's context, e.g. social/work requirements, will guide the clinician in seeking relevant information from the patient. Details on the patient's home situation are especially relevant; for example, elderly patients post distal radial fracture who may have to manage on their own. Does the patient's job involve sustained positions of wrist flexion or extension which might produce ischaemic tissue responses? Alternatively, does the patient undertake repetitive activities, e.g. typing, playing a musical instrument? This information may indicate direct and/or indirect mechanical influences on the wrist and hand and assist in reasoning possible cause of symptoms, directing treatment as well as assisting in appropriate goal setting.

An understanding of the patient's perspectives, attitudes and beliefs is important for appropriate person-centred management within a psychosocial framework. The clinician needs to be aware of, and sensitive to, the patient's feelings and modify her approach in order to develop a supportive rapport with the patient. The following types of questions can be useful in assessing psychosocial drivers of pain and behaviour which may be a risk factor in the development of chronicity:

- What do you understand to be the cause of your pain?
- What are you expecting will help you?
- What are you doing to cope with your pain?

Additionally there are a number of region-specific valid and reliable tools that can be used to measure patients' perceptions of their dysfunction and the impact on function, e.g. Michigan Hand Outcomes Questionnaire and Disabilities of the Arm, Shoulder and Hand (DASH) (Heras-Palou et al. 2003).

Body Chart

In order to be precise when mapping out the area of the symptoms it may be necessary to use an enlarged chart of the hand and wrist (Fig. 11.1).

Area of Current Symptoms

Lesions of the wrist and hand usually produce localized symptoms, so a thorough anatomical knowledge will help reason underlying structures. For example, pain into the thumb could be local to the CMC joint, or originate from tendon abductor pollicis longus (ABPL) or extensor pollicis brevis (EPB) as in de Quervain's disease or it could be as a result of sensitivity of the superficial radial nerve. In contrast, pain a few centimetres more proximal may be more indicative of intersection syndrome, where the first and second extensor compartments cross (Montechiarello et al. 2010). Once mapped on a body chart, ascertain which is the worst symptom and record where the patient feels the symptoms are coming from.

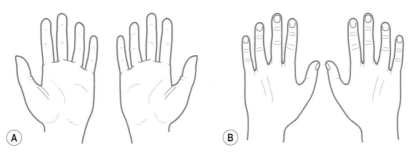

FIG. 11.1 ▪ Body chart for wrist and hand. (A) Palmar surface. (B) Dorsal surface.

Areas Relevant to the Region Being Examined

Symptoms in the wrist and hand may be referred from more proximal arthrogenic, myogenic or neurogenic structures in the lower cervical spine, upper thoracic spine, shoulder and/or elbow. Symptoms may also arise as a result of contributing factors, for example, poor proximal control of the scapula may result in compensatory increased loading on tendons at the wrist (Sueki et al. 2013). Therefore, the clinician should check all relevant areas for pain/stiffness reasoning the relevance to the patient's symptoms and mark unaffected areas with ticks (✓) on the body chart.

Quality of Symptoms

The quality of the symptoms may assist reasoning possible structures at fault, for example, a burning pain might support a hypothesis of a neural tissue source, especially if associated with altered sensation. Carpal instability or tears in TFCC may present with clunks/clicks with or without pain and the patient may report that the wrist feels vulnerable or loose (Christodoulou & Bainbridge 1999).

Intensity of Pain

The intensity of pain can be measured as shown in Chapter 2 and informs the clinician's clinical reasoning of severity, which may help to determine possible structures producing symptoms and also guides the extent and vigour of the physical examination.

Abnormal Sensation

Check for any altered sensation (such as paraesthesia or numbness) throughout the upper limb as well as locally around the wrist and hand. The distribution of any sensory changes will help to differentiate between lower and upper motor neuron lesions. For example, bilateral symptoms in both the hands and feet along with difficulties with fine motor activities, e.g. writing, could indicate cervical myelopathy and an upper motor neuron lesion. Symptoms into the ulnar side of the hand could emanate from a lesion at spinal root level C8–T1 or along the course of the ulnar nerve (lower motor neuron).

Constant or Intermittent Symptoms

Ascertain the frequency of symptoms, whether they are constant or intermittent. If symptoms are constant check whether there is variation in the intensity of symptoms, as constant unremitting pain may be indicative of a serious pathology. Whilst cancer is uncommon in the wrist and hand, more constant pain may be indicative of avascular necrosis, most commonly affecting the scaphoid postfracture or lunate (Kienbock's disease) (Wollstein et al. 2013). If associated with other symptoms, such as sensory, motor, vasomotor and/or trophic changes, incapacitating pain could indicate the development of chronic regional pain syndrome (CRPS type 1), which can be a complication post distal radial fractures (Davis & Baratz 2010).

Relationship of Symptoms

Determine the relationship between the symptomatic areas. This information will assist with reasoning the most likely cause of the patient's symptoms and so the focus of the physical examination. Questions to clarify the relationship might include:

- Do your symptoms come together or separately?
- If one symptomatic area becomes severe, what happens to the other symptomatic area?

■ Does giving way of your wrist occur with or without pain?

Behaviour of Symptoms

Aggravating Factors

Due to the functional importance of the hand in everyday life, patients may report significant limitations, especially if their dominant hand is affected. For each symptomatic area, ask patients what movements and/or positions aggravate their symptoms, if they are able to maintain an activity or position or do they have to stop or change position (severity)? How long does it take for symptoms to ease once the position or movement is stopped (irritability)? Irritability and severity are explained in Chapter 2.

The clinician should clinically reason how symptoms impact on function. For example, wrist extension provides a stable, close pack position for hand function, optimizing the length and tension of the long (extrinsic) flexor tendons. Loss of wrist extension range (20–30°) will impact on grip. Restricted forearm pronation and supination will limit optimal placing of the hand for activities such as opening doors, writing, turning a key in a lock. Weight-bearing activities, through the wrist, for example, typing on a keyboard, may provoke median nerve sensitivity through compression of the carpal tunnel. Limitation of thumb opposition/reposition and finger flexion/extension will impact on all functional activities. Cold intolerance commonly occurs after nerve injury and amputations, causing pain and vascular changes in cold weather (Novak & McCabe 2015).

Detailed information on each provocative activity helps refine reasoning of possible structures that may be at fault, the severity, irritability and the relationship between symptoms. The patient's most notable functional restrictions are highlighted with asterisks (*), to be explored in the physical examination and reassessed at subsequent treatment sessions to evaluate treatment intervention.

Easing Factors

For each symptomatic area, the clinician asks what movements and/or positions ease the patient's symptoms, how long it takes to ease them, whether they subside completely and what happens to other symptoms when this symptom is relieved. These questions help to confirm the relationship between the symptoms and determine their irritability. For example, symptoms from the wrist that are articular in nature may be relieved by holding the wrist in a semiflexed position out of close pack extension, whereas symptoms originating from neural tissue may be eased by certain cervical and upper-limb out-of-tension positions, e.g. ipsilateral cervical side flexion or shoulder girdle elevation.

Using clinical reasoning skills the clinician can then collate the information gained from aggravating and easing factors to formulate a hypothesis of the structure(s) which might be at fault. This information can be used to focus the physical examination, inform initial advice on how tasks could be modified and assist in identifying treatment goals. If the patient's symptoms do not fit a musculoskeletal presentation then the clinician needs to be alert to other possible serious causes.

Twenty-Four-Hour Behaviour of Symptoms

The clinician determines the 24-hour behaviour of symptoms by asking questions about night, morning and evening symptoms.

Night Symptoms. See Chapter 2 for details of questions. Patients with symptoms of neural origin such as carpal tunnel syndrome (CTS) often report symptoms being worse at night. Whilst asleep their blood pressure drops and their neural tissue becomes more ischaemic (Bland 2000).

Morning and Evening Symptoms. The clinician determines the pattern of the symptoms first thing in the morning, through the day and at the end of the day. Those with OA of the hands may report morning stiffness which eases with activity, whereas those with tendinopathies or neural tissue sensitivity may report increased symptoms with increased repetition or load through the day.

Past Medical History/Family History

Details of medical and family history are required so that precautions or contraindications to the physical examination and/or treatment can be identified (see Table 2.4). Details of any past medical history, such as major or long-standing illnesses, accidents or surgery relevant to the patient's condition, are obtained from the patient and/or medical notes. Details of past history may explain the development of current symptoms, e.g. a history of whiplash may be relevant if neural sensitization is a suspected cause of distal symptoms.

Special Questions

As mentioned in Chapter 2, the clinician must differentiate between conditions that are suitable for conservative treatment and other systemic, neoplastic and non-musculoskeletal conditions which require referral on to a medical practitioner.

For full details of all special questions see Chapter 2. Information from relevant questions for this region will contribute to an understanding of possible causes of wrist and hand symptoms.

General Health

Does the patient feel well? Does the patient suffer from any malaise, fatigue, fever, nausea, anxiety or depression? This will provide the clinician with an overview of the patient's health status, e.g. whether the patient smokes, how physically active he is, so contributing to clinical reasoning of the likely prognosis.

Serious Pathology

Does the patient have a history of serious pathology, such as cancer, tuberculosis (TB) or human immunodeficiency virus (HIV)? Malignant tumours of the wrist and hand are very rare. Although the hand is an atypical site for musculoskeletal TB, if suspected, patients should be asked about possible exposure to TB (Agarwal et al. 2005).

Inflammatory Arthritis

Patients are asked if they or a member of their family have been diagnosed as having an inflammatory condition. RA often initially presents in the small joints of the hands (Schnitzler 2005).

Thyroid Disease

Does the patient have a history of thyroid disease? Thyroid dysfunction is associated with a higher incidence of musculoskeletal conditions affecting the hand, such as Dupuytren's contracture, trigger finger and CTS (Cakir et al. 2003).

Dupuytren's Disease

Has the patient or anyone in the patient's family been diagnosed with Dupuytren's disease? There is evidence of an increased incidence of the disease with a positive family history. Other factors such as alcohol, smoking, diabetes, epilepsy and hypercholesterolaemia have also been implicated though none has been shown to be convincingly causative (Picardo & Khan 2012).

Osteoporosis

Has the patient been diagnosed with osteoporosis or does the patient have a history of frequent fractures? Distal radial fracture has been shown to be associated with an increased risk of hip fracture (Court-Brown & Caesar 2006). If osteoporosis is suspected then the vigour of the physical examination will need to be modified.

Diabetes Mellitus

There is evidence of a higher incidence of CTS, flexor tendon tenosynovitis and Dupuytren's disease in diabetics, which is related to the duration of the diabetes and the level of insulin dependence (Ballantyne & Hooper 2004). Due to vascular deficits, tissue healing is likely to be slower in diabetic patients (Gaston & Simpson 2007), so this is especially relevant to determining the prognosis and vigour of examination, for example, post fracture. Diabetic neuropathy affecting the hands may present with a glove distribution of thermal sensitivity deficits and so patients may also present with burns on their skin due to impaired sensation (Kalk 2005).

Radiograph and Medical Imaging

Has the patient been radiographed or had any other medical tests recently? Radiographs are commonly used to screen for or detect hand or joint fractures and dislocations. Scaphoid fractures are less easily detected on initial X-rays and protocols recommend suspected scaphoid fractures should be re-X-rayed 10 days post-injury (Baldassarre & Hughes 2013). Magnetic resonance imaging (MRI) or bone scans are useful in detecting subtle fractures, tears of the TFCC and scapholunate instabilities. Ultrasound is most appropriate for imaging tendons, tendon pulleys and ganglions. It should be noted that there can be poor correlation between imaging findings and patient-reported symptoms so a comprehensive history and thorough examination are key. Other tests may include blood tests required if systemic inflammatory conditions such as RA are suspected. These results will provide information that can inform the clinical reasoning of underlying causes of symptoms, guide rehabilitation and indicate likely prognosis.

Drug History

What medications are being taken by the patient? Are they for these presenting symptoms or other medical conditions? Are they effective? Use of anticoagulant and steroid medication would be an indication for precaution in the physical examination.

History of the Present Condition

For each symptomatic area, the clinician asks how long the symptoms have been present, whether there was a sudden or slow onset and whether there was a known cause that provoked the onset of the symptoms, such as a fall. The clinician may ask why and how the patient fell in order to identify likely structures that may have been injured. For example, a fall on the outstretched hand can produce fractures to distal radius/ulna commonly in older people, or scaphoid, ligamentous injury producing instability, more commonly seen in younger patients, or injury elsewhere in the kinetic chain at the elbow, shoulder or cervical spine. Was the injury a result of an assault with a knife or glass? Was the injury self-inflicted? The answer will prompt the clinician to consider whether the patient will require additional psychological support. If the onset was slow, can the development of symptoms be associated with a change in the patient's lifestyle, e.g. a new job or leisure activity or a change in sporting activity? Are there ongoing legal proceedings that may impact on the prognosis?

Is this the first episode or is there a history of wrist and hand problems? If so, how many episodes? When were they? What was the cause? What was the duration of each episode? And did the patient fully recover between episodes? If there have been no previous episodes, has the patient had any episodes of symptoms such as stiffness in the cervical spine, thoracic spine, shoulder, elbow, wrist, hand or any other relevant region? Prolonged posture or repeated movements can cause tissue impairments leading to less than optimal

movement patterns that can provoke tissue injury (Caldwell & Khoo-Summers 2010).

To confirm the relationship between the symptoms, the clinician asks what happened to other symptoms and when each symptom began. How symptoms have developed or changed over time will allow the clinician to stage the condition, which will inform prognosis.

In addition the clinician needs to ask if the patient has sought treatment to date, what it was and whether it helped? What has the patient been told and by whom? What does the patient believe is going on? Clarifying the patient's journey can help the clinician to understand the patient's context. Understanding and aligning beliefs about presenting symptoms allows management to be tailored to meet the needs of the individual patient.

Plan of the Physical Examination

It is useful at the end of the subjective examination to reconfirm briefly with patients the clinician's understanding of their main complaint, and offer them the opportunity to add anything that they may not have mentioned so far. The purpose and plan for the physical examination will need to be explained and the patient's consent obtained.

The information from the subjective examination helps the clinician to identify an initial primary hypothesis and alternative hypotheses as to the cause of a patient's symptoms. A physical examination planning form can help guide the clinician's reasoning in the development and testing of these initial hypotheses (see Fig. 2.9).

For ease of reference highlight with asterisks (*) important subjective findings and particularly one or more functional restrictions. These can then be reexamined at subsequent treatment sessions to evaluate treatment intervention.

It is helpful at the end of the subjective examination for the clinician to consider the following:

■ Are there any precautions and/or contraindications to elements of the physical examination that need to be explored further, such as neurological involvement, recent fracture, trauma, steroid therapy or rheumatoid conditions? There may also be certain contraindications to further examination and treatment, e.g. bilateral symptoms of cord compression.

- Based on subjective information the clinician reasons which structures are most likely to be at fault to develop a primary hypothesis with possible alternatives. It is helpful to consider arthrogenic, myogenic and neurogenic structures lying underneath the area of symptoms and those that refer into the wrist and hand region. For example, pain into the thumb could be referred from the cervical and thoracic spine or elbow or could be local, emanating from the CMC joint due to OA, or could originate from the tendon ABPL, EPB as in de Quervain's tendinopathy or be due to sensitivity of the dorsal sensory branch of the radial nerve. Using clinical reasoning skills, the clinician will need to prioritize and justify what 'must' be examined in the initial session and what 'should' or 'could' be followed up at subsequent sessions.
- Additional physical contributing factors that should be examined include posture and related functional activities such as gripping.
- What is the assessment of severity and irritability for each symptomatic area (see Chapter 2)? If severity is judged to be high, physical testing will be limited to testing to or just short of symptom reproduction. For those with high irritability the physical examination will also be limited to avoid exacerbating symptoms and the focus will shift to easing the patient's symptoms rather than provoking them. The patient will require rest periods between tests to avoid a build-up in symptoms. Alternatively, for patients with symptoms judged to be of low severity and irritability, physical testing will need to be more searching, requiring possible application of overpressures, repeated and combined movements to reproduce symptoms.

What are the pain mechanisms driving the patient's symptoms and how will this information impact on an understanding of the problem and subsequent decisions? What are the input mechanisms (sensory pathways)? For example, pain associated with sustained wrist and hand positions when typing may indicate ischaemic nociception. What are the processing mechanisms? How has the patient interpreted these symptoms? Is the patient worried? Is he demonstrating signs of catastrophization? What are the output mechanisms

in terms of the patient's response? Has the patient changed behaviours? For example, has the patient stopped or modified activity at work? Are these changes an adaptive or maladaptive response? Certainly this information will guide the clinician's language and allow for a more person-centred discussion with the patient. Patients' acceptance and willingness to be active participants in their management will depend on their perspective and subsequent behavioural response to their symptoms. If patients are demonstrating fear avoidance behaviours then the clinician's ability to understand, explain and teach them about their condition will be pivotal to achieving a successful outcome.

PHYSICAL EXAMINATION

The information from the subjective examination helps the clinician to plan an appropriate physical examination. The severity, irritability, ongoing pain mechanisms and primary working hypothesis and alternative hypotheses are the major factors that will influence the choice and priority of physical testing procedures.

Each significant physical test that either provokes or eases the patient's symptoms is highlighted in the patient's notes by an asterisk (*) for easy reference.

The order and detail of the physical tests described in this chapter should be appropriate for the patient being examined. The clinician should clinically reason selected tests to confirm or refute the hypotheses (primary and alternatives) under consideration. Issues of reliability, sensitivity and specificity (see Chapter 3) should also be considered when tests are selected so that findings can be interpreted appropriately. It is important that readers understand that the techniques included in this chapter are some of many and that those chosen are most clinically useful and include an indication of their level of support in the literature.

Observation

Informal Observation

Through the subjective examination the clinician observes the patient's reaction to the appearance of their wrist and hand as well as their ability and willingness to move their limb.

Formal Observation

Observation of Posture. The patient should be suitably undressed so that the clinician can observe the bony and soft-tissue contours of the spine, scapula, shoulder, elbow, wrist and hand, in a position relevant for that patient; for example, in sitting if symptoms are related to the use of computers (Caldwell & Khoo-Summers 2010). When the hand is in a relaxed posture the fingers of the hand naturally flex towards the tubercle of the scaphoid (Magee 2014).

Observation of Muscle Form. The clinician examines the muscle bulk and muscle tone of the patient, comparing left and right sides. It must be remembered that handedness and level and frequency of physical activity may well produce differences in muscle bulk between sides. Check for wasting of specific muscles, such as the first dorsal interosseous muscle supplied by the ulnar nerve, or opponens pollicis supplied by the median nerve, as this may indicate a peripheral nerve problem.

Observation of Soft Tissues. The clinician observes the skin creases, colour of the patient's skin, any swelling, increased hair growth on the hand, brittle fingernails, infection of the nail bed, sweating or dry palm, shiny skin, scars and bony deformities, and takes cues for further examination. These changes could be indicative of a range of conditions, for example, peripheral nerve injury, peripheral vascular disease, diabetes mellitus, Raynaud's disease, CRPS 1 (Magee 2014).

Impaired alignment of the wrist and hand results in suboptimal movement patterns often impacting on function. Common deformities of the hand include the following:

- Boutonnière deformity of fingers or thumb: the proximal interphalangeal joint (PIPJ) is flexed and the distal interphalangeal joint (DIPJ) is hyperextended (Fig. 11.2). The central slip of the extensor tendon is damaged following trauma or RA so the lateral bands displace in a palmar direction, producing flexion of PIPJ (Eddington 1993).
- Bouchard's nodes are calcific spurs over the dorsum of the PIPJs indicative of OA.

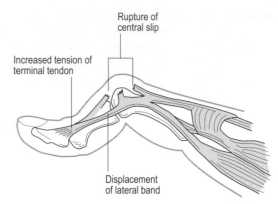

FIG. 11.2 ■ Boutonnière deformity. *(From Eddington 1993, with permission.)*

- Claw hand: the little and ring fingers are hyperextended at the MCPJ and flexed at the interphalangeal joints. This condition is due to ulnar nerve palsy.
- Club nails, where there is excessive soft tissue under the nail, are indicative of respiratory or cardiac disorders.
- Dupuytren's contracture of the palmar fascia produces a fixed flexion deformity of the MCPJ and PIPJ, particularly affecting the ring or little finger and is seen more commonly in men in the 50–70-years age group.
- Heberden's nodes are calcific spurs over the dorsum of the DIPJs and are indicative of OA.
- Mallet finger: rupture of the terminal extensor tendon at the DIPJ is usually a result of trauma, producing a flexed distal phalanx.
- Swan-neck deformity of fingers: the PIPJ is hyperextended due to damage to the volar plate or intrinsic muscle contracture and the MCPJ and DIPJ are flexed (Fig. 11.3) (Eckhaus 1993).
- Ulnar drift associated with RA results in a translocation of the carpus towards the ulna, with deviation of the digits in an ulnar direction due to weakening of the metacarpophalangeal ligaments, resulting in bowstringing of the finger extensors.
- Zigzag deformity of the thumb is a result of a flexed CMC joint and failure of the deep anterior oblique ligament, resulting in hyperextension at MCPJ and reciprocal flexion at the interphalangeal joint. Unchecked ABPL further pulls the

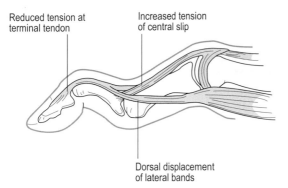

Reduced tension at terminal tendon

Increased tension of central slip

Dorsal displacement of lateral bands

FIG. 11.3 ■ Swan-neck deformity. *(From Eckhaus 1993, with permission.)*

thumb into an adducted position – a pattern of deformity associated with OA of the CMC joint (Batra & Kanvinde 2007).

Functional Testing

Some functional ability has already been tested by general observation of the patient during the subjective and physical examinations, e.g. the postures adopted during the subjective examination and the ease or difficulty of undressing prior to the physical examination. Any further functional testing can be carried out early in the examination. Clues for appropriate tests can be obtained from the subjective examination findings, particularly aggravating factors. Functional testing of the hand is very important and can include the ability to perform various power and precision (or pinch) grips, as well as more general activities, such as fastening a button, tying a shoelace, opening jars and writing. Analysis of the performance of these tests will guide further examination in identifying which physiological movements are affected.

Commonly documented dexterity tests can also be used to assess and measure outcomes such as the Purdue pegboard test (Blair et al. 1987), nine-hole peg test (Totten & Flinn-Wagner 1992) and Minnesota rate of manipulation test (Totten & Flinn-Wagner 1992).

Active Physiological Movements

The active physiological movements of the forearm, wrist and hand are shown in Table 11.1.

There are a number of different models proposed to explain the kinematics of the wrist complex

TABLE 11.1
Active Physiological Movements

Forearm pronation

Forearm supination

Wrist extension

Wrist flexion

Radial deviation

Ulnar deviation

Carpometacarpal and metacarpophalangeal joints of thumb:
- Flexion
- Extension
- Abduction
- Adduction
- Opposition

Distal intermetacarpal joints:
- Horizontal flexion
- Horizontal extension

Metacarpophalangeal joints (of the fingers):
- Flexion
- Extension
- Adduction
- Abduction

Proximal and distal interphalangeal joints:
- Flexion
- Extension

Possible modifications to physiological movements

Repeated

Speed altered

Combined movements and sequencing

Added compression or distraction

Sustained

Injuring movement

Differentiation tests

Functional movements

Identify any effect of the modifications of physiological movements on patient's signs and symptoms

Reassess all *asterisks

If necessary screen any proximal and distal regions that may refer to the area

Cervical spine

Thoracic spine

Shoulder

Wrist and hand

(Neumann 2010). Pronation and supination predominantly centre around the superior/inferior radioulnar joints, although there will be some contribution from the radiocarpal joint (Magee 2014). For wrist extension the ratio of relative contribution of radiocarpal to midcarpal is 60:40, with this being reversed in wrist flexion. Radial and ulnar deviation occurs through both radial and midcarpal joints. Due to the saddle joint of the first CMC joint and the thumb position 90° to the palm, the terminology for movement differs to the rest of the hand. Thumb flexion and extension take place parallel to the palm with adduction and abduction 90° to the palm (Fig. 11.4).

Having an understanding of the biomechanics of the wrist and hand complex can assist in clinically reasoning findings of active physiological movement and further assist in focusing testing.

Movements can be tested with the patient in supine or sitting with right and left sides compared. Range of movement for forearm and wrist can be measured using a goniometer. For finger range a specific finger goniometer or finger flexion tip measurement to palm crease might be easier. The choice of which active movements are to be tested will depend on the patient's reported aggravating and easing factors and the observation of functional tests. For example, if a patient has difficulty gripping then wrist extension and radial deviation should be examined. For each active physiological movement, the clinician notes the following:

- willingness of the patient to move
- range of movement available
- quality of movement, e.g. coordination, muscle activation patterning
- behaviour of pain through the range of movement.

The clinician establishes the patient's symptoms at rest, prior to each movement, and modifies/corrects any movement deviation to reason clinically its relevance to the patient's symptoms.

Symptom Modification

Modification of active movements can assist in differentiating the sources of symptoms (Hengeveld et al. 2014). For example, when supination reproduces the patient's wrist symptoms, differentiation between the inferior radioulnar joint and the radiocarpal joint can be useful in refining a working hypothesis of the underlying source of symptoms. The patient actively moves the forearm into supination just to the point where symptoms are produced. The clinician applies a passive supination force to the radius and ulna; if the symptoms are coming from the inferior radioulnar joint, then pain may increase. The inferior radioulnar joint is held in a supinated position whilst a supination

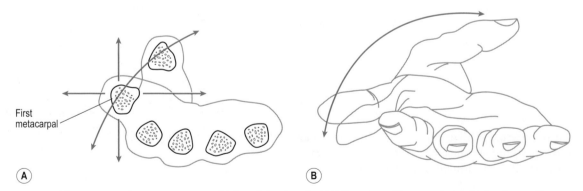

First metacarpal

(A)   (B)

FIG. 11.4 ■ Movement at the carpometacarpal joint of the thumb. (A) The arrows illustrate the multiple planes of movement that occur at the carpometacarpal joint of the thumb. Flexion/extension across the palm in a coronal plane about an anterior/posterior axis. Abduction/adduction away from the palm in a sagittal plane about a medial/lateral axis. (B) The arrow illustrates the movement of the thumb from reposition into opposition. Reposition is the normal anatomical position in the same plane as the the second metacarpal to a position of extension and abduction into a position of full opposition – flexion and medial rotation. *(From Fess & Philips 1987, with permission.)*

force to radiocarpal joint around the scaphoid and lunate is applied. If the symptoms are coming from the radiocarpal joint, then pain may increase. A pronation force to the scaphoid and lunate might then be expected to reduce symptoms (Fig. 11.5).

Mobilizations with movement (Hing et al. 2015) are sustained accessory glides applied to a joint during active or passive movement. Mobilizations with movement can serve as a useful diagnostic tool. For example, for a more specific method of exploring forearm pronation and supination, ask the patient actively to supinate or pronate the forearm while the clinician applies a sustained anterior or posterior force to the distal end of the ulna at the wrist. Fig. 11.6 demonstrates a

posteroanterior force to distal ulna as the patient actively supinates. An increase in painfree range or reduced pain on active supination or pronation is a positive examination finding, indicating a mechanical joint problem. This can then be applied as a mini treatment in order to confirm an articular cause.

Active movements demonstrating handling for application of overpressure are shown in Fig. 11.7 and these are applied to clear the joint.

It may be necessary to examine the cervical spine, thoracic spine, shoulder and elbow to determine their relevance to the patient's symptoms; they may be the source of the symptoms, or they may be contributing to the symptoms (see relevant regional chapter).

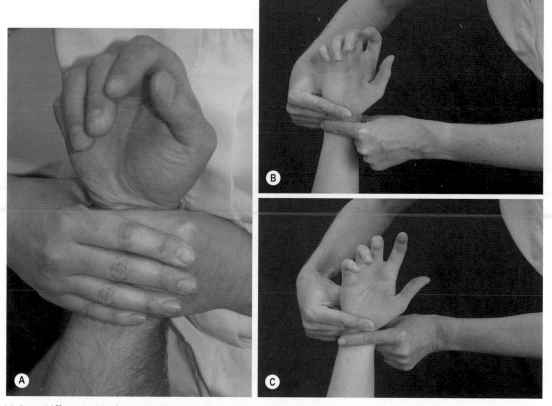

FIG. 11.5 ■ Differentiation between the superior/inferior radioulnar joint with radiocarpal joint and midcarpal joints. The patient supinates the forearm to the onset of symptoms. The clinician then: (A) applies a supination force to the radius and ulna; (B) releases the radius and ulna and applies a supination force around the proximal row of carpal bones to affect the radiocarpal joint; and (C) supination of the radius and ulnar is maintained and a pronation force is applied to the proximal carpal row. The clinician determines the effect of each overpressure on the symptoms. The symptoms would be expected to increase when the supination force is applied to the symptomatic level; further examination of accessory movements of individual bones may then identify a symptomatic joint.

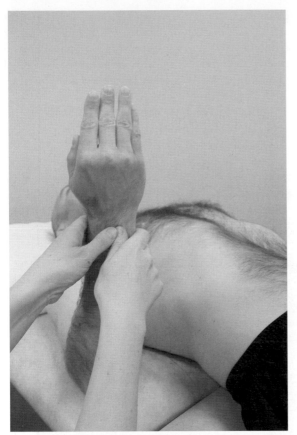

FIG. 11.6 ■ Mobilization with movement for supination. A posteroanterior force is applied to the ulna as the patient actively supinates.

Passive Physiological Movements

All active movements can be examined passively. The clinician feels through range for restriction and/or reproduction of symptoms and assesses end-feel of the joint. For the wrist and hand the clinician needs to consider carefully the starting position to account for the long flexors and extensors of the wrist; for example, to test articular range of wrist extension the fingers will need to be flexed.

Joint Integrity Tests

At the wrist, ligamentous instability can occur most often with lunate extending dorsally on scaphoid dorsal intercalated segment instability (DISI) or lunate rotating in a palmar/volar direction on triquetrum

volar intercalated segment instability (VISI). Instabilities are suspected if the patient has sustained trauma, reports clunking or weakness or has increased range/ symptoms on passive movement tests or point tenderness over specific ligaments on palpation. It should be noted that the integrity tests described are not sufficiently robust when used in isolation to diagnose an instability (Prosser et al. 2011; Valdes & LaStayo 2013). Instabilities can be confirmed using MRI as routine radiographs may appear normal (Taleisnik 1988; Trail et al. 2007).

Watson (Scaphoid Shift) Test

To test for a dorsal intercalated segment instability (DISI) the clinician applies a posteriorly directed glide to the distal pole of the scaphoid while passively moving the wrist from a position of ulnar deviation and slight extension to radial deviation and slight flexion (Fig. 11.8). Posterior subluxation of the scaphoid, over the dorsal rim of the radius produces a 'clunk' and reproduction of the patient's pain indicates instability of the scaphoid (Watson et al. 1988). Results of the test must be interpreted with care as a painless clunk is found in normal wrists (Easterling & Wolfe 1994). This test is estimated to be moderately accurate in detecting instability (Prosser et al. 2011).

Midcarpal Shift Test

With the patient's wrist in neutral and forearm pronated, a palmar force is applied to the distal portion of capitate and the wrist is axially loaded and deviated in an ulnar direction. The test is positive if a painful 'clunk' is felt, indicating a tear of the arcuate ligament, and the manoeuvre reproduces the patient's symptoms (Prosser et al. 2011; Valdes & LaStayo 2013). Several studies have identified sensitivity as 64% and specificity 45% for this test (La Stayo & Howell 1995; Prosser et al. 2011).

Lunotriquetral Ballottement (Reagan's) Test

This tests for instability at the joint between the lunate and triquetral bones occurring due to a loss of integrity of the lunotriquetral ligament volar intercalated segment instability (VISI). Excessive movement, crepitus or pain with anterior and posterior glide of the lunate on the triquetrum indicates a positive test (Magee 2014). This test has limited evidence to

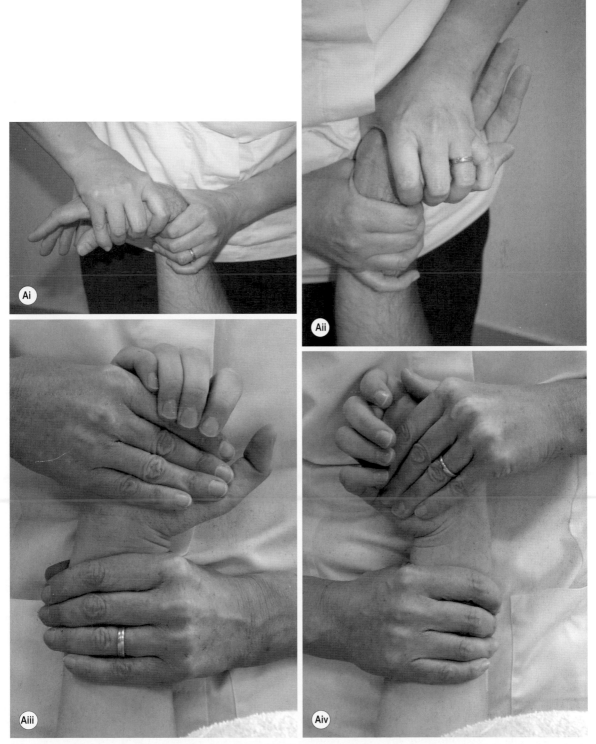

FIG. 11.7 ■ (A) Overpressures to the wrist and hand. (Ai) Flexion. The wrist and hand are grasped by both hands and taken into flexion. (Aii) Extension. The right hand supports the patient's forearm and the left hand takes the wrist and hand into extension. (Aiii) Radial deviation. The left hand supports just proximal to the wrist joint while the right hand moves the wrist into radial deviation. (Aiv) Ulnar deviation. The right hand supports just proximal to the wrist joint while the left hand moves the wrist into ulnar deviation.

Continued

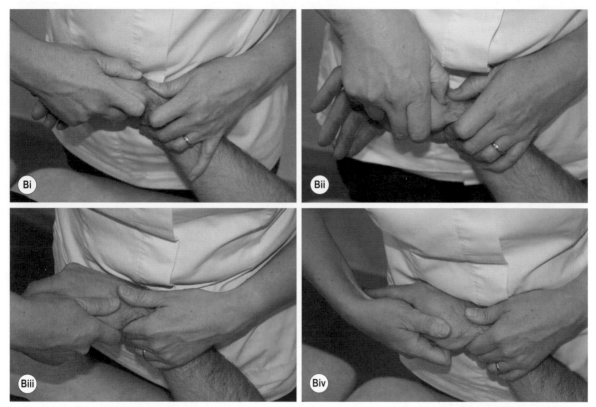

FIG. 11.7, cont'd ■ (B) Carpometacarpal joint of thumb. For all these movements, the hands are placed immediately proximal and distal to the joint line. (Bi) Flexion. The left hand supports the trapezium while the right hand takes the first metacarpal into flexion. (Bii) Extension. The left hand supports the trapezium while the right hand takes the first metacarpal into extension. (Biii) Abduction and adduction. The left hand supports the trapezium while the right hand takes the first metacarpal into abduction and adduction. (Biv) Opposition. The right hand supports the trapezium while the left hand takes the first metacarpal across the palm into opposition.

FIG. 11.7, cont'd ■ (C) Distal intermetacarpal joints. (Ci) Horizontal flexion. The right thumb is placed in the centre of the palm at the level of the metacarpal heads. The left hand cups around the back of the metacarpal heads and moves them into horizontal flexion. (Cii) Horizontal extension. The thumbs are placed in the centre of the dorsum of the palm at the level of the metacarpal heads. The fingers wrap around the anterior aspect of the hand and pull the metacarpal heads into horizontal extension. (D) Metacarpophalangeal joints. (Di) Flexion. The left hand supports the metacarpal while the right hand takes the proximal phalanx into flexion. (Dii) Extension. The right hand supports the metacarpal while the left hand takes the proximal phalanx into extension. (Diii) Abduction and adduction. The right hand supports the metacarpal while the left hand takes the proximal phalanx into abduction as shown.

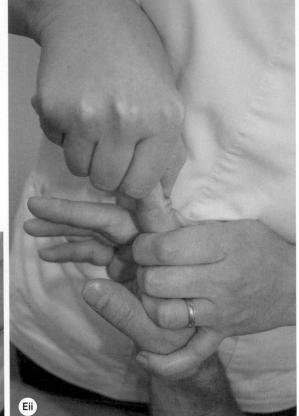

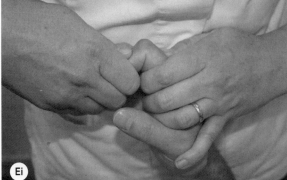

FIG. 11.7, cont'd ■ (E) Proximal and distal interphalangeal joints. (Ei) Flexion. The left hand supports the metacarpophalangeal joint in extension while the right hand takes the proximal interphalangeal joint into flexion. (Eii) Extension. The left hand supports the metacarpophalangeal joint in extension while the right hand takes the proximal interphalangeal joint into extension.

identify robustness but this injury is often associated with TFCC tears (Hattam & Smeatham 2010).

Triangular Fibrocartilaginous Complex Load Test

The TFCC, a complex stabilizing structure of the inferior radioulnar joint, is vulnerable to tearing or degenerative changes. This load-bearing test resembles the meniscal test of the knee (Fig. 11.9). The patient's forearm is stabilized and, as if shaking hands, the clinician places her hand in the patient's palm. An axial compression load is then applied to the patient's hand while ulnar deviation is added (Hattam & Smeatham 2010). Localized pain, apprehension and/or a click would indicate a positive test. A positive test combined

with a history of pain on pronation, ulnar deviation and gripping, with crepitus and tenderness over the TFCC, would increase suspicion of a TFCC lesion (Bulstrode et al. 2002).

Ligamentous Instability Test for the Joints of the Thumb and Fingers

Excessive movement when a varus or valgus force is applied to the joint is indicative of laxity of the collateral ligaments. To test the ulnar collateral ligament of the thumb, test with the MCPJ positioned in extension. When an incomplete rupture is present valgus stress testing reveals minimal or no instability (less than 30° of laxity or less than 15° more laxity than in the

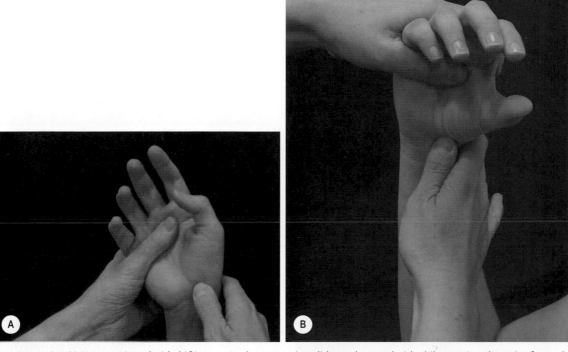

FIG. 11.8 ■ (A, B) Watson (scaphoid shift) test. Apply a posterior glide to the scaphoid whilst moving the wrist from ulnar deviation and slight extension to radial deviation and slight flexion.

non-injured thumb). When a complete rupture of the ulnar collateral ligament and accessory collateral ligament is present, valgus stress testing with the MCPJ positioned in extension reveals a lack of an end-feel and marked laxity – more than 30° or more than 15° more laxity than in the non-injured thumb (Tang 2011).

Axial Compression Test (Grind Test)

OA of the CMC joint is the most common site of degenerative joint disease of the hand and is characterized by sharp pain on gripping activities. Diagnosis can be staged from I to IV using radiology classification (Eaton & Glickel 1987).

The clinician stabilizes the radial side of the patient's hand with one hand whilst the other hand grips the shaft of the first metacarpal. An axial load with rotation is applied down the shaft. The test is positive if pain is elicited. This is a provocative test and so needs

to be applied with care (Hattam & Smeatham 2010) (Fig. 11.10).

Muscle Tests

Muscle tests include examining muscle strength, length, isometric muscle testing and some other muscle tests. Selection is clinically reasoned based on the patient's subjective examination as well as observations of posture and movement (Kendall et al. 2010; Hislop et al. 2013). See Chapter 3 for details of muscle testing.

Muscle Strength

Manual muscle testing may be carried out for the following muscle groups:

- elbow: flexors and extensors
- forearm: pronators and supinators
- wrist joint: flexors, extensors, radial deviators and ulnar deviators

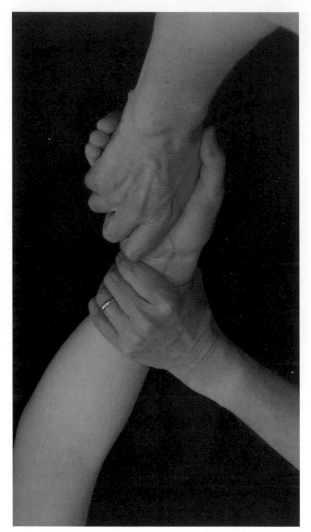

FIG. 11.9 ■ Triangular fibrocartilaginous complex load test. The patient's forearm is stabilized and, as if shaking hands, the clinician places her hand in the patient's palm. An axial compression load is then applied to the patient's hand while ulnar deviation is added.

- thenar eminence: flexors, extensors, adductors, abductors and opposers
- hypothenar eminence: flexors, extensors, adductors, abductors and opposers
- finger: flexors, extensors, abductors and adductors.

Grip strength can be measured using a dynamometer to provide some baseline quantitative data on which

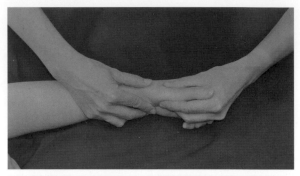

FIG. 11.10 ■ Axial compression test (grind test). The clinician stabilizes the radial side of the patient's hand with one hand whilst the other hand grips the shaft of the first metacarpal. An axial load with rotation is applied down the shaft. The test is positive if pain is elicited. This is a provocative test and so needs to be applied with care.

to evaluate progress. Left and right sides can be compared but variance due to hand dominance will need to be accounted for. A range of pinch-grip strengths can also be measured using a pinch meter (Magee 2014).

Muscle Length

Tenodesis Action. To test the normal balance in the extrinsic flexor and extensor muscle length with the wrist flexed, the fingers and thumb will extend; with the wrist extended, the fingers will flex towards the palm and the thumb opposers towards the index finger (Neumann 2010).

Intrinsic Muscle Tightness. To test for intrinsic muscle tightness the MCPJ is held in extension whilst the clinician passively flexes the interphalangeal joints. The test is repeated in MCP flexion; if interphalangeal flexion is full in this position restriction is due to the intrinsic tightness. If restricted range remains unchanged then the restriction is likely to be capsular.

Extrinsic Muscle Tightness. With the wrist in neutral the clinician compares the range of passive PIPJ movement with the MCPJs positioned in flexion and then in extension. If the PIPJ can be passively flexed while the MCP is extended but not when the MCPJ is flexed, this indicates extrinsic extensor tightness. Conversely, extrinsic flexor tightness is where there is a greater range of PIPJ extension with the MCPJs in flexion than with the MCPJs in extension.

The clinician may test the length of other muscles (Kendall et al. 2010; Hislop et al. 2013). Descriptions of the tests for muscle length are given in Chapter 3.

Isometric Muscle Testing

Test forearm pronation and supination, wrist flexion, extension, radial and ulnar deviation, finger and thumb flexion, extension, abduction and adduction and thumb opposition in different parts of the physiological range depending on subjective clues to provoking activities. The clinician observes the quality of the muscle contraction to hold the position, the adoption of substitution strategies as well as the reproduction of the patient's symptoms.

Muscles are palpated for trigger points (see Chapter 2).

Other Muscle/Tendon Tests

Tests for De Quervain's Disease. De Quervain's disease, a stenosing tenosynovitis of the ABPL and EPB tendons in the first dorsal compartment, usually presents with pain over the tip of the ulnar styloid associated with gripping activities. However there is some confusion regarding the two tests commonly described to assess for de Quervain's disease (Goubau et al. 2014). For the Eichhoff test (often mistakenly named the Finkelstein test) patients are asked to oppose their thumb across their palm and clench their fist whilst the clinician passively deviates their wrist into ulnar deviation (Goubau et al. 2014). This test has been associated with false positives in normal wrists. The Finkelstein test is a passive test, whereby, with the patient's thumb flexed across the palm, the clinician fixes the lower forearm with one hand and then gently passively takes the wrist into ulnar deviation (Fig. 11.11) (Elliott 1992).

It is argued this passive test stresses local articular structures as well as loading tendons in the first compartment (Magee 2014). It is possibly this variation in description and application that has resulted in these tests not being supported in the literature (Valdes & LaStayo 2013). Alternative tests are being developed (Goubau et al. 2014) and diagnostic criteria have been proposed to improve diagnostic accuracy, combining testing with signs such as local swelling and pain on resisted thumb extension (Batteson et al. 2008).

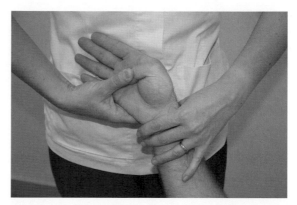

FIG. 11.11 ■ Finkelstein test. The patient flexes the thumb and the clinician guides the patient's wrist passively into ulnar deviation of the wrist. (Handling as described by Elliott 1992.)

Sweater Finger Sign Test. Loss of DIPJ flexion when a fist is made is a positive test indicating a ruptured flexor digitorum profundus (FDP) tendon. The ring finger is most commonly affected (Magee 2014).

Test for Flexor Digitorum Superficialis (FDS). The clinician holds all of any three fingers in extension and asks the patient actively to flex the MCPJ and PIPJ of the remaining finger. The DIPJ should be flail as the FDP has been immobilized. If the FDS is inactive, the finger will flex strongly at the DIPJ as well as at the PIPJ and MCPJ, indicating activity of FDP. If the finger does not flex at all, neither flexor is active. Be aware that a proportion of the population does not have an effective FDS to the little finger, so the test is then invalidated for this digit (Townley et al. 2010).

Neurological Testing

This includes neurological integrity testing, sensorimotor tests and some other nerve tests.

Integrity of the Nervous System

Keeping in mind the onset, description and distribution of symptoms, the clinician will use clinical reasoning to justify a neurological examination.

Dermatomes/Peripheral Nerves. Light touch and pain sensation of the upper limb are tested using cotton wool and pinprick respectively, as described in

Chapter 3. Following trauma or compression it is vital to assess the cutaneous sensation. Knowledge of the cutaneous distribution of nerve roots (dermatomes) and peripheral nerves (radial [C5–T1], median [C5–T1] and ulnar [C7–T1]) enables the clinician to distinguish sensory loss due to a spinal nerve root or brachial plexus lesion from that of a peripheral nerve lesion. There is overlap but areas shown to be 'constant' in injured patients are: radial nerve – dorsum of hand near apex of the anatomical snuffbox, median – tip of the index finger, ulnar – tip of little finger (Magee 2014). The cutaneous nerve distribution and dermatome areas are shown in Chapter 3.

Stereognosis is also tested by placing objects in the patient's hand and recording the time taken to recognize objects by touch alone. Indepth testing of two-point discrimination can also identify variance from published normal values (Magee 2014).

Myotomes/Peripheral Nerves. The following myotomes can be tested (see Chapter 3 for further details):

- C5: shoulder abduction
- C6: elbow flexion
- C7: elbow extension
- C8: thumb extension
- T1: finger adduction.

A working knowledge of the muscular distribution of nerve roots (myotomes) and peripheral nerves enables the clinician to differentiate motor loss due to a root lesion from that of a peripheral nerve lesion. The peripheral nerve distributions are shown in Chapter 3.

Reflex Testing

Deep tendon reflexes are not usually tested in the forearm, wrist and hand. The following deep tendon reflexes can be tested (see Chapter 3):

- C5–C6: biceps
- C7: triceps and brachioradialis.

The Hoffman reflex, the upper-limb equivalent of the Babinski test, can be tested if an upper motor neuron dysfunction is suspected. The clinician 'flicks' the terminal phalanx of the index, middle or ring finger and, in a positive test, the reflex flexion of the other distal phalanx will be observed (Magee 2014).

Neurodynamic Tests

The upper-limb neurodynamic tests (ULNT 1, 2a, 2b and 3) may be carried out in order to ascertain the degree to which neural tissue is responsible for the production of the patient's wrist and hand symptom(s). These tests are described in detail in Chapter 3.

Other Nerve Tests

Median Nerve. The median nerve can be palpated indirectly at the wrist between palmaris longus medially and flexor carpi radialis laterally.

Compression of the median nerve, under the flexor tendons in the retinaculum, results in CTS, the most common, peripheral, nerve compression neuropathy (Clark et al. 2011). Compression can result from fracture, tendonitis and diabetes; degenerative and inflammatory joint disease. CTS is also commonly seen in pregnant women due to fluid retention. Symptoms typically include burning pain, pins and needles, weakness and night pain, although no universally accepted diagnostic criteria exist. The use of Tinel's and Phalen's tests were supported in a review by Valdes and LaStayo (2013) and when used in combination raise the likelihood of detecting CTS.

TINEL'S SIGN (AT THE WRIST). With the patient's wrist in neutral the clinician taps the midpoint of the carpal tunnel at the wrist using a percussion hammer. Paraesthesia or numbness in the sensory distribution of the median nerve would indicate a positive test. Specificity and sensitivity values vary for this test (specificity 55–100%, sensitivity 38–100%: Brüske et al. 2002; specificity 30%, sensitivity 65%: El Miedany et al. 2008) and so the test should be used in conjunction with other tests (Hattam & Smeatham 2010).

PHALEN'S WRIST FLEXION TEST. With the patient's elbow in full extension and forearm in pronation the patient's wrist is held in full flexion for 1 minute. Paraesthesia in the distribution of the median nerve indicates a positive test (Amirfeyz et al. 2005).

MODIFIED CARPAL COMPRESSION TEST. A blood pressure cuff is wrapped around the wrist and inflated to 100 mm/Hg for 30 seconds. A 8 cm long 8 mm diameter wooden pencil-like object can be lay along the median nerve under the cuff to apply a more direct pressure to the median nerve during the test (Tekeoglu et al. 2007). This is a useful alternative to Phalen's test, whereby the range of movement at the wrist may be restricted or painful (González del Pino et al. 1997).

Ulnar Nerve. The ulnar nerve is superficial at the wrist and can be palpated in Guyon's (pisohamate) canal between pisiform and the hook of hamate. The nerve can be injured following fractures or ganglions or due to mechanical compression when cycling or typing (Baker et al. 2007).

FROMENT'S SIGN FOR ULNAR NERVE PARALYSIS. The patient holds a piece of paper between the index finger and thumb in a lateral key grip, and the clinician attempts to pull it away. Flexion at the interphalangeal joint of the thumb due to paralysis of adductor pollucis (Froment's sign) and clawing of the little and ring fingers are apparent as a result of paralysis of the interossei and lumbrical muscles and the unopposed action of the extrinsic extensors and flexors will indicate ulnar nerve paralysis (Magee 2014).

Radial Nerve. The radial nerve is palpable at the terminal parts of the radial sensory nerve in the anatomical snuffbox at the wrist (Butler 2000).

Tests for Circulation and Swelling

If it is suspected that the patient's circulation is compromised the pulses of the radial and ulnar arteries at the wrist should be palpated.

Allen Test for the Radial and Ulnar Arteries at the Wrist

The clinician applies pressure to the radial and ulnar arteries at the wrist and the patient is then asked to open and close the hand a few times and then to keep it open. To test the patency of each artery, release the pressure over the radial artery and then repeat the process for the ulnar artery. The hand should flush within 5 seconds on release of the pressure (Magee 2014).

Figure-of-Eight Measurement

This simple test is a reliable and valid method of measuring swelling in the hand (Pellecchia 2003). With the patient's wrist/hand in neutral position a measuring tape is placed on the distal ulnar styloid and brought horizontally along the palmar aspect of the wrist. The tape is brought diagonally across the dorsum of the hand and over the fifth MCPJ line, across the anterior surface of the MCPJs, then across the back of the hand to where the tape began and the measurement is recorded in centimetres. This value can be compared to the measurement for the other hand (Magee 2014).

Palpation

The extent of palpation will depend on the clinician's clinical reasoning and working hypotheses. A good anatomical knowledge and systematic approach will ensure palpation is logical and focused. Palpation findings can be recorded on a body chart (see Fig. 2.3) and/or palpation chart (see Fig. 3.35).

The clinician notes the following:

- the temperature of the area
- localized skin moisture
- the presence of oedema or effusion.
- Palmar/anterior surface: palpate tendons for tenderness, crepitus: flexor carpi radialis, flexor pollucis longus, FDS, FDP, palmaris longus, flexor carpi ulnaris. Check ulnar and radial pulses, palmar fascia for thickening, thenar and hypothenar eminences for tone/bulk, flexion creases, longitudinal and transverse arches of the hand. The hook of hamate – pisohamate /Guyon's canal – is a possible site of ulnar nerve compression. Assess the gap between flexor carpi ulnaris and distal ulnar styloid for TFCC tears and ulnotriquetral ligament tears.
- Dorsal/posterior surface: palpate the radial styloid, which should project more distally than the ulnar. This normal variance can be lost post Colles fracture, resulting in excessive loading on the TFCC. Palpate ABPL and EPB/extensor pollucis longus each side of the anatomical snuffbox; tenderness in the floor of the snuffbox can indicate scaphoid fracture, avascular necrosis or radial nerve sensitivity. Palpate the extensor tendons; check for increased or decreased prominence of carpal bones – scaphoid (through snuffbox or tubercle anteriorly), lunate, triquetral, pisiform, trapezium, trapezoid, capitate (located as a dip when the wrist is flexed) and hamate.

Accessory Movements

Wrist and hand accessory movements are shown (Fig. 11.12) and listed in Table 11.2; however it is not necessary to test all of those listed, as selection will be based on clinical reasoning of findings so far in the physical examination. Where are symptoms located? Which movements are symptomatic and/or restricted? For example, if wrist extension is limited then examination will initially primarily focus on the radiocarpal joint. These accessory tests will be selected in order to refine the clinician's working hypothesis and can be further refined, for example, using the Kaltenborn tests to explore the intercarpal joints in more detail. There are 10 parts to the Kaltenborn test, although it is not necessary to complete all parts of the test. For example, if the patient's symptoms are focused around the thumb the clinician will focus accessory testing on the radial side of the wrist and hand, exploring parts 1, 2, 5 and 6 of the Kaltenborn test (Table 11.3) in addition to the CMC joint, PIPJ and interphalangeal accessory joint, testing to identify the source of the symptoms. Although intercarpal movement is minimal a small study comparing judgements of two experienced clinicians found there to be good intrarater reliability in identifying hyper- and hypomobile joints using the Kaltenborn test (Staes et al. 2009).

A palpation chart and movement diagrams can be used to record findings (see Chapter 3).

At the end of the physical examination the clinician reassesses all the physical asterisks (movements or tests that have been found to reproduce the patient's symptoms) in order to establish the effect of the accessory

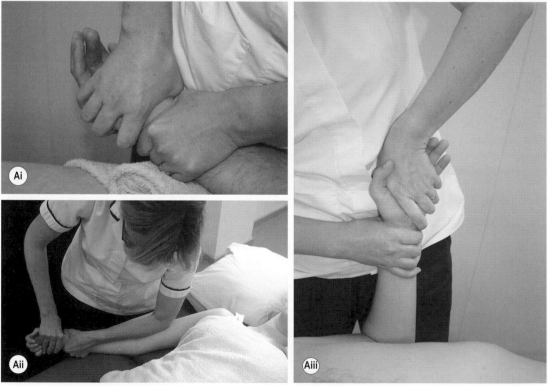

FIG. 11.12 ■ Wrist and hand accessory movements. (Ai) Anteroposterior and posteroanterior. Anteroposterior shown: the left hand grasps around the distal end of the radius and ulna and the right grasps the hand at the level of the proximal carpal row. The right hand then glides the patient's hand anteriorly to posteriorly. (Aii) Medial and lateral transverse. Medial shown: the left hand grasps around the distal radius and ulna and the right hand grasps the proximal carpal row, then glides the patient's hand medially. (Aiii) Longitudinal cephalad. The right hand grasps around the distal radius and ulna and the left hand applies a longitudinal cephalad force to the wrist through the heel of the hand.

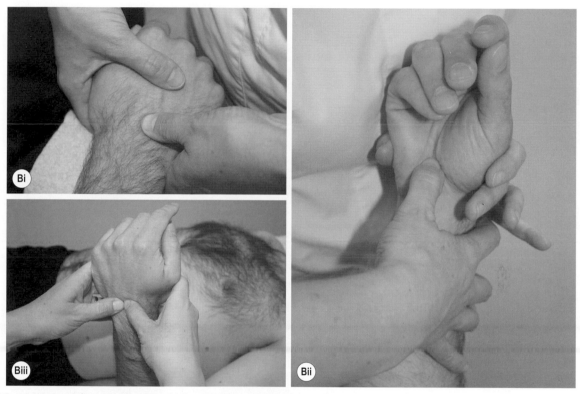

FIG. 11.12, cont'd ■ (B) Intercarpal joints. (Bi) Anteroposterior and posteroanterior. Thumb pressure can be applied to the anterior or posterior aspect of each carpal bone to produce an anteroposterior or posteroanterior movement, respectively. A posteroanterior pressure to the lunate is shown here. (Bii) Horizontal flexion. The right thumb is placed in the centre of the anterior aspect of the wrist and the left hand cups around the carpus to produce horizontal flexion. (Biii) Horizontal extension. The thumbs are placed in the centre of the posterior aspect of the wrist and the fingers wrap around the anterior aspect of the carpus to produce horizontal extension.   *Continued*

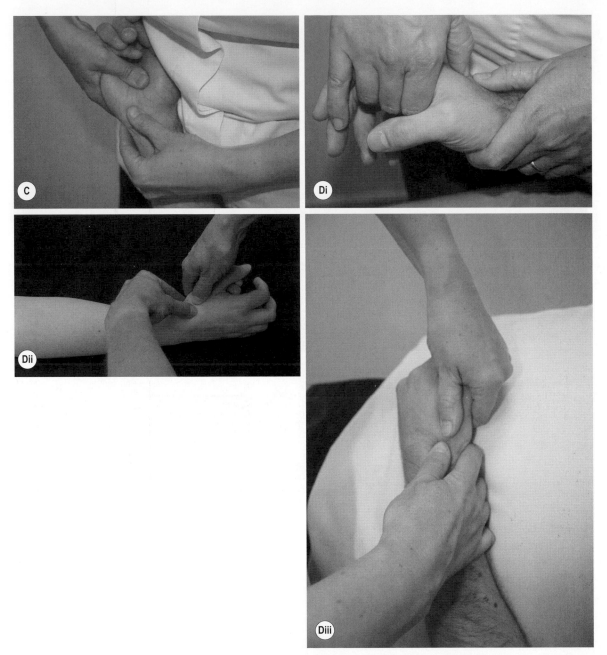

FIG. 11.12, cont'd ■ (C) Pisotriquetral joint. Medial and lateral transverse, longitudinal caudad and cephalad and distraction. Shown here, the right hand stabilizes the hand and the left hand grasps the triquetral bone and applies a medial and lateral transverse force to the bone. (D) Carpometacarpal joints. Fingers – the left hand grasps around the relevant distal carpal bone while the right hand grasps the proximal end of the metacarpal. (Di) Anteroposterior and posteroanterior. Posteroanterior shown: the right hand glides the metacarpal anteriorly. (Dii) Anteroposterior and posteroanterior. The left hand glides the thumb metacarpal anteriorly and posteriorly. (Diii) Medial and lateral rotation. The left hand rotates the thumb metacarpal medially and laterally.

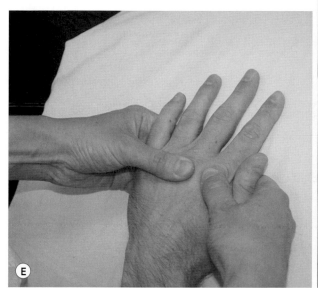

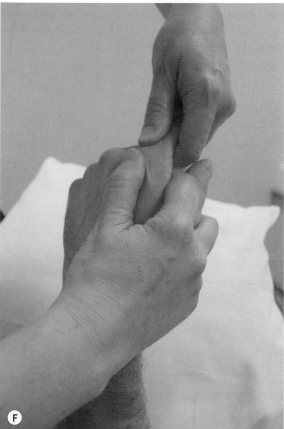

FIG. 11.12, cont'd ■ (E) Proximal and distal intermetacarpal joints of the fingers – anteroposterior and posteroanterior. The finger and thumb of each hand gently pinch the anterior and posterior aspects of adjacent metacarpal heads and apply a force in opposite directions to glide the heads anteriorly and posteriorly. (F) Anteroposterior and posteroanterior. The left hand glides the proximal phalanx anteriorly and posteriorly.

movements on the patient's signs and symptoms. If the patient's symptoms have improved or range has increased then this is a good indication that the patient's problem is predominantly articular and mechanical and the patient is likely to respond well to manual therapy. The clinician highlights important findings from the physical examination with an asterisk (*). These findings are reassessed at, and within, subsequent treatment sessions to evaluate the effects of treatment on the patient's condition.

Completion of the Examination

On completion of the physical examination, the clinician will need to collate the information to evaluate and revisit how findings compare with expected findings, based on the clinician's initial primary working hypothesis and alternative hypotheses. Throughout the physical examination the clinician will have been revisiting and refining the hypotheses categories (adapted from Jones & Rivett 2004):

- What can the patient do and what is the patient unable to do? How are these symptoms impacting on the patient's life?
- What are the patient's beliefs and are they helpful or unhelpful in terms of driving behaviours?
- What are the mechanisms of symptoms (include anatomy, biomechanics, mechanism of injury, pain mechanism, stages of tissue healing, tissues at fault). Are they arthrogenic/myogenic/neurogenic?

TABLE 11.2
Accessory Movements

Radiocarpal Joint

↕	Anteroposterior
↕	Posteroanterior
◄► Med	Medial transverse
►◄ Lat	Lateral transverse
◄►► Ceph	Longitudinal cephalad
◄►► Caud	Longitudinal caudad

Intercarpal Joints

↕	Anteroposterior
↕	Posteroanterior
↕↕	Anteroposterior/posteroanterior gliding
HF	Horizontal flexion
HE	Horizontal extension
◄►► Ceph	Longitudinal cephalad
◄►► Caud	Longitudinal caudad

Pisotriquetral Joint

◄► Med	Medial transverse
►◄ Lat	Lateral transverse
◄►► Ceph	Longitudinal cephalad
◄►► Caud	Longitudinal caudad
Dist	Distraction

Carpometacarpal Joints

Fingers

↕	Anteroposterior
↕	Posteroanterior
◄► Med	Medial transverse
►◄ Lat	Lateral transverse
↻	Medial rotation
↺	Lateral rotation

Thumb

↕	Anteroposterior
↕	Posteroanterior
◄► Med	Medial transverse
►◄ Lat	Lateral transverse
◄►► Ceph	Longitudinal cephalad
◄►► Caud	Longitudinal caudad
↻	Medial rotation
↺	Lateral rotation

Proximal and Distal Intermetacarpal Joints

↕	Anteroposterior
↕	Posteroanterior
HF	Horizontal flexion
HE	Horizontal extension

Metacarpophalangeal, Proximal and Distal Interphalangeal Joints of Fingers and Thumb

↕	Anteroposterior
↕	Posteroanterior
◄► Med	Medial transverse
►◄ Lat	Lateral transverse
◄►► Ceph	Longitudinal cephalad
◄►► Caud	Longitudinal caudad
↻	Medial rotation
↺	Lateral rotation

Choice of application and modifications to the above joints

Start position of the joint:
  Speed of force application
  Direction of the applied force
  Point of application of applied force

Identify any effect of accessory movements on patient's signs and symptoms

Reassess all *asterisks

If necessary screen any proximal and distal regions that may refer to the area

Cervical spine

Thoracic spine

Shoulder

Wrist and hand

TABLE 11.3
Ten-Point Movement Test for the Carpal Bones (Kaltenborn 2002)

Movements Around the Capitate

1. Fix the capitate and move the trapezoid
2. Fix the capitate and move the scaphoid
3. Fix the capitate and move the lunate
4. Fix the capitate and move the hamate

Movements on the Radial Side of the Wrist

5. Fix the scaphoid and move the trapezoid and trapezium

Movements of the Radiocarpal Joint

6. Fix the radius and move the scaphoid
7. Fix the radius and move the lunate
8. Fix the ulna and move the triquetrum

Movements on the Ulnar Side of the Wrist

9. Fix the triquetrum and move the hamate
10. Fix the triquetrum and move the pisiform

- What are the physical impairments and associated structures/tissue sources driving the patient's symptoms?
- Does this patient's problem have any other contributing factors that may be influencing the onset or maintenance of symptoms? For example, environmental, psychosocial, behavioural, physical or heredity factors.
- Are there any precautions/contraindications to treatment and management? This includes the severity and irritability of the patient's symptoms and the underlying cause(s) of the patient's symptoms.
- Where will initial management/treatment be focused?
- Assessing prognosis – this can be affected by factors such as the stage and cause of symptoms, the patient's expectations, personality and lifestyle. Included in the prognosis should be an initial estimate of the percentage improvement for the patient, the number of treatments required to achieve this and the time period over which it will occur.

Before the patient leaves the clinician:

- explains the findings of the physical examination and how these findings relate to the subjective assessment, offering some initial advice if appropriate
- allows the patient sufficient opportunity to discuss thoughts and beliefs which may well have changed over the course of the examination
- revisits the patient's initial expectations and through collaboration with the patient identifies an agreed treatment strategy in order to achieve agreed goals
- warns the patient of possible exacerbation up to 24–48 hours following the examination
- requests the patient to report details on the behaviour of the symptoms following examination at the next attendance.

For guidance on treatment and management principles, the reader is directed to the companion textbook (Petty & Barnard 2017).

ACKNOWLEDGEMENTS

The author would like to thank Professor Karen Beeton PhD, MPhty, BSc(Hons) FCSP, FMACP for her ongoing support.

REFERENCES

Agarwal, S., et al., 2005. Disseminated tuberculosis presenting with finger swelling in a patient with tuberculous osteomyelitis: a case report. Ann. Clin. Microbiol. Antimicrob. 4, 18.

Amirfeyz, R., et al., 2005. Hand elevation test for assessment of carpal tunnel syndrome. J. Hand Surg. Br. 30, 361–364.

Baker, N., et al., 2007. Kinematics of the fingers and hands during computer keyboard use. Clin. Biomech. (Bristol, Avon) 22, 34–43.

Baldassarre, R., Hughes, T., 2013. Investigating suspected scaphoid fractures. Br. Med. J. 346, 1370–1371.

Ballantyne, J.A., Hooper, G., 2004. The hand and diabetes. Curr. Orthop. 18, 118–125.

Batra, S., Kanvinde, R., 2007. Osteoarthritis of the thumb trapeziometacarpal joint. Curr. Orthop. 21, 135–144.

Batteson, R., et al., 2008. The de Quervain's screening tool: validity and reliability of a measure to support clinical diagnosis. Musculoskeletal Care 6, 168–180.

Blair, S.J., et al., 1987. Evaluation of impairment of the upper extremity. Clin. Orthop. Relat. Res. 221, 42–58.

Bland, J.D., 2000. The value of the history in the diagnosis of carpal tunnel syndrome. J. Hand Surg. Br. 25, 445–450.

Brüske, J., et al., 2002. The usefulness of the Phalen test and the Hoffmann-Tinel sign in the diagnosis of carpal tunnel syndrome. Acta Orthop. Belg. 68, 141–145.

Bulstrode, C., et al., 2002. Oxford textbook of orthopaedics and trauma. Oxford University Press, Oxford.

Butler, D., 2000. The sensitive nervous system. Neuro Orthopaedic Institute, Adelaide.

Cakir, M., et al., 2003. Musculoskeletal manifestations in patients with thyroid disease. Clin. Endocrinol. (Oxf) 59, 162–167.

Caldwell, C., Khoo-Summers, L., 2010. Movement system impairment syndromes of the wrist and hand. In: Sahrmann, S.A. (Ed.), Movement system impairment syndromes of the extremities, cervical and thoracic spines. Mosby, St Louis, MO, pp. 165–236.

Christodoulou, L., Bainbridge, L.C., 1999. Clinical diagnosis of triquetrolunate injuries. J. Hand Surg. Br. 24, 598.

Clark, D., et al., 2011. Often atypical? The distribution of sensory disturbance in carpal tunnel syndrome. Ann. R. Coll. Surg. Engl. 93, 470–473.

Court-Brown, C.M., Caesar, B., 2006. Epidemiology of adult fractures: a review injury. Int. J. Care Injured 37, 691–697.

Davis, D.I., Baratz, M., 2010. Soft tissue complications of distal radius fractures. Hand Clin. 26, 229–235.

Easterling, M.D., Wolfe, S.W., 1994. Scaphoid shift in the uninjured wrist. J. Hand Surg. Am. 19A, 604–606.

Eaton, R.G., Glickel, S.Z., 1987. Trapeziometacarpal osteoarthritis. Staging as a rationale for treatment. Hand Clin. 3, 455–471.

Eckhaus, D., 1993. Swan-neck deformity. In: Clark, G.L., et al. (Eds.), Hand rehabilitation, a practical guide. Churchill Livingstone, Edinburgh (Chapter 16).

Eddington, L.V., 1993. Boutonnière deformity. In: Clark, G.L., et al. (Eds.), Hand rehabilitation, a practical guide. Churchill Livingstone, Edinburgh (Chapter 17).

Elliott, B.G., 1992. Finkelstein's test: a descriptive error that can produce a false positive. J. Hand Surg. Am. 17B, 481–482.

El Miedany, Y., et al., 2008. Clinical diagnosis of carpal tunnel syndrome: old tests, new concepts. Joint Bone Spine 75, 451–457.

Fess, E., Philips, C., 1987. Hand splinting, principles and methods. C.V. Mosby, St Louis, MO.

Gaston, M.S., Simpson, A.H., 2007. Inhibition of fracture healing. J. Bone Joint Surg. Br. 89-B, 1553–1560.

González del Pino, J., et al., 1997. Value of the carpal compression test in the diagnosis of carpal tunnel syndrome. J. Hand Surg. Br. 22, 38–41.

Goubau, J.F., et al., 2014. The wrist hyperflexion and abduction of the thumb (WHAT) test: a more specific and sensitive test to diagnose de Quervain's tenosynovitis than the Eichhoff's test. J. Hand Surg. Eur. Vol. 39, 286–292.

Hattam, P., Smeatham, A., 2010. Special tests in musculoskeletal examination. An evidence-based guide for clinicians. Churchill Livingstone Elsevier, Edinburgh (Chapter 4).

Hengeveld, E., Banks, K., 2014. Maitland's peripheral manipulation, fifth ed. Butterworth-Heinemann Elsevier, London.

Heras-Palou, C., et al., 2003. Outcome measurement in hand surgery: report of a consensus conference. Br. J. Hand Ther. 8, 70–80.

Hing, W., et al., 2015. The Mulligan concept of manual therapy. Churchill Livingstone, Sydney.

Hislop, H., et al., 2013. Daniels and Worthingham's muscle testing: techniques of manual examination and performance testing, ninth ed. W.B. Saunders, Philadelphia.

Jones, M.A., Rivett, D.A., 2004. Clinical reasoning for manual therapists. Butterworth-Heinemann, Edinburgh.

Kalk, W.J., 2005. Endocrinology. In: Shamley, D. (Ed.), Pathophysiology: an essential test for the allied professions. Elsevier Butterworth Heinemann, Edinburgh.

Kaltenborn, F.M., 2002. Manual mobilization of the joints, vol. I, sixth ed. The extremities. Norli, Oslos.

Kendall, F.P., et al., 2010. Muscles testing and function, fifth ed. Lippincott Williams and Wilkins, Baltimore.

La Stayo, P., Howell, J., 1995. Clinical provocative tests used in evaluating wrist pain: a descriptive study. J. Hand Ther. 8, 10–17.

Magee, D.J., 2014. Orthopedic physical assessment, sixth ed. Saunders Elsevier, Philadelphia.

Montechiarello, S., et al., 2010. The intersection syndrome: ultrasound findings and their diagnostic value. J. Ultrasound 13, 70–73.

Neumann, D.A., 2010. Kinesiology of the musculoskeletal system. Foundations for rehabilitation, second ed. Mosby Elsevier, St Louis, MO (Chapter 7).

Novak, C., McCabe, S., 2015. Prevalence of cold sensitivity in patients with hand pathology. Hand 10, 173–176.

Pellecchia, G.L., 2003. Figure-of-eight method of measuring hand size: reliability and concurrent validity. J. Hand Ther. 16, 300–304.

Petty, N.J., Barnard, K., 2017. Principles of neuromusculoskeletal treatment and management: a handbook for therapists, third ed. Elsevier, Edinburgh.

Picardo, N.E., Khan, W.S., 2012. Advances in the understanding of the aetiology of Dupuytren's disease. Surgeon 10, 151–158.

Prosser, R., et al., 2011. Provocative wrist tests and MRI are of limited diagnostic value for suspected wrist ligament injuries: a cross-sectional study. J. Physiother. 57, 247–253.

Schnitzler, C., 2005. Bone and joint disorders. In: Shamley, D. (Ed.), Pathophysiology: an essential test for the allied professions. Elsevier Butterworth Heinemann, Edinburgh.

Staes, F., et al., 2009. Reliability of accessory motion testing at the carpal joints. Man. Ther. 14, 292–298.

Sueki, D.G., et al., 2013. A regional interdependence model of musculoskeletal dysfunction: research, mechanisms, and clinical implications. J. Man. Manip. Ther. 21, 90–102.

Taleisnik, J., 1988. Carpal instability. J. Bone Joint Surg. 70A, 1262–1268.

Tang, P., 2011. Collateral ligament injuries of the thumb metacarpophalangeal joint. J. Am. Acad. Orthop. Surg. 19, 287–296.

Tekeoglu, I., et al., 2007. The pneumatic compression test and modified pneumatic compression test in the diagnosis of carpal tunnel syndrome. J. Hand Surg. Eur. Vol. 32, 697–699.

Totten, P., Flinn-Wagner, S., 1992. Functional evaluation of the hand. In: Stanley, B., Tribuzi, S. (Eds.), Concepts in hand rehabilitation. F.A. Davis, New York, p. 128.

Townley, W.A., et al., 2010. Congenital absence of flexor digitorum superficialis: implications for assessment of little finger lacerations. J. Hand Surg. Eur. Vol. 35, 417–418.

Trail, I.A., et al., 2007. Twenty questions on carpal instability. J. Hand Surg. Am. 32, 240–255.

Valdes, K., LaStayo, P., 2013. The value of provocative tests for the wrist and elbow: a literature review. J. Hand Ther. 26, 33–43.

Watson, H.K., et al., 1988. Examination of the scaphoid. J. Hand Surg. Am. 13A, 657–660.

Wollstein, R., et al., 2013. A hand therapy protocol for the treatment of lunate overload or early Kienbock's disease. J. Hand Ther. 26, 255–260.

12

EXAMINATION OF THE LUMBAR REGION

CHRIS WORSFOLD

CHAPTER CONTENTS

The lumbar spine consists of the five largest vertebrae in the spine, connecting the ribcage to the pelvis and supporting the body weight, whilst also permitting movement.

Common conditions relevant to this region include nerve root, intervertebral disc and facet joint disorders. Narrowing of the spinal foramen and canal may occur (stenosis). It is important to note that these latter structural changes are not strongly associated with pain and disability and are commonly found in asymptomatic subjects (Brinjikji et al. 2015). The majority of low-back disorders have no diagnosis and the term 'non-specific low-back pain' is used. As a result, it is considered important – to direct physiotherapy management – that low-back disorders are classified into subgroups, based upon the hypothesized mechanism of the underlying disorder.

Serious pathology can occur in the lumbar spine – 1–2% of low-back pain presentations (Henschke et al. 2009): inflammatory disease (e.g. ankylosing spondylitis), abdominal aortic aneurysm, tumour and, very rarely, infection can all refer pain to the lumbar region and can mimic benign conditions. In view of these 'musculoskeletal masqueraders' it is strongly suggested that a high index of suspicion is maintained throughout the history and physical examination of the lumbar spine, with the clinician screening for 'red-flag' signs and symptoms of serious pathology (see Table 2.5). Additionally, a rare but devastating condition, cauda equina syndrome, caused by disc pathology compressing the lower section of the spinal cord (the cauda equina), can occur in the context of severe sciatica occurring in approximately 2% of cases of herniated lumbar discs (Gitelman et al. 2008).

The lumbar spine is defined here as the region between T12 and the sacrum and includes the joints and their surrounding soft tissues. Note that the order of the subjective questioning and the physical tests described below can be altered as appropriate for the patient being examined.

Further details of the questions asked during the subjective examination and the tests carried out in the physical examination can be found in Chapters 2 and 3, respectively.

SUBJECTIVE EXAMINATION

Patients' Perspectives on Their Experience

This includes the patient's perspectives, experience and expectations, age, employment, home situation and details of any leisure activities. In order to treat the patient appropriately, it is important that the condition is managed within the context of the patient's social and work environment.

Psychosocial factors need to be assessed, as they will strongly influence the recovery and treatment response. Screening for psychosocial risk can be divided into the following five factors (O'Sullivan et al. 2015):

1. cognitive: negative beliefs (e.g. 'slipped discs' and 'trapped nerves'), catastrophizing (e.g. thinking the worst) and fear of movement (e.g. believing that 'pain indicates damage')
2. social and cultural: may influence pain beliefs and stress load
3. work-related: compensation and work absenteeism
4. lifestyle: sleep, rest, workload, stress and exercise levels; deconditioning secondary to activity avoidance
5. individual: patient goals, preferences, expectations and readiness for change.

To elucidate psychosocial factors more formally the clinician may ask the following five questions, taken from the nine-item Keele STarT Back Screening Tool, a quick and simple prognostic questionnaire that helps clinicians identify modifiable risk factors (biomedical, psychological and social) for back pain disability (Hill et al. 2008).

1. Do you agree that it's not really safe for a person with a condition like yours to be physically active?
2. Have worrying thoughts been going through your mind a lot of the time?
3. Is your back pain terrible and do you feel it's never going to get any better?
4. Have you not enjoyed all the things you used to enjoy?
5. How bothersome has your back pain been in the last 2 weeks?

Body Chart

The following information concerning the type and area of the current symptoms can be recorded on a body chart (see Fig. 2.3).

Area of Current Symptoms

Be exact when mapping out the area of the symptoms. Lesions in the lumbar spine can refer symptoms over a large area – symptoms are commonly felt around the spine, abdomen, groin and lower limbs. Occasionally, symptoms may be felt in the thoracic spine. Ascertain which is the worst symptom and record the patient's interpretation of where he feels the symptoms are coming from.

Areas Relevant to the Region Being Examined

All other relevant areas are checked for symptoms; it is important to ask about pain or stiffness, as this may be relevant to the patient's main symptom. Mark unaffected areas with ticks (✓) on the body chart. Check for symptoms in the cervical spine, thoracic spine, abdomen, groin and lower limbs, some of which may suggest a systemic condition.

Quality of Pain

Establish the quality of the pain; descriptors such as 'burning' or 'electric shock'-type pains suggest symptoms arising from nerve tissue.

Intensity of Pain

The intensity of pain can be measured using, for example, a visual analogue scale, as shown in Fig. 2.5. A pain diary may be useful for patients with chronic low-back pain to determine the pain patterns and triggering factors over a period of time.

Abnormal Sensation

Check for any altered sensation over the lumbar spine and other relevant areas. Common abnormalities are paraesthesia and numbness with dermatomal reduction in sensation suggesting nerve root compression.

Constant or Intermittent Symptoms

Establish the frequency of the symptoms and whether they are constant or intermittent. If symptoms are constant, check whether there is variation in the intensity of the symptoms, as constant unremitting pain may be indicative of sinister pathology such as cancer.

Relationship of Symptoms

If there is more than one area of symptoms, determine the relationship between symptomatic areas – do they come together or separately? For example, the patient could have thigh pain without lumbar spine pain, or the pains may always be present together. It is possible that there may be two separate sources of symptoms.

Behaviour of Symptoms

Aggravating Factors

For each symptomatic area a series of questions can be asked:

- What movements and/or positions bring on or make the patient's symptoms worse?
- How long does it take before symptoms are aggravated?
- Is the patient able to maintain this position or movement?
- What happens to other symptoms when this symptom is produced or made worse?
- How do the symptoms affect function, e.g. sitting, standing, lying, bending, walking, running, walking on uneven ground and up and down stairs, washing, driving, lifting and digging, work, sport and social activities? Further detail about these activities may need to be gathered. For example, the patient may complain that driving aggravates the symptoms; this position implicates both the lumbar spine (flexion) and neural tissue (slumped position combined with knee extension) and signposts to the clinician those tests that need to be focused upon during the physical examination, e.g. lumbar flexion and the slump test.

No improvement in pain with rest is a classic feature of inflammatory back pain (Harris et al. 2012). It is

important to differentiate inflammatory from mechanical back pain as early as possible as the management of the two conditions is very different. Symptoms of lower-extremity pain or paraesthesia, occurring with or without back pain but especially in positions of lumbar extension, are suggestive of acquired lumbar spinal stenosis. Walking is commonly limited in acquired lumbar spinal stenosis due to neurogenic claudication in the extended lumbar spine (Genevay & Atlas 2010).

The clinician may ask the patient about theoretically known aggravating factors for structures that could be a source of the symptoms. However, this evidence is not conclusive as functional movements invariably stress other parts of the body. Common aggravating factors for the lumbar spine are flexion (e.g. when putting shoes and socks on), sitting, standing, walking, standing up from a sitting position, driving and coughing/sneezing. These movements and positions can increase symptoms because they stress various structures in the lumbar spine (Table 12.1). Aggravating factors for other regions, which may need to be queried if they are suspected to be a source of the symptoms, are shown in Table 2.2.

Easing Factors

For each symptomatic area a series of questions can be asked to help determine what eases the symptoms:

- What movements and/or positions ease the patient's symptoms?
- How long does it take before symptoms are eased? If symptoms are constant but variable it is important to know what the baseline is and how long it takes for the symptoms to reduce to that level.
- What happens to other symptoms when this symptom is eased?

Improvement in symptoms with movement and exercise could be suggestive of inflammatory back pain (Harris et al. 2012). The clinician asks the patient about theoretically known easing factors for structures that could be a source of the symptoms. Commonly suggested aggravating and found easing factors for the lumbar spine are shown in Table 12.1. A review paper suggests that there is little difference in intradiscal pressure between sitting and standing, and this should

TABLE 12.1

Effect of Position and Movement on Pain-Sensitive Structures of the Lumbar Spine (Jull 1986)

Activity	Symptoms	Possible Structural and Pathological Implications
Sitting		Compressive forces (White & Panjabi 1990) High intradiscal pressure (Nachemson 1992)
Sitting with extension	Decreased	Intradiscal pressure reduced Decreased paraspinal muscle activity (Andersson et al. 1977)
	Increased	Greater compromise of structures of lateral and central canals Compressive forces on lower zygapophyseal joints
Sitting with flexion	Decreased	Little compressive load on lower zygapophyseal joints Greater volume lateral and central canals Reduced disc bulge posteriorly
	Increased	Very high intradiscal pressure Increased compressive loads upper and mid zygapophyseal joints
Prolonged sitting	Increased	Gradual creep of tissues (Kazarian 1975)
Sit to stand	Increased	Creep, time for reversal, difficulty in straightening up Extension of spine, increase in disc bulge posteriorly
Standing	Increased	Creep into extension
Walking	Increased	Shock loads greater than body weight Compressive load (vertical creep) (Kirkaldy-Willis & Farfan 1982) Compressive loads decrease disc height (Hutton et al. 1999; Adams et al. 2000) Leg pain – neurogenic claudication, intermittent claudication
Driving	Increased	Sitting: compressive forces Vibration: muscle fatigue, increased intradiscal pressure, creep (Pope & Hansson 1992) Increased dural tension sitting with legs extended Short hamstrings: pulls lumbar spine into greater flexion
Coughing/sneezing/straining	Increased	Increased pressure subarachnoid space Increased intradiscal pressure Mechanical 'jarring' of sudden uncontrolled movement

be considered when looking at Table 12.1 (Claus et al. 2008). The clinician can then analyse the position or movement that eases the symptoms to help determine the structure at fault.

Aggravating and easing factors will help to determine the irritability of the patient's symptoms. These factors may help to determine the areas at fault and identify functional restrictions and also the relationship between symptoms. The severity can be determined by the intensity of the symptoms and whether the symptoms are interfering with normal activities of daily living, such as work and sleep. This information can be used to determine the direction of the physical examination as well as the aims of treatment and any advice that may be required. The most relevant subjective information should be highlighted with an asterisk (*), explored in the physical examination and

reassessed at subsequent treatment sessions to evaluate treatment intervention.

Twenty-Four-Hour Behaviour of Symptoms

The clinician determines the 24-hour behaviour of symptoms by asking questions about night, morning and evening symptoms.

Night Symptoms. Although severe night pain is a recognized red flag, it should be noted that night symptoms are common in back pain (Harding et al. 2004). It is necessary to establish whether the patient is being woken and kept awake by the symptoms. Patients complaining of needing to sleep upright or get up should raise some concern, e.g. patients with inflammatory back pain often experience a worsening of symptoms when resting at night, and complain of waking during the second half of the night due to pain and discomfort (Harris et al. 2012).

The following questions may be asked:

- Do you have any difficulty getting to sleep?
- Do your symptoms wake you at night? If so:
  - Which symptoms?
  - How many times in a night?
  - How many times in the past week?
  - What do you have to do to get back to sleep?
- If sleep is an issue, further questioning may be useful to determine management.

Morning and Evening Symptoms. The clinician determines the pattern of the symptoms first thing in the morning, through the day and at the end of the day. Morning stiffness that lasts more than 2 hours is suggestive of an inflammatory condition such as ankylosing spondylitis. Stiffness lasting only 30 minutes or less is likely to be mechanical and degenerative in nature. Patients with these symptoms may also report increased symptoms at the end of the day and at night time. This may warrant further investigation.

Stage of the Condition

In order to determine the stage of the condition, the clinician asks whether the symptoms are getting better, getting worse or remaining unchanged.

Special Questions

Special questions must always be asked, as they may identify certain precautions or contraindications to the physical examination and/or treatment (see Table 2.4). As mentioned in Chapter 2, the clinician must differentiate between conditions that are suitable for conservative management and systemic, neoplastic and other non-neuromusculoskeletal conditions (such as abdominal aortic aneurysm), which require referral to a medical practitioner. The reader is referred to Box 2.2 for details of various serious pathological processes which can mimic neuromusculoskeletal conditions (Grieve 1994).

Neurological Symptoms

Neurological symptoms may include pins and needles, numbness and weakness. These symptoms need to be mapped out on the body chart.

Has the patient experienced symptoms of cauda equina compression (i.e. compression below L1), indicating cauda equina syndrome: saddle anaesthesia/paraesthesia, sexual or erectile dysfunction, loss of vaginal sensation, bladder and/or bowel sphincter disturbance (loss of control, retention, hesitancy, urgency or a sense of incomplete evacuation) (Lavy et al. 2009)? These symptoms may be due to interference of S3 and S4 (Grieve 1981). Prompt imaging and surgical attention are required to prevent permanent sphincter paralysis (Lavy et al. 2009).

Has the patient experienced symptoms of spinal cord compression (i.e. compression above the L1 level, which may include the cervical and thoracic cord and brain), such as bilateral tingling in hands or feet and/or disturbance of gait? Are there motor, sensory or tonal changes in all four limbs? Does the patient report coordination changes, including gait disturbance?

Family History

Has the patient (or a member of the family) been diagnosed as having rheumatoid arthritis? Has the patient (or a member of the family) been diagnosed as having an inflammatory condition (such as rheumatoid arthritis)?

History of the Present Condition

For each symptomatic area, the clinician needs to know how long the symptom has been present, whether there was a sudden or slow onset and whether there was a known cause that provoked the onset of the symptom. If the onset was slow, the clinician finds out if there has been any change in the patient's lifestyle, e.g. a new job or hobby or a change in sporting activity. Inflammatory back pain usually begins in the third decade of life and is unlikely to have an onset after 45 years. Note that it is important to determine the patient's age at the onset of the back pain as opposed to noting the patient's current age as she may have been experiencing back pain for several years. Inflammatory back pain has an insidious onset and patients are likely to have been experiencing back pain for >3 months (Harris et al. 2012).

To confirm the relationship between the symptoms, the clinician asks what happened to other symptoms when each symptom began. Has the patient had previous similar episodes? If so, did she have treatment for this? What was the outcome?

Past Medical History

The following information is obtained from the patient and/or the medical notes:

- The details of any relevant medical history. Visceral structures are capable of masquerading as musculoskeletal conditions; for example, the pelvic organs, bowel and kidneys can refer to lumbar spine and sacral regions. Any relevant history related to these organs is important to help differentiate the cause of symptoms. For further information refer to the chapter on masqueraders by Grieve (1994).
- The history of any previous episodes: How many? When were they? What was the cause? What was the duration of each episode? Did the patient fully recover between episodes? Does the patient perceive the current condition to be better, the same or worse in relation to other previous episodes? If there have been no previous attacks, has the patient had any episodes of stiffness in the lumbar spine, thoracic spine or any other relevant region? Check for a history of trauma or recurrent minor trauma.
- Ascertain the results of any past treatment for the same or similar problem. Past treatment records may be obtained for further information.

General Health

Ascertain the general health of the patient – find out if the patient suffers from any malaise, fatigue, fever, nausea or vomiting, stress, anxiety or depression.

Weight Loss

Has the patient noticed any recent unexplained weight loss?

Serious Pathology

Does the patient have a previous history of serious pathology such as cancer? In all, 1% of new back pain visits to family doctors are cancer, but only 10% of these cancers are new cases; 90% are recurrences of cancers from other parts of the body, i.e. metastases. Thus a previous history of cancer is probably the most

useful red flag in low-back pain, and a high index of suspicion must be maintained in these cases (Henschke et al. 2013).

Cardiovascular Disease

Is there a history of cardiac disease, e.g. angina?

Blood Pressure

If the patient has raised blood pressure, is it controlled with medication?

Respiratory Disease

Does the patient have a history of lung pathology, including asthma? How is it controlled?

Diabetes

Does the patient suffer from diabetes? If so, is it type 1 or type 2 diabetes? Is the patient's blood glucose controlled? How is it controlled? Through diet, tablet or injection? Patients with diabetes may develop peripheral neuropathy and vasculopathy, are at increased risk of infection and may take longer to heal than those without diabetes.

Epilepsy

Is the patient epileptic? When was the last seizure?

Osteoporosis

Has the patient had a dual-energy X-ray absorptiometry (DEXA) scan, been diagnosed with osteoporosis or sustained low-impact fractures?

Previous Surgery

Has the patient had previous surgery which may be of relevance to the presenting complaint?

Drug Therapy

What drugs are being taken by the patient? Has the patient been taking anticoagulants recently? Has the patient ever been prescribed long-term (6 months or more) medication/steroids? Sudden-onset low-back pain in patients who use steroids, are older than 74 years and have a history of recent trauma (e.g. a fall) is strongly indicative of osteoporotic fracture (Williams et al. 2013).

X-Ray and Medical Imaging

Has the patient been X-rayed or had any other medical tests recently? Routine spinal X-rays are no longer considered necessary prior to conservative treatment as they identify only the normal age-related degenerative changes, which do not necessarily correlate with the symptoms experienced by the patient (Clinical Standards Advisory Report 1994). X-rays may be indicated in the younger patient (under 20 years) with conditions such as spondylolisthesis or ankylosing spondylitis and in the older patient (over 55 years) where management is difficult (Royal College of Radiologists 2007). In cases where there is a suspected fracture due to trauma or osteoporosis, X-rays are indicated in the first instance. The medical tests may include blood tests, magnetic resonance imaging, discography or a bone scan.

Plan of the Physical Examination

When all this information has been collected, the subjective examination is complete. It is useful at this stage to highlight with asterisks (*), for ease of reference, important findings and particularly one or more functional restrictions. These can then be reexamined at subsequent treatment sessions to evaluate the treatment intervention.

In order to plan the physical examination, the following hypotheses need to be developed from the subjective examination:

- The regions and structures that need to be examined as a possible cause of the symptoms, e.g. lumbar spine, thoracic spine, cervical spine, sacroiliac joint, pubic symphysis, hip, knee, ankle and foot, muscles and nerves. Often it is not possible to examine all of these areas fully at the first attendance and so examination of the structures must be prioritized over subsequent treatment sessions.
- In what way should the physical tests be carried out? Will it be easy or hard to reproduce each symptom? Will it be necessary to use combined movements and repetitive movements to reproduce the patient's symptoms? Are symptoms severe and/or irritable?
- If symptoms are severe, physical tests may be carried out to just before the onset of symptom

production or just to the onset of symptom production; no overpressures will be carried out, as the patient would be unable to tolerate this.

- If symptoms are non-severe, physical tests will be carried out to reproduce symptoms fully and may include overpressures and combined movements.
- If symptoms are irritable, physical tests may be examined to just before symptom production or just to the onset of provocation, with fewer physical tests being examined to allow for a rest period between tests.
- If symptoms are non-irritable physical tests will be carried out to reproduce symptoms fully and may include overpressures and combined movements.

Other factors that need to be examined include working and everyday postures, leg length and muscle weakness.

Are there any precautions and/or contraindications to elements of the physical examination that need to be explored further, such as significant neurological involvement, recent fracture, trauma, steroid therapy or rheumatoid arthritis? There may also be certain contraindications to further examination and treatment, e.g. symptoms of cord compression.

A physical planning form can be useful for clinicians to help guide them through the clinical reasoning process (see Fig. 2.9).

PHYSICAL EXAMINATION

The information from the subjective examination helps the clinician to plan an appropriate physical examination (Jones & Rivett 2004). The severity, irritability and nature of the condition are the major factors that will influence the choice and priority of physical testing procedures. The first and overarching question the clinician might ask is: 'Is this patient's condition suitable for me to manage?' For example, a patient presenting with cauda equina compression symptoms may only need neurological integrity testing, prior to an urgent medical referral. The second question the clinician might ask is: 'Does this patient have a neuromusculoskeletal dysfunction that I may be able to help?' To answer that, the clinician needs to carry out a full physical examination; however, this may not be possible if the symptoms are severe and/or irritable. If the patient's symptoms are severe and/or irritable, the clinician aims to explore movements as much as possible, within a symptom-free range. If the patient has constant and severe and/or irritable symptoms, then the clinician aims to find physical tests that ease the symptoms. If the patient's symptoms are non-severe and non-irritable, then the clinician aims to find physical tests that reproduce each of the patient's symptoms.

Each significant physical test that either provokes or eases the patient's symptoms is highlighted in the patient's notes by an asterisk (*) for easy reference. The highlighted tests are often referred to as 'asterisks' or 'markers'.

The order and detail of the physical tests described below need to be appropriate to the patient being examined; some tests will be irrelevant, some tests will be carried out briefly, while it will be necessary to investigate others fully. It is important that readers understand that the techniques shown in this chapter are some of many; the choice depends mainly on the relative size of the clinician and patient, as well as the clinician's preference. For this reason, novice clinicians may initially want to try what is shown, but then quickly adapt to what is best for them.

Observation

Informal Observation

This should begin as soon as the clinician sees the patient for the first time. This may be in the reception or waiting area, or as the patient enters the treatment room, and should continue throughout the subjective examination. The clinician should be aware of the patient's posture, demeanour, facial expressions, gait and interaction with the clinician, as these may all give valuable information regarding possible pain mechanisms and the severity and irritability of the problem. O'Sullivan et al. (2015) described maladaptive and pain-provoking movement patterns using the example of a sprained ankle: a limp from a sprained ankle may be adaptive in the acute phase (allowing less painful ambulation), but would become maladaptive and pain provoking if it persists past natural tissue-healing time.

Formal Observation

The clinician observes the patient's spinal, pelvic and lower-limb posture in standing, from anterior, lateral and posterior views. The presence of a lateral shift, scoliosis, kyphosis or lordosis is noted. Any asymmetry in levels at the pelvis and shoulders is noted. Observation should include inspection of the muscle bulk, tone and symmetry. This may be related to the patient's handedness or physical activity, or may relate to the complaining symptom. Findings may lead the clinician to investigate muscle length/strength in the physical examination. Skin colour, areas of redness, swelling or sweating should be noted, as these may indicate areas of local pathology, or possibly a systemic or dermatological condition. The clinician should watch the patient performing simple functional tasks. Observation of gait, of sit-to-stand and dressing/undressing will help to give the clinician a good idea of how the patient is likely to move in the physical examination, and may help to highlight any problems such as hypervigilance and fear avoidance.

Active Physiological Movements

For active physiological movements, the clinician notes the:

- quality of movement
- range of movement
- behaviour of pain through the range of movement
- resistance through the range of movement and at the end of the range of movement
- provocation of any muscle spasm.

The active movements with overpressure listed are tested with the patient in standing and are shown in Fig. 12.1. Active physiological movements of the lumbar spine and possible modifications are shown in Table 12.2. The clinician usually stands behind the patient to be able to see the quality and range of movement. Before starting the active movements, the clinician notes any deformity or deviation in the patient's spinal posture or any muscle spasm. This may include scoliosis, a lateral shift, or a kyphotic or lordotic posture. Postural deformities can be corrected prior to starting the active movements to see if this changes the patient's symptoms. Symptom response through range is noted, and any deviation during movement can again be corrected to see if this changes the symptoms. Changes in pain response may help to guide the treatment. Pain through range may result from a number of causes, including instability or lack of control of movement, a structural deformity or fear of movement. Activation of the postural control muscles may help to decrease through-range pain, and this may suggest the use of muscle control exercises in the treatment programme. Equally, reassurance of the patient that movement is a good thing may also help to correct movement abnormalities.

Patients may exhibit a range of compensatory movement strategies, some of which may be a way to avoid pain (adaptive), but some of which are likely to be provocative (maladaptive). O'Sullivan (2006) describes typical movement patterns and related tests

as part of a subclassification system for patients with low-back pain.

Simple movements tested are:

■ flexion
■ extension
■ lateral flexion to the right
■ lateral flexion to the left
■ lateral glide to the left
■ lateral glide to the right
■ left rotation
■ right rotation.

At the end of range, if no symptoms have been produced and the problem is non-irritable, then overpressure may be applied in order to clear that single movement and to explore further for symptoms

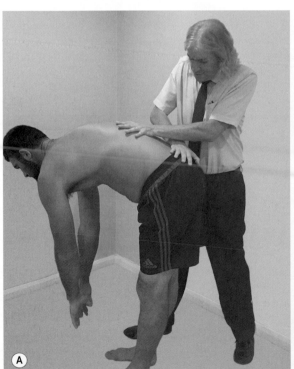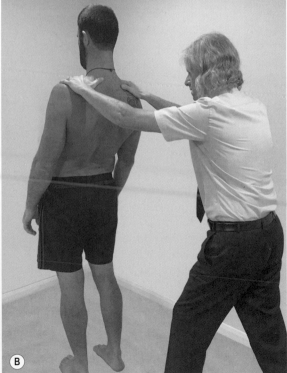

FIG. 12.1 ■ Overpressures to the lumbar spine. (A) Flexion. The hands are placed proximally over the lower thoracic spine and distally over the sacrum. Pressure is then applied through both hands to increase lumbar spine flexion. (B) Extension. Both hands are placed over the shoulders, which are then pulled down in order to increase lumbar spine extension. The clinician observes the spinal movement. *Continued*

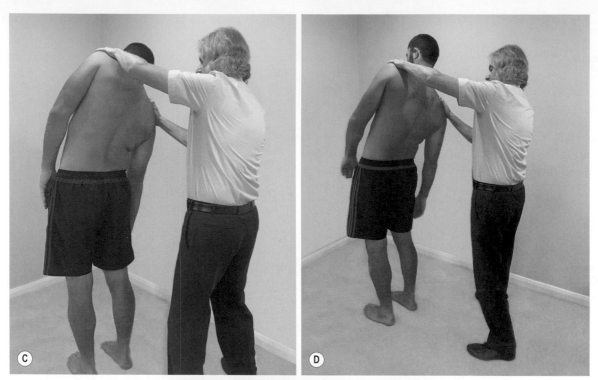

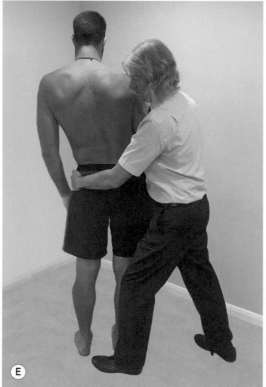

FIG. 12.1, cont'd ■ (C) Lateral flexion. Both hands are placed over the shoulders and a force is applied that increases lumbar lateral flexion. (D) Right extension quadrant. This movement is a combination of extension, right rotation and right lateral flexion. The hand hold is the same as for extension. The patient actively extends and the clinician maintains this position and passively rotates the spine and then adds lateral flexion overpressure. (E) Right side gliding in standing. The clinician guides the movement, displacing the hips away from the shoulders.

TABLE 12.2
Active Physiological Movements and Possible Modifications

Active Physiological Movements	Modifications
Lumbar spine	Repeated movements
Flexion	Speed altered
Extension	Combined movements
Left lateral flexion	(Edwards 1994, 1999), e.g.
Right lateral flexion	■ Flexion then lateral flexion
Left rotation	■ Extension then lateral flexion
Right rotation	■ Lateral flexion then flexion
	■ Lateral flexion then extension
Repetitive flexion in standing	Compression or distraction
Repetitive extension in standing	Sustained
Left side gliding in standing (SGIS)	Injuring movement
Left repetitive side gliding in standing (RSGIS)	Differentiation tests
Right SGIS	Function
Right RSGIS	
Flexion in lying	
Repetitive flexion in lying	
Extension in lying	
Repetitive extension in lying	
Sacroiliac joint: compression/distraction	
Hip medial/lateral rotation	
Knee flexion/extension	

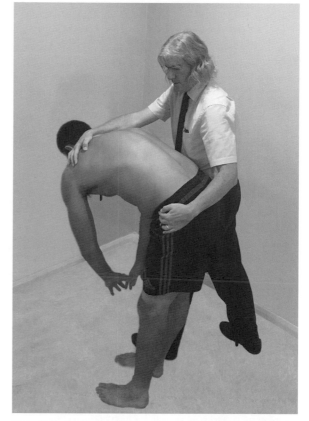

FIG. 12.2 ■ Combined movement of the lumbar spine. The patient moves into lumbar spine flexion and the clinician then maintains this position and passively adds right lateral flexion.

(Maitland et al. 2005). If this produces no symptoms and the clinician is still searching for the patient's pain, or is looking to screen the lumbar spine as a source of the pain, then these movements may be combined. The order in which the movements are combined will depend on the aggravating activities, and the patient's response to plane movements. An example of the combined movement of flexion, right lateral flexion and right rotation is shown in Fig. 12.2.

Hicks et al. (2003) examined the reliability of active movement testing and found good kappa values (mean 0.60 and 95% confidence intervals 0.43–0.73).

Movements may also be repeated to see the effect this has on the patient's symptoms. McKenzie and May (2003) suggest a classification of low-back pain based on presenting signs and symptoms, and the response of symptoms to movement (Table 12.3). There is evidence to suggest that if peripheral pain centralizes with repeated movements, then the prognosis for the patient is likely to be favourable. There is also evidence that patients respond well to treatment consisting of repeated movements in the direction that centralizes their pain (Long et al. 2004; Hefford 2008).

Additional tests may also be useful to help to differentiate the lumbar spine from the hip and sacroiliac joint in standing. For example, when trunk rotation in standing on one leg (causing rotation in the lumbar spine and hip joint) reproduces the patient's buttock pain, differentiation between the lumbar spine and hip joint may be required. The clinician can increase and decrease the lumbar spine rotation and the pelvic rotation in turn, to find out what effect each has on

TABLE 12.3

Operational Definitions for McKenzie Classification (McKenzie & May 2003)

Reducible Derangement

Centralization: in response to therapeutic loading strategies, pain is progressively abolished in a distal to proximal direction, and each progressive abolition is retained over time, until all symptoms are abolished, and if back pain only is present this moves from a widespread to a more central location and then is abolished. Or pain is decreased and then abolished during the application of therapeutic loading strategies. The change in pain location or decrease or abolition of pain remains better, and should be accompanied or preceded by improvements in the mechanical presentation (range of movement and/or deformity)

Irreducible Derangement

Peripheralization of symptoms: increase or worsening of distal symptoms in response to therapeutic loading strategies, and/or no decrease, abolition or centralization of pain

Dysfunction

Spinal pain only, and intermittent pain, and at least one movement is restricted, and the restricted movement consistently produces concordant pain at end-range, and there is no rapid reduction or abolition of symptoms, and no lasting production and no peripheralization of symptoms

Adherent Nerve Root

History of radiculopathy or surgery in the last few months that has improved, but is now unchanging, and symptoms are intermittent, and symptoms in the limb, including 'tightness', and tension test is clearly restricted and consistently produces concordant pain or tightness at end-range, and there is no rapid reduction or abolition of symptoms, and no lasting production of distal symptoms

Postural

Spinal pain only, and concordant pain only with static loading, and abolition of pain with postural correction, and no pain with repeated movements, and no loss of range of movement, and no pain during movement

the buttock pain. If the pain is emanating from the hip then the lumbar movements may have no effect, but pelvic movements may alter the pain; conversely, if the pain is emanating from the lumbar spine, then lumbar spine movements may alter the pain, but pelvic movement may have no effect. The hip can also be placed in a different position, in order to see how much it is contributing to the pain. It can be placed in a more or less provocative position, depending on the subjective aggravating factors and the irritability of the problem, and the pain response noted. Changes

to symptom response may guide the clinician towards a more indepth hip assessment, or may equally focus the clinician on the lumbar spine. Compression or distraction of the sacroiliac joints can be added at the same time to see if this helps to change symptoms. Changes in pain may help guide the clinician towards a more indepth assessment of the sacroiliac joints (see Chapter 13).

Some functional ability has already been tested by the general observation of the patient during the subjective and physical examinations, e.g. the posture adopted during the subjective examination and the ease or difficulty of undressing and changing position prior to the examination. Any further functional testing can be carried out at this point in the examination and may include lifting, sitting postures and dressing. Clues for appropriate tests can be obtained from the subjective examination findings, particularly aggravating factors. These may be particularly helpful if the pain is proving difficult to reproduce with the other tests described.

Passive Physiological Movements

Passive physiological intervertebral movements (PPIVMs), which examine the movement at each segmental level, may be a useful adjunct to passive accessory intervertebral movements (described later in this chapter) to identify segmental hypomobility and hypermobility (Grieve 1991). They can be performed with the patient in side-lying with the hips and knees flexed (Fig. 12.3) or in standing. The clinician palpates the gap between adjacent spinous processes to feel the range of intervertebral movement during flexion, extension, lateral flexion and rotation. It is usually not necessary to examine all directions of movement, only the movement that has been most provocative or most positive during active movement tests, or the movement that most closely fits the patient's aggravating activities, e.g. if a patient says he has most pain when bending to tie shoelaces, then flexion would be the logical PPIVM choice.

It may be necessary to examine other regions to determine their relevance to the patient's symptoms; they may be the source of the symptoms, or they may be contributing to the symptoms. The regions most likely are the sacroiliac joint, hip, knee, foot and ankle.

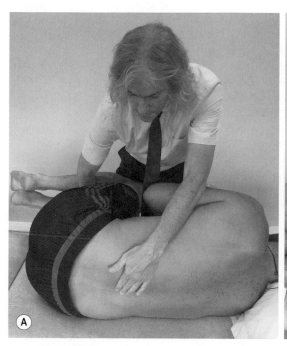
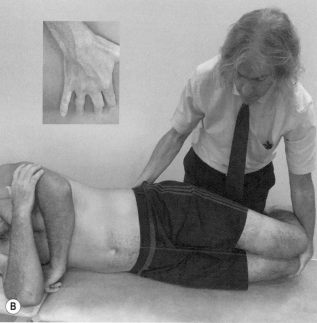

FIG. 12.3 ■ Flexion/extension passive physiological intervertebral movements (PPIVMs) of the lumbar spine. (A) Flexion PPIVM: palpate the interspinous space of the spinal level being assessed. Flex the patient's hips and feel for gapping at the interspinous space. Assess the same movement at other lumbar levels to give an indication of the relative segmental motion. (B) Extension PPIVM with inset showing right hand position: palpate the interspinous space of the spinal level being assessed. Extend the patient's hips and feel for the closing down or coming together of the spinous processes at the interspinous space. Assess the same movement at other lumbar levels to give an indication of the relative segmental motion. One leg may be used for this technique, depending on the relative size of the clinician and the patient.

Joint Integrity Tests

In side-lying with the lumbar spine in extension and hips flexed to 90°, the clinician pushes along the femoral shafts while palpating the interspinous spaces between adjacent lumbar vertebrae to feel for any excessive movement (Fig. 12.4). In the same position but with the lumbar spine in flexion, the clinician pulls along the shaft of the femur and again palpates the interspinous spaces to feel for any excessive movement. Observation of the quality of active flexion and extension can also indicate instability of the lumbar spine (see below). This test is described more fully by Maitland et al. (2005).

Muscle Tests

The muscle tests may include examining muscle strength, control, length and isometric muscle testing. Depending on the patient presentation, these tests may not be a priority on day 1 of the examination, but they may well be part of the ongoing patient management and rehabilitation. Assessment should be based on the subjective asterisks (movements or tests that have been found to reproduce the patient's symptoms). If the clinician thinks that the muscle is the main source of symptoms, or a strong contributing factor to the patient's problem, then the muscle control component should be examined on day 1. Patients may complain of a feeling of weakness, of a lack of control of movement, or catches of pain through movement, and these types of descriptions should alert the clinician to the importance of the muscle component of the patient presentation. Muscle may be both a source of symptoms and a contributing factor.

Muscle Strength

The clinician may test the trunk flexors, extensors, lateral flexors and rotators and any other relevant

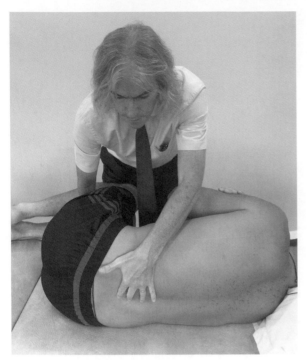

FIG. 12.4 ■ Joint integrity test for the lumbar spine. The fingers are placed in the interspinous space to feel the relative movement of the spinous processes as the clinician passively pushes and then pulls along the femoral shafts.

muscle groups, if these are indicated from the subjective examination. For details of these general tests readers are directed to Cole et al. (1988), Hislop and Montgomery (1995) or Kendall et al. (2010). There is good evidence to suggest that general exercise and strengthening exercises are likely to be of benefit for people with low-back pain (Van Tulder et al. 2005; Mercer et al. 2006; National Institute for Health and Clinical Excellence 2009).

Muscle Control

Muscular control of trunk movement may be relevant to the patient's pain and disability and should be considered in the assessment. There is good evidence to suggest that people with low-back pain have changes in their muscle activity, posture and movement and these can all be changed with the use of motor control approaches (Hides et al. 1994, 2008; Hodges & Richardson 1999; O'Sullivan et al. 2002; Richardson et al. 2004; Dankaerts et al. 2006; Hodges 2015). Indeed, the

improvements seen with motor control approaches carry over to function, can be maintained and are related to clinical improvement (Hodges 2015). It appears that patients with poorer activation of the deep trunk muscles at the commencement of treatment achieve better improvement in pain (Hodges 2015).

Hodges (2015) has described the formal assessment of lumbar motor control as being comprised of:

- Muscle activation: observing evidence of under- or overactivity, atrophy/hypertrophy of muscles. Lumbar multifidus has been found to atrophy in patients with low-back pain (Hides et al. 1994). Formal tests of independent activation of the anterior and posterior deep muscles to evaluate quality of control of deep muscles and evidence of overactive superficial muscles may be performed. More advanced testing of the deep muscles can be done in four-point kneeling, palpating the muscles whilst asking the patient to move either the trunk or individual limbs. These tests may transfer nicely into home exercise programmes if problems are identified. It is important to try to progress the patient to functional exercises as soon as possible.
- Posture: observing alignment in sitting and standing, correcting deviations and evaluating the response, e.g. correcting excessive pelvic tilt.
- Movement: observing strategies during physiological movements (e.g. bending forward), functional tasks (e.g. sit-to-stand) and formal movement tests (e.g. pelvic tilting). Tests in lying, standing and sitting, either on stable or unstable surfaces such as wobble boards or gym balls, may be of use, with the clinician looking to see how the patient controls and moves the trunk, as well as the pain response to such tests. These tests may also help the clinician determine any degree of fear of movement on the part of the patient. Luomajoki et al. (2007) demonstrated that tests of lumbopelvic movement control have a good to substantial inter- and intrarater reliability, with the best all-over reliability ($\kappa > 0.6$) shown for the waiter's bow, sitting knee extension, pelvic tilt and one-leg stand tests. These 'movement control' tests are described in Table 12.4 and

TABLE 12.4	
Movement Control (Mc) Tests **(Luomajoki et al. 2007)**	
MC test 1: Waiter's bow	**Instruction** Flexion of the hips in upright standing. Maintain lumbar lordosis **Compensatory Movements** ■ Flexion occurring in the lumbar spine ■ Less than 50° hip flexion
MC test 2: Sitting knee extension	**Instruction** Upright sitting with corrected lumbar lordosis. Extend one knee at a time **Compensatory Movements** ■ Movement of the lumbar spine ■ Patient unaware of movement in lumbar spine ■ Less than 30° knee extension
MC test 3: Pelvic tilt	**Instruction** Tilt pelvis backwards in upright standing **Compensatory Movements** ■ Thoracic flexion ■ Hip flexion ■ Absence of pelvic tilt ■ Lumbar spine extension
MC test 4: One-leg stand	**Instruction** Stand with feet one-third of trochanter distance apart. Move from normal standing to one leg standing. Perform both sides. Observe lateral movement of the belly button **Compensatory Movements** ■ Lateral transfer of belly button >10 cm ■ Difference between sides >2 cm

shown in Fig. 12.5. It is recommended that patients are rated by the same therapist, as intra-observer reliability is better than interobserver reliability. Carlsson and Rasmussen-Barr (2013) also found that the one-leg stand test has good reliability and recommend its use in clinical work.

O'Sullivan et al. (2006, 2015) describe a subclassifica-tion system for patients with low-back pain which explores functional movements and analyses the movement dysfunction. This system may help to determine aberrant movement patterns and altered

muscular control of the spine, which can be addressed in treatment.

Vleeming et al. (1990a, b) describe anterior and posterior muscle sling systems across the trunk which may help to control trunk movement and support the spine. These slings consists of large muscle groups that help to provide support, or 'force closure' across the trunk and pelvic joints, which are thought to help with the control of movement.

Muscle Length

The clinician may also choose to test the length of muscles which act on, or attach to, the trunk. Whilst shortened muscles may not necessarily be the source of symptoms, they may well contribute to movement dysfunction (Janda 1994). In the anterior and lateral muscle groups, the three hip flexor test may help to establish differences in muscle length. Ober's test may help with lateral muscle length and posteriorly the hamstrings and piriformis muscles may need to be assessed. Testing the length of these muscles is described in Chapter 3.

Neurological Tests

Neurological examination includes neurological integ-rity testing, tests for neural sensitization and other specific nerve tests.

Integrity of the Nervous System

As a general guide, a neurological examination is indi-cated if the patient has symptoms below the level of the buttock crease, or if complaining of numbness, pins and needles, weakness or any neurological symptoms.

Dermatomes/Peripheral Nerves

Light touch and pain sensation of the lower limb are tested using cotton wool and pinprick respectively, as described in Chapter 3. It is always useful to quantify any variations from the normal, as this can then be used as an asterisk and retested at a later date. For example, if sensation to light touch is 4/10 at initial assessment, but then 7/10 following treatment, this identifies an important marker of change for the clini-cian and the patient. Knowledge of the cutaneous dis-tribution of nerve roots (dermatomes) and peripheral nerves enables the clinician to distinguish the sensory

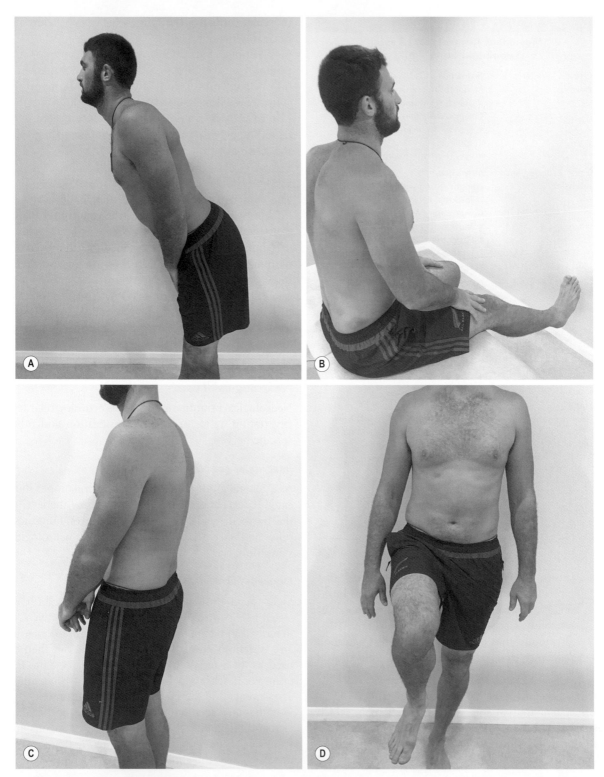

FIG. 12.5 ■ Movement control tests. (A) Waiter's bow. (B) Sitting knee extension. (C) Pelvic tilt. (D) One-leg stand.

loss due to a root lesion from that due to a peripheral nerve lesion. The cutaneous nerve distribution and dermatome areas are shown in Chapter 3. It should be remembered that these vary considerably from patient to patient, and also differ in textbooks, so they should be used only as a guide to the affected level or nerve.

It should be noted that sensation may be increased in certain conditions. The clinician should be aware of the possible different descriptions of these sensory variations, e.g. allodynia, hyperalgesia, analgesia and hyperpathia.

Myotomes/Peripheral Nerves

The following myotomes are tested in sitting or lying, or in a position of comfort for the patient. The clinician should take account of the patient's pain when testing muscle power, as pain will often inhibit full cooperation from the patient, and may lead to a false-positive test.

- L2–3–4: hip flexion
- L2–3–4: knee extension
- L4–5–S1: foot dorsiflexion and inversion
- L4–5–S1: extension of the big toe
- L5–S1: eversion foot, contract buttock, knee flexion
- L5–S1: toe flexion
- S1–S2: knee flexion, plantarflexion
- S3–S4: muscles of the pelvic floor, bladder and genital function.

A working knowledge of the muscular distribution of nerve roots (myotomes) and peripheral nerves enables the clinician to distinguish motor loss due to a root lesion from that due to a peripheral nerve lesion. The peripheral nerve distributions are shown in Chapter 3.

Reflex Testing

The following deep tendon reflexes are tested with the patient relaxed, usually in sitting or lying (see Chapter 3 for further details):

- L3–L4: knee jerk
- S1–S2: ankle jerk.

Neural Sensitization Tests

The following neural sensitization tests may be carried out in order to ascertain the degree to which neural

tissue is responsible for the production of the patient's symptoms. The choice of test should again be guided by the aggravating activities:

- passive neck flexion
- straight-leg raise (SLR)
- femoral nerve tension test in side-lying
- slump test.

Majlesi et al. (2008) found that the slump test was more sensitive (0.84) than the SLR (0.52) in patients with lumbar disc herniations confirmed on magnetic resonance imaging. However, the SLR was found to be a slightly more specific test (0.89) than the slump test (0.83).

Further tests may be added, in order to bias specific peripheral nerves, such as the sural nerve or common peroneal nerve, depending on the area of symptoms. These tests are described in detail in Chapter 3.

Nerves in the lower limb can be palpated at the following points:

- the sciatic nerve two-thirds of the way along an imaginary line between the greater trochanter and the ischial tuberosity
- the common peroneal nerve medial to the tendon of biceps femoris and also around the head of the fibula
- the tibial nerve centrally over the posterior knee crease medial to the popliteal artery; it can also be felt behind the medial malleolus, which is more noticeable with the foot in dorsiflexion and eversion
- the superficial peroneal nerve on the dorsum of the foot along an imaginary line over the fourth metatarsal; it is more noticeable with the foot in plantarflexion and inversion
- the deep peroneal nerve between the first and second metatarsals, lateral to the extensor hallucis tendon
- the sural nerve on the lateral aspect of the foot behind the lateral malleolus, lateral to the tendocalcaneus.

Other Nerve Tests

Plantar Response to Test for an Upper Motor Neuron Lesion (Walton 1989). Pressure applied from the heel along the lateral border of the plantar aspect of the foot produces flexion of the toes in the normal individual. Extension of the big toe with outward fanning of the other toes occurs with an upper motor neuron lesion.

Clonus. The patient's ankle is rapidly dorsiflexed by the clinician in order to elicit a stretch response in the calf. A normal response would be up to 2–4 beats of plantarflexion from the patient. More than this is suggestive of an upper motor neuron problem.

Coordination. Simple coordination tests can be used if the clinician suspects that there is an issue with control of movement. Finger–nose tests and heel–shin sliding tests done bilaterally may help to identify problems with coordination.

Cauda Equina Syndrome. Although there is no simple clinical test for this syndrome, any patient who complains of symptoms of cauda equina compression should have a full neurological examination. As the symptoms can include inability to urinate, loss of bladder control, faecal incontinence and/or saddle-area numbness, it necessarily follows that tests for saddle-area sensation and anal tone are critical to the diagnosis (Lavy et al. 2009). Clearly there is a requirement for training and assessment of clinical competence prior to testing and if the clinician is not trained to undertake these tests, then she should refer the patient immediately to a clinician who can carry out these tests. If the clinician is in any doubt as to the presence of cauda equina syndrome then urgent referral for further testing must be instigated without delay.

Miscellaneous Tests

Vascular Tests

If the patient's circulation is suspected of being compromised, the pulses of the femoral, popliteal and dorsalis pedis and posterior tibial arteries are palpated. The state of the vascular system can also be determined by the response of symptoms to dependence and elevation of the lower limbs. The clinician should be vigilant for male patients over the age of 65 who complain of diffuse low-back pain which is not mechanical in nature. Abdominal aortic aneurysms may present as low-back pain. The clinician should

clearly ask about any vascular history when exploring the patient's past medical history.

Leg Length

True leg length is measured from the anterior superior iliac spine to the medial or lateral malleolus. Apparent leg length is measured from the umbilicus to the medial or lateral malleolus. A difference in leg length of up to 1–1.3 cm is considered normal. If there is a leg length difference then test the length of individual bones, the tibia with knees bent and the femurs in standing. Ipsilateral posterior rotation of the ilium (on the sacrum) or contralateral anterior rotation of the ilium will result in a decrease in leg length (Magee 2014).

Palpation

The clinician palpates the lumbar spine and any other relevant areas. It is useful to record palpation findings on a body chart (see Fig. 2.3) and/or palpation chart (see Fig. 3.35).

The clinician notes the following:

- the temperature of the area
- localized increased skin moisture
- the presence of oedema or effusion
- mobility and feel of superficial tissues, e.g. ganglions, nodules and the lymph nodes in the femoral triangle
- the presence or elicitation of any muscle spasm
- tenderness of bone, trochanteric and psoas bursae (palpable if swollen), ligaments, muscle (Baer's point, for tenderness/spasm of iliacus, lies a third of the way down a line from the umbilicus to the anterior superior iliac spine), tendon, tendon sheath, trigger points (see Fig. 3.36) and nerve
- increased or decreased prominence of bones
- pain provoked or reduced on palpation.

Passive Accessory Intervertebral Movements

It is useful to use the palpation chart and movement diagrams (or joint pictures) to record findings. These are explained in detail in Chapter 3.

The clinician notes the:

- quality of movement
- range of movement

- resistance through the range and at the end of the range of movement
- behaviour of pain through the range
- provocation of any muscle spasm.

Lumbar spine (L1–L5) accessory movements are listed in Table 12.5. A central posteroanterior, unilateral posteroanterior and transverse glide are shown in Fig. 12.6. Lumbar spine accessory movements may need to be examined with the patient in flexion, extension, lateral flexion, rotation or a combination of these positions. Fig. 12.7 shows right unilateral posteroanterior glide being performed in left lateral flexion. Following accessory movements to the lumbar region, the clinician reassesses all the physical asterisks (movements or tests that have been found to reproduce the patient's symptoms) in order to establish the effect of the accessory movements on the patient's signs and symptoms. Accessory movements can then be tested for other regions suspected to be a source of, or contributing to, the patient's symptoms. Again, following accessory movements to any one region, the clinician reassesses all the asterisks. Regions that

may be examined are the sacroiliac, hip, knee, foot and ankle.

If the clinician feels that the symptoms may be difficult to reproduce, then s/he may choose to do the accessory movements in a more provocative position, which will be dependent on the aggravating active movements or provocative functional activities. Conversely, if the patient's condition is severe and irritable, the clinician may choose a non-provocative position for the accessory movements, or may choose to omit them completely from the initial examination.

Hicks et al. (2003) examined the reliability of passive movement testing, palpation and provocation tests for the identification of lumbar segmental instability and found poor kappa values for segmental passive tests (κ range 0.02–0.26) but better reliability (κ range 0.25–0.55) for passive pain provocation tests. Hidalgo et al. (2014) also found that a combination of pain provocative tests demonstrated acceptable inter-examiner reliability in identifying the main pain provocative movement pattern and the level of lumbar segment involvement.

TABLE 12.5

Accessory Movements, Choice of Application and Reassessment of the Patient's Asterisks

Accessory Movements	Choice of Application	Identify Any Effect of Accessory Movements on Patient's Signs and Symptoms
Lumbar spine (L1–L5)		
Central posteroanterior Unilateral posteroanterior Transverse Unilateral anteroposterior	Start position, e.g. ■ In flexion ■ In extension ■ In lateral flexion ■ In flexion and lateral flexion	Reassess all asterisks
Sacrum		
Posteroanterior pressure over base, body and apex Anterior gapping test Posterior gapping test	■ In extension and lateral flexion Speed of force application Direction of the applied force Point of application of applied force	
Coccyx		
Posteroanterior		
?Sacroiliac joint	As above	Reassess all asterisks
?Hip	As above	Reassess all asterisks
?Knee	As above	Reassess all asterisks
?Foot and ankle	As above	Reassess all asterisks

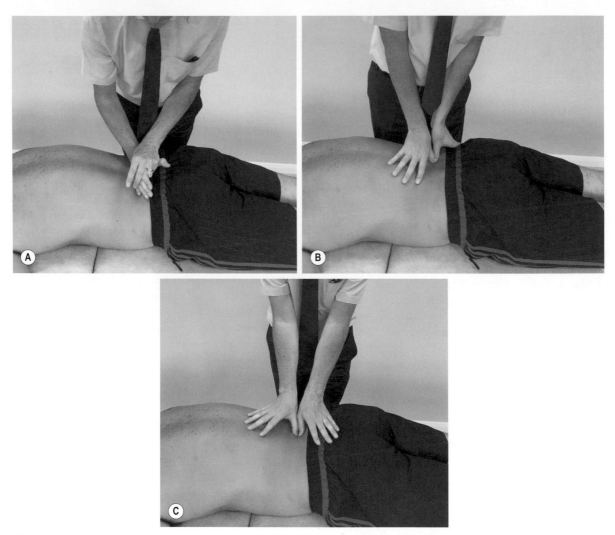

FIG. 12.6 ■ Lumbar spine accessory movements. (A) Central posteroanterior. The pisiform grip is used to apply a posteroanterior pressure on the spinous process. (B) Unilateral posteroanterior. Thumb pressure is applied to the transverse process. (C) Transverse. Thumb pressure is applied to the lateral aspect of the spinous process.

COMPLETION OF THE EXAMINATION

This completes the examination of the lumbar spine. The subjective and physical examinations produce a large amount of information which needs to be recorded accurately and quickly. It is important, however, that the clinician does not examine in a rigid manner, simply following the suggested sequence outlined in the chart. Each patient presents differently and this needs to be reflected in the examination process. The therapist needs to be flexible in approach depending on how the patient presents. It is vital at this stage to highlight important findings from the examination with an asterisk (*). These findings must be reassessed at, and within, subsequent treatment sessions to evaluate the effects of treatment on the patient's condition.

On completion of the physical examination the clinician:

■ explains the findings of the physical examination to the patient. Any questions patients may have

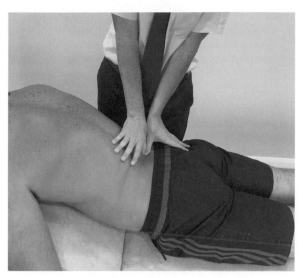

FIG. 12.7 ■ Right unilateral posteroanterior pressure in extension.

regarding their illness or injury should be addressed at this stage

- evaluates the findings, formulates a clinical diagnosis and writes up a problem list
- in conjunction with the patient, determines the objectives of treatment, including clear, timed goals
- warns the patient of possible exacerbation up to 24–48 hours following the examination
- requests the patient to report details on the behaviour of the symptoms following examination at the next attendance.

For guidance on treatment and management principles, the reader is directed to the companion textbook (Petty & Barnard 2017).

REFERENCES

Adams, M.A., et al., 2000. Mechanical initiation of intervertebral disc degeneration. Spine 25, 1625–1636.

Andersson, G.B.J., et al., 1977. Intradiskal pressure, intra-abdominal pressure and myoelectric back muscle activity related to posture and loading. Clin. Orthop. Relat. Res. 129, 156–164.

Brinjikji, W., et al., 2015. Systematic literature review of imaging features of spinal degeneration in asymptomatic populations. AJNR Am. J. Neuroradiol. 36, 811–816.

Carlsson, H., Rasmussen-Barr, E., 2013. Clinical screening tests for assessing movement control in non-specific low-back pain. A systematic review of intra- and inter-observer reliability studies. Man. Ther. 18, 103–110.

Claus, A., et al., 2008. Sitting versus standing: does intradiscal pressure cause disc degeneration or low back pain? J. Electromyogr. Kinesiol. 18, 550–558.

Clinical Standards Advisory Report, 1994. Report of a CSAG committee on back pain. HMSO, London.

Cole, J.H., et al., 1988. Muscles in action, an approach to manual muscle testing. Churchill Livingstone, Edinburgh.

Dankaerts, W., et al., 2006. Altered patterns of superficial trunk muscle activation during sitting in non-specific chronic low back pain patients: importance of subclassification. Spine 31, 2017–2023.

Edwards, B.C., 1994. Combined movements in the lumbar spine: their use in examination and treatment. In: Boyling, J.D., Palastanga, N. (Eds.), Grieve's modern manual therapy, second ed. Churchill Livingstone, Edinburgh, p. 745.

Edwards, B.C., 1999. Manual of combined movements: their use in the examination and treatment of mechanical vertebral column disorders, second ed. Butterworth-Heinemann, Oxford.

Genevay, S., Atlas, S., 2010. Lumbar spinal stenosis. Best Pract. Res. Clin. Rheumatol. 24, 253–265.

Gitelman, A., et al., 2008. Cauda equina syndrome: a comprehensive review. Am. J. Orthop. 37, 556–562.

Grieve, G.P., 1981. Common vertebral joint problems. Churchill Livingstone, Edinburgh.

Grieve, G.P., 1991. Mobilisation of the spine, fifth ed. Churchill Livingstone, Edinburgh.

Grieve, G.P., 1994. The masqueraders. In: Boyling, J.D., Palastanga, N. (Eds.), Grieve's modern manual therapy, second ed. Churchill Livingstone, Edinburgh, p. 745.

Harding, I., et al., 2004. Is the symptom of night pain important in the diagnosis of serious spinal pathology in a back pain triage clinic? Spine J. 4, S30.

Harris, C., et al., 2012. Differentiating inflammatory and mechanical back pain: challenge your decision making. National Association of Ankylosing Spondylitis. Abbott, London.

Hefford, C., 2008. McKenzie classification of mechanical spinal pain: profile of syndromes and directions of preference. Man. Ther. 13, 75–81.

Henschke, N., et al., 2009. Prevalence of and screening for serious spinal pathology in patients presenting to primary care settings with acute low back pain. Arthritis Rheumatol. 60, 3072–3080.

Henschke, N., et al., 2013. Red flags to screen for malignancy in patients with low-back pain. Cochrane Database Syst. Rev. (2), CD008686.

Hicks, G.E., et al., 2003. Interrater reliability of clinical examination measures for identification of lumbar segmental instability. Arch. Phys. Med. Rehabil. 8412, 1858–1864.

Hidalgo, B., et al., 2014. Intertester agreement and validity of identifying lumbar pain provocative movement patterns using active and passive accessory movement tests. J. Manipulative Physiol. Ther. 37, 105–115.

Hides, J.A., et al., 1994. Evidence of lumbar multifidus muscle wasting ipsilateral to symptoms in patients with acute/subacute low back pain. Spine 19, 165–172.

Hides, J., et al., 2008. Multifidus size and symmetry among chronic LBP and healthy asymptomatic subjects. Man. Ther. 13, 43–49.

Hill, J.C., et al., 2008. A primary care back pain screening tool: identifying patient subgroups for initial treatment. Arthritis Rheumatol. 59, 632–641.

Hislop, H., Montgomery, J., 1995. Daniels and Worthingham's muscle testing, techniques of manual examination, seventh ed. W.B. Saunders, Philadelphia.

Hodges, P., 2015. The role of motor control training. In: Jull, G., et al. (Eds.), Grieve's modern musculoskeletal physiotherapy, fourth ed. Elsevier, Edinburgh.

Hodges, P.W., Richardson, C.A., 1999. Altered trunk muscle recruitment in people with low back pain with upper limb movement at different speeds. Arch. Phys. Med. Rehabil. 80, 1005–1012.

Hutton, W.C., et al., 1999. Altered trunk muscle recruitment in people with low back pain with upper limb movement at different speeds. Aviat. Space Environ. Med. 74, 73–78.

Janda, V., 1994. Muscles and motor control in cervicogenic disorders: assessment and management. In: Grant, R. (Ed.), Physical therapy of the cervical and thoracic spine, second ed. Churchill Livingstone, Edinburgh, p. 195.

Jones, M.A., Rivett, D.A., 2004. Clinical reasoning for manual therapists. Butterworth-Heinemann, Edinburgh.

Jull, G.A., 1986. Examination of the lumbar spine. In: Grieve, G.P. (Ed.), Modern manual therapy of the vertebral column. Churchill Livingstone, Edinburgh, p. 547.

Kazarian, L.E., 1975. Creep characteristics of the human spinal column. Orthop. Clin. North. Am. 6, 3–18.

Kendall, F.P., et al., 2010. Muscles testing and function, 5th ed. Lippincott Williams and Wilkins, Baltimore.

Kirkaldy-Willis, W.H., Farfan, H.F., 1982. Instability of the lumbar spine. Clin. Orthop. Relat. Res. 165, 110–123.

Lavy, C., et al., 2009. Cauda equina syndrome. Br. Med. J. 338, 881–884.

Long, A., et al., 2004. Does it matter which exercise? A randomized controlled trial of exercise for low back pain. Spine 29, 2593–2602.

Luomajoki, H., et al., 2007. Reliability of movement control tests in the lumbar spine. BMC Musculoskelet. Disord. 8, 90.

Magee, D.J., 2014. Orthopedic physical assessment, 6th ed. Saunders Elsevier, Philadephia.

Maitland, G.D., et al., 2005. Maitland's vertebral manipulation, 7th ed. Butterworth-Heinemann, Edinburgh.

Majlesi, J., et al., 2008. The sensitivity and specificity of the Slump and the straight leg raising tests in patients with lumbar disc herniation. J. Clin. Rheumatol. 14, 87–91.

McKenzie, R.A., May, S.J., 2003. The lumbar spine: mechanical diagnosis and therapy. Spinal Publications New Zealand, Waikanae, New Zealand.

Mercer, C., et al., 2006. Clinical guidelines for the physiotherapy management of persistent low back pain. Chartered Society of Physiotherapy, London.

Nachemson, A., 1992. Lumbar mechanics as revealed by lumbar intradiscal pressure measurements. In: Jayson, M.I.V. (Ed.), The lumbar spine and back pain, fourth ed. Churchill Livingstone, Edinburgh, p. 157.

National Institute for Health and Clinical Excellence 2009 Guidelines for the early management of persistent non specific low back pain. Available online at: www.nice.org.wk/CG88.

O'Sullivan, P., 2006. Classification of lumbopelvic disorders – why is it essential for management? Man. Ther. 11, 169–170.

O'Sullivan, P., et al., 2002. The effect of different standing and sitting postures on trunk muscle activity in a pain-free population. Spine 27, 1238–1244.

O'Sullivan, P., et al., 2015. Multidimensional approach for the targeted management of low back pain. In: Jull, G., et al. (Eds.), 2015 Grieve's modern musculoskeletal physiotherapy, fourth ed. Elsevier, Edinburgh.

Petty, N.J., Barnard, K., 2017. Principles of musculoskeletal treatment and management: a handbook for therapists, third ed. Churchill Livingstone, Edinburgh.

Pope, M.H., Hansson, T.H., 1992. Vibration of the spine and low back pain. Clin. Orthop. Relat. Res. 279, 49–59.

Richardson, C., et al., 2004. Therapeutic exercise for lumbopelvic stabilization. A motor control approach for the treatment and prevention of low back pain, second ed. Churchill Livingstone, Edinburgh.

Royal College of Radiologists, 2007. Making the best use of a department of clinical radiology. Guidelines for doctors, sixth ed. Royal College of Radiologists, London.

Van Tulder, M., et al. 2005 Back Pain Europe: European Guidelines on the management of persistent low back pain. Available online at: http://www.backpaineurope.org.

Vleeming, A., et al., 1990a. Relation between form and function in the sacroiliac joint. Part 1. Clinical anatomical aspects. Spine 15, 130–132.

Vleeming, A., et al., 1990b. Relation between form and function in the sacroiliac joint. Part II. Biomechanical aspects. Spine 15, 133–136.

Walton, J.H., 1989. Essentials of neurology, sixth ed. Churchill Livingstone, Edinurgh.

White, A.A., Panjabi, M.M., 1990. Clinical biomechanics of the spine, second ed. J.B. Lippincott, Philadelphia.

Williams, C.M., et al., 2013. Red flags to screen for vertebral fracture in patients presenting with low-back pain. Cochrane Database Syst. Rev. (1), CD008643.

13

EXAMINATION OF THE PELVIS

BILL TAYLOR ■ HOWARD TURNER

CHAPTER CONTENTS

INTRODUCTION TO THE PELVIC REGION

The pelvic region is a complex region closely connected to the lumbar spine. As well as assessing the pelvis as a source of symptoms, consideration can be given to the role the pelvis may play in relation to symptoms elsewhere. It is mechanically linked to the lumbar spine and there is some evidence of neuromuscular interactions. It is important to differentiate pelvic girdle pain and dysfunction from low-back pain and dysfunction in order to be as accurate and effective with treatment as possible.

To assess the pelvic girdle it is essential to have a full knowledge of the anatomy and an understanding of its main functions, which include movement, stability, urination and defecation and sexual function.

The pelvic girdle consists of two innominate bones and one sacrum. There are three joints, two joints posteriorly between the ilial portion of the innominate and the sacrum forming the sacroiliac joints (SIJ) and the one anteriorly between the pubic bone portions of the innominates forming the symphysis pubis (Fig. 13.1).

The main ligaments of the SIJ are the ventral SIJ ligaments, interosseous ligaments, long dorsal SIJ ligament, sacrotuberous, sacrospinous and iliolumbar ligament, as shown in Fig. 13.2.

The nerve supply of the SIJ has been reported as being inconsistent and various authors report contributions from ventral rami of L5 to S4. This widespread pattern of innervation may well be the reason for such wide variations in the clinical pain patterns reported by patients with SIJ pain (Lee 2010).

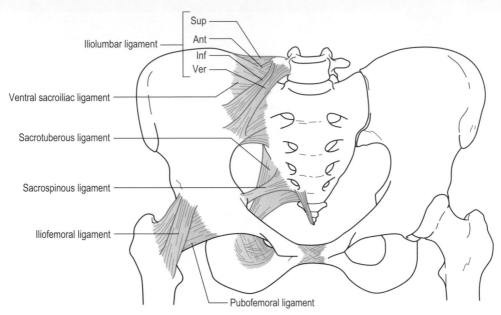

FIG. 13.1 ■ The ligaments of the pelvic girdle viewed from the anterior aspect. *Ant*, anterior; *Inf*, inferior; *Sup*, superior; *Ver*, vertical. *(From Lee 2010, with permission.)*

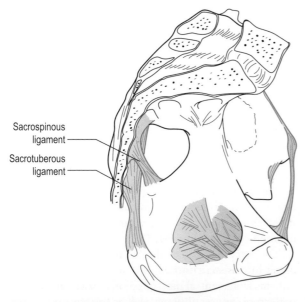

FIG. 13.2 ■ Sagittal section of the pelvic girdle illustrating the anchoring effects on the sacral base. *(From Lee 2010, with permission.)*

The anterior joint, the symphysis pubis, consists of a fibrocartilaginous disc, with hyaline cartilage covering the osseous surfaces.

The supporting ligaments include superior, anterior and posterior ligaments and the inferior arcuate ligament (Fig. 13.3). The pubic symphysis is supplied by the pudendal (S2–S3–S4) and/or genitofemoral nerve (L1–L2) and/or ilioinguinal/iliohypogastric nerves (L1–L2).

The SIJs and symphysis pubis are subject to large forces and are required to meet the contradictory demands of mobility and stability.

Certain aspects of the structure of the SIJ optimize its capacity to resist shear: its surfaces have a higher friction coefficient than other joints in the body, the sacrum is wedge-shaped in a way that means body weight produces some joint compression and the joint surfaces have interlocking ridges and grooves and a twisted, propeller-type shape after the second decade that helps stabilize the joint. These structural components have been characterized as elements of form

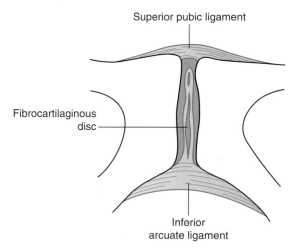

Superior pubic ligament

Fibrocartilaginous disc

Inferior arcuate ligament

FIG. 13.3 ■ A coronal section through the pubic symphysis. *(From Lee 2010, with permission.)*

closure (Vleeming et al. 1997). It is evident, however, that form closure of the SIJ is not adequate to control independently the forces to which the joint is subjected: additional joint compression is required. This has been termed force closure.

Force closure of the SIJ arises from the activity of muscle contraction and from tension in the ligamentous support system. When a combination of sacral nutation (anterior sacral rotation in the sagittal plane) and innominate posterior rotation occurs, the ligaments are tensioned maximally and the joint surfaces are drawn together and compressed. When the opposite combination occurs the ligaments are mostly de-tensioned and the joint decompressed.

Muscle contraction supports stability by either directly or indirectly producing joint compression. Muscles that cross the joint, for example, gluteus maximus, piriformis and the transverse and oblique abdominals, are able to compress the joint directly.

The diagnosis and classification of pelvic pain are controversial and attempts have been made to classify pelvic girdle pain disorders following a mechanism-based paradigm within a biopsychosocial framework (O'Sullivan & Beales 2007a). This classification system acknowledges the often complex and multifactorial nature of pelvic dysfunction which can be associated with reduced or increased force closure of the pelvic girdle, the effect this may have on pain-sensitive pelvic

structures and the interaction of passive coping strategies, faulty belief systems and anxiety and depression. O'Sullivan and Beales (2007b) hypothesize that a motor control system can become dysfunctional in response to pain or may itself produce pain due to abnormal tissue strain. This can result in ongoing peripheral pain sensitization.

When patients present to physiotherapy it is usually because they find they are functionally limited due to pain or stiffness in one or more of their everyday activities. The level of limitation can range from being immobilized and unable to walk, to a reduced ability to work or play sport.

Examination of the pelvic region is not performed in isolation and will always include an assessment of the lumbar spine (see Chapter 12). If the patient complains of any symptoms suggestive of hip in origin a modified assessment of the hip may well be required (see Chapter 14). It is not unusual for there to be concomitant symptoms in the hip and the SIJ, which will need to be assessed and treated independently. The frequency of isolated SIJ pain, reported to be as high as 15% in people with chronic low back and pelvic pain below L5/S1 (Dreyfuss et al. 2004), makes it important to develop skills in the assessment and differential diagnosis of this region.

During pregnancy the point prevalence of pelvic girdle pain – pain between the posterior iliac crest and the gluteal fold – is around 20%, but estimates of incidence range up to 76% (Vleeming 2008). Estimates of postpartum pelvic girdle pain range from 1% to 43% depending on definition (Elden et al. 2016). No study has evaluated prevalence using validated test procedures.

SUBJECTIVE EXAMINATION

When you begin interviewing patients it is often useful to follow a specific order of subjective questioning and the physical tests, as described below. Once you become more proficient with your interview technique the order can become more fluid and personalized to the patient being examined.

Further details of the questions asked during the subjective examination and the tests carried out in the physical examination can be found in Chapters 2 and 3, respectively.

Patients' Perspective on Their Experience

Social and family history relevant to the onset and progression of the patient's condition can be useful in the management of ongoing pelvic pain. This includes the patient's perspectives, experience and expectations, age, employment, home situation and details of any leisure activities. This information may indicate mechanical influences on the pelvis. In order to treat the patient appropriately, it is important that the condition is managed within the context of the patient's social and work environment.

There are a number of patients whose pain may persist beyond the expected point of tissue healing. These patients will require a different approach to a traditional assessment. The following questions may be helpful in evaluating the psychosocial risk factors, or 'yellow flags' for poor treatment outcome (Waddell & Burton 2004):

- Have you had time off work in the past with back pain?
- What do you understand to be the cause of your back pain?
- What are you expecting will help you?
- How is your employer/coworkers/family responding to your back pain?
- What are you doing to cope with your back pain?
- Do you think you will return to work? When?

Although these questions are suggested for patients with low-back pain (Waddell & Burton 2004), they may also be relevant to patients with pelvic pain.

Body Chart

The information gathered concerning the type and area of current symptoms can be recorded on a body chart (see Fig. 2.3).

Area of Current Symptoms

Be exact when mapping out the area of the symptoms. Guided SIJ anaesthetic injection studies show that pain from the SIJ presents very similarly to pain referred into the lower limb from the lumbar spine – it can refer to the buttock, the groin, the anterior and posterior thigh and into the calf and foot (Schwarzer et al. 1995; Dreyfuss et al. 1996; van der Wurff et al. 2006; Visser et al. 2013). Pain over the posterior superior iliac spine (PSIS) and sacral sulcus is the most common area of symptoms – 80–100% of patients who respond to SIJ injection had pain over their PSIS – but pain in that location is not diagnostic of SIJ-mediated pain (Dreyfuss et al. 1996; van der Wurff et al. 2006).

Extraarticular sources of pain, e.g. the dorsal sacroiliac, or long dorsal, ligament, for example, are relatively common sources of postpartum pelvic pain (Vleeming et al. 2002) and chronic pelvic pain (Dreyfuss et al. 1996; Fortin et al. 1999).

Ischial pain can be referred from the pelvic floor (Pastore & Katzman 2012). Pain is often unilateral with mechanical SIJ problems, though it is classically bilateral in ankylosing spondylitis. Referral into the lower leg and foot is uncommon but can be present (Schwarzer et al. 1995; Dreyfuss et al. 1996; Visser et al. 2013).

Areas Relevant to the Region Being Examined

All other relevant areas are checked for symptoms. It is important to ask about pain or even stiffness, as this may be relevant to the patient's main symptom. This could include the foot, knee, hip, lumbar spine and the pelvic floor.

Mark unaffected areas with ticks (✓) on the body chart.

Quality of Symptoms

Establishing the quality of the pain can be helpful in trying to identify which structure may be at fault, as different structures can produce their own specific type of pain. This is described in further detail in Chapter 2. It is important to assess the severity, irritability and nature of the patient's pain.

Intensity of Pain

The intensity of pain and pain patterns can be assessed using numerical or visual analogue scales and a pain diary, as shown in Chapter 2.

Abnormal Sensation

Check for any altered sensation over the lumbar spine and SIJ, hip and upper thigh. Common abnormalities are paraesthesia, numbness and weakness.

These symptoms need to be mapped out on the body chart.

Constant or Intermittent Symptoms

Ascertain the frequency of the symptoms, whether they are constant or intermittent. Constant pain means that it is present every minute the patient is awake and the patient is never free from pain. If symptoms are constant, check whether there is any variation in the intensity of the symptoms, as constant unremitting pain may be indicative of a sinister pathology.

Relationship of Symptoms

If there is more than one area of symptoms, determine the relationship between the symptomatic areas. Does the pelvic pain occur first and then the referred pain or do they always happen together? For example, the patient could have buttock pain without SIJ pain, or the pains may always be present together. It is possible that there may be two separate sources of symptoms.

Behaviour of Symptoms

Aggravating Factors

For each symptomatic area a series of questions may be asked:

- Are the symptoms constant or intermittent?
- What makes or brings on the patient's symptoms?
- How long does it take before symptoms are aggravated?
- If there is a primary and a secondary symptom, what happens when the primary symptom is produced or made worse?
- How long does it take for symptoms to settle once they are aggravated?
- Is the patient able to maintain this position or movement?
- How do the symptoms affect function? For example, sitting, standing, lying, bending, walking, running, walking on uneven ground and up and down stairs, washing, driving, lifting and digging, work, sport and social activities.

The clinician may ask the patient about functional activities for structures that could be a source of symptoms. However, this questioning does not provide conclusive evidence as functional movements invariably stress other parts of the body, and the activities listed below will also stress the lumbar spine and hips.

Commonly cited aggravating factors for the SIJ are standing on one leg, turning over in bed, getting in or out of bed, sloppy standing with uneven weight distribution through the legs, habitual work stance, stepping up on the affected side and walking (Huijbregts 2004). Injection studies do not demonstrate any particular aggravating or easing factors that are specific to SIJ pain and/or studies using pain provocation test procedures show that these aggravating activities are just as commonly associated with the lumbar spine (Young et al. 2003; Dreyfuss et al. 2004; Visser et al. 2013). For aggravating factors for other regions, which may need to be asked if they are suspected to be a source of the symptoms, see Table 2.2.

Easing Factors

For each symptomatic area a series of questions can be asked to help determine what eases the symptoms:

- What movements and/or positions ease the patient's symptoms?
- How long does it take before symptoms are eased? If symptoms are constant but variable it is important to know what the baseline is and how long it takes for the symptoms to reduce to that level.
- What happens to other symptoms when this symptom is eased?
- What else can you do to ease symptoms?

Analysis of the aggravating and easing factors helps determine the irritability of the presenting condition.

Although no particular aggravating or easing factors have been found to be associated with the proven presence of SIJ pain (Young 2003; Dreyfuss et al. 2004; Visser et al. 2013), the therapist might postulate on activities and interventions that make a difference to SIJ compression. In some people compression of the pelvis makes their symptoms better and in others it makes symptoms worse. The most direct way to apply compression is to wear an SIJ compression belt, and some patients will intuitively replicate its effect by wearing their normal belt lower.

The clinician can ask the patient about theoretically known easing factors for structures that could be a source of the symptoms. For example, symptoms from the SIJ may be eased by crook-lying, sitting with the pelvis posteriorly tilted, stooping forwards in standing.

The effect of pelvic compression and/or applying a sacroiliac stabilization belt might suggest a degree of functional instability, e.g. in pregnant women (Ostgaard et al. 1994) or athletic or groin pain patients (Mens et al. 2006) testing compression forces on the pelvis can be further explored in the physical examination.

Analysis of these factors will help to determine the potential areas at fault and identify functional restrictions and also the relationship between symptoms. The severity can be determined by the intensity of the symptoms and whether the symptoms are interfering with normal activities of daily living, such as work and sleep. This information can be used to determine the direction of the physical examination as well as the aims of treatment and any advice that may be required. The most relevant subjective information should be highlighted with an asterisk (*), explored in the physical examination and reassessed at subsequent treatment sessions to evaluate treatment intervention.

Twenty-Four-Hour Behaviour of Symptoms

The clinician determines the 24-hour behaviour of symptoms by asking questions about night, morning and evening symptoms.

Night Symptoms. Although severe night pain is a recognized red flag, it should be noted that night symptoms are common in back pain (Harding et al. 2004). It is necessary to establish whether the patient is being woken and kept awake by the symptoms. Patients complaining of needing to sleep upright or get up should raise some concern.

The following questions may be asked:

- Do you have any difficulty getting to sleep (particularly related to your pain)?
- Do your symptoms wake you at night? Which symptoms?
- How many times in a night?
- How many times in the past week?
- What do you have to do to get back to sleep?
- If sleep is an issue, further questioning may be useful to determine management, e.g. positioning, advice regarding medication, hot/cold application.

SIJ patients often report turning in bed as being painful and difficult to perform. They have trouble initiating the turning movement. This may be made easier if the therapist applies a compressive load across the pelvic girdle compressing the SIJs bilaterally, indicating an issue with force closure through the pelvic girdle (Van der Wurff et al. 2000a, b).

Morning and Evening Symptoms. The clinician determines the pattern of the symptoms first thing in the morning, through the day and at the end of the day. Stiffness on rising lasting >1 hour is often a sign of arthropathy (Yazici et al. 2004). In ankylosing spondylitis, the cardinal and often earliest sign is erosion of the SIJs, which is often manifested by pain and stiffness around the SIJ and lumbar spine for the first few hours in the morning (Solomon et al. 2010). Stiffness lasting only 30 minutes or less is more likely to be mechanical in nature (Suresh 2004).

Stage of the Condition

In order to determine whether the condition is in the acute inflammatory stage or subacute stage it is necessary to assess whether there is an inflammatory component of the presentation. This is often indicated by constant pain, which can be aggravated by mechanical stress but is difficult to ease.

Special Questions

Special questions must always be asked, as they may identify certain precautions or contraindications to the physical examination and/or treatment, as mentioned in Chapter 2. The clinician must screen for any features of the patient's presentation that suggest a non-musculoskeletal origin, for example, visceral or systemic conditions (Goodman & Snyder 2013).

General Health

Ascertain the general health of the patient – find out if the patient is suffering from any malaise, fatigue, fever, nausea or vomiting, stress, anxiety or depression.

Obstetric History

Due to an increased incidence of pelvic pain in women postpartum, a full obstetric history should be taken. Is the patient pregnant? How many children has she given birth to? When was she last pregnant? Has she had caesarean sections? Did she suffer trauma to her pelvic floor during delivery through instrumental deliveries with forceps and ventouse? Did she have episiotomies and/or tears?

It is common for low-back and pelvic pain to be associated with pregnancy, although the underlying mechanism remains unclear. A number of factors have been proposed and have included an increase in the load on the lumbar spine because of weight gain, hormonal changes causing hypermobility of the SIJ and pubic symphysis (Hagen 1974) and an increase in the abdominal sagittal diameter (Ostgaard et al. 1993). Little evidence supports the hypothesis that the pain is related to alteration in posture (Bullock et al. 1987; Ostgaard et al. 1993).

If the patient is pregnant, she may develop associated symptoms as early as week 18 (Bullock et al. 1987). There are presently no studies showing a causal relationship between relaxin and reduced stability in the pelvic girdle. Indeed, studies have shown there is no relationship between relaxin and pelvic girdle pain (Petersen et al. 1994; Hansen 1996). Relaxin is not detectable after 3 months postpregnancy and unlikely to be the cause of symptoms (Sapsford et al. 1999).

Neurological Symptoms

Symptoms of cauda equina compression (i.e. compression below L1) include saddle anaesthesia/paraesthesia, sexual or erectile dysfunction, loss of vaginal sensation, bladder and/or bowel sphincter disturbance (loss of control, retention, hesitancy, urgency or a sense of incomplete evacuation) (Lavy et al. 2009). These symptoms may be due to interference of S3 and S4 (Jull et al. 2015). Prompt referral for a surgical opinion is required to prevent permanent sphincter paralysis (Lavy et al. 2009).

Has the patient experienced symptoms of spinal cord compression, such as bilateral tingling in hands or feet and/or disturbance of gait? Are there motor and sensory tone changes in all four limbs? Does the patient report coordination changes, including gait disturbance?

History of the Present Condition

The main information to be gathered during this part of the exam is the history of the presenting condition, especially the mode of onset. Was it sudden or did it come on gradually? Was there a history of trauma? It is commonly assumed that there is often a traumatic

event causing SIJ pain; however, only 40% of patients have been found to relate a traumatic incident to the onset of symptoms (Dreyfuss et al. 1996; Visser et al. 2013).

For each symptomatic area, the clinician needs to know how long the symptom has been present, whether there was a sudden or insidious onset and whether there was a specific incident that caused the onset of the symptom, such as a fall or another trauma. If the onset was slow, the clinician finds out if there has been any change in the patient's lifestyle, e.g. a new job or hobby or a change in sporting activity.

Past Medical History

The following information is obtained from the patient and/or the medical notes:

- Relevant medical history: pelvic inflammatory disease or fractures of the lower limbs. Visceral structures are capable of masquerading as musculoskeletal conditions; for example, the pelvic organs, including testes, ovaries and uterus, can refer to the sacral region. Any relevant history related to these organs is important to help differentiate the cause of symptoms.
- The history of any previous episodes: How many? When were they? What was the cause? What was the duration of each episode? Did the patient fully recover between episodes? Does the patient perceive the current condition to be better, the same or worse in relation to previous episodes s/he may have experienced? Has the patient had any episodes of stiffness in the lumbar spine, thoracic spine or any other relevant region? Check for a history of trauma or recurrent minor trauma.
- Ascertain the results of any past treatment for the same or a similar problem. Past treatment records may be obtained for further information.

Radiography and Medical Imaging

Routine spinal radiographs are not considered necessary prior to conservative treatment as they only identify the normal age-related degenerative changes, which do not necessarily correlate with the symptoms experienced by the patient (Clinical Standards Advisory Report 1994). Bone single-photon emission computed tomography (SPECT) imaging has been shown to be useful in diagnosing sacroiliitis in patients with even mild SIJ joint changes (Yong-il Kim et al. 2015).

Radiographs may be indicated in the younger patient (under 20 years) with conditions such as spondylolisthesis or ankylosing spondylitis and in the older patient (over 55 years), where they have not responded to conservative treatment (Royal College of Radiologists 2007). In cases of suspected ankylosing spondylitis, radiographs of the SIJs may not show significant changes until the patient has had ankylosing spondylitis for 6–9 years. In cases where there is a suspected fracture due to trauma or osteoporosis radiographs are indicated in the first instance. Other medical tests may include blood tests, magnetic resonance imaging, myelography, discography or a bone scan.

Plan of the Physical Examination

When all this information has been collected, the subjective examination is complete. It is useful at this stage to highlight with asterisks, for ease of reference, important findings and particularly one or more functional restrictions. These can then be reexamined at subsequent treatment sessions to evaluate treatment intervention.

In order to plan the physical examination, the following hypotheses need to be developed from the subjective examination:

- Are there any precautions and/or contraindications to elements of the physical examination, such as neurological involvement, recent fracture, trauma, steroid therapy or active rheumatoid arthritis? Absolute contraindications to further examination and treatment include symptoms of spinal cord or cauda equina syndrome.
- The regions and structures that need to be examined as a possible cause of the symptoms, e.g. SIJ, pubic symphysis, lumbar spine, thoracic spine, hip, knee, ankle and foot, muscles and nerves. Often it is not possible to examine fully at the first attendance and so examination of the structures must be prioritized and assessed at subsequent treatment sessions.
- How should the physical tests be carried out? Will it be difficult to reproduce each symptom?

Will it be necessary to use combined movements or repetitive movements to reproduce the patient's symptoms? Are symptoms severe and/or irritable? With severe symptoms, physical tests may be carried out to just before or at the point of symptom reproduction; no overpressures will be carried out. If symptoms are non-severe, physical tests may be carried out to reproduce symptoms fully and may include overpressures. If symptoms are irritable, physical tests may be carried out to just before or at the point of symptom provocation, with fewer physical tests being examined to allow for a rest period between tests. If symptoms are non-irritable physical tests may be carried out to reproduce symptoms fully and may include overpressures.

A physical planning sheet can be useful for clinicians to help guide them through the clinical reasoning process (see Fig. 2.9).

PHYSICAL EXAMINATION

The information from the subjective examination helps the clinician to plan an appropriate physical examination. The severity, irritability and nature of the condition are the major factors that will influence the choice and priority of physical testing procedures. It is necessary to determine whether the patient has a musculoskeletal dysfunction that is suitable for physical treatment. The nature of the patient's condition will have a large impact on the extent of the physical examination. If the patient's symptoms are severe and/or irritable, the aim of the assessment is to explore movements as much as possible, within a symptom-free range. If the patient has constant and severe and/or irritable symptoms, then the clinician aims to find physical tests that ease the symptoms. If the patient's symptoms are non-severe and non-irritable, then the clinician aims to find physical tests that reproduce each of the patient's symptoms.

As previously stated, each significant physical test that either provokes or eases the patient's symptoms is highlighted in the patient's notes by an asterisk.

The order and detail of the physical tests described below will vary according to each individual. Some tests will be irrelevant, some tests will be carried out briefly, while others will need to be fully investigated. The assessment techniques described are not an exhaustive list of available assessment procedures but have been chosen as they show some degree of reliability and validity. While it would always be the first choice to choose a valid and reliable assessment tool it may be necessary to modify a test depending on the relative physical match of the therapist and patient.

Observation

Informal Observation

This should begin as soon as the clinician meets the patient for the first time. It can often be advantageous to greet the patient in the waiting room. Has the patient chosen to sit or remained standing? A general idea of global function can be made while the patient is sitting or standing. Does the patient have difficulty moving from sitting to standing? Does the patient have an efficient gait pattern? The clinician should be alert to the patient's demeanour, facial expressions and verbal interaction as these may all give valuable information regarding the severity and irritability of the condition.

Formal Observation

The clinician observes the patient's spinal, pelvic and lower-limb posture in standing, from anterior, lateral and posterior views. The presence of any deformity of the spine is noted, e.g. scoliosis, lateral shift. Any asymmetry in levels at the pelvis, particularly of the iliac crests, the posterior and anterior superior iliac spine (ASIS), is noted. For example, the level of the greater trochanters compared with the level of the iliac crests can be examined in standing, to estimate any leg length discrepancy and whether it is accommodated for or accentuated by asymmetrical hemipelvis size. The iliac crest heights can then be assessed in sitting to see if there is any reason to explore correcting sitting asymmetry as well as, or instead of, leg length asymmetry.

Any anomalies should be noted and referred to later in the assessment of mobility.

Observation should also include assessment of the muscle bulk, tone and symmetry. The patient's handedness or physical activity must be taken into account. Findings may lead the clinician to investigate muscle length and strength in the physical examination. Skin colour, areas of redness, swelling or sweating should be noted, as these may indicate areas of local pathology, or possibly a systemic or dermatological condition.

Functional Testing

Some functional ability has already been tested by the general observation of the patient during the initial meeting and subjective and physical examinations, e.g. the postures adopted during the subjective examination and the ease or difficulty of undressing prior to the examination. Any further functional testing can be carried out at this point in the examination and may include gait analysis and functional activities such as turning over on the examination plinth, sitting to standing, lifting or sport-specific activities. Functional assessment will give the therapist a good idea of whether the patient is willing to move and may help to highlight problems such as hypervigilance and fear avoidance. The Pelvic Girdle Questionnaire is a pelvic-specific assessment tool which can be useful in assessing symptoms and dysfunction in the pelvic girdle (Stuge et al. 2011).

Active Physiological Movements

There are no isolated active physiological movements at the SIJ since the pelvic girdle moves with the lumbar spine. Between the iliac articular surfaces the sacrum nutates (anteriorly rotates) and counternutates (posteriorly rotates) (Kapandji 2008). These sacral movements occur conjunctly with movement of the spine and hip joints. The ilia move, as bones in space, on top of the bilateral femoral heads, anteriorly rotating in flexion and posteriorly in extension. SIJ movements are therefore tested indirectly or conjoined with the active physiological movements of the lumbar spine and hip joints, while the SIJ is palpated by the clinician (Kapandji 2008).

Standing Hip Flexion Test (Gillet Test) (Fig. 13.4) (Greenman 1996)

The standing hip flexion test examines the ability of the low back, pelvis and hip to transfer load unilaterally, the hip to flex, the lumbar spine to rotate and the pelvis to allow intrapelvic torsion. The innominate is palpated with one hand while the sacrum is palpated at either the spinous process of S2 or ipsilateral inferior lateral angle. The patient stands on her left leg and flexes her right hip to 90° and there should be a palpable posterior rotation of the innominate relative to the ipsilateral sacrum. The left PSIS should remain level with S2 or S2 should drop slightly for a negative test. If the left PSIS moves superiorly relative to S2 (i.e. left anterior innominate rotation) the test is positive (Hungerford & Gilleard 2007). Note also any change in axis of the femoral head and any loss of control of either side of the pelvis (Lee 2015). The test should be repeated three times to maximize consistency. This test has been shown to have good intertester reliability (Hungerford & Gilleard 2007).

Active Straight-Leg Raise (ASLR) Test (Fig. 13.5A) (Mens et al. 2001, 2002)

The ASLR has been validated as a clinical test for assessing load transfer between the trunk and the lower extremity in patients with peripartum pelvic girdle pain. In supine, the patient is asked to lift one leg at a time to around 30° of hip flexion or 20 cm off the bed. The pain response is noted, and the patient is asked to rate the effort involved in lifting each leg. A six-point scale for each leg is advised: 0–5, where 0 is 'no effort' and 5 relates to an inability to lift the leg (Mens et al. 2001). The test should then be repeated with the therapist applying pressure medially over both ilia, or after the application of a sacroiliac stabilisation belt, and any change in the pain and perceived effort noted. Compression of the SIJ's in this way can make it easier or harder for the patient to lift the leg. This is the basis of some models of subgrouping in patients with pelvic pain (O'Sullivan & Beales 2007a; Hungerford 2014); the therapist should note the presence of any trunk rotation as the test is performed and evaluate whether this is affected by the application of pelvic compression. The therapist should also note any compensatory strategies such as breath holding, and intervention may involve relaxation of muscle activity. An optimal ASLR test means the only joint moving is the hip joint whilst the thorax, lumbar spine and pelvis remain still. During the test the clinician should observe any compensatory strategies such as breath holding.

In cases where the pelvis and trunk rotate significantly as the leg is lifted, the therapist should discriminate the effect of pelvic compression from the effect of manually reducing the amount of rotation that occurs. Compression assesses the pelvis and controlling the rotation is more likely to assess lumbar spine rotational control.

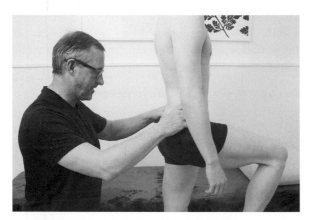

FIG. 13.4 ■ Standing hip flexion (Gillet) test.

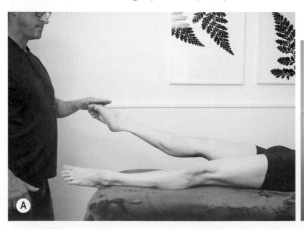
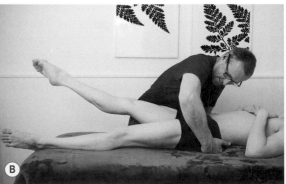

FIG. 13.5 ■ (A) Active straight-leg raise test. (B) Active straight-leg raise test with posterior compression.

When the test is positive, compression of the SIJs by applying pressure medially over both ilia can make it either easier or harder for the patient to lift the leg (Fig. 13.5B). If compression makes the leg easier to lift it is considered to be a sign of a motor control deficit of the pelvic stabilizing muscles leading to a loss of force closure. Rehabilitation, in that case, may include motor control activation strategies.

If compression makes the leg harder to lift it is considered to be a sign of excessive recruitment of the pelvic stabilizing muscles causing excessive force closure, and intervention may involve relaxation of muscle activity. The ASLR is an appropriate reassessment of those rehabilitation strategies and of manual therapy interventions.

Muscle Tests

The muscle tests may include examining muscle strength, control, length and isometric muscle testing of the muscles of the trunk and hip; readers are referred to relevant chapters for further details.

During pregnancy the rectus abdominis muscle can be stretched so far from the midline that it becomes separated from the linea alba – a condition known as diastasis recti abdominis (Boissonnault & Blaschak 1988). The inter recti distance varies along its length from the xiphoid to the pubic symphysis. What is considered abnormal may differ below as compared with above the umbilicus (Axer et al. 2001; Beer et al. 2009).

Abdominal wall assessment involves manual assessment of the inter recti distance, via digital assessment, from the xiphisternum to the symphysis pubis. Reliable measurements can also be made using ultrasound imaging (Coldron et al. 2008). These techniques are specialized (Lee 2015).

Muscle Strength

Manual muscle testing can be used to test the strength of hip adductors/abductors, flexor/extensors and internal/external rotators (see Chapter 14).

Assessment of the abdominal and pelvic floor muscles is essential to assess the core stability of the pelvic girdle and the lumbopelvic cylinder. The pelvic floor is known to work in conjunction with transversus abdominis (TrA), multifidus and the abdominals to produce effective force closure of the pelvic girdle.

Abdominal wall assessment can be performed via palpation and ultrasound imaging.

It can sometimes be difficult to palpate the TrA if there is increased tone in the muscle and fascia, as it lies beneath external and internal oblique. In order to palpate the TrA effectively the therapist must follow a strict protocol, as described by Lee (2015). The therapist palpates the abdominal wall with both thumbs 7 cm medial to and slightly inferior to each ASIS. With gentle pressure the therapist sinks her thumbs down to the fascia of external oblique, and then the fibres of the internal oblique. Next a transverse traction is applied to the TrA fascia laterally.

The TrA is known to contract with the pelvic floor. In order to assess the contraction of TrA a cue is used that initiates a pelvic floor contraction.

Cues can be specific to individual patients. Commonly used cues are:

- Slowly and gently squeeze pelvic floor muscles as if to stop urine flow.
- Slowly and gently draw your vagina/testicles up into your body.
- Imagine a line from a point on your anus to a point on your pubic bone; slowly and gently connect the points.

A normal response is a deep light tension felt in the TrA fascia and the abdomen will hollow and the thumbs will move deeper and laterally.

Abnormal responses include absent response to cues, asymmetrical response and activation of external oblique (Lee 2015).

Muscle Length

The clinician tests the length of muscles; in particular, those thought prone to shortening (Sahrmann 2002; Lee 2015). A description of muscle length tests is given in Chapter 3. Special consideration may be given to quadratus lumborum, piriformis, hip flexors and hamstrings. Muscle length tests may not be sensitive enough to identify all possible strategies that might be employed by a patient with excessive force closure. There are no validated tests available to employ in this regard but clinically simple palpation is rewarding. If the patient is relaxed, his muscles should be relaxed and feel relaxed. Palpation may reveal tightness or rigidity or tenderness which can be hypothesized as an indication of excessive recruitment. This may affect the abdominals or back muscles, the gluteals or deep hip rotators such as piriformis, obturators or quadratus femoris, the hip flexors or adductors or pelvic floor. With so many muscles having some involvement in stabilization of the area, maintenance of high levels of co-contraction can be widespread (O'Sullivan & Beales 2007a).

The Pelvic Floor

The pelvic floor is often overlooked in the assessment of the pelvic region.

Increased muscle tone and/or decreased muscle strength can play a significant role in the control and function of the pelvic girdle (Pastore et al. 2012).

Many of the pelvic floor muscles can be palpated externally and pelvic floor function can be assessed along with the abdominals and trunk muscles. Further assessment might well require internal digital examination. Due to the intimate nature of this type of examination additional specialist training and specific patient consent will be required.

Neurological Tests

The neurological integrity examination is detailed in Chapter 3.

Nerve Tissue Palpation

Several nerves in the pelvic region can be palpated:

- Genitofemoral nerve (L1–L2) passes along the inguinal ligament, parallel to the spermatic cord in the male and the round ligament in the female. Due to the sensitive nature of this nerve's location, specific consent must be sought from the patient before assessment.
- Ilioinguinal nerve (L1) can be palpated just medial to the ASIS as it emerges through the abdominals to run down the inguinal ligament. Injury of this nerve can cause pain over the inguinal ligament and testicular/labial pain (McCrory & Bell 1999; Comin et al. 2013).
- Sciatic nerve (L4–S3) can be palpated indirectly. With the patient in prone lying, palpate two-thirds of the way along an imaginary line between the greater trochanter and the ischial tuberosity. Clinically this is useful when it is suspected the

patient may have piriformis syndrome (McCrory & Bell 1999).

- Posterior femoral cutaneous nerve of the thigh (S1–S3) passes through the sciatic foramen, below the piriformis muscle and passes down the buttock and thigh medial to the sciatic nerve. It can be palpated between the heads of the hamstring muscles at the level of the ischium.
- Pudendal nerve (S2–S4) has three main branches: rectal, perineal and vaginal, and penile/clitoral. These nerves are usually palpated rectally in the male and vaginally in the female. Specific consent from the patient is required and specialist training is required before attempting to assess this area.

Pain Provocation Tests

Pain provocation tests are designed to stress the SIJ mechanically and so provoke pain and determine whether the SIJ is a source of symptoms. They have been shown to have some reliability, but validity and specificity have been questioned.

Various authors have proposed different combinations of tests (Laslett & Williams 1994; Van der Wurff et al. 2000a, b; Laslett et al. 2005; Robinson et al. 2007; Stuber 2007). Of five reliable tests, using the criteria that three or more should reproduce the patient's pain, sensitivity of 94% and specificity of 78% were achieved (Young 2003; Laslett et al. 2005; van der Wurff et al. 2006; Laslett 2008). The tests used in these studies include the distraction test, compression test, thigh thrust test or P4 test, Gaenslen's test, sacral thrust test and FABER (flexion/abduction/external rotation) test (Laslett & Williams 1994; Laslett et al. 2005; Stuber 2007).

Thigh Thrust Test/Posterior Shear Test/Posterior Pelvic Pain Provocation (P4) (Fig. 13.6) (Laslett et al. 2005)

With the patient in supine and 90 degrees flexion, the clinician applies a longitudinal cephalad force through the femur to produce an anteroposterior shear at the SIJ. Variations include the use of a hand under the sacrum to stabilize the sacrum, and stabilization of the opposite innominate via pressure on the opposite ASIS. The test is positive if it reproduces

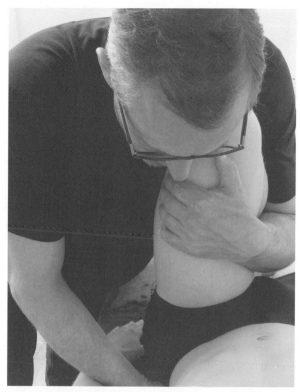

FIG. 13.6 ■ Posterior shear/thigh thrust test.

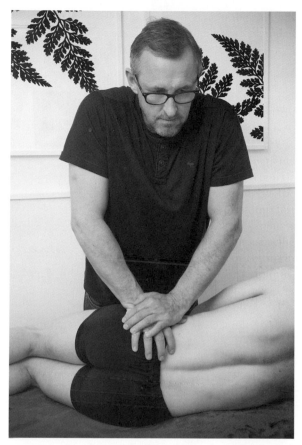

FIG. 13.7 ■ Compression test/posterior gapping.

the patient's symptoms. The test has a sensitivity of 88% (Laslett et al. 2005). The test also stresses the hip.

Compression Test/Posterior Gapping (Fig. 13.7) (Laslett et al. 2005)

With the patient in supine or side-lying, the clinician applies a force that attempts to push the left and right ASIS towards each other. The pressure must be applied to the very anterolateral edge of the ASIS. The test is positive if it reproduces the patient's symptoms. It has a specificity of 81% (Laslett et al. 2005).

Distraction/Anterior Gapping Test (Laslett & Williams 1994; Hengeveld & Banks 2005; Magee 2014)

This test assesses the right and left SIJ simultaneously.

Vertically oriented pressure is applied to the ASIS processes directed posteriorly and laterally, distracting the SIJ (Laslett & Williams 1994).

Gaenslen's/Pelvic Torsion Test (Fig. 13.8)

In supine with the patient close to the edge of the plinth, the leg nearest the edge of the bed is extended whilst the opposite hip is fully flexed and overpressure is applied. This test is repeated on the other side of the plinth with the opposite leg. The test is positive if it reproduces the patient's symptoms. This test has been shown to be the least sensitive and specific of the pain provocation tests (Laslett et al. 2005).

Sacral Thrust Test (Fig. 13.9) (Laslett & Williams 1994; Laslett et al. 2005)

This tests the right and left SIJ simultaneously. In prone, vertically directed force is applied to the midline of the sacrum at the apex of the curve of the sacrum, directed anteriorly, producing a posterior shearing force at the SIJs with the sacrum nutated.

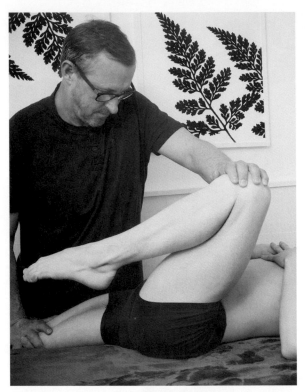

FIG. 13.8 ■ Pelvic torsion/Gaenslen's test.

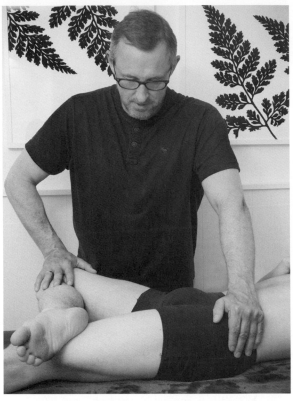

FIG. 13.10 Flexion/abduction/external rotation (FABER) test.

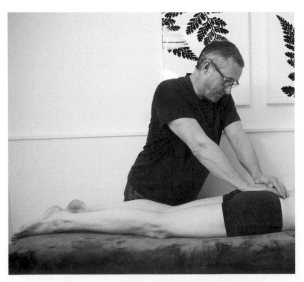

FIG. 13.9 ■ Sacral thrust technique.

FABER Test (Fig. 13.10) (van der Wurff et al. 2006)

With the patient in supine, the therapist places the patient's hip into full flexion, abduction and external rotation, whilst stabilizing the opposite pelvis via vertical pressure through the opposite ASIS.

Palpation

Assuming local tenderness is directly attributable to a particular underlying tissue can result in spurious clinical decisions. Hence, while palpation may help identify the general area, it has poor specificity. The clinician palpates over the pelvis, including the sacrum, SIJs, pubic symphysis and any other relevant areas. Palpation around the pubic symphysis can only be performed after a clear explanation and specific consent has been obtained. It is useful to record palpation findings on a body chart (see Fig. 2.3) and/or palpation chart (see Fig. 3.35).

The clinician notes the following:

- the temperature of the skin
- localized increased skin moisture
- the presence of oedema, which is not common but can be seen
- mobility and feel of superficial tissues, e.g. ganglions, nodules and lymph nodes in the femoral triangle
- the presence or elicitation of any muscle hypertonicity or spasm, especially piriformis, obturator internus, quadratus lumborum
- tenderness of bone, e.g. ASIS, pubis, greater trochanter and psoas bursae (palpable if swollen).

Palpation of the Long Dorsal Ligament
(Vleeming 2008)

The long dorsal ligament runs from the PSIS almost vertically down to the inferior portion of the lateral edge of the sacrum. It is a tender area to palpation in pregnancy-related and postpartum pelvic pain (Vleeming et al. 2002) and chronic pelvic pain (Dreyfuss et al. 1996; Fortin et al. 1999). Tenderness is not specific to SIJ-mediated pain (sensitivity: 85–95%; specificity: 10–15%) (Schwarzer et al. 1995; Dreyfuss et al. 1996; Fortin et al. 1999). Palpation of tenderness in this area therefore does not prove the presence of SIJ pain but absence of tenderness is a strong indication that the SIJ is not a source of pain. Where there is tenderness, further differentiation of pelvic and lumbar spine is indicated.

Passive Accessory Movements

The ileum is capable of small amounts of translation relative to the sacrum (Kapandji 2008). The direction is variable and depends on the orientation of the joint surfaces. To test motion in the right anteroposterior direction the patient lies in crook-lying, muscles relaxed. The therapist stands on the side to be tested: the therapist's right hand is placed over the ASIS using a lumbrical grip; the left palpates the movement in the sacral sulcus, when an anteroposterior force is applied (Fig. 13.11).

To test the motion in the right craniocaudal direction the patient lies in the same position, with the therapist on the right side: the therapist's right hand applies a longitudinal force along the femur whilst the

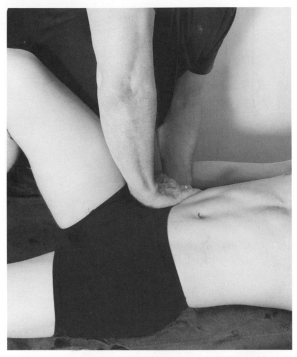

FIG. 13.11 ■ Anteroposterior glide of sacroiliac joint.

left hand palpates the movement in the sacral sulcus when a craniocaudal force is applied (Fig. 13.12).

COMPLETION OF THE EXAMINATION

The subjective and physical examinations produce a large amount of information, which needs to be recorded accurately. As stated, it is vital to highlight important findings from the examination with an asterisk, which will be reassessed within and at subsequent treatment sessions to evaluate the effects of treatment on the patient's condition.

On completion of the physical examination the clinician:

- explains the findings of the physical examination to the patient. Any questions patients may have regarding their illness or injury should be addressed at this stage
- evaluates the findings, formulates a clinical diagnosis and writes up a problem list
- in conjunction with the patient, determines the objectives of treatment, including clear, timed goals

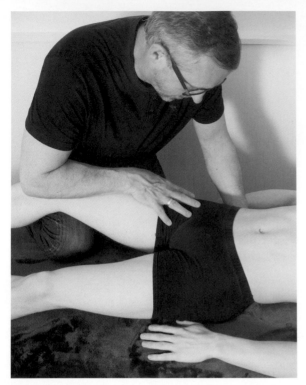

FIG. 13.12 ■ Craniocaudal glide of sacroiliac joint. *(Adapted from Lee 2015.)*

- warns the patient of possible exacerbation up to 24–48 hours following the examination
- requests the patient to report details on the behaviour of the symptoms following examination at the next attendance.

For guidance on treatment and management principles, the reader is directed to the companion textbook (Petty & Barnard 2017).

REFERENCES

Axer, H., et al., 2001. Collagen fibers in linea alba and rectus sheaths. General scheme and morphological aspects. J. Surg. Res. 96, 127–134.

Beer, G.M., et al., 2009. The normal width of the linea alba in nulliparous women. Clin. Anat. 22, 706.

Boissonnault, J., Blaschak, M., 1988. Incidence of diastasis recti abdominis during childbearing years. Phys. Ther. 68, 1082–1086.

Bullock, J.E., et al., 1987. The relationship of low back pain to postural changes during pregnancy. Aust. J. Physiother. 33, 10–17.

Clinical Standards Advisory Report, 1994. Report of a CSAG committee on back pain. London: HMSO.

Coldron, Y., et al., 2008. Postpartum characteristics of rectus abdominis on ultrasound imaging. Man. Ther. 13, 112–121.

Comin, J., et al., 2013. Radiofrequency denervation of the inguinal ligament for the treatment of 'sportsman's hernia': a pilot study. Br. J. Sports Med. 47, 380–386.

Dreyfuss, P., et al., 1996. The value of medical history and physical examination in diagnosing sacroiliac joint pain. Spine 21, 2594–2602.

Dreyfuss, P., et al., 2004. Sacroiliac joint pain. J. Am. Acad. Orthop. Surg. 12, 255–265.

Elden, H., et al., 2016. Predictors and consequences of long-term pregnancy-related pelvic girdle pain: a longitudinal follow-up study. BMC Musculoskelet. Disord. 17, 276.

Fortin, J.D., et al., 1999. Sacroiliac joint innervation and pain. Am. J. Orthop. 28, 687–690.

Goodman, C.C., Snyder, T.K., 2013. Differential diagnosis for physical therapists, fifth ed. Elsevier, St Louis, MO.

Greenman, P.E., 1996. Principles of manual medicine, second ed. Williams & Wilkins, Baltimore.

Hagen, R., 1974. Pelvic girdle relaxation from an orthopaedic point of view. Acta Orthop. Scand. 45, 550–563.

Hansen, A., 1996. Relaxin is not related to symptom-giving pelvic girdle relaxation in pregnant women. Acta Obstet. Gynecol. Scand. 75, 245–249.

Harding, I., et al., 2004. Is the symptom of night pain important in the diagnosis of serious spinal pathology in a back pain triage clinic? Spine J. 4, S30.

Hengeveld, E., Banks, K. (Eds.), 2005. Maitland's peripheral manipulation, fourth ed. Butterworth-Heinemann, Oxford.

Huijbregts, P., 2004. Sacroiliac joint dysfunction; evidence based diagnosis. Reh. Med. 8, 14–37.

Hungerford, B., 2014. Sacroiliac joint – pelvis series. In Touch issue 1.

Hungerford, B., Gilleard, W., 2007. The pattern of intrapelvic motion and lumbopelvic muscle recruitment alters in the presence of pelvic girdle pain. In: Vleeming, A., et al. (Eds.), Movement, stability, and lumbopelvic pain: integration and research. Churchill Livingstone, Edinburgh, pp. 361–376.

Jull, G., et al., 2015. Grieve's modern musculoskeletal physiotherapy. Elsevier, Edinburgh.

Kapandji, I.A., 2008. The physiology of the joints, sixth ed. Churchill Livingstone, Edinburgh.

Laslett, M., 2008. Evidence-based diagnosis and treatment of the painful sacroiliac joint. J. Man. Manip. Ther. 16, 142–152.

Laslett, M., et al., 2005. Diagnosis of sacroiliac joint pain: validity of individual provocation tests and composites of tests. Man. Ther. 10, 207–218.

Laslett, M., Williams, M., 1994. The reliability of selected pain provocation tests for sacroiliac joint pathology. Spine 19, 1243–1249.

Lavy, C., et al., 2009. Cauda equina syndrome. Br. Med. J. 338, 881–884.

Lee, D., 2010. The pelvic girdle: an integration of clinical expertise and research, fourth ed. Churchill Livingstone, Edinburgh.

Lee, D., 2015. The pelvic girdle. An approach to the examination and treatment of the lumbo-pelvic-hip region, second ed. Churchill Livingstone, Edinburgh.

Magee, D.J., 2014. Orthopedic physical assessment. Elsevier Health Sciences, Philadelphia.

McCrory, P., Bell, S., 1999. Nerve entrapment syndromes as a cause of pain the hip, groin and buttock. Sports Med. 27, 261–274.

Mens, J.M.A., et al., 2001. Reliability and validity of the active straight leg raise test in posterior pelvic pain since pregnancy. Spine 26, 1167–1171.

Mens, J.M., et al., 2002. Validity of the active straight leg raise test for measuring disease severity in patients with posterior pelvic pain after pregnancy. Spine 27, 196–200.

Mens, J.M., et al., 2006. The mechanical effect of a pelvic belt in patients with pregnancy-related pelvic pain. Clin. Biomech. (Bristol, Avon) 21, 122–127.

Ostgaard, H.C., et al., 1993. Influence of some biomechanical factors in low-back pain in pregnancy. Spine 18, 61–65.

Ostgaard, H.C., et al., 1994. Reduction of back and posterior pelvic pain in pregnancy. Spine 19, 894–900.

O'Sullivan, P.B., Beales, D.J., 2007a. Diagnosis and classification of pelvic girdle pain disorders, part 1: a mechanism based approach within a biopsychosocial framework. Man. Ther. 12, 86–97.

O'Sullivan, P.B., Beales, D.J., 2007b. Diagnosis and classification of pelvic girdle pain disorders, part 2: illustration of the utility of a classification system via case studies. Man. Ther. 12, e1–e12.

Pastore, A.E., Katzman, W.B., 2012. Recognizing myofascial pelvic pain in the female patient with chronic pelvic pain. J. Obstet. Gynecol. Neonatal Nurs. 41, 680–691.

Petersen, L.K., et al., 1994. Normal serum relaxin in women with disabling pelvic pain during pregnancy. Gynecol. Obstet. Invest. 38, 21–23.

Petty, N.J., Barnard, K., 2017. Principles of neuromusculoskeletal treatment and management: a handbook for therapists, third ed. Churchill Livingstone, Edinburgh.

Robinson, H.S., et al., 2007. The reliability of selected motion and pain provocation tests for the sacroiliac joint. Man. Ther. 12, 72–79.

Royal College of Radiologists, 2007. Making the best use of a department of clinical radiology. Guidelines for doctors, sixth ed. Royal College of Radiologists, London.

Sahrmann, S.A., 2002. Diagnosis and treatment of movement impairment syndromes. Mosby, St Louis.

Sapsford, R., et al., 1999. Women's health – a textbook for physiotherapists. W.B. Saunders, London.

Schwarzer, A.C., et al., 1995. The spine in chronic low back pain. Spine 20, 31.

Solomon, L., et al., 2010. Apley's system of orthopaedics and fractures, ninth ed. Arnold, London.

Stuber, K.J., 2007. Specificity, sensitivity and predictive values of clinical tests of the sacroiliac joint: a systematic review of the literature. J. Can. Chiropr. Assoc. 51, 30–41.

Stuge, B., et al., 2011. The pelvic girdle questionnaire: a condition-specific instrument for assessing activity limitations and symptoms in people with pelvic girdle pain. Phys. Ther. 91, 1096–1108.

Suresh, E., 2004. Diagnosis of early rheumatoid arthritis: what the non-specialist needs to know. J. R. Soc. Med. 97, 421–424.

van der Wurff, P., et al., 2000a. Clinical tests of the sacroiliac joint. A systematic review. Part 1: reliability. Man. Ther. 5, 30–36.

van der Wurff, P., et al., 2000b. Clinical tests of the sacroiliac joint. A systematic review. Part 2: validity. Man. Ther. 5, 89–96.

van der Wurff, P., et al., 2006. Intensity mapping of pain referral areas in sacroiliac joint pain patients. J. Manipulative Physiol. Ther. 29, 190–195.

Visser, L.H., et al., 2013. Sciatica-like symptoms and the sacroiliac joint: clinical features and differential diagnosis. Eur. Spine J. 22, 1657–1664.

Vleeming, A., 2008. European guidelines for the diagnosis and treatment of pelvic girdle pain. Eur. Spine J. 17, 794–819.

Vleeming, A., et al. (Eds.), 1997. Movement, stability and low back pain, the essential role of the pelvis. Churchill Livingstone, Edinburgh.

Vleeming, A., et al., 2002. Possible role of the long dorsal sacroiliac ligament in women with peripartum pelvic pain. Acta Obstet. Gynecol. Scand. 81, 430–436.

Waddell, G., Burton, K.A., 2004. Concepts of rehabilitation for the management of common health problems. London: Department of Work and Pensions.

Yazici, Y., et al., 2004. Stiffness in patients with rheumatoid arthritis is associated more strongly with functional disability than with joint swelling and erythrocyte sedimentation rate. J. Rheumatol. 31, 1723–1726.

Yong-il, K., et al., 2015. The usefulness of bone SPECT/CT imaging with volume of interest analysis in early axial spondyloarthritis. BMC Musculoskelet. Disord. 16, 9.

Young, S., et al., 2003. Correlation of clinical examination characteristics with three sources of chronic low back pain. Spine J. 3, 460–465.

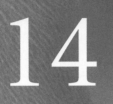

14

EXAMINATION OF THE HIP REGION

KIERAN BARNARD

CHAPTER CONTENTS

INTRODUCTION

The hip is a large, congruent and stable joint. The hip region may become symptomatic due to intraarticular or extraarticular pathology. Intraarticular pathology may be of traumatic origin, for example, in the case of a fractured neck of femur, or may present more gradually. Hip pain of insidious onset may represent, for example, degenerative pathology such as osteoarthritis or femoroacetabular impingement (FAI) caused by morphological changes within the hip joint. Although clinically both hip osteoarthritis and FAI may lead to groin pain, the presentation is often quite different. Osteoarthritis is often characterized by stiffness in the hip when moving from a static position, particularly first thing in the morning when getting out of bed. FAI however often causes pain during flexion and twisting movements. Typically osteoarthritis affects the older population whilst FAI is more likely to affect the young adult.

Extraarticular pathology may also present as an acute or more insidious onset. Acute trauma when accelerating or twisting during sport might represent an adductor muscle strain if felt in the groin or a hamstring injury if felt in the buttock or upper thigh. Overuse or biomechanical stresses may cause extraarticular symptoms of more gradual onset. For example, persistent medial torsion of the femur due to reduced endurance of the hip abductors and lateral rotators may in time cause a gluteal tendinopathy, leading to lateral hip pain during walking or running. The clinician must also be mindful of less common conditions such as inflammatory or infective pathologies, for example rheumatoid or septic arthritis.

This chapter will outline the questions asked and the core physical tests necessary to perform a thorough examination of the hip region. The order of the subjective questioning and the physical tests described below can be altered as appropriate for the patient being examined. The reader is directed to Chapters 2 and 3, respectively, for further details on the principles of the subjective and physical examinations.

SUBJECTIVE EXAMINATION

Patients' Perspectives and Experiences

Patients' perspectives and experiences may be relevant to the onset and progression of their problem and are therefore recorded. The patient's age, employment, home situation and details of any leisure activities are also recorded. Factors from this information may indicate direct and/or indirect mechanical influences on the hip. In order to treat the patient appropriately, it is important the condition is managed within the context of the patient's social and work environment.

The clinician may ask the following types of questions to elucidate psychosocial factors:

- Have you had time off work in the past with your pain?
- What do you understand to be the cause of your pain?
- Are you worried about the cause of your pain?
- What are you expecting will help you?
- How is your employer/coworkers/family responding to your pain?
- What are you doing to cope with your pain?
- Do you think you will return to work? When?
- What does the future hold for you in relation to your pain?

Early identification of psychosocial risk factors is important as the presence of such factors may be an important component in the development of chronic musculoskeletal disability (Nicholas et al. 2011).

Body Chart

The following information concerning the type and area of current symptoms can be recorded on a body chart (see Fig. 2.3).

Area of Current Symptoms

Be meticulous when mapping out the area of the symptoms. Lesions of the hip joint commonly refer symptoms into the groin, anterior thigh and knee. Ascertain which is the worst symptom and record where the patient feels the symptoms are coming from.

Areas Relevant to the Region Being Examined

Symptoms around the hip may be referred from more proximal anatomy, including arthrogenic, myogenic or neurogenic structures in the region of the lumbar spine or sacroiliac joints. Groin and medial thigh pain, for example, may be referred from the upper lumbar spine or may result from a peripheral neuropathy affecting the obturator nerve. Symptoms may also arise as a result of contributing factors such as weak hip lateral rotators or a pronated foot leading to medial femoral torsion. It is important therefore to include all areas of symptoms. Check all relevant areas including the lumbar spine, sacroiliac joint, knee and ankle joints for symptoms including pain or even stiffness, as this may be relevant to the patient's main symptom. Be sure to negate all possible areas that might refer or contribute to symptoms. The clinician marks unaffected areas with ticks (✓) on the body chart.

Quality of Pain

Establish the quality of the pain, e.g. is the pain sharp, aching, throbbing?

Intensity of Pain

The intensity of pain can be measured using, for example, a pain-rating scale, as shown in Chapter 2.

Abnormal Sensation

Check for any altered sensation, such as paraesthesia or numbness, over the hip and other relevant areas.

Constant or Intermittent Symptoms

Ascertain the frequency of the symptoms, whether they are constant or intermittent. If symptoms are constant, check whether there is variation in the intensity of the symptoms, as constant unremitting pain may be indicative of serious pathology.

Relationship of Symptoms

Determine the subjective relationship between symptomatic areas – do they come on together or separately? For example, the patient could have lateral thigh pain without back pain, or the pains may always be present together. Questions to clarify the relationship might include:

- Do you ever get your back pain without your thigh pain?
- Do you ever get your thigh pain without your back pain?
- If symptoms are constant: Does your thigh pain change when your back pain gets worse?

Behaviour of Symptoms

Aggravating Factors

For each symptomatic area, establish what movements and/or positions aggravate the patient's symptoms, i.e. what brings them on (or makes them worse)? Is the patient able to maintain this position or movement (severity)? What happens to symptoms? And how long does it take for symptoms to ease once the position or movement is stopped (irritability)? The principles of severity and irritability are discussed in Chapter 2.

If a subjective relationship has already been established, it is helpful firstly to ask about the aggravating factors affecting the hypothesized source, e.g. lumbar spine, and follow-up by establishing the aggravating factors affecting areas dependent on the source, e.g. the groin. If the aggravating factors for the two areas are the same or similar, this may further strengthen the hypothesis that there is a relationship between the two areas of symptoms.

Specific structures in the region of the hip may be implicated by correlating the area of symptoms with certain aggravating factors. For example, groin pain which is aggravated by putting on shoes (flexion) may be more indicative of an arthrogenic hip joint problem than, for example, a femoral nerve peripheral neuropathy.

It is important for the clinician to be as specific as possible when hunting for aggravating factors. Where possible, break the movement or activity down as this may provide clues for what to expect during the physical examination. 'What is it about …?' is a useful question to ask. Groin pain aggravated by 'gardening', for example, does not offer as much information as groin pain aggravated by 'weeding a flower bed' (flexion) or 'pruning a high hedge' (extension).

The clinician ascertains how the symptoms affect function, such as static and active postures, e.g. sitting, standing, lying, bending, walking, running, walking on uneven ground and up and down stairs, driving, work,

sport and social activities. Note details of the training regimen for any sports activities. The clinician finds out if the patient is left- or right-handed as there may be increased stress on the dominant side.

Detailed information on each of the above activities is useful in order to help determine the structure(s) at fault and identify functional restrictions. This information can be used to determine the aims of treatment and any advice that may be required. The most notable functional restrictions are highlighted with asterisks (*), explored in the physical examination and reassessed at subsequent treatment sessions to evaluate treatment intervention.

Easing Factors

For each symptomatic area, the clinician asks what movements and/or positions ease the patient's symptoms, how long it takes for them to ease completely (if symptoms are intermittent) or back to the base level (if symptoms are constant) and what happens to other symptoms when this symptom is relieved. These questions help to confirm the relationship between the symptoms as well as determine the level of irritability.

Occasionally, particularly with symptoms that are irritable or with a patient who is catastrophizing, it is difficult to establish clear and distinct aggravating factors. When this is the case it may be worth starting with the easing factors and working backwards. For example, if sitting down eases symptoms, it may be worth asking: 'Does that mean that standing makes your groin pain worse?'

At this point the clinician synthesizes the information gained from the aggravating and easing factors and has a working hypothesis of the structure(s) which might be at fault. Beware of, and do not dismiss, symptoms which do not conform to a mechanical pattern as this may be a sign of serious pathology.

Twenty-Four-Hour Behaviour of Symptoms

The clinician determines the 24-hour behaviour of symptoms by asking questions about night, morning and evening symptoms.

Night Symptoms. It is important to establish whether the patient has pain at night. If so, does the patient have difficulty getting to sleep? How many times does the patient wake per night? How long does it take to get back to sleep?

It is crucial to establish whether the pain is position-dependent. The clinician may ask: 'Can you find a comfortable position in which to sleep?' or 'What is the most/least comfortable position for you?' Pain which is position-dependent is mechanical; pain which is not position-dependent and unremitting is non-mechanical and should arouse suspicion of more serious pathology.

Position-dependent pain may give clues as to the structure(s) at fault; for example, patients with trochanteric pain syndrome often have trouble sleeping and lying on the symptomatic side.

Morning and Evening Symptoms. The clinician determines the pattern of the symptoms first thing in the morning, through the day and at the end of the day. This information may provide clues as to the pain mechanisms driving the condition and the type of pathology present. For example, early-morning pain and stiffness lasting for more than half an hour may indicate inflammatory-driven pain.

Special Questions

Hip-specific special questions may help in the generation of a clinical hypothesis. Such questions may include the following movements..

Squatting

Groin pain on squatting may implicate intraarticular pathology as a source of symptoms.

Locking/Catching

Locking, clicking and/or catching in the groin may be associated with FAI (Philippon et al. 2013).

Crepitus

Crepitus with groin pain in the older patient may indicate degenerative change.

Neurological Symptoms

During the subjective examination it is important to keep the hypothesis as open as possible. If, when questioning the patient and reviewing the body chart, a neurological lesion may be a possibility, establish with precision areas of pins and needles, numbness or weakness.

Has the patient experienced symptoms of spinal cord compression (compression of the spinal cord to L1 level), including bilateral tingling in hands or feet and/or disturbance of gait? Has the patient experienced symptoms of cauda equina compression (i.e. compression below L1)? Symptoms of cauda equina include perianal sensory loss and sphincter disturbance, with or without urinary retention. As well as retention, bladder symptoms may include reduced urine sensation, loss of desire to empty the bladder and a poor urine stream (Lavy et al. 2009). These symptoms may indicate compression of the sacral nerve roots and prompt surgical attention is required to prevent permanent disability.

History of the Present Condition

For each symptomatic area the clinician needs to know how long the symptom has been present, whether there was a sudden or slow onset and whether there was a known cause that provoked the onset of the symptom. If the onset was slow, the clinician finds out if there has been any change in the patient's lifestyle, e.g. a new job or hobby or a change in sporting activity or training schedule. The stage of the condition is established: are the symptoms getting better, staying the same or getting worse?

The clinician ascertains whether the patient has had this problem previously. If so, how many episodes has s/he had? When were they? What was the cause? What was the duration of each episode? And did the patient fully recover between episodes? If there is no previous history, has the patient had any episodes of pain and/or stiffness in the lumbar spine, knee, foot, ankle or any other relevant region?

To confirm the relationship between the symptoms, the clinician asks what happened to other symptoms when each symptom began. Symptoms which came on at the same time may indicate that the areas of symptoms are related. This evidence is further strengthened if there is a subjective relationship (symptoms come on at the same time or one is dependent on the other) and if the aggravating factors are the same or similar.

Has there been any treatment to date? The effectiveness of any previous treatment regime may help to guide patient management. Has the patient seen a specialist or had any investigations which may help with clinical diagnosis, such as blood tests, X-ray or magnetic resonance imaging (MRI)?

The mechanism of injury gives the clinician some important clues as to the injured structure around the hip, particularly in the acute stage, when a full physical examination may not be possible. For example, sudden buttock pain on sprinting may implicate the hamstring origin, whilst groin pain during extreme flexion activities such as hurdling or martial arts might implicate FAI pathology.

Past Medical History

A detailed medical history is vitally important to identify certain precautions or contraindications to the physical examination and/or treatment (see Table 2.4). As mentioned in Chapter 2, the clinician must differentiate between conditions that are suitable for conservative treatment and systemic, neoplastic and other non-musculoskeletal conditions, which require referral to a medical practitioner.

The following information is routinely obtained from patients.

General Health

The clinician ascertains the state of the patient's general health and finds out if the patient suffers from any malaise, fatigue, fever, nausea or vomiting, stress, anxiety or depression.

Weight Loss

Has the patient noticed any recent unexplained weight loss?

Serious Pathology

Does the patient have a history of serious pathology, such as cancer, tuberculosis, osteomyelitis or human immunodeficiency virus (HIV)?

Inflammatory Arthritis

Has the patient been diagnosed as having an inflammatory condition such as rheumatoid arthritis or polymyalgia rheumatica? Does the patient have any features of a systemic inflammatory process such as psoriasis, dry eyes (iritis) or irritable-bowel problems?

Family History

Is there any relevant family history such as serious pathology or inflammatory arthritis?

Cardiovascular Disease

Is there a history of cardiac disease, e.g. angina? Does the patient have a pacemaker? If the patient has raised blood pressure, is it controlled with medication?

Respiratory Disease

Does the patient have a history of lung pathology? How is it controlled?

Diabetes

Does the patient suffer from diabetes? If so, is it type 1 or type 2 diabetes? Is the patient's blood glucose controlled? How is it controlled? Is it through diet, tablet or injection? Patients with diabetes may develop peripheral neuropathy and vasculopathy, are at increased risk of infection and may take longer to heal than those without diabetes.

Epilepsy

Is the patient epileptic? When was the last seizure?

Thyroid Disease

Does the patient have a history of thyroid disease? Hypothyroidism can cause proximal muscle myopathy in 29–75% of patients (Anwar & Gibofsky 2010). Symptoms may include proximal muscle weakness, stiffness and cramping.

Osteoporosis

Has the patient had a dual-energy X-ray absorptiometry (DEXA) scan, been diagnosed with osteoporosis or sustained frequent fractures?

Previous Surgery

Has the patient had previous surgery which may be of relevance to the presenting complaint?

Drug History

What medications are being taken by the patient? Has the patient ever been prescribed long-term (6 months or more) medication? Particular attention may need to be paid to the following.

Steroids. Long-term use of steroids for conditions such as polymyalgia rheumatica or chronic lung disease may lead to an increased risk of osteoporosis.

Anticoagulants. Anticoagulant medication such as warfarin prescribed for conditions such as atrial fibrillation may cause an increased risk of bleeding and bruising.

Non-Steroidal Anti-Inflammatory Drugs (NSAIDs). NSAIDs such as ibuprofen have systemic effects which may lead to gastrointestinal bleeding in some patients. Use of such medications should not be encouraged if they do not appear to be positively influencing the condition. Inflammatory nociceptive pain may however be relieved by NSAIDs.

Plan of the Physical Examination

When all this information has been collected, the subjective examination is complete. It is useful at this stage to highlight with asterisks (*), for ease of reference, important findings and particularly one or more functional restrictions. These can then be reexamined at subsequent treatment sessions to evaluate treatment intervention.

In order to plan the physical examination, the following hypotheses are developed from the subjective examination:

- Is each area of symptoms severe and/or irritable (see Chapter 2)? Will it be necessary to stop short of symptom reproduction, to reproduce symptoms partially or fully? If symptoms are severe, physical tests are carried out to just short of symptom production or to the very first onset of symptoms; no overpressures will be carried out, as the patient would be unable to tolerate this. If symptoms are irritable, physical tests need to be performed to just short of symptom production or just to the onset of symptoms with fewer physical tests being performed to allow for rest period between tests.
- What are the predominant pain mechanisms which might be driving the patient's symptoms? What are the active 'input mechanisms' (sensory pathways): are symptoms the product

of a mechanical, inflammatory or ischaemic nociceptive process? What are the 'processing mechanisms': how has the patient processed this information? What are his or her thoughts and feelings about the pain? Finally, what are the 'output mechanisms': what is the patient's physiological, psychological and behavioural response to the pain? Clearly establishing which pain mechanisms may be causing and/or maintaining the condition will help the clinician manage both the condition and patient appropriately. The reader is directed to Gifford (1998), Jones et al. (2002) and Thacker (2015) for further reading.

- What are the possible arthrogenic, myogenic and neurogenic structures which could be causing the patient's symptoms: what structures could refer to the area of pain? And what structures are underneath the area of pain? For example, medial thigh pain could theoretically be referred from the lumbar spine or the sacroiliac joint. The structures directly under the medial thigh could also be implicated, for example the hip joint, the adductor muscles or the obturator nerve.
- In addition, are there any contributing factors which could be maintaining the condition? These could be:
  - physical, such as weak hip lateral rotators causing medial femoral torsion
  - environmental, for instance, driving for a living
  - psychosocial, such as fear of serious pathology
  - behavioural, for instance, excessive rest in an attempt to help the area heal.
- The clinician decides, based on the evidence, which structures are most likely to be at fault and prioritizes the physical examination accordingly. It is helpful to organize structures into ones that 'must', 'should' and 'could' be tested on day 1 and over subsequent sessions. This will develop the clinician's clinical reasoning and avoid a recipe-based hip assessment. Where possible it is advisable to clear an area fully. For example, if the clinician feels the lumbar spine needs to be excluded on day 1, s/he needs to assess this area fully, leaving no stone unturned, to implicate or negate this area as a source of symptoms. This

approach will avoid juggling numerous potential sources of symptoms for several sessions, which may lead to confusion.

■ Another way to develop the clinician's reasoning is to consider what to expect from each physical test. Will it be easy or hard to reproduce each symptom? Will it be necessary to use combined movements or repetitive movements? Will a particular test prove positive or negative? Will the pain be direction-specific? Synthesizing evidence from the subjective examination and in particular the aggravating and easing factors will provide substantial evidence as to what to expect in the physical examination.

■ Are there any precautions and/or contraindications to elements of the physical examination that need to be explored further, such as neurological involvement, recent fracture, trauma, steroid therapy or rheumatoid arthritis? There may also be certain contraindications to further examination and treatment, e.g. symptoms of spinal cord or cauda equina compression.

A physical planning form can be useful for clinicians to help guide them through the clinical reasoning process (see Fig. 2.9).

PHYSICAL EXAMINATION

The information from the subjective examination helps the clinician to plan an appropriate physical examination. The severity, irritability and nature of the condition are the major factors that will influence the choice and priority of physical testing procedures. The first and overarching question the clinician might ask is: 'Is this patient's condition suitable for me to manage as a therapist?' For example, a patient presenting with cauda equina compression symptoms may only need neurological integrity testing, prior to an urgent medical referral. The nature of the patient's condition has had a major impact on the physical examination. The second question the clinician might ask is: 'Does this patient have a musculoskeletal dysfunction that I may be able to help?' To answer that, the clinician needs to carry out a full physical examination; however, this may not be possible if the symptoms are severe and/or irritable. If the patient's

symptoms are severe and/or irritable, the clinician aims to explore movements as much as possible, within a symptom-free range. If the patient has constant and severe and/or irritable symptoms, then the clinician aims to find physical tests that ease the symptoms. If the patient's symptoms are non-severe and non-irritable, then the clinician aims to find physical tests that reproduce each of the patient's symptoms.

Each significant physical test that either provokes or eases the patient's symptoms is highlighted in the patient's notes by an asterisk (*) for easy reference. The highlighted tests are often referred to as 'asterisks' or 'markers'.

The order and detail of the physical tests described below need to be appropriate to the patient being examined; some tests will be irrelevant, some tests will be carried out briefly, while it will be necessary to investigate others fully. It is important for the reader to understand that not all physical tests are equal and that the reliability, sensitivity and specificity will vary markedly between tests (see Chapter 3). The author has chosen to present the most clinically useful tests according to the literature. None of these physical tests should however take the place of a thorough subjective examination. A good subjective history when examining the hip region is crucial in helping to determine the diagnosis in the vast majority of cases (Reiman & Thorborg 2014). The clinician needs to have a clear clinical hypothesis after the subjective examination and the purpose of the physical examination is to confirm or refute this hypothesis.

Observation

Informal Observation

The clinician needs to observe the patient in dynamic and static situations; the quality of lower-limb and general movement is noted, as are the postural characteristics and facial expression. Informal observation will have begun from the moment the clinician begins the subjective examination and will continue to the end of the physical examination.

Formal Observation

Observation of Posture. The clinician examines the patient's spinal and lower-limb posture from anterior, lateral and posterior views in standing and where necessary in functional positions related to the patient's complaint. Specific observation of the pelvis involves noting its position in the sagittal, coronal and horizontal planes: in the sagittal plane, there may be excessive anterior or posterior pelvic tilt; in the coronal plane there may be a lateral pelvic tilt; and in the horizontal plane there may be rotation of the pelvis. These abnormalities will be identified by observing the relative position of the iliac crest, the anterior and posterior iliac spines, skin creases (particularly the gluteal creases) and the position of the pelvis relative to the lumbar spine and lower limbs. In addition, the clinician notes whether there is even weight bearing through the left and right leg. The clinician passively corrects any asymmetry to determine its relevance to the patient's problem.

Observation of Muscle Form. The clinician observes the muscle bulk and muscle tone of the patient, comparing left and right sides. It must be remembered that the level and frequency of physical activity as well as the dominant side may well produce differences in muscle bulk between sides. Some muscles are thought to shorten under stress, while other muscles weaken, producing muscle imbalance (see Table 3.7). Patterns of muscle imbalance are thought to produce the postures mentioned above.

Observation of Soft Tissues. The clinician observes the quality and colour of the patient's skin and any area of swelling or presence of scarring, and takes cues for further examination.

Observation of Balance. Balance is provided by vestibular, visual and proprioceptive information. This rather crude and non-specific test is conducted by asking the patient to stand on one leg with the eyes open and then closed. If the patient's balance is as poor with the eyes open as with the eyes closed, this suggests a vestibular or proprioceptive dysfunction (rather than a visual dysfunction). The test is carried out on the affected and unaffected sides; if there is greater difficulty maintaining balance on the affected side, this may indicate some proprioceptive dysfunction.

As well as monitoring the ability of the patient to balance on one leg, the clinician also pays close attention to the patient's pelvis. A pelvis that drops on the unsupported side indicates abductor weakness on the standing leg and is known as a positive Trendelenburg sign (Fig. 14.1). A positive Trendelenburg sign is a common finding in patients who have undergone hip joint arthroplasty, and hip abductor function may be particularly compromised when the surgeon has employed a lateral approach to the hip (Berstock et al. 2015). Abductor weakness leads to increased adduction and altered pelvic kinematics during gait and may be associated with gluteal tendinopathy (Grimaldi & Fearon 2015; Grimaldi et al. 2015; Allison et al. 2016).

Observation of Gait. Analyse gait on even/uneven ground, slopes, stairs and running. Note the stride length and weight-bearing ability. Inspect the feet, shoes and any walking aids. The typical gait patterns that might be expected in patients with hip pain are the gluteus maximus gait, the Trendelenburg gait and the short-leg gait (see Chapter 3 for further details).

Observation of Function. If possible, meticulously examine a functional task related to the patient's presenting complaint, such as squatting, pivoting or climbing stairs. Does pain occur at any phase of that particular movement, e.g. taking weight through the leg when stepping up? It may be possible at this stage to modify the activity to see if symptoms change by, for example, adjusting pelvic rotation. The reader is directed to the section on symptom modification, below, to explore this concept further.

Active Physiological Movements

Active physiological movements of the hip include flexion, extension, abduction, adduction, medial rotation and lateral rotation (Table 14.1). All movements may be performed bilaterally in supine, with the exception of extension, which may be more readily appreciated in prone. Movements are overpressed if symptoms allow (Fig. 14.2).

The clinician establishes the patient's symptoms at rest, prior to each movement, and passively corrects any movement deviation to determine its relevance to the patient's symptoms. The following are noted:

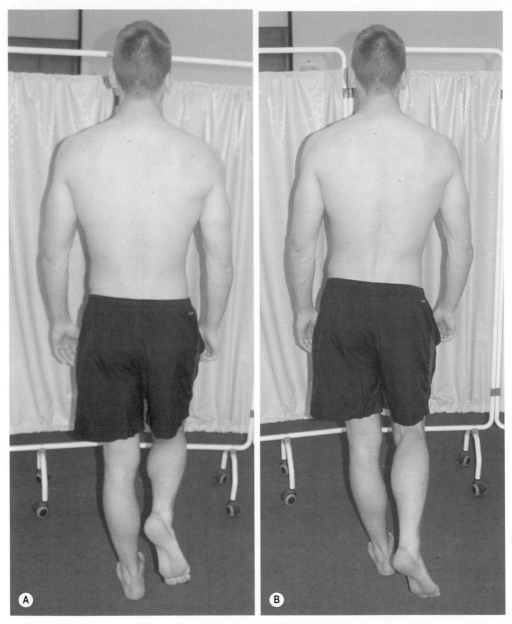

FIG. 14.1 ■ Trendelenburg test. (A) The patient stands on the affected leg. (B) Positive test indicated by the pelvis dropping on the unsupported side.

TABLE 14.1
Active Physiological Movements With Possible Modifications

Active Physiological Movements	Modifications
Flexion	Repeated
Extension	Speed altered
Abduction	Combined, e.g.
Adduction	■ Flexion with rotation
Medial rotation	■ Rotation with flexion
Lateral rotation	Compression or distraction, e.g.
?Lumbar spine	■ Through greater tuberosity
?Sacroiliac joint	with flexion
?Knee	Sustained
?Ankle and foot	Injuring movement
	Differentiation tests
	Functional ability

- quality of movement
- range of movement
- behaviour of pain through the range of movement
- resistance through the range of movement and at the end of the range of movement
- provocation of any muscle spasm.

In a similar way to the manipulation of a symptomatic physical task (see the section on symptom modification, below), the thoughtful clinician may be able to manipulate physiological movements to help differentiation between tissues. For example, when trunk rotation with the patient standing on one leg (causing rotation in the lumbar spine and hip joint) reproduces the patient's buttock pain, differentiation between the lumbar spine and hip joint may be required. The clinician can increase and decrease the lumbar spine rotation and the pelvic rotation in turn, to find out what effect each movement has on the buttock pain. If the pain is coming from the hip then the lumbar spine movements will have no effect on the pain, but pelvic movements will alter the pain; conversely, if the pain is coming from the lumbar spine then lumbar spine movements will affect the pain but pelvic movement will have no effect.

It may be necessary to examine other regions to determine their relevance to the patient's symptoms; they may be the source of the symptoms, or they may be contributing to the symptoms. The most likely regions are the lumbar spine, sacroiliac joint, knee, foot and ankle. These regions can be quickly screened; see Chapter 3 for further details. Contrary to what the name might suggest, however, performing a clearing test on the lumbar spine, for example, does not fully negate this region as a source of symptoms and if there is any doubt the clinician is advised to assess the suspected area fully (see relevant chapter).

Passive Physiological Movements

All the active movements described above can be examined passively with the patient usually in supine, comparing left and right sides. In the presence of osteoarthritis, the clinician may expect a limitation to flexion, abduction and internal rotation, slight limitation of extension and no limitation of lateral rotation (Cyriax 1982).

Comparison of the response of symptoms to the active and passive movements can help to determine whether the structure at fault is non-contractile (articular) or contractile (extraarticular) (Cyriax 1982). If the lesion is non-contractile, such as liga ment, then active and passive movements will be painful and/or restricted in the same direction. If the lesion is in a contractile tissue (i.e. muscle) then active and passive movements are painful and/or restricted in opposite directions. For example, a hip adductor strain may be painful during active adduction and passive abduction. Such patterns are however theoretical and a muscle strain may be more readily assessed by contracting muscle isometrically where there will be little or no change in the length of non-contractile tissue.

Tests for Intraarticular Structures

As well as testing the active and passive physiological range, the clinician may employ specific tests to bias different structures around the hip. The reliability, sensitivity and specificity of these tests are variable. The author has chosen to present the most clinically useful tests according to the literature. The intraarticular tests include tests for hip impingement and fracture.

Hip Impingement

FAI is a morphological hip condition leading to groin pain during flexion and twisting movements,

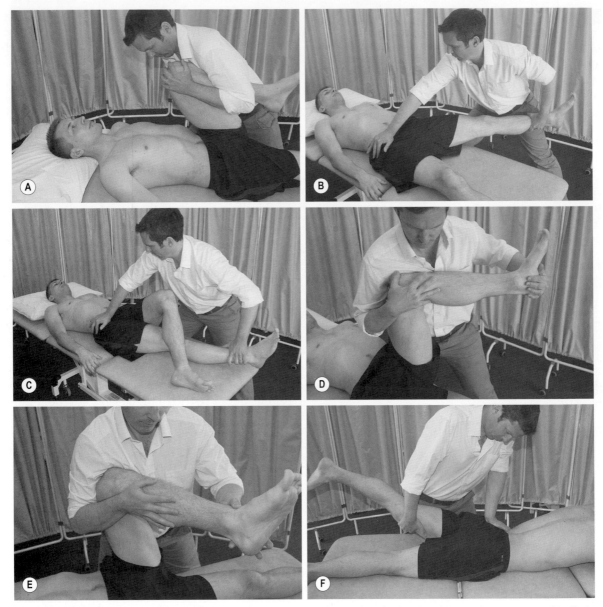

FIG. 14.2 ■ Overpressures to the hip joint. (A) Flexion. Both hands rest over the knee and apply overpressure to hip flexion. (B) Abduction. The right hand stabilizes the pelvis while the left hand takes the leg into abduction. (C) Adduction. With the left leg crossed over the right leg, the right hand stabilizes the pelvis and the left hand takes the leg into adduction. (D) Medial rotation. The clinician's trunk and right hand support the leg. The left hand and trunk then move to rotate the hip medially. (E) Lateral rotation. The clinician's trunk and right hand support the leg. The left hand and trunk then move to rotate the hip laterally. (F) Extension. In prone, the left hand supports the pelvis whilst the right hand takes the leg into extension.

typically in young adults. Despite there being a lack of clarity as to the exact morphological changes leading to the condition (Agricola & Weinans 2016) and the most appropriate examination and treatment strategies (Reiman & Thorborg 2014), pain is thought to arise from the femoral head abutting the acetabular rim during movement. The condition may be caused by an abnormality in the shape of the femoral head (known as a 'cam' deformity), abnormal morphology of the acetabulum (known as a pincer deformity), or a combination of the two (Diamond et al. 2014). The condition may lead to osteoarthritic change (Agricola & Weinans 2016). Three tests which appear to be clinically useful according to recent systematic reviews are presented below (Reiman et al. 2015a; Pacheco-Carrillo & Medina-Porqueres 2016). In general terms these tests are sensitive but not specific, so the clinician should be mindful of false positives.

Internal Rotation Over Pressure (IROP)

With the patient lying in supine, the affected hip is flexed to 90°. The clinician stabilizes at the pelvis and internally rotates the hip to the end of range with some overpressure (Fig. 14.3). The IROP test is deemed positive if the patient's pain is reproduced. The IROP test has a sensitivity of greater than 80% (Maslowski et al. 2010; Pacheco-Carrillo and Medina-Porqueres 2016) but a specificity as low as 17%.

Flexion Adduction Internal Rotation (FADDIR)

The patient lies supine with one knee flexed. The clinician fully flexes the hip and then adducts and internally rotates the femur (Fig. 14.4). This movement approximates the anterior aspect of the femoral neck with the acetabulum. The test is positive if it reproduces pain, clicking, catching or locking. The sensitivity of the FADDIR has been reported as excellent – 94% (with MRI arthrogram as a reference), with a poor specificity of 8% (Reiman et al. 2015b).

Flexion Abduction External Rotation (FABER)

The FABER test has also been found to be a sensitive test in detecting FAI, at 82%, but again the test lacks specificity, at 25% (Maslowski et al. 2010). With the patient lying supine, the foot of the symptomatic leg is placed on the knee of the asymptomatic leg. The clinician then stabilizes the pelvis and adds some gentle downward pressure to the knee (Fig. 14.5). A positive test is indicated by reproduction of the patient's ipsilateral hip pain (Pacheco-Carrillo & Medina-Porqueres 2016). As well as the presence of FAI, a positive FABER test may also indicate iliopsoas spasm or sacroiliac joint dysfunction (Magee 2014).

Fracture

Some tests have been advocated in the diagnosis of fracture and stress fracture to the femur. Indeed, the two tests presented below show good discriminative ability (Reiman et al. 2015b).

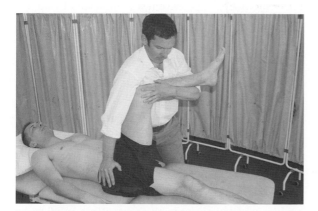

FIG. 14.3 ■ Internal rotation over pressure (IROP). The clinician stabilises at the pelvis and internally rotates the hip to the end of range with some overpressure.

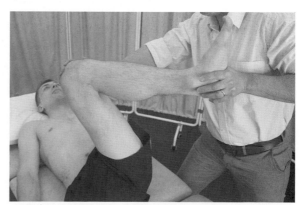

FIG. 14.4 ■ Flexion, adduction, internal rotation (FADDIR). The clinician fully flexes the hip and then adducts and internally rotates the femur.

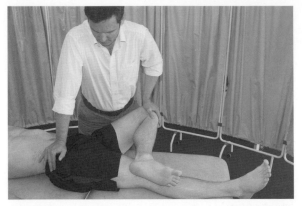

FIG. 14.5 ■ Flexion, abduction, external rotation (FABER) test. The foot of the symptomatic leg is placed on the knee of the asymptomatic leg so the symptomatic leg lies in a flexed, abducted and externally rotated position. The clinician then stabilizes the pelvis and adds some gentle downward pressure to the knee.

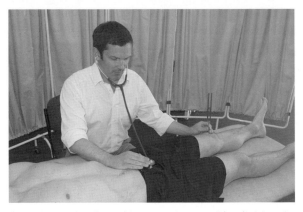

FIG. 14.6 ■ Patellar pubic percussion test. The clinician sits or stands by the symptomatic leg and places a stethoscope over the pubic symphysis. The patella of the leg being tested is then tapped or a tuning fork is used and the sound is noted.

Patellar Pubic Percussion Test

In this test, the clinician sits or stands by the symptomatic leg and places a stethoscope over the pubic symphysis. The patella of the leg being tested is then tapped or a tuning fork is used and the sound is noted (Fig. 14.6). The quality of the sound is then compared to the contralateral side. If the sound is duller ipsilaterally, then the test is considered positive. The sensitivity and specificity may be as high as 95% and 86%, respectively (Reiman et al. 2013, 2015b).

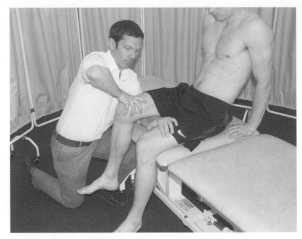

FIG. 14.7 ■ Fulcrum test. The patient sits on the treatment couch with the clinician on the symptomatic side. The clinician's hand rests on the asymptomatic thigh with the patient's symptomatic thigh resting on the clinician's forearm. The patient leans back slightly and the clinician places a downward pressure on the symptomatic side at the knee.

Fulcrum Test

Another test which has shown good sensitivity and specificity in the diagnosis of fracture is the fulcrum test. The patient sits on the treatment couch with the clinician on the symptomatic side. The clinician's hand rests on the asymptomatic thigh with the patient's symptomatic thigh resting on the clinician's forearm. The patient leans back slightly and the clinician places a downward pressure on the symptomatic side at the knee (Fig. 14.7). A positive test is indicated by apprehension and the reproduction of symptoms. Sensitivity and specificity have been reported at 93% and 75%, respectively (Reiman et al. 2013, 2015b).

Tests for Extraarticular Structures

Tests for symptoms emanating from extraarticular structures will now be presented. These have been categorized as tests for gluteal tendinopathy and sports-related groin pain.

Gluteal Tendinopathy

It is now acknowledged that lateral hip pain is more multifactorial than once thought. What used to be termed 'trochanteric bursitis' is now described as 'trochanteric pain syndrome' or simply 'lateral hip pain'.

It is now widely recognized that the primary source of lateral hip pain is gluteal tendinopathy (Grimaldi & Fearon 2015; Grimaldi et al. 2015).

Resisted External Derotation Test

The resisted external derotation test has demonstrated good sensitivity (88%) and excellent specificity (97.3%) in the diagnosis of gluteal tendinopathy (Reiman et al. 2013, 2015b). The patient lies in supine with the symptomatic hip at 90° of flexion. The clinician fully externally rotates the hip and the patient is asked to return the leg actively to neutral against the clinician's resistance (Fig. 14.8). A positive test is indicated by the reproduction of pain (Reiman et al. 2015b).

Sustained Single-Leg Stance

Grimaldi and Fearon (2015) recommend the single-leg stance as a valid and simple test in the diagnosis of gluteal tendinopathy. They point out that several variations of the test are described in the literature. They recommend a simple one-leg stance on the symptomatic side for 30 seconds with the clinician offering balance support at the fingertips, as suggested by Lequesne et al. (2008; Fig. 14.9). Those with poorer hip abductor endurance may develop an adducted hip during this test, increasing the compressive load over the lateral hip and causing pain. The test is positive if pain is reproduced within the 30-second period. Lequesne et al. (2008) found the test to have excellent sensitivity and specificity at 100% and 97.3%, respectively, in the identification of gluteal tendinopathy.

Sports-Related Chronic Groin Pain

Whilst sports-related hip injuries are varied (Reiman et al. 2013), the aim of the following tests is to place stress across the common adductor origin and pubic symphysis (Reiman et al. 2015b). In so doing it may be possible to establish if this region may be the source of the patient's symptoms. In general terms these tests are specific with moderate sensitivity.

Double Adductor Test

The patient lies supine with the legs extended. The clinician lifts the legs passively into slight flexion and asks the patient to adduct maximally against manual

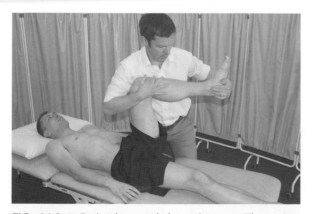

FIG. 14.8 ■ Resisted external derotation test. The patient lies in supine with the symptomatic hip at 90° of flexion. The clinician fully externally rotates the hip and the patient is asked actively to return the leg to neutral against the clinician's resistance.

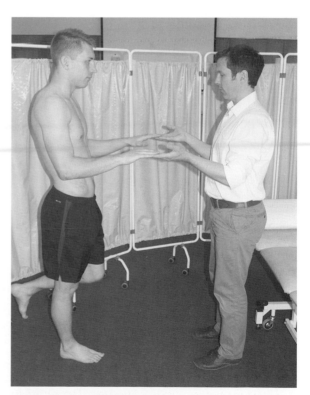

FIG. 14.9 ■ Sustained single-leg stance. The patient stands on the symptomatic leg for 30 seconds with the clinician offering balance support at the fingertips.

resistance (Fig. 14.10). A positive test is indicated by the reproduction of the patient's symptoms (Reiman et al. 2013). The sensitivity for this test is 54% and the specificity is 93% (Reiman et al. 2015b).

Squeeze Test

Similarly to the double adductor test, in this test the patient contracts the adductors of both hips simultaneously. This time the knee is flexed to 45° and the patient is asked to squeeze the clinician's clenched fist, which is placed between the patient's knees (Fig. 14.11). A positive test is indicated by the reproduction of the patient's symptoms (Reiman et al. 2013). The diagnostic accuracy of the squeeze test is similar to the double adductor test, with a sensitivity of 43% and a specificity of 91% (Reiman et al. 2015b).

Muscle Tests

Muscle tests include those examining muscle strength, control and length and isometric muscle testing.

Muscle Strength

For a true appreciation of a muscle's strength, the clinician tests the muscle isotonically through the available range. During the physical examination of the hip, it may be appropriate to test the hip flexors, extensors, abductors, adductors, medial and lateral rotators and any other relevant muscle group.

Greater detail may be required to test the strength of muscles, in particular those thought prone to become weak; that is, rectus abdominis, gluteus maximus, medius and minimus, vastus lateralis, medialis and intermedius, tibialis anterior and the peronei (Jull & Janda 1987; Sahrmann 2002). Testing the strength of these muscles is described in Chapter 3.

Muscle Control

The relative strength of muscles is considered to be more important than the overall strength of a muscle group (Janda 1994, 2002; White & Sahrmann 1994; Sahrmann 2002). Relative strength is assessed indirectly by observing posture, as already mentioned, by the quality of active movement, noting any changes in muscle recruitment patterns and by palpating muscle activity in various positions.

Muscle Length

The clinician may test the length of muscles, in particular those thought prone to shortening (Janda

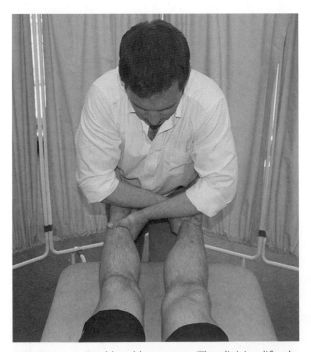

FIG. 14.10 ■ Double adductor test. The clinician lifts the legs passively into slight flexion and asks the patient to adduct maximally against manual resistance.

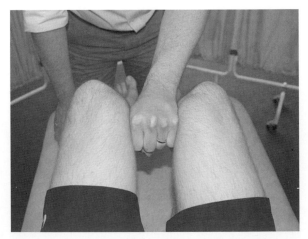

FIG. 14.11 ■ Squeeze test. With the knees flexed to 45°, the patient is asked to squeeze the clinician's clenched fist which is placed between the patient's knees.

1994); that is, erector spinae, quadratus lumborum, piriformis, iliopsoas, rectus femoris, tensor fasciae latae, hamstrings, tibialis posterior, gastrocnemius and soleus (Jull & Janda 1987; Sahrmann 2002). Testing the length of these muscles is described in Chapter 3.

Isometric Muscle Testing

Isometric muscle testing may help to differentiate whether symptoms are arising from contractile or non-contractile tissue. Isometric testing is described in detail in Chapter 3.

It may be appropriate to test the hip joint flexors, extensors, abductors, adductors, medial and lateral rotators (and other relevant muscle groups) in a resting position and, if indicated, in different parts of the physiological range. The clinician notes the strength and quality of the contraction, as well as any reproduction of the patient's symptoms.

Neurological Tests

Neurological examination includes neurological integrity testing and neurodynamic tests.

Integrity of the Nervous System

The integrity of the nervous system is tested if the clinician suspects that the symptoms are emanating from the spine or from a peripheral nerve.

Dermatomes/Peripheral Nerves. Light touch and pain sensation of the lower limb are tested using cotton wool and pinprick, respectively, as described in Chapter 3. Knowledge of the cutaneous distribution of nerve roots (dermatomes) and peripheral nerves enables the clinician to distinguish the sensory loss due to a root lesion from that due to a peripheral nerve lesion. The cutaneous nerve distribution and dermatome areas are shown in Chapter 3.

Myotomes/Peripheral Nerves. The following myotomes are tested (see Chapter 3 for further details):

- L2: hip flexion
- L3: knee extension
- L4: foot dorsiflexion and inversion
- L5: extension of the big toe
- S1: eversion of the foot, contract buttock, knee flexion

- S2: knee flexion, toe standing
- S3–S4: muscles of pelvic floor, bladder and genital function.

A working knowledge of the muscular distribution of nerve roots (myotomes) and peripheral nerves enables the clinician to distinguish the motor loss due to a root lesion from that due to a peripheral nerve lesion. The peripheral nerve distributions are shown in Chapter 3.

Reflex Testing. The following deep tendon reflexes are tested (see Chapter 3):

- L3–L4: knee jerk
- S1: ankle jerk.

Neurodynamic Tests

The following neurodynamic tests may be carried out in order to ascertain the degree to which neural tissue is responsible for the production of the patient's symptom(s):

- passive neck flexion
- straight-leg raise
- passive knee bend
- slump.

These tests are described in detail in Chapter 3.

Miscellaneous Tests

Vascular Tests

If the circulation is suspected of being compromised, the clinician palpates the pulses of the femoral, tibial, popliteal and dorsalis pedis arteries. The clinician then checks for skin and temperature changes and capillary refill of the nail beds. The state of the vascular system can also be determined by the response of symptoms to positions of dependence and elevation of the lower limbs.

Leg Length

True leg length, which tends to be congenital, is measured from the anterior superior iliac spine to the medial or lateral malleolus. Apparent leg length, which results from compensatory change such as a pronated foot or spinal scoliosis, is measured from the umbilicus to the medial or lateral malleolus. A difference in leg length of up to 1–1.5 cm is considered normal (Magee 2014).

Palpation

The clinician palpates the hip region and any other relevant area. It is useful to record palpation findings on a body chart (see Fig. 2.3) and/or palpation chart (see Fig. 3.35).

The clinician notes the following:

- the temperature of the area
- localized increased skin moisture
- the presence of oedema. This can be measured using a tape measure and left and right sides compared
- mobility and feel of superficial tissues, e.g. ganglions, nodules, lymph nodes in the femoral triangle
- the presence or elicitation of any muscle spasm
- tenderness of bone (the greater trochanter may be tender because of trochanteric bursitis and the ischial tuberosity because of ischiogluteal bursitis); inguinal area tenderness may be due to iliopsoas bursitis, ligaments, muscle (Baer's point, for tenderness/spasm of iliacus, lies a third of the way down a line from the umbilicus to the anterior superior iliac spine), tendon, tendon sheath, trigger points (shown in Fig. 3.36) and nerve.

Palpable nerves which may be relevant to assessment of the hip region are as follows:

- The sciatic nerve can be palpated two-thirds of the way along an imaginary line between the greater trochanter and the ischial tuberosity with the patient in prone.
- The common peroneal nerve can be palpated medial to the tendon of biceps femoris and also around the head of the fibula.
- The tibial nerve can be palpated centrally over the posterior knee crease medial to the popliteal artery; it can also be felt behind the medial malleolus, which is more noticeable with the foot in dorsiflexion and eversion.
- Increased or decreased prominence of bones
- Pain provoked or reduced on palpation.

Accessory Movements

It may be useful to use the palpation chart and movement diagrams (or joint pictures) to record findings. These are explained in detail in Chapter 3.

The clinician notes the following:

- quality of movement
- range of movement
- resistance through the range and at the end of the range of movement
- behaviour of pain through the range
- provocation of any muscle spasm.

Hip joint accessory movements are shown in Fig. 14.12 and are listed in Table 14.2. Following accessory movements to the hip region, the clinician reassesses all the physical asterisks (movements or tests that have been found to reproduce the patient's symptoms) in order to establish the effect of the accessory movements on the patient's signs and symptoms. Accessory movements can then be tested for other regions suspected to be a source of, or contributing to, the patient's symptoms. Again, following accessory movements to any one region, the clinician reassesses all the asterisks. Regions likely to be examined are the lumbar spine, sacroiliac joint, knee, foot and ankle (Table 14.2).

Symptom Modification

It can be extremely useful to examine a symptomatic physical task specific to the patient's complaint. This functional task can then be modified and the patient's symptomatic response can be closely monitored. A suitable functional task may be replicated in the clinical setting and can often be identified when asking the patient about the aggravating factors. It may be useful to examine a functional task early in the assessment; this is for three reasons:

1. The task will provide a useful initial snapshot of the patient's problem.
2. It may be possible to manipulate the task to aid the clinical diagnosis and highlight possible treatment options (see the worked example below).
3. The task will provide a useful physical marker (*).

By manipulating the functional task in various ways to bias different tissues (which need not be time

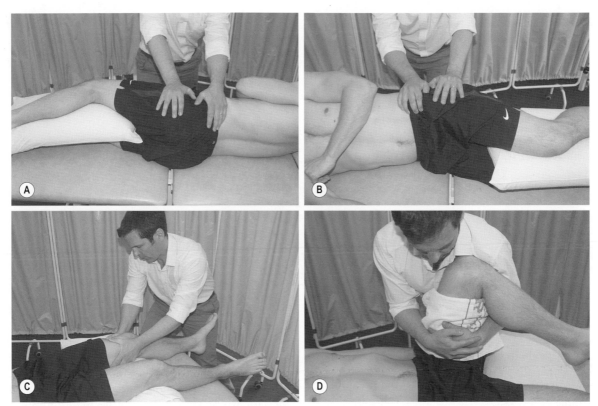

FIG. 14.12 ▪ Hip joint accessory movements. (A) Anteroposterior. With the patient in side-lying, pillows are placed between the patient's legs to position the hip joint in neutral. The left hand is then placed posterior on the iliac crest to stabilize the pelvis while the heel of the right hand applies an anteroposterior pressure over the anterior aspect of the greater trochanter. (B) Posteroanterior. With the patient in side-lying, pillows are placed between the patient's legs to position the hip joint in neutral. The right hand grips around the anterior aspect of the anterior superior iliac spine to stabilize the pelvis while the left hand applies a posteroanterior force to the posterior aspect of the greater trochanter. (C) Longitudinal caudad. The hands grip just proximal to the medial and lateral femoral epicondyles and pull the femur in a caudad direction. (D) Lateral transverse. The hip is flexed and a towel is placed around the upper thigh. The clinician clasps the hands together on the medial aspect of the thigh and pulls the leg laterally.

consuming), useful information may be gleaned as to the likely clinical diagnosis as well as the most appropriate way to manage the condition. Although the worked example below highlights the art of clinical reasoning in practice, it is important to emphasize that modifications to symptomatic tasks are not standardized tests and will therefore lack a degree of validity and reliability. There is a tradeoff here: on the one hand the clinician is being very patient-focused and examining the specific problem that prompted the patient to seek help in the first place, but on the other hand there is a lack of standardization. It is worth noting, however, that, even well-known orthopaedic

tests may lack robust diagnostic accuracy or reliability. It may be wise to use both approaches in a clinical context as both have relative strengths and add to the clinical picture. As always, the clinician is encouraged to synthesize information from the whole subjective and physical examination to reach a reasoned view of the patient's condition, rather than placing too much emphasis on any one test.

A Worked Example of Symptom Modification: Trochanteric Pain

The causes of pain emanating from the trochanteric region are often multifactorial. A combination of

TABLE 14.2

Accessory Movements, Choice of Application and Reassessment of the Patient's Asterisks

Accessory Movements	Modifications	Identify Any Effect of Accessory Movements on Patient's Signs and Symptoms
Hip joint ↕ Anteroposterior ↕ Posteroanterior ←→ Caud Longitudinal caudad ←→ Lat Lateral transverse	Start position, e.g. ■ In flexion ■ In extension ■ In medial rotation ■ In lateral rotation (medial or lateral) ■ In flexion and medial rotation ■ In extension and lateral rotation Speed of force application Direction of the applied force Point of application of applied force	Reassess all asterisks
?Lumbar spine ?Sacroiliac joint ?Knee ?Foot and ankle	As above	Reassess all asterisks

factors may lead to abnormal tensile load being placed on the lateral hip structures (Grimaldi & Fearon 2015; Grimaldi et al. 2015). Possible factors which may contribute to the generation of trochanteric pain may include:

- sitting with the hip adducted or legs crossed (Grimaldi et al. 2015)
- 'hanging' off one hip whilst standing with the hip in adduction (Grimaldi et al. 2015)
- poor gluteal abductor strength (Allison et al. 2015)
- crossing the midline during gait/running (Grimaldi et al. 2015)
- an adducted foot strike which may cause hip adduction (Lack et al. 2014).

Because of the wide range of factors which may influence the generation of trochanteric pain functionally, a multifactorial approach to its assessment and management needs to be adopted. If the patient complains of pain during the transition from sitting to standing, for example, it may be useful for the clinician to observe this specific activity during the assessment. The clinician closely monitors the symptomatic response to the task. If sitting to standing reproduces symptoms immediately then symptom modification may begin. If not, the clinician may need to think of ways of provoking the symptoms, for example, standing from a lower chair or repeated movements.

Once the task has been observed and confirmed to be symptomatic, the clinician may attempt to modify the task whilst closely monitoring the symptomatic response. It may help for clinicians to think systematically and ask themselves: 'How can I influence the load placed on the lateral structures of the hip?'

It may first be worth the clinician checking to see if the hip on the symptomatic side is starting the movement from an adducted position. If so, the hip position could be corrected and the patient could be asked to repeat the movement (Fig. 14.13). If symptoms improve and the patient is able to maintain a neutral hip position without excessive adduction then this simple exercise could be the start of a graded exercise programme. If the patient is unable to maintain a neutral position through the sit-to-stand movement, some abductor activity could be facilitated with the addition of a resistance band around the knees (Fig. 14.14). The patient is instructed to maintain resistance on the band throughout the movement. Again, if this helps, a sit-to-stand exercise with the addition of a resistance band could be a useful starting point for rehabilitation, perhaps with some isolated abductor-strengthening exercises if the abductors have been found to be weak on muscle testing.

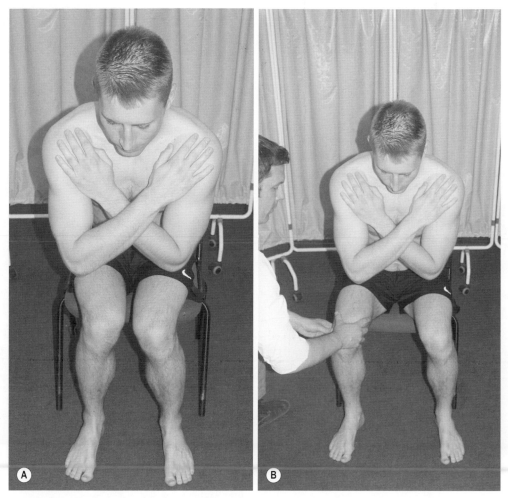

FIG. 14.13 ■ (A) The patient's hip starts in an adducted position. (B) The clinician manually repositions the hip to neutral prior to the patient standing.

If the pain occurs towards the top of the sit-to-stand motion, with or without the presence of a Trendelenburg sign, the clinician may encourage facilitation of the hip abductors in standing. This may be achieved by asking the patient to squeeze the hip abductors on the ipsilateral side whilst simultaneously hitching the pelvis up slightly on the contralateral side. Some contralateral support may be helpful initially (Fig. 14.15). Again the symptomatic response of the patient is closely monitored.

In relation to distal control of movement, because pronation of the foot may contribute to an adducted hip, and a foot orthotic may reduce hip adduction during functional tasks (Lack et al. 2014), the clinician may wish to correct the patient's foot position where appropriate and monitor the symptomatic response (Fig. 14.16). If this relieves the patient's symptoms, the insertion of an orthotic into the patient's shoe may be trialled.

This example has sought to demonstrate how methodically manipulating a functional task in various ways may help to determine the tissues which may be contributing to symptoms and may also help to direct appropriate management strategies. In practice, a multifactorial problem requires a multifactorial management approach and it may be that several strategies

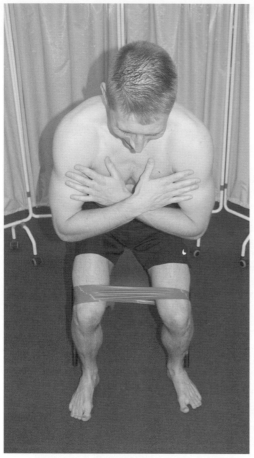

FIG. 14.14 ■ The patient goes from sitting to standing with a resistance band placed around the knees to facilitate the hip abductors.

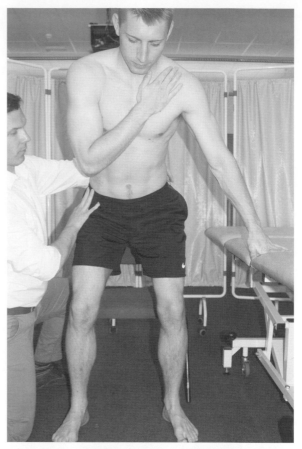

FIG. 14.15 ■ The patient is asked to squeeze the hip abductors on the ipsilateral side whilst simultaneously hitching the pelvis up slightly on the contralateral side. Some support is used in this example.

may need to be combined into one coherent management plan. When thinking about symptom modification, it may be helpful for clinicians to ask themselves: 'Which myogenic, arthrogenic or neurogenic structures may be contributing to this patient's problem?' The clinician is encouraged to think functionally, methodically and creatively, whilst at the same time closely monitoring the patient's symptomatic response to the intervention.

COMPLETION OF THE EXAMINATION

Once all of the above tests have been carried out, the examination of the hip region is complete. The subjective and physical examinations produce a large amount of information which needs to be recorded accurately and quickly. It is vital at this stage to highlight important findings from the examination with an asterisk (*). These findings are reassessed at, and within, subsequent treatment sessions to evaluate the effects of treatment on the patient's condition.

The physical testing procedures which specifically indicate joint, nerve or muscle tissues, as a source of the patient's symptoms, are summarized in Table 3.9.

On completion of the physical examination, the clinician:

■ warns the patient of possible exacerbation up to 24–48 hours following the examination

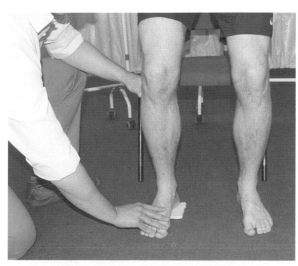

FIG. 14.16 ■ An orthotic is placed under the patient's foot to correct pronation.

- requests the patient to report details on the behaviour of the symptoms following examination at the next attendance
- explains the findings of the physical examination and how these findings relate to the subjective assessment. Any misconceptions patients may have regarding their illness or injury need to be addressed
- evaluates the findings, formulates a clinical diagnosis and writes up a problem list
- determines the objectives of treatment
- devises an initial treatment plan

In this way, the clinician will have developed the following hypotheses categories (adapted from Jones & Rivett 2004):

- function: abilities and restrictions
- patient's perspective on his/her experience
- source of symptoms. This includes the structure or tissue that is thought to be producing the patient's symptoms, the nature of the structure or tissues in relation to the healing process and the pain mechanisms
- contributing factors to the development and maintenance of the problem. There may be environmental, psychosocial, behavioural, physical or heredity factors

- precautions/contraindications to treatment and management. This includes the severity and irritability of the patient's symptoms and the nature of the patient's condition
- management strategy and treatment plan
- prognosis – this can be affected by factors such as the stage and extent of the injury as well as the patient's expectations, personality and lifestyle.

For guidance on treatment and management principles, the reader is directed to the companion textbook (Petty & Barnard 2017).

REFERENCES

Agricola, R., Weinans, H., 2016. What is femoroacetabular impingement? Br. J. Sports Med. 50, 196–197.

Allison, K., et al., 2015. Hip abductor muscle weakness in individuals with gluteal tendinopathy. Med. Sci. Sports Exerc. 48, 346–352.

Allison, K., et al., 2016. Kinematics and kinetics during walking in individuals with gluteal tendinopathy. Clin. Biomech. (Bristol, Avon) 32, 56–63.

Anwar, S., Gibofsky, A., 2010. Musculoskeletal manifestations of thyroid disease. Rheum. Dis. Clin. North Am. 36, 637–646.

Berstock, J.R., et al., 2015. A systematic review and meta-analysis of complications following the posterior and lateral surgical approaches to total hip arthroplasty. Ann. R. Coll. Surg. Engl. 97, 11–16.

Cyriax, J., 1982. Textbook of orthopaedic medicine – diagnosis of soft tissue lesions, eighth ed. Baillière Tindall, London.

Diamond, L.E., et al., 2014. Physical impairments and activity limitations in people with femoroacetabular impingement: a systematic review. Br. J. Sports Med. 49, 230–242.

Gifford, L.S., 1998. Pain, the tissues and the nervous system: a conceptual model. Physiotherapy 84, 27–36.

Grimaldi, A., et al., 2015. Gluteal tendinopathy: a review of mechanisms, assessment and management. Sports Med. 45, 1107–1119.

Grimaldi, A., Fearon, A., 2015. Gluteal tendinopathy: integrating pathomechanics and clinical features in its management. J. Orthop. Sports Phys. Ther. 45, 910–922.

Janda, V., 1994. Muscles and motor control in cervicogenic disorders: assessment and management. In: Grant, R. (Ed.), Physical therapy of the cervical and thoracic spine, second ed. Churchill Livingstone, New York, p. 195.

Janda, V., 2002. Muscles and motor control in cervicogenic disorders. In: Grant, R. (Ed.), Physical therapy of the cervical and thoracic spine, third ed. Churchill Livingstone, New York, p. 182.

Jones, M.A., et al., 2002. Conceptual models for implementing biopsychosocial theory in clinical practice. Man. Ther. 7, 2–9.

Jones, M.A., Rivett, D.A., 2004. Clinical reasoning for manual therapists. Butterworth-Heinemann, Edinburgh.

Jull, G.A., Janda, V., 1987. Muscles and motor control in low back pain: assessment and management. In: Twomey, L.T., Taylor, J.R. (Eds.), Physical therapy of the low back. Churchill Livingstone, New York, p. 253.

Lack, S., et al., 2014. The effect of anti-pronation foot orthoses on hip and knee kinematics and muscle activity during a functional step-up task in healthy individuals: a laboratory study. Clin. Biomech. (Bristol, Avon) 29, 177–182.

Lavy, C., et al., 2009. Cauda equina syndrome. Br. Med. J. 338, 881–884.

Lequesne, M., et al., 2008. Gluteal tendinopathy in refractory greater trochanter pain syndrome: diagnostic value of two clinical tests. Arthritis Rheum. 59, 241–246.

Magee, D.J., 2014. Orthopedic physical assessment. Elsevier Health Sciences, Philadelphia.

Maslowski, E., et al., 2010. The diagnostic validity of hip provocation maneuvers to detect intra-articular hip pathology. PM&R 2, 174–181.

Nicholas, M.K., et al., 2011. Early identification and management of psychological risk factors ('yellow flags') in patients with low back pain: a reappraisal. Phys. Ther. 91, 737–753.

Pacheco-Carrillo, A., Medina-Porqueres, I., 2016. Physical examination tests for the diagnosis of femoroacetabular impingement. A systematic review. Phys. Ther. Sport 21, 87–93.

Petty, N.J., Barnard, K.J., 2017. Principles of musculoskeletal treatment and management: a handbook for therapists, third ed. Churchill Livingstone, Edinburgh.

Philippon, M.J., et al., 2013. Arthroscopic hip labral repair. Arthrosc. Tech. 2, e73–e76.

Reiman, M.P., et al., 2013. Diagnostic accuracy of clinical tests of the hip: a systematic review with meta-analysis. Br. J. Sports Med. 47, 893–902.

Reiman, M.P., et al., 2015a. Diagnostic accuracy of clinical tests for the diagnosis of hip femoroacetabular impingement/labral tear: a systematic review with meta-analysis. Br. J. Sports Med. 49, 811.

Reiman, M.P., et al., 2015b. Physical examination tests for hip dysfunction and injury. Br. J. Sports Med. 49, 357–361.

Reiman, M.P., Thorborg, K., 2014. Invited clinical commentary. Clinical examination and physical assessment of hip-related pain in athletes. Int. J. Sports Phys. Ther. 9, 737–755.

Sahrmann, S.A., 2002. Diagnosis and treatment of movement impairment syndromes. Mosby, St Louis.

Thacker, M., 2015. Louis Gifford – revolutionary: the mature organism model, an embodied cognitive perspective of pain. In Touch 152, 4–9.

White, S.G., Sahrmann, S.A., 1994. A movement system balance approach to musculoskeletal pain. In: Grant, R. (Ed.), Physical therapy of the cervical and thoracic spine, second ed. Churchill Livingstone, Edinburgh, p. 339.

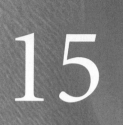

15

EXAMINATION OF THE KNEE REGION

KIERAN BARNARD

INTRODUCTION

The knee is a large and complex region made up of the tibiofemoral, patellofemoral and superior tibiofibular joints with their surrounding soft tissues. It is a common site for traumatic injury. For example, significant varus or valgus force to the knee may cause injury to the collateral ligaments, forceful pivoting over a fixed foot may cause injury to the anterior cruciate ligament (ACL) or menisci and acute pain behind the knee on rapid acceleration may be due to a musculotendinous hamstring injury. Traumatic knee injuries often occur, although not exclusively, during sport.

The knee may also become symptomatic in the presence of overuse or biomechanical stresses such as anterior knee pain or patellar tendinopathy. For example, persistent medial torsion of the femur due to reduced endurance of the hip abductors and lateral rotators may in time cause anterior knee symptoms as a result of a valgus knee pattern during walking or running.

Other symptomatic conditions may be more insidious. The knee is a common site for osteoarthritic degenerative change which may become symptomatic over time and the clinician must also be mindful of other less common conditions such as inflammatory on infective pathologies, for example, rheumatoid or septic arthritis.

This chapter will outline the questions asked and the core physical tests necessary to perform a thorough examination of the knee. The order of the subjective questioning and the physical tests described below can be altered as appropriate for the patient being examined. The reader is directed to Chapters 2 and 3, respectively, for further details on the principles of the subjective and physical examinations.

SUBJECTIVE EXAMINATION

Patients' Perspectives on Their Experiences

Patients' perspectives and experiences may be relevant to the onset and progression of their problem and are therefore recorded. The patient's age, employment, home situation and details of any leisure activities are also recorded. Factors from this information may indicate direct and/or indirect mechanical influences on the knee. In order to treat the patient appropriately, it is important that the condition is managed within the context of the patient's social and work environment.

The clinician may ask the following types of questions to elucidate psychosocial factors:

- Have you had time off work in the past with your pain?
- What do you understand to be the cause of your pain?
- Are you worried about the cause of your pain?
- What are you expecting will help you?
- How is your employer/coworkers/family responding to your pain?
- What are you doing to cope with your pain?
- Do you think you will return to work? When?
- What does the future hold for you in relation to your pain?

Early identification of psychosocial risk factors is important as the presence of such factors may be an important component in the development of chronic musculoskeletal disability (Nicholas et al. 2011).

Observation of the Patient's Attitudes and Feelings

The age, gender and ethnicity of patients and their cultural, occupational and social backgrounds will all affect their attitudes and feelings towards themselves, their condition and the clinician. The clinician needs to be aware of and sensitive to these attitudes, and empathize and communicate appropriately so as to develop a rapport with the patient and thereby enhance the patient's compliance with the treatment.

Body Chart

The following information concerning the type and area of the current symptoms can be recorded on a body chart (see Fig. 2.3).

Area of Current Symptoms

Be meticulous when mapping out the area of the symptoms. A lesion in the knee joint complex may refer symptoms proximally to the thigh or distally to the foot and ankle. Ascertain which is the worst symptom and record where the patient feels the symptoms are coming from.

Areas Relevant to the Region Being Examined

Symptoms around the knee complex may be referred from more proximal anatomy, including arthrogenic, myogenic or neurogenic structures in the region of the lumbar spine, pelvis or hip. For example, anterior knee pain may be referred from the lumbar spine or may result from a peripheral neuropathy affecting the femoral nerve. Symptoms may also arise as a result of contributing factors affecting the foot and/or ankle complex; for example, pronation of the foot may cause excessive medial rotation of the tibia and femur which may in turn lead to increased stress on the lateral patella (Barton et al. 2010). It is important therefore to include all areas of symptoms. Check all relevant areas, including the lumbar spine, pelvis, hip, foot and ankle, for symptoms including pain or even stiffness, as this may be relevant to the patient's main symptom. Be sure to negate all possible areas that might refer or contribute to the area of pain. Mark unaffected areas with ticks (✓) on the body chart.

Quality of Pain

Establish the quality of the pain, e.g. is the pain sharp, aching, throbbing?

Intensity of Pain

The intensity of pain can be measured using, for example, a pain-rating scale, as shown in Chapter 2.

Depth of Pain

Does the patient feel it is on the surface or deep inside? If appropriate, distinguish between pain felt underneath the patella and that felt in the tibiofemoral joint.

Abnormal Sensation

Check for any altered sensation (such as paraesthesia or numbness) over the knee and other relevant areas.

Constant or Intermittent Symptoms

Ascertain the frequency of the symptoms, whether they are constant or intermittent. If symptoms are constant, check whether there is variation in the intensity of the symptoms, as constant unremitting pain may be indicative of serious pathology.

Relationship of Symptoms

Determine the subjective relationship between symptomatic areas – do they come on together or separately? For example, the patient could have knee pain without back pain, or the pains may always be present together. Questions to clarify the relationship might include:

- Do you ever get your back pain without your knee pain?
- Do you ever get your knee pain without your back pain?
- If symptoms are constant: Does your knee pain change when your back pain gets worse?

Behaviour of Symptoms

Aggravating Factors

For each symptomatic area, establish what movements and/or positions aggravate the patient's symptoms, i.e. what brings them on (or makes them worse)? Is the patient able to maintain this position or movement (severity)? What happens to and how long does it take for symptoms to ease once the position or movement is stopped (irritability)? The principles of severity and irritability are discussed in Chapter 2.

If a subjective relationship has already been established, it is helpful firstly to ask about the aggravating factors affecting the hypothesized source, e.g. lumbar spine, and follow up by establishing the aggravating factors affecting areas dependent on the source, e.g. the knee. If the aggravating factors for the two areas are the same or similar, this may further strengthen the hypothesis that there is a relationship between the two areas of symptoms.

If the knee is suspected, specific knee structures may be implicated by correlating the area of symptoms with certain aggravating factors. For example, anterior knee pain which is aggravated by climbing up and down stairs may implicate the patellofemoral joint

(Petersen et al. 2014), whereas pain whilst squatting may implicate the menisci (McHale et al. 2014).

It is important for the clinician to be as specific as possible when hunting for aggravating factors. Where possible, break the movement or activity down as this may provide clues for what to expect during the physical examination. 'What is it about …?' is a useful question to ask. Knee pain aggravated by 'driving' does not offer as much information as knee pain aggravated by 'pushing the clutch' (extension), 'changing pedals' (twisting) or 'long distances on a motorway' (sustained flexion). Aggravating factors for other regions, which may need to be queried if they are suspected to be a source of the symptoms, are shown in Table 2.2.

The clinician ascertains how the symptoms affect function, such as: static and active postures, e.g. sitting, standing, lying, bending, walking, running, walking on uneven ground and up and down stairs, driving, work, sport and social activities. Note details of the training regimen for any sports activities. The clinician finds out if the patient is left- or right-handed as there may be increased stress on the dominant side.

Detailed information on each of the above activities is useful in order to help determine the structure(s) at fault and identify functional restrictions. This information can be used to determine the aims of treatment and any advice that may be required. The most notable functional restrictions are highlighted with asterisks (*), explored in the physical examination and reassessed at subsequent treatment sessions to evaluate treatment intervention.

Easing Factors

For each symptomatic area, the clinician asks what movements and/or positions ease the patient's symptoms, how long it takes for them to ease completely (if symptoms are intermittent) or back to the base level (if symptoms are constant) and what happens to other symptoms when this symptom is relieved. These questions help to confirm the relationship between the symptoms as well as determine the level of irritability.

Occasionally, particularly with symptoms that are irritable or with a patient who is catastrophizing, it is difficult to establish clear and distinct aggravating factors. When this is the case it may be worth starting with the easing factors and working backwards. For example, if knee extension eases symptoms, it may be worth asking: 'Does that mean that bending your knee makes your pain worse?'

At this point the clinician synthesizes the information gained from the aggravating and easing factors and has a working hypothesis of the structure(s) which might be at fault. Beware of, and do not dismiss, symptoms which do not conform to a mechanical pattern as this may be a sign of serious pathology.

Twenty-Four-Hour Behaviour of Symptoms

The clinician determines the 24-hour behaviour of symptoms by asking questions about night, morning and evening symptoms.

Night Symptoms. It is important to establish whether the patient has pain at night. If so, does s/he have difficulty getting to sleep? How many times does s/he wake at night? How long does it take to get back to sleep?

It is crucial to establish whether the pain is position-dependent. The clinician may ask: 'Can you find a comfortable position in which to sleep?' or 'What is the most/least comfortable position for you?' Pain which is position-dependent is mechanical; pain which is not position-dependent and unremitting is non-mechanical and should arouse suspicion of more serious pathology.

Position-dependent pain may give clues as to the structure(s) at fault; for example, patients with an injury to the medial meniscus often have trouble sleeping and lying with the symptomatic side uppermost as it compresses that side.

Morning and Evening Symptoms. The clinician determines the pattern of the symptoms first thing in the morning, through the day and at the end of the day. This information may provide clues as to the pain mechanisms driving the condition and the type of pathology present. For example, early-morning pain and stiffness lasting for more than half an hour may indicate inflammatory-driven pain.

Special Questions

Knee-specific special questions may help in the generation of a clinical hypothesis. Such questions may include the following:

Swelling

Does the knee swell? If so, the clinician needs to establish whether the swelling occurred immediately after the injury (within 2 hours) or whether it took some hours or days to form. Immediate swelling, particularly after a pop or click within the knee, may indicate bleeding (haemarthrosis) suggestive of significant trauma or rupture and is distinct from swelling occurring within hours of an injury, which is more suggestive of the build-up of inflammatory exudate (Wagemakers et al. 2010).

Giving Way

Giving way of the knee may be suggestive of either ligamentous instability or an inability of the surrounding musculature, particularly the quadriceps, to support the knee adequately. Ligamentous instability is normally the result of trauma, whilst giving way of muscular origin is more complex and may be due to weakness as a result of disuse, pain inhibition, joint effusion (Torry et al. 2000) or ligamentomuscular reflex inhibition (Solomonow 2009). Correlating giving way with the wider clinical picture may therefore provide useful information. For example, falling to the floor without warning and a history of trauma may represent mechanical instability whilst giving way without trauma and in the presence of pain and/or swelling may represent a muscular cause.

Locking

If locking is present, it is important to distinguish between true and 'pseudo'-locking. True locking might represent an intraarticular derangement such as a meniscal tear, whilst pseudo-locking may simply represent an unwillingness to move the knee due to pain. Qualifying locking by asking, 'Does your knee get stuck so you can't bend or straighten it?' may be helpful.

Crepitus

If crepitus is associated with pain it may help to build a clinical picture. For example, crepitus anteriorly when descending stairs may suggest patellofemoral pain.

Neurological Symptoms

During the subjective examination it is important to keep the hypothesis as open as possible. If, when questioning the patient and reviewing the body chart, a neurological lesion may be a possibility, establish with precision areas of pins and needles, numbness or weakness.

Has the patient experienced symptoms of spinal cord compression (compression of the spinal cord to L1 level), including bilateral tingling in hands or feet and/or disturbance of gait? Has the patient experienced symptoms of cauda equina compression (i.e. compression below L1)? Symptoms of cauda equina include perianal sensory loss and sphincter disturbance, with or without urinary retention. As well as retention, bladder symptoms may include reduced urine sensation, loss of desire to empty the bladder and a poor urine stream (Lavy et al. 2009). These symptoms may indicate compression of the sacral nerve roots and prompt surgical attention is required to prevent permanent disability.

History of the Present Condition

For each symptomatic area the clinician needs to know how long the symptom has been present, whether there was a sudden or slow onset and whether there was a known cause that provoked the onset of the symptom. If the onset was slow, the clinician finds out if there has been any change in the patient's lifestyle, e.g. a new job or hobby or a change in sporting activity or training schedule. The stage of the condition is established by asking whether the symptoms are getting better, staying the same or getting worse.

The clinician ascertains whether the patient has had this problem previously. If so, how many episodes has s/he had? When were they? What was the cause? What was the duration of each episode? And did the patient fully recover between episodes? If there is no previous history, has the patient had any episodes of pain and/ or stiffness in the lumbar spine, hip, knee, foot, ankle or any other relevant region?

To confirm the relationship between the symptoms, the clinician asks what happened to other symptoms when each symptom began. Symptoms which came on at the same time may indicate that the areas of symptoms are related. This evidence is further strengthened if there is a subjective relationship (symptoms come on at the same time or one is dependent on the other) and if the aggravating factors are the same or similar.

Has there been any treatment to date? The effectiveness of any previous treatment regime may help to guide patient management. Has the patient seen a specialist or had any investigations which may help with clinical diagnosis, such as blood tests, X-ray or magnetic resonance imaging (MRI)?

The mechanism of injury gives the clinician some important clues as to the injured structure in the knee, particularly in the acute stage, when a full physical examination may not be possible. For example, pain on twisting, catching one's foot or rising from a crouched position may indicate a meniscal injury (Drosos & Pozo 2004; McHale et al. 2014), whilst an ACL rupture may be suspected following an injury that involved rotation of the body on a fixed foot followed by immediate swelling (Wagemakers et al. 2010). Such an injury may be (but not always) accompanied by a pop or cracking sound (Casteleyn et al. 1988). The possible diagnoses suspected from the mechanism of injury are given in Table 15.1.

Past Medical History

A detailed medical history is vitally important to identify certain precautions or contraindications to the physical examination and/or treatment (see Table 2.4). As mentioned in Chapter 2, the clinician must differentiate between conditions that are suitable for conservative treatment and systemic, neoplastic and other non-musculoskeletal conditions, which require referral to a medical practitioner.

The following information is routinely obtained from patients.

General Health

The clinician ascertains the state of the patient's general health and finds out if the patient suffers from any malaise, fatigue, fever, nausea or vomiting, stress, anxiety or depression.

Weight Loss. Has the patient noticed any recent unexplained weight loss?

Serious Pathology. Does the patient have a history of serious pathology such as cancer, tuberculosis, osteomyelitis or human immunodeficiency virus (HIV)?

TABLE 15.1
The Possible Diagnoses Suspected From the Mechanism of Injury (Adapted From Magee 1997; Hayes et al. 2000)

Mechanism of Injury	Possible Structures Injured	Comments
Hyperflexion	Posterior horn of medial and/or lateral meniscus ACL	May complain of locking
Prolonged flexion	Posterior horn of medial and/or lateral meniscus	Particularly in older patients. May complain of locking
Hyperextension	Anterior tibial and/or femoral condyles PCL, ACL Posterior capsule Fat pad	Cruciate injury may result from tibial translation anteriorly (ACL) or posteriorly (PCL)
Valgus	Lateral tibial and/or femoral condyles MCL, ACL, PCL	Cruciate injury with severe force
Varus	Medial tibial and/or femoral condyles LCL, ITB	Uncommon
Flexion valgus without rotation	Lateral tibial and/or femoral condyles MCL Patellar subluxation/dislocation	
Flexion valgus with rotation	Lateral tibial and/or femoral condyles MCL, ACL Medial and/or lateral menisci Patellar subluxation/dislocation	Common injury. Immediate swelling (haemarthrosis) with a pop may suggest ACL rupture. Meniscal injury may present with locking
Flexion varus without rotation	Medial tibial and/or femoral condyles ACL, posterolateral corner Medial and/or lateral menisci	Meniscal injury may present with locking
Extension with valgus	Anterolateral tibial and/or femoral condyles MCL, PCL Posteromedial corner	
Extension with varus	Anteromedial tibial and/or femoral condyles ACL Posterolateral corner Popliteal tendon	May lead to unstable posterolateral corner injury
Flexion with posterior tibial translation (dashboard injury)	PCL posterior dislocation with severe force resulting in posterior instability ± patellar, proximal tibial and/or tibial plateau fracture	Most common mechanism for isolated PCL injury

ACL, anterior cruciate ligament; ITB, iliotibial band; LCL, lateral collateral ligament; MCL, medial collateral ligament; PCL, posterior cruciate ligament;

Inflammatory Arthritis. Has the patient been diagnosed as having an inflammatory condition such as rheumatoid arthritis or polymyalgia rheumatica? Does the patient have any features of a systemic inflammatory process such as psoriasis, dry eyes (iritis) or irritable-bowel problems?

Family History

Is there any relevant family history such as serious pathology or inflammatory arthritis?

Cardiovascular Disease

Is there a history of cardiac disease, e.g. angina? Does the patient have a pacemaker? If the patient has raised blood pressure, is it controlled with medication?

Respiratory Disease

Does the patient have a history of lung pathology? How is it controlled?

Diabetes

Does the patient suffer from diabetes? If so, is it type 1 or type 2 diabetes? Is the patient's blood glucose controlled? How is it controlled: through diet, tablet or injection? Patients with diabetes may develop peripheral neuropathy and vasculopathy, are at increased risk of infection and may take longer to heal than those without diabetes.

Epilepsy

Is the patient epileptic? When was the last seizure?

Thyroid Disease

Does the patient have a history of thyroid disease? Hypothyroidism can cause proximal muscle myopathy in 29–75% of patients (Anwar & Gibofsky 2010). Symptoms may include proximal muscle weakness, stiffness and cramping.

Osteoporosis

Has the patient had a dual-energy X-ray absorptiometry (DEXA) scan, been diagnosed with osteoporosis or sustained frequent fractures?

Previous Surgery

Has the patient had previous surgery which may be of relevance to the presenting complaint?

Drug History

What medications are being taken by the patient? Has the patient ever been prescribed long-term (6 months or more) medication? Particular attention may need to be paid to the following.

Steroids. Long-term use of steroids for conditions such as polymyalgia rheumatica or chronic lung disease may lead to an increased risk of osteoporosis.

Anticoagulants. Anticoagulant medication such as warfarin prescribed for conditions such as atrial fibrillation may cause an increased risk of bleeding and bruising.

Non-Steroidal Anti-Inflammatory Drugs (NSAIDs). NSAIDs such as ibruprofen have systemic effects which may lead to gastrointestinal bleeding in some patients. Use of such medications is not encouraged if they do not appear to be positively influencing the condition. Inflammatory nociceptive pain may however be relieved by NSAIDs.

Plan of the Physical Examination

When all this information has been collected, the subjective examination is complete. It is useful at this stage to highlight with asterisks (*), for ease of reference, important findings and particularly one or more functional restrictions. These can then be reexamined at subsequent treatment sessions to evaluate treatment intervention.

In order to plan the physical examination, the following hypotheses are developed from the subjective examination:

- Is each area of symptoms severe and/or irritable (see Chapter 2)? Will it be necessary to stop short of symptom reproduction, to reproduce symptoms partially or fully? If symptoms are severe, physical tests are carried out to just short of symptom production or to the very first onset of symptoms; no overpressures will be carried out, as the patient would be unable to tolerate this. If symptoms are irritable, physical tests are performed to just short of symptom production or just to the onset of symptoms, with fewer physical tests being performed to allow for a rest period between tests.

- What are the predominant pain mechanisms which might be driving the patient's symptoms? What are the active 'input mechanisms' (sensory pathways): are symptoms the product of a mechanical, inflammatory or ischaemic nociceptive process? What are the 'processing mechanisms': how has the patient processed this information, what are his or her thoughts and feelings about the pain? Finally, what are the 'output mechanisms': what is the patient's physiological, psychological and behavioural response to the pain? Clearly establishing which pain mechanisms may be causing and/or maintaining the condition will help the clinician manage both the condition and the patient appropriately. The reader is directed to Gifford (1998), Jones et al. (2002) and Thacker (2015) for further reading.

- What are the possible arthrogenic, myogenic and neurogenic structures which could be causing the patient's symptoms, i.e. what structures could refer to the area of pain and what structures are underneath the area of pain? For example, medial knee pain could theoretically be referred from the lumbar spine, the sacroiliac joint, the hip, the quadriceps and the hip adductors. The structures directly under the medial knee could also be implicated, for example, the medial collateral ligament (MCL), the medial meniscus, the medial compartment joint surfaces, the medial facet of the patellofemoral joint, the pes anserine tendon and the saphenous nerve.
- In addition, are there any contributing factors which could be maintaining the condition? These could be:
  - physical, e.g. weak hip lateral rotators causing medial femoral torsion
  - environmental, e.g. driving for a living
  - psychosocial, e.g. fear of serious pathology
  - behavioural, e.g. excessive rest in an attempt to help the area heal.
- The clinician decides, based on the evidence, which structures are most likely to be at fault and prioritizes the physical examination accordingly. It is helpful to organize structures into ones that 'must', 'should' and 'could' be tested on day 1 and over subsequent sessions. This will develop the clinician's clinical reasoning and avoid a recipe-based knee assessment. It is advisable where possible to clear an area fully. For example, if the clinician feels the lumbar spine needs to be excluded on day 1, s/he will fully assess this area leaving no stone unturned to implicate or negate this area as a source of symptoms. This approach will avoid juggling numerous potential sources of symptoms for several sessions, which may lead to confusion.
- Another way to develop the clinician's reasoning is to consider what to expect from each physical test. Will it be easy or hard to reproduce each symptom? Will it be necessary to use combined movements or repetitive movements? Will a particular test prove positive or negative? Will the pain be direction-specific? Synthesizing evidence from the subjective examination and in particular the aggravating and easing factors will provide substantial evidence as to what to expect in the physical examination.
  - Are there any precautions and/or contraindications to elements of the physical examination that need to be explored further, such as neurological involvement, recent fracture, trauma, steroid therapy or rheumatoid arthritis? There may also be certain contraindications to further examination and treatment, e.g. symptoms of spinal cord or cauda equina compression.

A physical planning form can be useful for clinicians to help guide them through the clinical reasoning process (see Fig. 2.9).

PHYSICAL EXAMINATION

The information from the subjective examination helps the clinician to plan an appropriate physical examination. The severity, irritability and nature of the condition are the major factors that will influence the choice and priority of physical testing procedures. The first and overarching question the clinician might ask is: 'Is this patient's condition suitable for me to manage as a clinician?' For example, a patient presenting with cauda equina compression symptoms may only need neurological integrity testing prior to an urgent medical referral. The nature of the patient's condition has had a major impact on the physical examination. The second question the clinician might ask is: 'Does this patient have a musculoskeletal dysfunction that I may be able to help?' To answer that, the clinician needs to carry out a full physical examination; however, this may not be possible if the symptoms are severe and/or irritable. If the patient's symptoms are severe and/or irritable, the clinician aims to explore movements as much as possible, within a symptom-free range. If the patient has constant and severe and/or irritable symptoms, then the clinician aims to find physical tests that ease the symptoms. If the patient's symptoms are non-severe and non-irritable, then the clinician aims to find physical tests that reproduce each of the patient's symptoms.

Each significant physical test that either provokes or eases the patient's symptoms is highlighted in the patient's notes by an asterisk (*) for easy reference. The highlighted tests are often referred to as 'asterisks' or 'markers'.

The order and detail of the physical tests described below need to be appropriate to the patient being examined; some tests will be irrelevant, some tests will be carried out briefly, while it will be necessary to investigate others fully. It is important for the reader to understand that not all physical tests are equal and that the reliability, sensitivity and specificity will vary markedly between tests (see Chapter 3). The author has chosen to present the most clinically useful tests according to the literature. None of these physical tests should however take the place of a thorough subjective examination. The clinician needs to have a clear clinical hypothesis after the subjective examination and the purpose of the physical examination is to confirm or refute this hypothesis.

Observation

Informal Observation

The clinician needs to observe the patient in dynamic and static situations; the quality of movement is noted, as are the postural characteristics and facial expression. Informal observation will have begun from the moment the clinician begins the subjective examination and will continue to the end of the physical examination.

Formal Observation

This is particularly useful in helping to determine the presence of intrinsic predisposing factors.

Observation of Posture. The clinician examines the patient's lower-limb posture in standing and where necessary in functional positions related to the patient's complaint. Abnormalities include internal femoral rotation, enlarged tibial tubercle (seen in Osgood–Schlatter disease), genu varum/valgum/recurvatum, medial/lateral tibial torsion and excessive foot pronation. Genu valgum and genu varum are identified by measuring the distance between the ankles and the distance between the femoral medial epicondyles respectively. Normally, medial tibial torsion is associated with genu varum and lateral tibial torsion with genu valgum (Magee 2014).

Internal femoral rotation due to insufficient gluteal function is a common finding with patients with patellofemoral pain and can cause squinting of the patella and an increased Q angle. There may be abnormal positioning of the patella, such as a medial/lateral glide, a lateral tilt, an anteroposterior tilt, a medial/lateral rotation or any combination of these positions. An enlarged fat pad is usually associated with hyperextension of the knees and poor quadriceps control, particularly eccentric inner range (0–20° of flexion).

The clinician can palpate the talus medially and laterally; both aspects will normally be equally prominent in the midposition of the subtalar joint. If the medial aspect of the talus is more prominent, this suggests that the subtalar joint is in pronation. The position of the calcaneus and talus can be examined: if the subtalar joint is pronated the calcaneus would be expected to be everted. Any abnormality will require further examination, as described in the section on palpation, below. In addition, the clinician notes whether there is even weight bearing through the left and right legs. The clinician passively corrects any asymmetry to determine its relevance to the patient's problem.

It is worth remembering that pure postural dysfunction rarely influences one region of the body in isolation and it may be necessary to observe the patient more fully for a full postural examination.

The clinician examines dynamic postures related to the patient's presenting complaint such as squatting, walking or climbing stairs. If the aggravating factors suggest pain occurs when weight bearing and walking, for example, the clinician observes that particular activity meticulously and if possible tries to establish at which phase of the gait cycle pain occurs. Observation of gait may reveal, for example, excessive pelvic rotation (about a horizontal plane) associated with anterior pelvic tilt. This may be due to hyperextension of the knees and limited extension and external rotation of the hip. It may be possible at this stage to modify the activity to see if symptoms change by, for example, adjusting pelvic rotation. The reader is directed to the section on symptom modification, below, to explore this concept further.

Observation of Muscle Form. The clinician observes the muscle bulk and muscle tone of the patient, comparing left and right sides. It must be remembered that the level and frequency of physical activity as well as the dominant side may well produce differences in muscle bulk between sides. Some muscles are thought to shorten under stress, while other muscles weaken, producing muscle imbalance (see Table 3.7).

Observation of Soft Tissues. The clinician observes the quality and colour of the patient's skin, any area of swelling, joint effusion or presence of scarring, and takes cues for further examination.

Observation of Balance. Balance is provided by vestibular, visual and proprioceptive information. This rather crude and non-specific test is conducted by asking the patient to stand on one leg with the eyes open and then closed. If the patient's balance is as poor with the eyes open as with the eyes closed, this suggests a vestibular or proprioceptive dysfunction (rather than a visual dysfunction). The test is carried out on the affected and unaffected sides; if there is greater difficulty maintaining balance on the affected side, this may indicate some proprioceptive dysfunction.

Observation of Gait. Analyse gait on even/uneven ground, slopes, stairs and running. Note the stride length and weight-bearing ability. Inspect the feet, shoes and any walking aids.

Joint Effusion Tests

The clinician firstly checks for a knee joint effusion, which may not be necessary if a large effusion is obvious. It is important to distinguish between soft-tissue swelling, which may be localized and superficial, for example, in the presence of a low-grade MCL sprain, and swelling within the joint, which may represent a more significant intraarticular injury, e.g. an ACL rupture.

Patellar Tap Test

With the patient lying supine, the clinician adds pressure across the suprapatellar pouch with one hand which will squeeze fluid under the patella. With the other hand the clinician applies a light downward force to the patella which, in the presence of an effusion, will feel as if it is 'floating' and may 'tap' against the underlying femoral condyles. Data on the reliability of the patella tap is conflicting so the test needs to be used with caution. Interobserver reliability may range from poor to good, whilst intraobserver reliability appears to be poor (Maricar et al. 2015).

Sweep Test

This test is also known as the brush or stroke test. Interobserver reliability of this test for the presence or absence of an effusion appears to be moderate to excellent (Maricar et al. 2015). With the patient lying supine, the clinician uses the palm of one hand to sweep fluid proximally up the medial side of the knee into the suprapatellar pouch. The other hand is then used to sweep distally down the lateral side of the knee. In the presence of an effusion a small bulge of fluid appears on the medial side of the knee.

Joint Integrity Tests

For all of the joint integrity tests below, a positive test is indicated by excessive movement relative to the unaffected side.

Collateral Stability Tests

The collateral stability tests examine the integrity of the medial and lateral structures of the knee. They comprise the valgus and varus stress tests.

Valgus Stress Tests. With the patient supine, the clinician palpates the medial joint line of the knee and applies a valgus force to 'gap' the medial aspect of the knee. The clinician may perform this test with the knee in full extension and in 20–30° flexion (Fig. 15.1); the clinician compares the left- and right-knee range of movement; excessive movement would be considered a positive test. If the test is positive in slight flexion but negative in full extension, a partial MCL tear is suspected, whilst a test which is positive in both flexion and extension may suggest a complete MCL rupture with possible posteromedial corner and anterior and/or posterior cruciate ligament injury (Kurzweil & Kelley 2006).

As well as the pure tests described above, it may be beneficial to explore valgus stress testing with and/or through varying degrees of flexion, extension and rotation. Although moving away from the more standardized tests may reduce the validity and reliability of the technique, in some patients, thinking outside the narrow confines of the tests as described may help the clinician reproduce mild symptoms or establish a

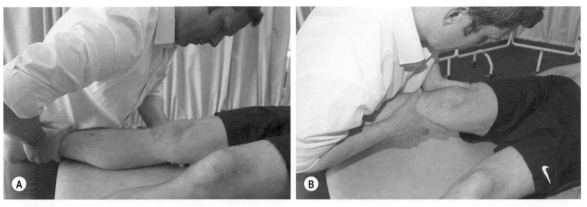

Fig. 15.1 ■ Valgus stress test with the knee in (A) extension and (B) some flexion.

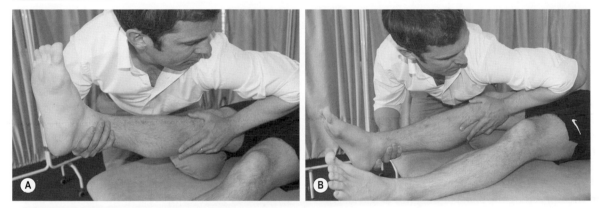

Fig. 15.2 ■ Varus stress test with the knee in (A) extension and (B) some flexion.

physical marker. Such variations may even be helpful as treatment techniques.

Varus Stress Tests. With the patient supine, the clinician palpates the lateral joint line and applies a varus force to 'gap' the lateral aspect of the knee. The clinician may perform this test with the knee in full extension and in 20–30° flexion (Fig. 15.2). The clinician compares the left- and right-knee range of movement; excessive movement would be considered a positive test. If the test is positive in slight flexion, as well as the lateral collateral ligament, the test may suggest injury to the posterolateral capsule, arcuate–popliteus complex, iliotibial band (ITB) and biceps femoris tendon. A positive test in full extension may implicate the lateral collateral ligament, posterolateral capsule,

the arcuate–popliteus complex, anterior and posterior cruciate ligaments and lateral gastrocnemius muscle (Magee 2014).

Again, as with the valgus stress test, in some patients it may be helpful to explore this test with and/or through varying degrees of flexion, extension and rotation.

Anterior Stability Tests

The anterior stability tests principally examine the integrity of the ACL. Several recent systematic reviews have examined the literature pertaining to the diagnostic accuracy and reliability of physical tests for the integrity of the ACL (Swain et al. 2014; Lange et al. 2015; Leblanc et al. 2015; Anderson et al. 2016). The tests presented include the Lachman test, the anterior

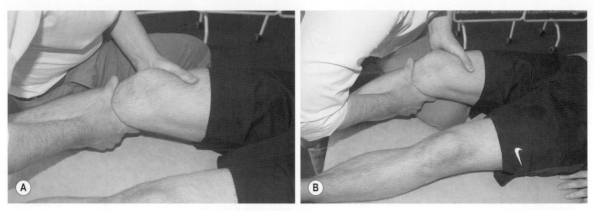

Fig. 15.3 ■ (A) Lachman test. The clinician stabilizes the femur with the left hand and with the right hand applies a postero-anterior force to the tibia. (B) Modified Lachman test. The patient's knee rests over the clinican's thigh and is stabilized by the left hand. The right hand applies a posteroanterior force to the tibia.

drawer test and the pivot shift. Because these tests have different strengths and weaknesses, the clinician is advised to use the tests in combination.

Lachman Test. The Lachman test is primarily a test for the integrity of the ACL, although the posterior oblique ligament and the arcuate–popliteus complex may also be stressed (Magee 2014). With the patient in supine and with the knee flexed (0–30°), the clinician stabilizes the femur and applies a posteroanterior force to the tibia along the plane of the joint (Fig. 15.3A). A positive test is indicated by a soft end-feel and excessive motion. The Lachman test appears to have the highest intrarater reliability of all the ACL tests, although the interrater reliability appears less clear (Lange et al. 2015). Despite this, a positive Lachman test has consistently been shown to be the strongest physical indicator of ACL rupture (Jonsson et al. 1982; Katz & Fingeroth 1986; Mitsou & Vallianatos 1988; Ostrowski 2006; Swain et al. 2014; Leblanc et al. 2015; Anderson et al. 2016). The sensitivity of the test appears reasonable in the detection of partial ruptures (68%), good in the detection of all rupture types (89%) and excellent in the detection of complete ruptures (96%: Leblanc et al. 2015). The specificity of the test also seems reasonable at 78.1% (Beldame et al. 2011). The test has its disadvantages, however, as it can be technically difficult, especially if the clinician has small hands or the patient has a particularly large leg. In such circumstances, one modification which may help is for

the patient to rest the knee over the clinician's thigh, as shown in Fig. 15.3B. This will stabilize the knee, take some of the leg's weight and allow the patient's muscles to relax fully.

Anterior Drawer Test. The anterior drawer test is similar to the Lachman test but is carried out with the knee flexed to 90°. This test is easier to perform than the Lachman test but appears inferior. The reliability of the test is uncertain (Lange et al. 2015), the sensitivity appears poor compared to the Lachman at 55%, although the specificity appears good at 92% (Benjaminse et al. 2006). The clinician applies the same posteroanterior force to the tibia along the plane of the joint, feeling the movement of the tibia anteriorly and any contraction of the hamstring muscle group, which may oppose the movement (Fig. 15.4). Sitting on the patient's foot may help to stabilize the leg. A positive test, indicated by a soft end-feel and excessive motion, may indicate injury to the ACL, posterior oblique ligament, arcuate–popliteus complex, posteromedial and posterolateral joint capsules, MCL and the ITB (Magee 2014). Again, exploring this test with other angles of knee flexion, and with internal or external tibial rotation, may be relevant and necessary for some patients. Varying the anterior drawer test to include internal and external tibial rotation is known as the Slocum test. With the addition of internal tibial rotation, excessive movement on the lateral aspect of the knee is thought to indicate anterolateral instability, whilst

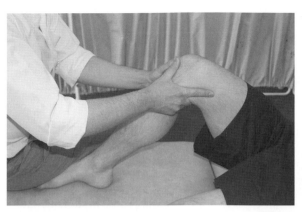

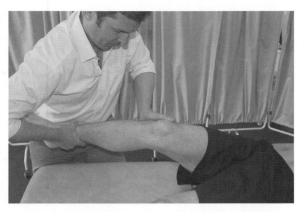

Fig. 15.4 ■ Anterior drawer test. With the knee at around 90° flexion the clinician sits lightly on the patient's foot to stabilize the leg. The fingers grasp around the posterior aspect of the calf to apply the posteroanterior force, while the thumbs rest over the anterior joint line to feel the movement.

Fig. 15.5 ■ Lateral pivot shift. The clinician applies an adduction stress to the lower leg with the left hand and the right hand passively moves the knee from extension to flexion, while maintaining the medial rotation of the lower leg.

excessive movement of the medial aspect of the knee with the addition of lateral rotation may represent anteromedial instability.

Pivot Shift Test. A further test for anterolateral stability and ACL integrity is the pivot shift test. This test exploits the fact that the ITB acts as a flexor in flexion and an extensor in extension. The patient lies supine with the hip slightly flexed and medially rotated and with the knee flexed. In the first part of the test, the lower leg is medially rotated at the knee and the clinician moves the knee into extension while applying a posteroanterior force to the fibula. The tibia subluxes anteriorly when there is anterolateral instability as the ITB draws the tibia anteriorly. In the second part of the test, the clinician applies an adduction stress to the lower leg and passively moves the knee from extension to flexion while maintaining the medial rotation of the lower leg (Fig. 15.5). A positive test is indicated if at about 20–40° of knee flexion the tibia 'jogs' backward as the ITB draws the tibia posteriorly (reduction of the subluxation). This will often reproduce the patient's feeling of the knee 'giving way'.

Although a difficult test to master, the pivot shift test is the most specific of all ACL integrity tests. In the awake patient, the specificity has been reported at 81% and when the patient is anaesthetized the specificity may be as high as 98% (van Eck et al. 2013). The sensitivity is reasonable but inferior to the Lachman, at

86% for complete ruptures (Leblanc et al. 2015). The reliability of the test is difficult to determine from the available studies (Lange et al. 2015).

Posterior Stability Tests

The posterior stability tests examine the integrity of the posterior structures of the knee, including the posterior cruciate ligament and the posterolateral corner. The tests presented are the posterior drawer test and the dial test.

Posterior Drawer Test. Although a commonly performed test, the true diagnostic accuracy of the posterior drawer test is yet to be established (Kopkow et al. 2013). The test is typically carried out with the knee flexed to 90°. The clinician first inspects the knee to check the tibia is not sagging posteriorly and then applies an anteroposterior force to the tibia (Fig. 15.6). A positive test is indicated by excessive motion due to injury of one or more of the following structures: posterior cruciate ligament, arcuate–popliteus complex, posterior oblique ligament and ACL (Magee 2014). If the clinician inadvertently performs the test on a tibia which is already sagging posteriorly, due to injury of the aforementioned structures, the test may appear falsely negative.

As mentioned in previous tests, exploring the posterior drawer test in different angles of knee flexion, and with internal or external tibial rotation, may be

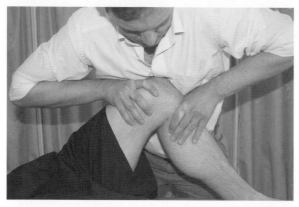

Fig. 15.6 ■ Posterior drawer test. With the knee at around 90° flexion, the right hand supports the knee and the web space of the left hand applies an anteroposterior force to the tibia.

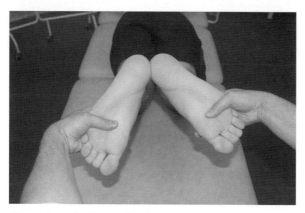

Fig. 15.7 ■ Dial test. The clinician externally rotates both tibia at both 30° and 90°.

relevant and necessary for some patients. The addition of external tibial rotation during the posterior drawer test may be useful to check for posterolateral instability, which would be indicated by excessive movement at the lateral aspect of the tibia (Bonadio et al. 2014).

Dial Test. A further test to assess for posterolateral instability is the dial test (Fig. 15.7). During this test the patient may lie supine or prone and the clinician externally rotates the tibia at both 30° and 90°. Increased rotation compared with the uninjured side at 30° but not 90° may indicate posterolateral corner instability, whilst increased rotation at 30° and 90° may indicate injury to both the posterolateral corner and posterior

cruciate ligament (Magee 2014). The reliability and validity of the dial test are uncertain so the test should be used with caution and reference should be made to the subjective history when diagnosing posterolateral instability.

Meniscal Tests

Not all meniscal tears are the same. Radial tears, meniscal root tears and flap tears can have a devastating effect on meniscal function, yet degenerate tears, particularly in the middle-aged or older person, appear to be an entirely normal finding in asymptomatic knees (Guermazi et al. 2012). Randomized controlled trials indicate that osteoarthritis and degenerate meniscal tears may respond no better to arthroscopic intervention than to sham surgery or conservative management (Moseley et al. 2002; Kirkley et al. 2008; Herrlin et al. 2013; Sihvonen et al. 2013), even in the presence of mechanical symptoms (Sihvonen et al. 2016). Although the following tests may be useful in detecting meniscal lesions, a degree of caution is advised because not all meniscal tears are symptomatic. The tests presented are the McMurray test, the Thessaly test and joint line tenderness.

McMurray Test

During the McMurray test, the medial meniscus is typically tested using a combination of knee flexion/extension with lateral rotation of the tibia whilst compressing the medial compartment. The clinician palpates the medial joint line and passively flexes and then laterally rotates the knee so that the posterior part of the medial meniscus is rotated with the tibia – a 'snap' of the joint may occur if the meniscus is torn. The knee is then moved from this fully flexed position to 90° flexion, so the whole of the posterior part of the meniscus is tested (Fig. 15.8). A positive test occurs if the clinician feels a click, which may be heard, indicating a tear of the medial meniscus (McMurray 1942). The test is then repeated to bias the lateral meniscus, this time using a combination of knee flexion/extension with medial rotation of the tibia whilst compressing the lateral compartment (Fig. 15.9). A recent systematic review has calculated the sensitivity of the McMurray test to be 61% with a specificity of 84% (Smith et al. 2015).

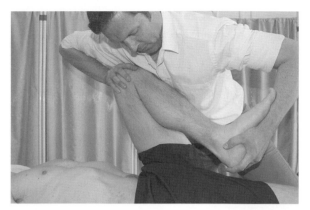

Fig. 15.8 ■ Medial meniscus. The right hand supports the knee and palpates the medial joint line. The left hand laterally rotates the lower leg and moves the knee from full flexion to extension.

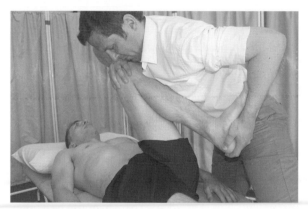

Fig. 15.9 ■ Lateral meniscus. The right hand supports the knee and palpates the lateral joint line. The left hand medially rotates the lower leg and moves the knee from full flexion to extension.

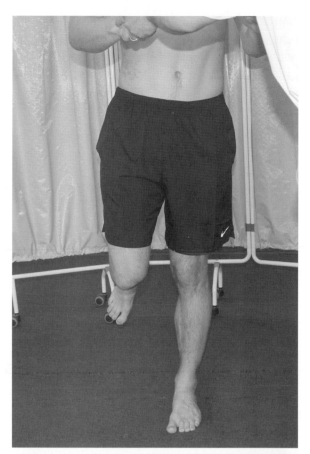

Fig. 15.10 ■ Thessaly test. With the patient standing on one leg with support at the hands for balance, the clinician guides the patient around to full external rotation and then full internal rotation at the knee. This movement is repeated three times at 5° of flexion and three further times at 20° of flexion.

Clinicians vary in performing this test; they may, for example, internally and externally rotate the tibia while moving the knee from full flexion to extension. The key is to explore both the medial and lateral compartments fully. It is worth noting that tears most commonly occur at the posterior horns of the menisci. Most positive findings during the McMurray test therefore occur towards end-of-range flexion when the menisci are maximally loaded.

Thessaly Test

The Thessaly test is a relatively new orthopaedic test (Karachalios et al. 2005) with a fairly high sensitivity (75%) and specificity (87%: Smith et al. 2015). The Thessaly test is performed at 5° and 20° of flexion. The patient is asked to stand on the symptomatic leg with the arms outstretched and support from the clinician at the hands. The clinician guides the patient around to full external rotation and then full internal rotation at the knee (Fig. 15.10). This movement is repeated three times at 5° of flexion and three further times at 20° for flexion. A positive test is indicated by the reproduction of medial or lateral joint line pain, or a sense of locking or catching (Karachalios et al. 2005). The Thessaly test is a valid quick and easy test that does not require significant skill to perform on the part of the clinician.

Joint Line Tenderness

Palpation of the medial and lateral joint lines should not be overlooked when suspicious of a meniscal tear. Although joint line palpation is used as an adjunct to, and not a replacement for, the McMurray or the Thessaly test, it is of note that joint line tenderness in itself has a sensitivity of 83% and a specificity of 83% (Smith et al. 2015). Such tenderness could of course also be emanating from structures other than the meniscus, e.g. the MCL, but the index of suspicion may be heightened if, for example, valgus stress testing were negative and the MCL proximal and distal to the joint line was painfree.

Patellofemoral Tests

Unfortunately no patellofemoral tests have demonstrated significant diagnostic accuracy (Nijs et al. 2006; Cook et al. 2012). The Clarke and Fairbank tests are presented below for completeness but patellofemoral pain is primarily a diagnosis made during the subjective assessment. The clinician is encouraged to explore symptom modification in the diagnosis and management of patellofemoral pain as the condition is invariably multifactorial (see the section on symptom modification, below).

Clarke Test

The Clarke test is of limited value as this test is often provocative to some degree in the asymptomatic population. Thankfully, patellofemoral pain usually offers the clinician strong subjective clues from which to build a clinical hypothesis, such as pain descending stairs, and provocation tests should be seen as the icing on the cake of the assessment.

The Clarke test is possibly the most widely used patellofemoral provocation test together with palpation of the patellar facets, which can be partially palpated by gliding the patella medially and laterally. With the patient lying supine or in long sitting and the knee in full extension, the clinician places the web space of one hand just superior to the patella and applies a gentle downward and caudad force (Fig. 15.11). The patient is then instructed to contract the quadriceps by pushing the back of the knee into the bed. The test is positive if pain is reproduced. As the test is often painful in the absence of patellofemoral dysfunction,

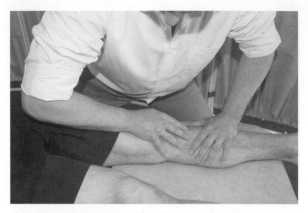

Fig. 15.11 ▪ Clarke test. The clinician places the web space of the right hand just superior to the patella and applies a gentle downward and caudad force. The patient then contracts the quadriceps.

the clinician needs to be aware of the falsely positive test and when positive it is helpful to ask the patient, 'Was that your pain?'

Fairbank's Apprehension Test

This is considered a test for patellar subluxation or dislocation. It is typically carried out with the patient's knee in 30° of flexion; the clinician passively moves the patella laterally and a positive test is indicated by pain, apprehension of the patient and/or excessive movement (Nijs et al. 2006). There may also be a reflex contraction of the quadriceps in the presence of instability. It may be necessary and relevant for some patients to test the patellar glide with the knee in other angles of knee flexion.

Active Physiological Movements

Active physiological movements of the knee include flexion, extension, medial rotation of the tibia and lateral rotation of the tibia (Table 15.2). The primary movements of flexion and extension are tested bilaterally with the patient in supine. Movements of flexion and extension are overpressed if symptoms allow (Fig. 15.12). Tibial rotation can be readily tested with the patient in sitting, although clinically it is unusual to find an isolated rotation dysfunction.

The clinician establishes the patient's symptoms at rest, prior to each movement, and passively corrects any movement deviation to determine its relevance to the patient's symptoms. The following are noted:

- quality of movement
- range of movement
- behaviour of pain through the range of movement
- resistance through the range of movement and at the end of the range of movement
- provocation of any muscle spasm.

In a similar way to the manipulation of a symptomatic physical task (see the section on symptom modification, below), the thoughtful clinician may be able to manipulate physiological movements to help differentiate between tissues. For example, when knee flexion in prone reproduces the patient's anterior knee pain, differentiation between knee joint, anterior thigh muscles and neural tissues may be required. Adding a compression force through the lower leg will stress the knee joint without particularly altering the muscle length or neural tissue. If symptoms are increased, this would suggest that the knee joint (patellofemoral or tibiofemoral joint) may be the source of the symptoms.

It may be necessary to examine other regions to determine their relevance to the patient's symptoms; they may be the source of the symptoms, or they may be contributing to the symptoms. The most likely regions are the lumbar spine, sacroiliac joint, hip, foot and ankle. These regions can be quickly screened; see Chapter 3 for further details. Contrary to what their name might suggest, however, performing a clearing test on the lumbar spine, for example, does not fully negate this region as a source of symptoms and if there is any doubt the clinician is advised to assess the suspected area fully (see relevant chapter).

Passive Physiological Movements

All of the active movements described above can be examined passively with the patient in supine, comparing left and right sides. Comparison of the response of symptoms to the active and passive movements can help to determine whether the structure at fault is non-contractile (articular) or contractile (extra-articular) (Cyriax 1982). If the lesion is non-contractile,

TABLE 15.2	
Active Physiological Movements With Possible Modifications	

Active Physiological Movements	Modifications
Knee flexion	Repeated
Knee extension	Speed altered
Medial rotation of the knee	Combined, e.g.
Lateral rotation of the knee	■ Flexion with internal rotation
?Lumbar spine	Compression or distraction
?Sacroiliac joint	Sustained
?Hip	Injuring movement
?Foot and ankle	Differentiation tests
	Function

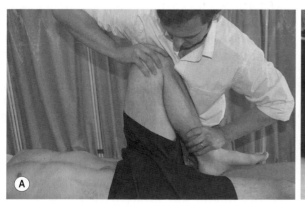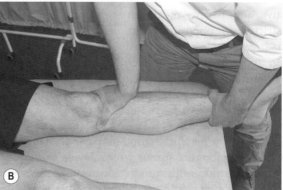

Fig. 15.12 ■ Overpressures to the knee. (A) Flexion. One hand supports the knee while the other hand applies overpressure to flexion. (B) Extension. One hand stabilizes the tibia while the other hand lifts the lower leg into extension.

Reflex Testing. The following deep tendon reflexes are tested and are shown in Chapter 3:

- L3–L4: knee jerk
- S1: ankle jerk.

Neurodynamic Tests

The following neurodynamic tests may be carried out in order to ascertain the degree to which neural tissue is responsible for the production of the patient's symptom(s):

- passive neck flexion
- straight-leg raise
- passive knee bend
- slump.

These tests are described in detail in Chapter 3.

Palpable nerves around the knee region are as follows:

- The common peroneal nerve can be palpated medial to the tendon of biceps femoris and also around the head of the fibula.
- The tibial nerve can be palpated centrally over the posterior knee crease medial to the popliteal artery; it can also be felt behind the medial malleolus, which is more noticeable with the foot in dorsiflexion and eversion.

Miscellaneous Tests

Vascular Tests

If the circulation is suspected of being compromised, the clinician palpates the pulses of the femoral, tibial, popliteal and dorsalis pedis arteries. The clinician then checks for skin and temperature changes, and capillary refill of the nail beds. The state of the vascular system can also be determined by the response of symptoms to positions of dependence and elevation of the lower limbs.

Leg Length

True leg length, which tends to be congenital, is measured from the anterior superior iliac spine to the medial or lateral malleolus. Apparent leg length, which results from compensatory change, such as a pronated foot or spinal scoliosis, is measured from the umbilicus to the medial or lateral malleolus. A difference in leg length of up to 1–1.5 cm is considered normal (Magee 2014).

Palpation

The clinician palpates the knee region and any other relevant areas. It is useful to record palpation findings on a body chart (see Fig. 2.3) and/or palpation chart (see Fig. 3.35).

The clinician notes the following:

- the temperature of the area
- localized increased skin moisture
- the presence of oedema or effusion – the clinician examines with the patellar tap and sweep test to assess if joint effusion is present. The circumference of the limb or joint can be measured with a tape measure and left and right sides compared
- mobility and feel of superficial tissues, e.g. ganglions, nodules, scar tissue
- the presence or elicitation of any muscle spasm
- tenderness of bone (the upper pole of the patella and the femoral condyle may be tender in plica syndrome, while the undersurface of the patella may be tender with patellofemoral joint problems), bursae (prepatellar, infrapatellar), ligaments, muscle, tendon, tendon sheath, trigger points (shown in Fig. 3.36) and nerve
- increased or decreased prominence of bones – observe the position of the patella in terms of glide, lateral tilt, anteroposterior tilt and rotation on the femoral condyles (see below). The quadriceps (Q) angle can be measured. It is the angle formed by the intersection of the line of pull of the quadriceps muscle and the patellar tendon measured through the centre of the patella. The normal outer value is considered to be in the region of 15°. An increased Q angle has been proposed to lead to an increased lateralization force on the patella, which may lead to pain or dislocation; however, this measure does not appear as useful as once thought. Indeed, the literature suggests an increased Q angle does not adequately 'distinguish between pathological and non-pathological knees' (Smith et al. 2013)
- pain provoked or reduced on palpation.

Increased or Decreased Prominence of Bones

The optimal position of the patella is thought to be one in which the patella is parallel to the femur in the frontal and sagittal planes and the patella is midway between the two condyles of the femur when the knee is slightly flexed (Grelsamer & McConnell 1998). Patellofemoral pain has been linked to increased lateralization of the patella leading to increased stress on the lateral facet (Heino Brechter & Powers 2002; Farrokhi et al. 2011; Lack et al. 2015). Often these stresses result from biomechanical causes such as a pronated foot or weak proximal musculature causing internal rotation of the femur and tibia. Such forces may alter the tracking of the patella, causing increased lateral translation, tilt and rotation (Herrington 2008; Draper et al. 2009; Wilson et al. 2009; Souza et al. 2010; Lack et al. 2015). The reader is directed to the section on symptom modification, below, to explore further the assessment of patellofemoral pain. There is evidence to suggest that assessment of patellar position, particularly by an experienced clinician, has good intratester reliability and moderate to good criterion validity when compared to MRI (McEwan et al. 2007; Smith et al. 2009).

In terms of the position of the patella, the following may be noted:

■ The base of the patella normally lies equidistant (±5 mm) from the medial and lateral femoral epicondyles when the knee is flexed 20°. If the patella lies closer to the medial or lateral femoral epicondyle, it is considered to have a medial or lateral glide respectively. The clinician also needs to test for any lateral glide of the patella on quadriceps contraction. The clinician palpates the left and right base of the patella and the vastus medialis obliquus (VMO) and vastus lateralis with thumbs and fingers, respectively, while the patient is asked to extend the knee. In some cases the patella is felt to glide laterally, indicating a dynamic problem, and VMO may be felt to contract after vastus lateralis; VMO is normally thought to be activated simultaneously with, or slightly earlier than, vastus lateralis. Quite a large difference will be needed to enable the clinician to feel a difference in the timing of muscle contraction.

■ The lateral tilt is calculated by measuring the distance of the medial and lateral borders of the patella from the femur. The patella is considered to have a lateral tilt, for example, when the distance is decreased on the lateral aspect and increased on the medial aspect such that the patella faces laterally. A lateral tilt is considered to be due to a tight lateral retinaculum (superficial and deep fibres) and ITB. When a passive medial glide is first applied (see below), the patellar tilt may be accentuated, indicating a dynamic tilt problem implicating a tight lateral retinaculum (deep fibres).

■ The anteroposterior tilt is calculated by measuring the distance from the inferior and superior poles of the patella to the femur. Posterior tilt of the patella occurs if the inferior pole lies more posteriorly than the superior pole and may lead to fat pad irritation and inferior patellar pain. Dynamic control of a posterior patellar tilt is tested by asking the patient to brace the knee back and observing the movement of the tibia. With a positive patellar tilt the foot moves away from the couch and the proximal end of the tibia is seen to move posteriorly; this movement is thought to pull the inferior pole of the patella into the fat pad.

■ Rotation is the relative position of the long axis of the patella to the femur, and is normally parallel. The patella is considered to be laterally rotated if the inferior pole of the patella is placed laterally to the long axis of the femur. A lateral or medial rotation of the patella is considered to be due to tightness of part of the retinaculum. The most common abnormality seen in patellofemoral pain is both a lateral tilt and a lateral rotation of the patella, which is thought to be due to an imbalance of the medial (weakness of VMO) and lateral structures (tightness of the lateral retinaculum and/or weakness of vastus lateralis) of the patella (McConnell 1996).

■ Testing the length of the lateral retinaculum. With the patient in side-lying and the knee flexed approximately 20°, the clinician passively glides the patella in a medial direction. The patella will normally move sufficiently to expose the lateral femoral condyle; if this is not possible then tightness of the superficial retinaculum is suspected. The deep retinaculum is tested as above, but with the addition of an anteroposterior force to the medial border of the patella. The lateral border of the patella is normally able to move anteriorly away from the femur; inability may suggest tightness of the deep retinaculum.

Accessory Movements

It may be useful to use the palpation chart and movement diagrams (or joint pictures) to record findings. These are explained in detail in Chapter 3.

The clinician notes the following:

- quality of movement
- range of movement
- resistance through the range and at the end of the range of movement
- behaviour of pain through the range
- provocation of any muscle spasm.

Patellofemoral joint (Fig. 15.14), tibiofemoral joint (Fig. 15.15) and superior tibiofibular joint (Fig. 15.16) accessory movements are listed in Table 15.3. All movements can be explored in various degrees of flexion/extension and medial/lateral tibial rotation. The clinician reassesses all the physical asterisks (movements or tests that have been found to reproduce the patient's symptoms) following accessory movements, in order to establish the effect of the accessory movements on the patient's signs and symptoms. Accessory movements can then be tested for other regions suspected to be a source of, or contributing to, the patient's symptoms. Again, following accessory movements, the clinician reassesses all the asterisks. Regions likely to be examined are the lumbar spine, sacroiliac joint, hip, foot and ankle (Table 15.3).

Symptom Modification

It can be extremely useful to examine a symptomatic physical task specific to the patient's complaint. This functional task can then be modified and the patient's symptomatic response can be closely monitored. A suitable functional task may be replicated in the clinical setting and can often be identified when asking the patient about the aggravating factors. It may be useful to examine a functional task early in the assessment; this is for three reasons:

1. The task will provide a useful initial snapshot of the patient's problem.
2. It may be possible to manipulate the task to aid the clinical diagnosis and highlight possible treatment options (see the worked example below).
3. The task will provide a useful physical marker (*).

By manipulating the functional task in various ways to bias different tissues (which need not be time consuming), useful information may be gleaned as to the likely clinical diagnosis as well as the most appropriate way to manage the condition. Although the worked example below highlights the art of clinical reasoning in practice, it is important to emphasize that modifications to symptomatic functional tasks are not standardized tests and will therefore lack a degree of validity and reliability. There is a tradeoff here: on the one hand the clinician is being very patient-focused and examining the specific problem that prompted the patient to seek help in the first place, but on the other hand there is a lack of standardization. It is worth noting however that, even well-known orthopaedic tests may lack robust diagnostic accuracy or reliability. It may be wise to use both approaches in a clinical context as both have relative strengths and add to the clinical picture. As always, the clinician is encouraged to synthesize information from the whole subjective and physical examination to reach a reasoned view of the patient's condition, rather than placing too much emphasis on any one test.

A Worked Example of Symptom Modification: Anterior Knee Pain

Anterior knee pain is multifactorial (Lankhorst et al. 2012; Barton et al. 2015), leading to abnormal patellar stresses during functional tasks (Draper et al. 2009; Wilson et al. 2009; Souza et al. 2010; Farrokhi et al. 2011). Factors which may contribute to the generation of anterior knee pain may include:

- Local factors – these may include tight retinacular tissue or altered timing of the VMO

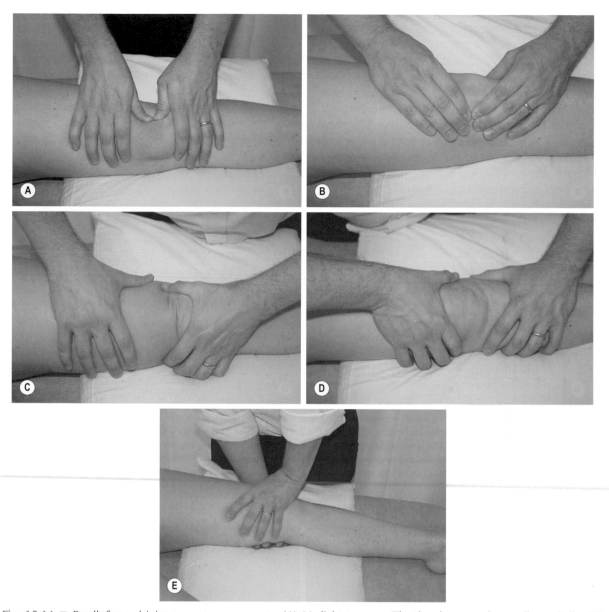

Fig. 15.14 ■ Patellofemoral joint accessory movements. (A) Medial transverse. The thumbs move the patella medially. (B) Lateral transverse. The fingers move the patella laterally. (C) Longitudinal cephalad. The left hand pushes the patella in a cephalad direction. (D) Longitudinal caudad. The right hand pushes the patella in a caudad direction. (E) Compression. The left hand rests over the anterior aspect of the patella and pushes the patella towards the femur.

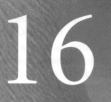

16

EXAMINATION OF THE FOOT AND ANKLE

ANDREA MOULSON

CHAPTER CONTENTS

THE FOOT AND ANKLE: AN OVERVIEW

The foot and ankle are a complex of 26 bones, a variable number of sesamoids (usually two) with 34 joints and over 100 muscles, tendons and ligaments, all supplied by three different peripheral nerves – the tibial, common peroneal and saphenous nerves. The main joints of the foot and ankle include the inferior tibiofibular, talocrural, subtalar, midtarsal, tarsometatarsal, intermetatarsal, metatarsophalangeal and interphalangeal joints and, classically, the foot is divided into the forefoot, midfoot and hindfoot (Table 16.1). The foot and ankle form part of the whole-body kinetic chain and combine flexibility with stability to facilitate two principal functions: propulsion and support. For propulsion, the foot and ankle act as a complex flexible lever; for support, it acts as a rigid structure that supports the entire body weight. Aligned with these functions the foot and ankle must also adapt to uneven terrain and provide for shock absorption during the gait cycle and other activities of daily living.

There are many musculoskeletal pathologies that can impact on the normal function of the foot and ankle; symptoms can arise from local sources or can be referred from other areas of the body or indeed may be the result of more systemic, preexisting conditions. Trauma is relatively common and can potentially result in significant dysfunction. For example, an ankle inversion sprain can cause fractures of the lateral malleolus or base of the fifth metatarsal, osteochondral defects affecting the talus, disruption of the inferior tibiofibular joint and lateral ligamentous complex

TABLE 16.1

Functional Units of the Foot

Rearfoot	Midfoot	Forefoot
Talocrural joint	Talonavicular joint	Tarsometatarsal joints
Subtalar joint	Calcaneocuboid joint	Metatarsophalangeal joint
		Interphalangeal joints

with resultant ankle instability. Alternatively, patients can present with traumatic or overuse tendinopathies such as tibialis posterior tendon dysfunction or Achilles tendinopathy or neural tissue sensitization associated with trauma, surgery, overuse, overload or entrapment. Other insidious-onset conditions, such as plantar fasciosis, metatarsalgia or Morton's neuroma, can significantly impact on activities of daily living, whilst more proximal conditions, such as lumbar spine dysfunction, can refer pain distally into the foot and ankle. Alternatively, systemic inflammatory conditions, such as rheumatoid arthritis (RA), ankylosing spondylosis (AS), gout and degenerative joint conditions such as osteoarthritis (OA), mean pain and the associated deformities can impact on the normal function of the foot and ankle. Other metabolic disorders such as diabetes may also significantly affect the foot, causing peripheral neuropathy, vascular compromise and specific disease such as Charcot disease. Hereditary predisposition to certain conditions has also been recognized, such as a familial link to hallux valgus and other lesser-toe deformities. In addition, other less commonly encountered upper motor neuron and lower motor neuron conditions, such as traumatic brain injury, stroke, spinal cord injury, cerebral palsy and Charcot–Marie–Tooth disease, can all have a significant impact on foot and ankle function. These examples are by no means exhaustive, but highlight the diversity of conditions which can affect the region.

In light of the foot and ankle's functional significance patients with specific conditions (or postsurgery) may be managed by a dedicated foot and ankle therapy team which could include orthopaedic consultants, physiotherapists, chiropodists and podiatrists with additional skills, including surgery, wound management, injections and orthotic provision. A thorough working knowledge of anatomy and biomechanics and an appreciation of the functional role of the foot and ankle will help inform clinical reasoning, ensuring that the initial examination is efficient and management strategies seek to optimize all aspects of functional restoration.

SUBJECTIVE EXAMINATION

Further details of the questions asked during the subjective examination and the tests carried out in the physical examination can be found in Chapters 2 and 3, respectively.

The order of subjective questioning and the physical tests described below needs to be justified through sound clinical reasoning and altered as appropriate for the patient being examined.

Patients' Perspectives on Their Experience

Most patients will seek treatment because they have symptoms and/or functional limitations which are impacting on their activities of daily living, for example, pain, paraesthesia, swelling and/or difficulty with weight-bearing activities. Sometimes patients experience difficulty finding comfortable footwear or the aesthetic appearance of the foot alone or in combination with other symptoms is troublesome, and this may affect patient psychological well-being. Examples of this maybe progressive hallux valgus or claw/hammer-toe deformities. An understanding of the patient's primary concerns and context, e.g. social/work requirements, will guide the clinician in seeking relevant information from the patient. Examples of this might include: does the patient's job involve significant weight-bearing activities with loads, such as for manual workers? This may stimulate mechanical nociceptive pain or inflammation and may have implications for fitness to work. Alternatively, does the patient find the use of orthotics beneficial? This may indicate that biomechanical factors contribute toward symptom production. Does the patient find periods of inactivity aggravate symptoms when first standing up? This type of 'start-up' pain is common for tendinopathies and plantar fasciosis. Gleaning the patient's individual perspective will aid in reasoning possible sources of symptoms, directing treatment as well as assisting in appropriate goal setting.

An understanding of the patient's perspectives, attitudes and beliefs is also important for appropriate management within a biopsychosocial framework. The clinician needs to be aware of, and sensitive to, the patient's feelings and empathize and communicate appropriately so as to develop a supportive rapport with the patient. The following types of questions can be useful in assessing psychosocial drivers of pain and behaviour, which may be risk factors in the development of persistent symptoms.

- What do you understand to be the cause of your pain/symptoms?
- What are you hoping/expecting will help you?
- What are you able to do to cope with your pain/symptoms?

Additionally there are a number of valid and reliable self-reported outcome tools that can be used to measure the impact of symptoms on function and patient perceptions of their dysfunction and to measure the effect of interventions over time, e.g. Foot and Ankle Ability Measure (FAAM), Foot Function Index (FFI), Foot Health Status Questionnaire (FHSQ), Lower Extremity Function Scale (LEFS) and Sports Ankle Rating System Quality of Life measure – see Martin and Irrgang (2007) for an overview.

Social History

Social and family history that is relevant to the onset and progression of the patient's problem is recorded. This includes the patient's age, employment, home situation and details of any leisure activities. With sporting pursuits it can be helpful to check if the patient is planning to engage in any competitions or events to understand existing motivations towards continuing exercise programmes. Factors from this information may indicate direct and/or indirect mechanical influences on the foot and ankle and their frequency. It is helpful to have a working knowledge of these demands and to equate these to tissue loading/healing processes for injuries for which this is a consideration for returning to activity.

In order to treat the patient appropriately, it is important that the condition is managed within the context of the patient's social and work environment.

This can serve as an area for both creativity on the part of the clinician and a helpful reminder for timing of completing home exercises for the patient. Taking the stairs instead of a lift and performing exercises when on a rest break can be useful so that home programmes are less onerous.

The clinician may ask the following types of questions to elucidate these factors:

- Have you had time off work in the past with your symptoms?
- What are your symptoms preventing you from currently doing?
- How is your employer/coworkers/family responding to your symptoms?
- Do you think you will return to work? When?

Early identification of psychosocial risk factors is important as these may play a role in the development of persistent musculoskeletal disability (Nicholas et al. 2011).

Body Chart

The following information concerning the type and area of current symptoms can be recorded on a body chart (see Fig. 2.3).

Area of Current Symptoms

Be exact when mapping out the area of the symptoms. It is often useful to ask the patient to use one finger to point to where they have predominant symptoms. Dysfunctions in the foot and ankle tend to produce local symptoms, so a thorough anatomical knowledge will help reason underlying structures and pain mechanisms. For example, with stress fractures of the tibia or metatarsal, the area of pain indicated tends to be very specific (Fetzer & Wright 2006; Young & McAllister 2006), whilst plantar fasciosis is the most common cause of plantar medial heel pain (Martin et al. 2014). However, this can become more complex. For example, posteromedial ankle pain could be attributable to the local talocrural joint, as a result of impingement or joint degeneration, or could originate from the tendon of tibialis posterior, flexor digitorum longus or flexor hallucis longus, or it could be as a result of sensitivity of the tibial nerve in the tarsal tunnel, or even vascular structures such as the tibial artery. If the patient is able to tell you, ascertain the worst symptom and record both where the patient feels the symptoms are coming from and the patient's underlying thoughts as to the cause of these.

Areas Relevant to the Region Being Examined

Symptoms in the foot and ankle may be referred from more proximal arthrogenic, myofascial or neural sources such as the lumbar spine and proximal lower-limb structures (Uth 1999; Nelson & Hall 2011). Symptoms may also arise as a result of contributing factors, for example, poor proximal control of the pelvis, hip or knee or as a result of dysfunctional foot biomechanics, which may result in compensatory pathological loads on tendons at the foot and ankle (Sueki et al. 2013). Check all relevant areas for pain/stiffness; use reasoning relevance to the patient's symptoms and mark unaffected areas with ticks (✓) on the body chart.

Quality of Symptoms

The quality of the symptoms may assist reasoning possible structures at fault. For example, paraesthesia might support a hypothesis of a neural tissue source, especially if associated with burning or electric shock-type pain. Functional or mechanical ligamentous instability of the lateral ligament complex may result in 'giving way' of the ankle with or without pain and patients may report they 'don't trust their ankle' (van Rijn et al. 2008; O'Loughlin et al. 2009). Alternatively descriptions of stiffness are often indicative of degenerative changes, for example, hallux rigidus in the first metatarsophalangeal joint (MTPJ) or OA of the talocrural joint. Prolonged stiffness may also indicate more systemic disorders if associated with other signs and symptoms of inflammatory/reactive disease, e.g. RA, Reiter's, gout, AS.

Intensity of Pain

The intensity of pain can be measured using a visual analogue scale or numerical rating scale, as discussed in Chapter 2. This informs clinical reasoning related to severity, and helps to determine possible structures producing symptoms. This also serves as one of a number of subjective markers to monitor progress.

Abnormal Sensation

Check for any altered sensation (such as paraesthesia, anaesthesia, hypoaesthesia, hyperaesthesia and allodynia) throughout the lower limb as well as locally around the foot and ankle. The distribution of any sensory changes will help to differentiate between dermatomal distribution from spinal nerve roots, symptoms of peripheral nerve origin and upper motor neuron lesions. For example, bilateral paraesthesia/anaesthesia in both hands and feet associated with weakness/heaviness in the legs, difficulty walking and difficulties with fine-motor activities, e.g. writing, could indicate cervical myelopathy (Cook & Cook 2016).

Constant or Intermittent Symptoms

Ascertain the frequency of the symptoms and whether these are constant or intermittent. If symptoms are constant, check whether there is variation in the intensity of the symptoms as constant symptoms (especially progressive unremitting pain) may require further investigation to exclude more serious pathology such as neoplastic disease. Whilst cancer is uncommon in the foot and ankle, more constant pain may be indicative of inflammatory disorders such as gout and RA. If associated with other symptoms, such as sensory, motor, vasomotor and/or trophic changes, incapacitating pain could indicate the development of chronic regional pain syndrome, which can be a complication post fracture, minor injury or surgery (Rewhorn et al. 2014; Kim 2016).

Relationship of Symptoms

Determine the relationship between the symptomatic areas. This information will assist with reasoning the most likely cause of the patient's symptoms and so focus the physical examination. Questions to clarify the relationship might include:

- Do your symptoms come together or separately?
- If one symptomatic area becomes severe what happens to the other symptomatic area?

Establish the Depth of the Pain

Determine whether symptoms are felt on the surface or deep inside. This information will assist with reasoning the most likely source of the patient's symptoms and so focus the physical examination. For example, after an ankle inversion injury deep anterolateral or anteromedial ankle pain in conjunction with pain on weight bearing may indicate the presence of an osteochondral lesion, whilst more superficial symptoms may support superficial soft-tissue involvement (van Dijk et al. 1996; O'Loughlin et al. 2010).

Behaviour of Symptoms

Aggravating Factors

Due to the functional importance of the foot and ankle in everyday life, patients may report significant limitations. For each symptomatic area, ask patients what movements and/or positions aggravate their symptoms, if they are able to maintain an activity or position or whether they have to stop or change position (severity). How long does it take for symptoms to ease once the position or movement is stopped (irritability)? Irritability and severity are explained in Chapter 2. These questions help to confirm the relationship between the symptoms and serve as subjective/physical markers to gauge progress.

In addition, it is wise to question the patient about common aggravating factors for the anatomical structures within this region to try to 'rule in' or 'rule out' structures which may form part of the clinical presentation. Common aggravating factors for the foot and ankle are weight-bearing activities such as stair climbing, squatting, walking and running, especially on uneven ground. Clinically specific examples may include the effect of shoe wear versus barefoot walking – patients with Morton's neuroma or hallux valgus tend to prefer barefoot (Vanore et al. 2003; Adams 2010). Patients with plantar fasciosis or tendinopathy often describe classic 'start-up' pain, and so specific questioning regarding this can be useful (Martin et al. 2014). Alternatively, patients demonstrating neural mechanosensitivity may find slump positions such as driving provocative or limited (Pahor & Toppenberg 1996). Questioning can be further developed in relation to known patterns of clinical prediction rules for specific pathologies. For example, anterolateral ankle impingement has been shown to demonstrate the following features: anterolateral joint tenderness and recurrent swelling, pain with forced dorsiflexion

and eversion, pain with single-leg squat, pain with activities and possible absence of ankle instability (Liu et al. 1997). Thorough knowledge of specific pathologies and classic presentations is therefore essential to direct efficient subjective questioning and use of physical examination tests.

Aggravating factors for other regions, which may need to be queried if suspected as a source of the symptoms, are shown in Table 2.2.

Detailed information on each activity helps refine reasoning of possible structures that may be at fault, the severity, irritability and relationship between symptoms. This information can be used to explain symptoms and advise patients in understandable, non-threatening terms. In addition, it serves to determine both a treatment plan and the formulation of agreed goals. The most notable functional restrictions are highlighted with asterisks (*), explored in the physical examination and reassessed at subsequent treatment sessions to evaluate treatment intervention.

Easing Factors

For each symptomatic area, the clinician asks what movements and/or positions ease the patient's symptoms, how long it takes to ease them, whether symptoms subside completely and what happens to other symptoms when one symptom is relieved. These questions help to confirm the relationship between symptoms and helps the clinician judge irritability and therefore how difficult or easy it may be to relieve the patient's symptoms in the physical examination. Along with a knowledge of relevant biomechanics and functional movement this helps the clinician to reason why an activity might improve symptoms. For example, running may aggravate local ankle or first MTPJ OA due to the increased range of dorsiflexion required and greater impact forces, whereas walking may be symptom-free.

Using clinical reasoning skills the clinician can then collate the information gained from aggravating and easing factors to formulate a hypothesis of the structure(s) which might be at fault. This information can be used to focus the physical examination, the aims of treatment and any advice that may be required. If the patient's symptoms do not fit a musculoskeletal presentation then the clinician needs to be alert to other, possibly more serious causes.

Twenty-Four-Hour Behaviour of Symptoms

The clinician determines the 24-hour behaviour of symptoms by asking questions about night, morning and evening symptoms.

Night Symptoms. See Chapter 2 for questions and further details. Whilst night pain may raise suspicions regarding serious pathology, it is useful to consider alternative thought processes as well. For example, patients with OA may describe night pain as the disease progresses and becomes more severe (Abhishek & Doherty 2013), and night pain in this group may be one indication for potential surgery.

Morning and Evening Symptoms. The clinician determines the pattern of the symptoms first thing in the morning, through the day and at the end of the day. This information may provide clues as to the pain mechanisms driving the condition and the type of pathology present. For example, early-morning pain and stiffness may indicate inflammatory pain. Localized medial plantar heel pain on the initial weight-bearing steps in the morning is commonly attributed to plantar fasciosis; although 'start up' pain is also reported with symptoms relating to other tendinopathies such as Achilles and tibialis posterior pathology (Patla & Abbot 2000; Chiodo & Gomez-Tristan 2012). The pattern of symptoms may also be a helpful reassessment marker to establish the effectiveness of treatment and management.

Stage of the Condition

In order to determine the stage of the condition, the clinician asks whether the symptoms are getting better, getting worse or remaining unchanged. Asking this allows one to question if symptoms are continuing beyond the expected timescale for recovery and, if so, to question possible factors to explain this.

Special Questions

Special questions must always be asked, as these may identify certain precautions or contraindications to the physical examination and/or treatment. As discussed in Chapter 2, the clinician must differentiate between conditions that are suitable for manual or manipulative therapy and systemic, neoplastic and other non-musculoskeletal conditions, which are not suitable for such treatment and require referral to a medical practitioner. Chapter 2 discusses special questions in detail, and hence only examples of the relevance of some of these questions to the foot and ankle are highlighted below.

General Health

Ascertain the general health of the patient. The clinician should be aware of the impact of a patient's lifestyle choices on health, such as smoking, alcohol intake, use of recreational drugs and levels of physical activity. The clinician asks about any feelings of general malaise or fatigue, fever, nausea or vomiting, stress, anxiety or depression. Simple examples of the relevance of such factors for the foot and ankle can be seen, with links being established between smoking and depression and an increased incidence of chronic regional pain syndrome in women after foot and ankle surgery (Rewhorn et al. 2014) and links between smoking and musculoskeletal disorders (Lee et al. 2013). Feeling unwell or tired is common with systemic, metabolic or malignant disease (Greenhalgh & Selfe 2010).

Weight Loss

Has the patient noticed any recent unexplained weight loss?

Serious Pathology

See Chapter 2 for further discussion of cancer, tuberculosis and human immunodeficiency virus (HIV). It is worth noting that malignant tumours of foot and ankle are rare (Kennedy et al. 2016). The foot and ankle are also atypical sites for musculoskeletal tuberculosis; if suspected, patients should be asked about possible exposure to tuberculosis (Korim et al. 2014).

Osteoporosis

Has the patient been diagnosed with osteoporosis or does the patient have a history of frequent fractures? Elderly women with a lower radial and calcaneal bone density than matched controls have been shown to have an increased risk of foot fracture (Hasselman et al. 2003). If osteoporosis is suspected then the vigour of the physical examination may need to be modified.

Inflammatory Arthritis

Patients should be asked if they or a member of their family has been diagnosed as having an inflammatory condition. RA often initially presents in the small joints of the feet and hands and can cause significant disability (Aletaha et al. 2010).

Cardiovascular Disease

Does the patient have a history of cardiovascular disease, e.g. hypertension, angina, previous myocardial infarction, stroke? Patients who develop symptoms of peripheral vascular disease usually present with intermittent claudication – an aching muscle pain that is brought on by exercise and rapidly relieved by rest. Symptoms are determined by the site of disease and can include aching in the calf and foot (Peach et al. 2012) and thus may mimic musculoskeletal disorders.

Respiratory Disease

Does the patient have any condition which affects breathing? If so, how is it managed?

Diabetes Mellitus

The foot and ankle are complex targets of this multisystem disease, and the effects of diabetes can manifest in a wide spectrum of pathology in the foot, from mild neuropathy to severe ulcerations, infections, vasculopathy, Charcot arthropathy and neuropathic fractures (Oji & Schon 2013). Due to vascular deficits tissue healing is likely to be slower in diabetic patients (Gaston & Simpson 2007) and hence can be especially relevant to determining the prognosis and vigour of examination. There is evidence of higher complication and infection rates in patients with diabetes who have sustained acute fractures or following planned foot and ankle surgery (Wukich et al. 2010, 2011). Diabetic neuropathy affecting the feet and hands typically presents with a stocking-and-glove distribution, beginning distally and spreading proximally, and can demonstrate a combination of diminished light touch sensation, proprioception, temperature awareness and pain perception. As a consequence diabetic patients may present with ulcerations and infections on their feet due to impaired sensitivity, resulting in pathological mechanical tissue stress (Oji & Schon 2013).

Neurological Symptoms if a Spinal Lesion Is Suspected

See Chapter 2 for discussions related to spinal cord compression, cauda equina syndrome and neuropathic pain presentations. Of note, spinal cord compression may also result in bilateral tingling in the hands or feet (Cook & Cook 2016) as well as other symptoms highlighted in Chapter 2 and thus may be pertinent to consider when assessing patients with altered lower-limb sensation.

Joint Hypermobility Syndrome

Has the patient been diagnosed with joint hypermobility syndrome? A positive history has to be clinically reasoned in the context of the patient's presenting symptoms and explored in the physical examination.

Drug History

What medications are being taken by the patient? Are these for other medical conditions or for the presenting symptoms? Are they effective? Use of anticoagulant and steroid medication would be an indication for caution in the physical examination and contraindicates some treatment modalities. Use of certain drugs may also have implications for the complexity and prognosis of any potential surgery.

Past Medical History

Details of any past medical history such as major or long-standing illnesses, accidents or surgery that are relevant to the patient's condition are obtained from the patient and/or medical notes, as these may explain the development of current symptoms. For example, a history of low-back pain may be relevant if neural sensitization is a suspected cause of distal symptoms, or a past history of ankle sprain or lower-limb fracture is relevant, as these may predispose the patient to post-traumatic arthritis.

Family History

Patients are asked if they or a member of their family have been diagnosed as having any conditions relevant to the presenting symptoms. For example, there is an acknowledged genetic predisposition to deformities such as hallux valgus (Perera et al. 2011) and inflammatory conditions such as RA and AS, whilst Charcot–Marie–Tooth disease is one of a group of hereditary disorders involving the peripheral nerves, which can result in progressive loss of muscle function and deformity in the feet and lower limbs (Botte & Franko 2013).

Radiography and Medical Imaging

Has the patient been radiographed or had any other medical tests recently? Radiographs are the cornerstone of diagnostic imaging and provide an often essential screening tool for many foot and ankle problems. When trauma is involved the Ottawa ankle rules provide guidelines for patients who certainly should be X-rayed (Bachmann et al. 2003). Magnetic resonance imaging (MRI) is routinely used in the evaluation of soft-tissue pathology of the foot and ankle, and is particularly useful for imaging osteochrondal lesions, bony and soft-tissue tumours, stress reactions, bone bruising, ligamentous damage, bursitis, fasciosis, tendinopathy/tendon tears and for the diabetic foot (Mohan et al. 2010; Pedowitz 2012). Ultrasound is used in patients with foot and ankle symptoms to examine soft tissues such as tendons, ganglions and neuromas, and is often the preferred imaging modality when Morton's neuroma or Achilles tendinosis is suspected (Pedowitz 2012; Bignotti et al. 2015). It is also useful for guiding aspirations and specific injections.

Computed tomography (CT) provides rapid imaging to help evaluate complex anatomy and pathology, and is used primarily for evaluating bone as opposed to soft tissue. The muliplanar nature of CT enhances its ability to detect disease not appreciable on plain radiographs (Haapamaki et al. 2005). SPECT-CT, a radionuclide bone scan with single-photon emission CT and CT, is a relatively new imaging modality which combines highly detailed CT with the functional information from a triple-phase radionuclide bone scan. SPECT-CT is becoming increasingly recognized as having high diagnostic accuracy, and is recommended for use in foot and ankle cases of diagnostic uncertainty and for the evaluation of chronic foot/ankle pain, especially in patients with previous surgery or in situ metal work (Mohan et al. 2010; Williams et al. 2012; Singh et al. 2013).

Other tests may include blood tests, required if systemic inflammatory conditions such as RA, AS or gout are suspected.

Results from careful questioning and additional tests will provide information that can inform clinical reasoning of underlying causes of symptoms, guide rehabilitation and indicate likely prognosis.

History of the Present Condition

For each symptomatic area, the clinician asks how long the symptoms have been present, whether there was a sudden or slow onset and whether there was a known cause that provoked the onset of the symptoms. If the patient is able to recall a traumatic onset, closer questioning as to the mechanism of injury may suggest structures which could have been injured and to what degree. Under the Ottawa ankle rules, determining whether a patient can weight bear, in conjunction with the presence of specific bony tenderness after an injury, is an accurate instrument for excluding fractures of the ankle and midfoot. The instrument has a sensitivity of almost 100% and a modest specificity and is used for adults and children over the age of 5 (Bachmann et al. 2003; Dowling et al. 2009). Alternatively, if there has been an insidious onset to symptoms, the clinician finds out if there has been any change in the patient's lifestyle, e.g. a new job or hobby, or a change in existing sporting activities, including alterations in footwear, equipment, surface or intensity. Sensitively determining recent or chronic weight gain can be useful in assessing the impact of additional biomechanical stresses, and certainly increased body mass index in the non-athletic population has been associated with conditions such as plantar fasciosis (Martin et al. 2014). The goal here is simply to work out what has happened or to build a picture of what has changed so as to understand fully why a patient is presenting with symptoms.

To confirm the relationship between the symptoms, the clinician asks what happened to other symptoms when each symptom began. Is this the first episode or is there a history of foot or ankle problems? If so, how many episodes? When were they? What was the cause? What was the duration of each episode? And did the patient fully recover between episodes? It may be that injuries sustained years previously are relevant, for example, previous ankle sprains or fractures have been shown to predict the development of osteochondral lesions and posttraumatic arthritis (Hirose et al. 2004; Valderrabano et al. 2006). If there have been no previous episodes, has the patient had any episodes of stiffness in the lumbar spine, hip or knee or any other relevant region?

In addition the clinician needs to ask if the patient has sought treatment to date, what it was and whether it helped. What has the patient been told and by whom? What does the patient believe is going on? Clarifying the patient's journey can help the clinician in understanding the patient's context and allows management to be tailored to meet the needs of the individual.

Plan of the Physical Examination

In order to plan the physical examination, the hypotheses generated from the subjective examination are considered (see Fig. 2.8). It is useful at the end of the subjective examination to reconfirm the patients main complaint, and offer them the opportunity to add anything that they may not have mentioned so far. The purpose and plan for the physical examination will need to be explained and the patient's consent obtained.

The information from the subjective examination helps the clinician to identify an initial primary hypothesis and alternative hypotheses as to the cause of a patient's symptoms. A physical examination planning form can help guide the clinician's reasoning in the development and testing of these initial hypotheses (see Fig. 2.9).

For ease of reference, highlight with asterisks (*) important subjective findings and particularly one or more functional restrictions. These can then be re-examined at subsequent treatment sessions to evaluate the treatment intervention. It is useful to communicate this to patients so they become proactive in monitoring progress.

In order to plan the physical examination, the following hypotheses need to be developed from the subjective examination:

- Based on subjective information the clinician decides which regions and structures are most likely to be the cause of symptoms. It is helpful to consider arthrogenic, myofascial, neural and other sources such as vascular structures lying underneath the area of symptoms and those that refer into the foot and ankle region. Using clinical reasoning skills, the clinician will need to

prioritize and justify what 'must' be examined in the initial session and what 'should' or 'could' be followed up at subsequent sessions, as it is not always possible to examine fully at the first attendance. Consider that a goal of the examination is to offer patients some explanation of their symptoms and also, where possible, to eliminate more sinister causes of symptoms or facilitate further investigations if suspected.

- Additional physical contributing factors should be examined as relevant, e.g. posture, foot biomechanics, related functional activities such as squatting, stairs or static/dynamic balance.
- If pain is a feature of the presentation, what are the pain mechanisms driving the patient's symptoms and how will this information impact on an understanding of the problem and subsequent assessment and management decisions? What are the input mechanisms (sensory pathways)? For example, pain associated with specific movements may indicate mechanical nociception. What are the central processing mechanisms? How has the patient interpreted these symptoms? Is the patient worried? What are the output mechanisms in terms of the patient's response? For example, has the patient changed working requirements or sporting participation and are these changes adaptive or maladaptive? Certainly this information might indicate an early assessment of specific functional activities and a deeper exploration of patient fears and concerns. Identifying and addressing these relevant factors may prove pivotal for a successful outcome. The reader is directed to Gifford (1998), Jones et al. (2002) and Thacker (2015) for further reading.
- What is the assessment of severity and irritability for each symptomatic area (see Chapter 2)? If severity is judged to be high, physical testing will be limited to testing to or just short of symptom reproduction. For those with high irritability the physical examination will also be contracted to avoid exacerbating symptoms and the focus may shift to easing the patient's symptoms rather than provoking them. The patient will require rest periods between tests to avoid build-up in symptoms. Alternatively, for patients with symptoms judged to be of low severity

and irritability, physical testing will need to be more searching and may require the use of overpressures, repeated and combined movements to reproduce symptoms.

■ Are there any precautions and/or contraindications to elements of the physical examination that need to be explored further, such as neurological involvement, recent fracture, trauma, steroid therapy or inflammatory conditions? There may also be certain contraindications to further examination and treatment, e.g. symptoms of spinal cord or cauda equina compression.

PHYSICAL EXAMINATION

The information from the subjective examination helps the clinician to plan an appropriate physical examination. The severity, irritability, ongoing pain mechanisms and primary working hypothesis and alternative hypotheses are the major factors that will influence the choice and priority and extent of physical testing procedures.

Each significant physical test that either provokes or eases the patient's symptoms is highlighted in the patient's notes by an asterisk (*) for easy reference.

The order and detail of the physical tests described below should be appropriate to the patient being examined. The clinician should select tests based on clinical reasoning of the hypotheses (primary and alternatives) under consideration. The aim is to confirm or refute the hypotheses. Issues of reliability, sensitivity and specificity (see Chapter 3) should also be considered when tests are selected so that findings can be interpreted appropriately. It is important that readers understand that the techniques shown in this chapter are some of many and that those chosen are clinically useful and supported with literature. Not all will be appropriate for every patient. Adaptations of the techniques, depending on patient presentation/size and therapist size and style of handling, are part of evolving and flexible practice.

Observation

Informal Observation

The clinician needs to observe the patient in dynamic and static situations; the quality of movement is noted, as are the postural characteristics and reactions. Informal observation will have begun from the moment the clinician sees the patient and begins the subjective examination and will continue to the end of the physical examination.

Formal Observation

Observation of Posture. The patient should be suitably dressed so that the clinician can observe the patient's bony and soft-tissue contours in standing, noting the posture of the feet, lower limbs, pelvis and spine. Observation of the foot and ankle can also be carried out in a non-weight-bearing position. General lower-limb abnormalities include uneven weight bearing through the legs and feet, internal femoral rotation and genu varum/valgum or recurvatum (hyperextension). It is worth noting the general foot posture and whether the foot has a particularly flattened or exaggerated medial longitudinal arch, as these may indicate pes planus or pes cavus, respectively. Further assessment of foot posture can be undertaken using the Foot Posture Index (FPI) (Redmond et al. 2006). The toes may be deformed, for example, claw toes, hammer toes, mallet toe and hallux valgus/rigidus. Further details of these abnormalities can be found in a standard orthopaedic textbook (Thordarson 2013; Magee 2014). Deviations observed in standing may be produced by a number of lower-limb factors, including tibial torsions and femoral anteversion or retroversion. Passive correction of observed deformity may give an idea of the ease by which this can be achieved and any associated impact on the lower limb and pelvis, but is not always indicative of the cause of any deformity.

Observation of Foot and Ankle Alignment. Multiple theories and approaches to the assessment of foot and lower-limb biomechanics have developed over time; some of these include subtalar joint neutral (Root et al. 1977), tissue stress theory (McPoil & Hunt 1995; Fuller & Kirby 2013), foot function approach (Harradine et al. 2006), treatment direction test (Vicenzino 2004), sagittal-plane approach (Dananberg 1986), subtalar joint axis location & rotational equilibrium theory of foot function (Kirby 2001) and the FPI (Redmond et al. 2006). These approaches are used by clinicians such as podiatrists, physiotherapists and orthotists to assess and manage foot and ankle symptoms and prescribe devices such as orthotics. Preferencing one method over another is controversial (Kirby 2015); however it is useful when beginning to assess foot and ankle biomechanics to use a systematic and relatively straightforward approach.

The FPI (Redmond et al. 2006) is one such approach and consists of six validated, criterion-based observations of the rearfoot and forefoot of a subject standing in a relaxed position. The rearfoot is assessed via palpation of the head of the talus, observation of the curves above and below the lateral malleoli and the extent of the inversion/eversion of the calcaneus. The observations of the forefoot consist of assessing the bulge in the region of the talonavicular joint, the congruence of the medial longitudinal arch and the extent of abduction/adduction of the forefoot on the rearfoot. The FPI has demonstrated concurrent and internal construct validity as well as high intra-rater reliability and moderate interrater reliability (Redmond et al. 2006; Keenan et al. 2007; Cornwall et al. 2008), and results in a score between −12 and +12 (where −12 indicates a highly supinated foot posture and +12 indicates a highly pronated foot posture; normative values of +4 in the adult population have been suggested) (Redmond et al. 2008). The FPI has demonstrated sensitivity to detect posturally pathological populations (Redmond et al. 2008), and research has suggested a link between FPI scores and lower-limb pathologies such as medial compartment knee OA, hip OA, chronic plantar heel pain and medial tibial stress syndrome (Yates & White 2004; Irving et al. 2007; Reilly et al. 2009), although this relationship is unclear and not fully established (Neal et al. 2014). Specific details of the FPI are freely available for clinical purposes at: http://www.leeds.ac.uk/medicine/FASTER/fpi.htm and knowledge and use of such tools or other methods of assessing lower-limb biomechanics can assist clinicians in supporting or refuting clinically reasoned hypotheses, communicating with colleagues, educating patients and can assist in management decision making such as referral for orthotics.

Observation of Muscle Form. The clinician observes the muscle bulk and muscle tone of the patient, comparing the left and right sides. It must be remembered that the level and frequency of physical activity as well as the dominant side may well produce differences in muscle bulk between sides. Some muscles are thought to shorten under stress while other muscles weaken, producing muscle imbalance (see Table 3.7).

Observation of Soft Tissues. The clinician observes the quality and colour of the patient's skin, any area of swelling, exostosis, callosities, joint effusion or presence of scarring or infection, and takes cues for further examination.

Common observations in the foot and ankle include the following:

- pes planus (flatfoot)
- pes cavus (high arch)
- hallux valgus: valgus alignment of the hallux at the MTPJ with prominent medial eminence ± pronation of the big toe. Often referred to as a bunion
- hallux rigidus: OA of the first MTPJ which may result in palpable bony osteophytes over the dorsal aspect of the first MTPJ
- hammer-toe deformity: affecting the lesser toes, the proximal interphalangeal joint has a flexion contracture with secondary extension at the MTPJ and distal interphalangeal joint. Can be fixed or flexible
- claw-toe deformity: affecting the lesser toes, the MTPJ is hyperextended, with flexion contracture at the proximal interphalangeal and distal interphalangeal joints. Can be fixed or flexible
- mallet-toe deformity: flexion contracture of the distal interphalangeal joint. Can be fixed or flexible
- bunionette (tailor's bunion): characterized by prominence of the lateral aspect of the fifth metatarsal head and medial deviation of the fifth toe at the MTPJ, often with associated callus
- Hagland's deformity or 'pump bump': an exostosis located on the posterolateral or posteromedial aspect of the calcaneus. Aetiology unclear but may be the result of overuse, trauma or excessive pressure (Magee 2014)
- intractable plantar keratosis: hyperkeratotic tissue proliferation (callus) on the plantar aspect of the foot, usually under the metatarsal head(s),

occurs usually as a result of excessive mechanical load

- posteromedial pitting oedema along the course of the tibialis posterior: this observation has been shown to be a highly specific and sensitive (100% and 86%, respectively) sign of tibialis posterior tendon dysfunction in comparison to MRI findings (DeOrio et al. 2011), and so may prompt further assessment of this structure following observation
- fusiform swelling locally in the Achilles tendon may indicate a reactive tendinopathy (Cook & Purdam 2009; Cook et al. 2016), and is usually observed in the midportion of the Achilles tendon
- oedema as a result of trauma/ankle sprain – swelling observed proximally to the ankle mortise may indicate syndesmotic injury of the inferior tibiofibular joint, whereas swelling distal to the lateral malleolus may indicate a lateral ligament complex injury, although this may spread into the foot if the capsule has been damaged (Dubin et al. 2011)
- adult acquired flatfoot deformity: commonly secondary to tibialis posterior tendon dysfunction, this ranges from a flexible deformity to a rigid deformity with advanced arthritis. Clinical observations can include hindfoot valgus, medial arch collapse, forefoot abduction with 'too-many-toes' sign and inability to perform double and single heel-rise tests (Zaw & Calder 2010).

Any clinical observation or test result should not be viewed in isolation; instead it needs to be placed within a clinically reasoned framework which is relevant to the patient's presenting signs and symptoms.

Functional Testing

Some functional ability has already been tested by general observation of the patient during the subjective and physical examinations, e.g. the observation of gait when walking into the appointment, postures adopted during the subjective examination and the ease or difficulty of sit-to-stand activities. Any further functional testing can be carried out early in the examination. Clues for appropriate tests can be obtained from the subjective examination findings, particularly aggravating factors, and might include activities such as walking, going up or down stairs, squatting, hopping or running.

Observation of Gait

Gait analysis is usually an essential component of the physical examination and it is useful to include walking forwards/backwards, on even/uneven ground and on toes, heels and outer and inner borders of feet, as well as slopes, up and down stairs and running. It is useful to observe gait in a logical manner from head to toe, or vice versa, observing each body segment for variations in the normal range. Look for asymmetries, e.g. head side flexion, arm swing, trunk rotation, uneven stride length from and differences in weight bearing. Each variation may indicate tight musculature, structural anomalies or functional movement patterns which may have altered through a habit, e.g. such as carrying a bag on one shoulder. Gait analysis serves as a physical measure, which may assist in the identification of contributing factors in presenting symptoms. More detailed guidance on gait analysis and methods of analysis can be found in Whittle et al. (2012b) and Magee (2014).

The gait cycle is defined as 'the time interval between two successive occurrences of one of the repetitive events of walking' (Whittle et al. 2012a, p. 32). It is often started at the point one foot touches the floor; this used to be referred to as heel strike but as it is not always the heel that strikes first it is now referred to as initial contact. The gait cycle consists of the following major events:

1. initial contact
2. opposite toe-off
3. heel rise
4. opposite initial contact
5. toe-off
6. feet adjacent
7. tibial vertical
8. initial contact – the gait cycle begins again.

The angle of heel contact with the ground is usually slightly varus. Marked variations from this may cause abnormal foot function, with compensation attained either in the foot across the midtarsal joint and first and fifth rays or more proximally in the ankle, knee (less often hip) and sacroiliac joints. Early heel lift may indicate tight posterior leg muscles which can be a cause of functional ankle equinus (Pascual Huerta 2014), where the range of dorsiflexion required for normal gait is lacking; this requires compensations throughout the foot, ankle and lower limb.

The degree of pronation of the foot during midstance is observed and noted. Pronation is a normal part of gait that allows the foot to become a shock absorber and mobile adapter. Prolonged pronation or failure/delayed supination of the subtalar joint during mid to late stance (often indicated by a prolonged or rigid valgus of the calcaneum and collapse of the medial longitudinal arch) may indicate tibialis posterior tendon dysfunction. This condition can lead to a progressive sequelae of flat-foot deformity, which may ultimately require significant surgical intervention (Zaw & Calder 2010). At heel lift the foot changes to a more rigid lever for toe-off. Limitation or alteration of normal function of the MTPJs may affect toe-off significantly and result in more proximal dysfunctions/compensations (Canseco et al. 2008; Nix et al. 2013). Abnormality of function at any phase of gait may cause symptoms, varying from low-grade and cumulative to acute, in other structures of the locomotor system.

Summary of Gait Analysis
- Systematically observe the alignment of each area from top to bottom during a number of gait cycles.
- Note any asymmetry from side to side.
- Note the point at which asymmetry occurs and consider why that might be.

Joint Integrity Tests

Osseous congruency, static ligamentous and capsular restraints and myofascial structures are the major contributors to stability at the ankle. Epidemiological research suggests there is a high incidence of ankle sprain injury, accounting for an estimated 300 000 admissions to UK emergency departments each year (Bridgman et al. 2003). Research suggests lateral ligament sprains are the most common injury, followed by syndesmotic (disruption of the inferior tibiofibular joint) and then medial ankle sprain (Doherty et al.

2014), with residual symptoms following acute ankle sprain reported at rates between 5% and 33% (van Rijn et al. 2008). Lateral ligament sprains consist of partial or complete disruption of the lateral ankle ligaments (anterior talofibular ligament [ATFL], calcaneofibular ligament [CFL] and posterior talofibular ligament [PTFL]), but the majority of injuries involve isolated ATFL disruption (Martin et al. 2013), followed by the CFL and, rarely, the PTFL. Differing mechanisms of injury are suggested for different ligamentous structures. For example, the ATFL is most likely to be damaged in positions of ankle plantarflexion and inversion, whereas the CFL is most vulnerable in positions of ankle dorsiflexion and inversion (Neumann 2002). Conversely, the most common position for syndesmotic injuries is ankle dorsiflexion and external rotation with a firmly planted foot (Sman et al. 2013). This subjective information can be combined with physical examination tests to support the clinical reasoning process. Joint integrity tests then form part of a reasoned examination.

Anterior Drawer Sign

This is a test of the amount of anterior talar translation in respect to the ankle mortise. The patient is usually positioned in sitting with 90° of knee flexion and ankle plantarflexion between 10° and 20°. The leg should be relaxed and unsupported. One hand of the examiner is placed on the anterior aspect of the distal tibia and fibula. The second hand grasps the posterior aspect of the calcaneus. The test is performed by applying a firm posteroanterior force to the calcaneus (and hence the talus) while the distal tibia/fibula is stabilized (Fig. 16.1). The test can also be performed in other positions, such as supine or prone, with slight flexion of the knee. Excessive anterior translation of the talus, compared to the uninvolved side, with a loose end-feel, indicates a reduction in the passive stabilizing function of the medial and lateral ligaments (Martin et al. 2013). Observation of a dimple or sulcus sign near the region of the ATFL may also indicate instability (Cook & Hegedus 2011). Martin et al.'s (2013) clinical practice guideline review of current evidence suggests the anterior drawer test has a sensitivity range of 58–80% and specificity 74–94%, with intertester reliability ranging between 0.5 and 1.0 (moderate to perfect) based on several studies (Raatikainen et al. 1992; van

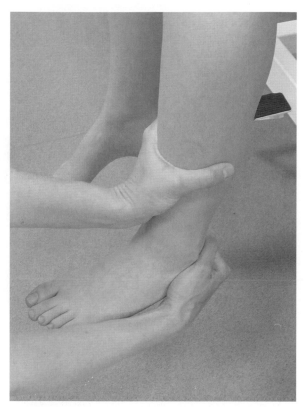

FIG. 16.1 ■ Anterior drawer sign. The left hand stabilizes the lower leg while the right hand applies a posteroanterior force to the talus, via the calcaneus.

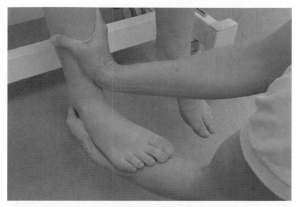

FIG. 16.2 ■ Talar tilt. The left hand grips around the calcaneum and talus and moves it into a small amount of inversion whilst the other hand stabilizes the lower leg.

Dijk et al. 1996; Hertel et al. 1999). The combination of pain with palpation of the ATFL, lateral haematoma and a positive anterior drawer on examination 5 days after injury has demonstrated a sensitivity of 96% and specificity of 84% to identify lateral ligament rupture (van Dijk et al. 1996).

Talar Tilt

The talar tilt is a test of the amount of talar inversion occurring within the ankle mortise. The patient is usually positioned in sitting with 90° of knee flexion, with the leg relaxed and unsupported and the ankle in a plantargrade position. One hand of the examiner is placed on the distal tibia and fibula while the second hand grasps the calcaneus and slowly moves it into inversion; a small amount of traction can be applied (Fig. 16.2). Increased adduction movement of the

calcaneus on the involved side compared to the uninvolved side, a reduced or absent end-feel and clicks/clunks suggest injury to the lateral ligament complex or that the calcaneofibular ligament (CFL) is injured. The test can also be performed in other positions, such as supine or prone. Sensitivity of 50% and specificity of 88% have been reported for this test (Hertel et al. 1999; Schwieterman et al. 2013).

Some research suggests that these tests individually are not sufficient to differentiate which of the lateral ligaments has been compromised and to what extent the lateral ligament complex has been damaged following trauma. It may therefore be wise to use these tests in combination with others to confirm an injury to the lateral ligaments; see Martin et al. (2013) and Kerkhoffs et al. (2012).

Cotton Test

The cotton test is a test of the integrity of the inferior tibiofibular syndesmosis. The patient is usually positioned in supine. The examiner stabilizes the distal tibia and fibula with one hand and applies a lateral translation force to the foot, via the calcaneus (Fig. 16.3). Increased translation of the foot on the involved side compared to the uninvolved side or a clunk/click may indicate syndesmotic instability. Sensitivity and specificity for this test have been reported as 25–29% and 71%, respectively (Beumer et al. 2002; Schwieterman et al. 2013; Sman et al. 2013).

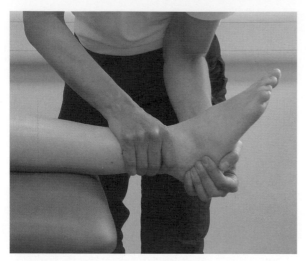

FIG. 16.3 ■ Cotton test. The right hand stabilizes the lower leg while the left hand applies lateral translation to the foot, via the calcaneus.

External Rotation Stress Test (Kleiger Test)

This is a test of the integrity of the inferior tibiofibular syndesmosis; it is pain provocative. The patient is usually positioned in sitting with 90° of knee flexion. The examiner stabilizes the tibia and fibula with one hand, in a manner which does not compress the distal tibiofibular syndesmosis. With the other hand, the examiner holds the foot in plantargrade and applies a passive lateral rotation stress to the foot and ankle (Fig. 16.4). The test can also be performed in other positions, such as supine or prone. A positive test is indicated if pain is produced over the anterior or posterior tibiofibular ligaments and the interosseous membrane and is indicative of a syndesmosis 'high ankle' injury. The specificity for this test has been reported between 85% and 99%, with sensitivity between 20% and 50% (Beumer et al. 2002; de Cesar et al. 2011; Schwieterman et al. 2013; Sman et al. 2013).

Squeeze Test

The squeeze test is a test of the integrity of the inferior tibiofibular syndesmosis; it is pain provocative. The patient is usually positioned in sitting with 90° of knee flexion or in supine with the knee in a small degree of flexion. The examiner applies a manual squeeze, pushing the fibula and tibia together, applying a force at the midpoint of the calf. The examiner then applies

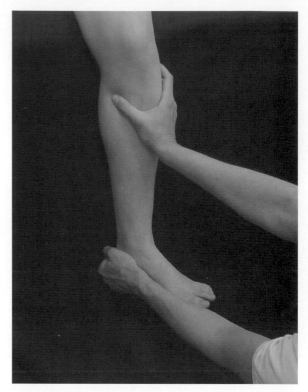

FIG. 16.4 ■ External rotation stress test. The right hand stabilizes the lower leg while the left hand holds the foot in plantargrade and applies a passive external rotation stress to the foot and ankle.

the same load at more distal locations moving toward the ankle (Fig. 16.5). Pain in the lower leg may indicate a syndesmotic injury (provided fracture and compartment syndrome have been ruled out). Sensitivity and specificity for this test have been reported as 30–100% and 14–93%, respectively (Nussbaum et al. 2001; Beumer et al. 2002; de Cesar et al. 2011; Schwieterman et al. 2013; Sman et al. 2013).

Active Physiological Movements

Movements can be tested with the patient in prone, supine or sitting with the right and left sides compared. The range of movement for the foot and ankle can be measured using a goniometer. For active physiological movements, the clinician notes the following:

■ willingness of the patient to move
■ quality of movement

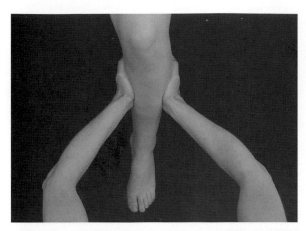

FIG. 16.5 ■ Squeeze test. Both hands apply a manual squeeze, pushing the tibia and fibula together at the midpoint of the calf.

- range of movement
- behaviour of pain through the range of movement
- resistance through the range of movement and at the end of the range of movement
- provocation of any protective muscle spasm.

A movement diagram can be used to depict this information (see Chapter 3). Active movements with overpressure to the foot and ankle are shown in Fig. 16.6. Overpressure at the end of the range can be applied to the whole foot. For differentiation purposes, the foot may be considered in functional units: the rearfoot, midfoot and forefoot. These are described in Table 16.1. Using a knowledge of the joint lines the various regions may be individually examined with localized overpressure at the end of range. The clinician establishes the patient's symptoms at rest, prior to each movement, and notes the effect of passively correcting any movement deviation to determine its relevance to the patient's symptoms. Active physiological movements of the foot and ankle and possible modifications are shown in Table 16.2.

Numerous differentiation tests (Hengeveld & Banks 2014) can be performed; the choice depends on the patient's signs and symptoms. For example, when lateral ankle pain is reproduced on inversion, inversion consists of rearfoot, midfoot and forefoot movement along with a degree of adduction. The clinician takes the foot into inversion and, if symptomatic, the foot can be taken to a position short of symptoms and overpressure applied to each region and the effect on reproducing symptoms noted. In this way the possible source of symptoms can be clinically reasoned and localized.

Other regions may need to be examined to determine their relevance to the patient's symptoms as they may be contributing to symptoms. The most likely regions are the lumbar spine, sacroiliac joint, hip and knee. The joints within these regions can be tested fully (see relevant chapter) or partially with the use of screening tests (see Chapter 3 for further information).

Some functional ability has already been tested by general observation of the patient during the subjective and physical examination, e.g. the postures adopted during the subjective examination and the ease or difficulty of undressing and changing position prior to the examination. Any further functional testing can be carried out at this point in the examination and may involve further gait analysis over and above that carried out in the observation section earlier. Clues for appropriate tests can be obtained from the subjective examination findings, particularly aggravating factors.

Weight-Bearing Lunge Test

This is a test to measure the range of functional dorsiflexion of the foot and ankle. The patient is in weight bearing and is asked to place one foot perpendicular to a wall, and then gently to lunge the ipsilateral knee to the wall, keeping the hips in a neutral position. The foot is then progressively moved away from the wall until the knee barely touches the wall; however the foot should remain flat to the floor, without the heel lifting and should not deviate laterally or medially (Fig. 16.7). The distance from the wall to the big toe is then measured in centimetres. Left and right sides are compared, and differences may indicate restriction in dorsiflexion as a result of talocrural joint stiffness (Hoch & McKeon 2011). Results of a recent systematic review demonstrate that there is a strong level of evidence for good inter- and intra-clinician reliability of the test to measure ankle dorsiflexion range of motion and reasonable responsiveness of the

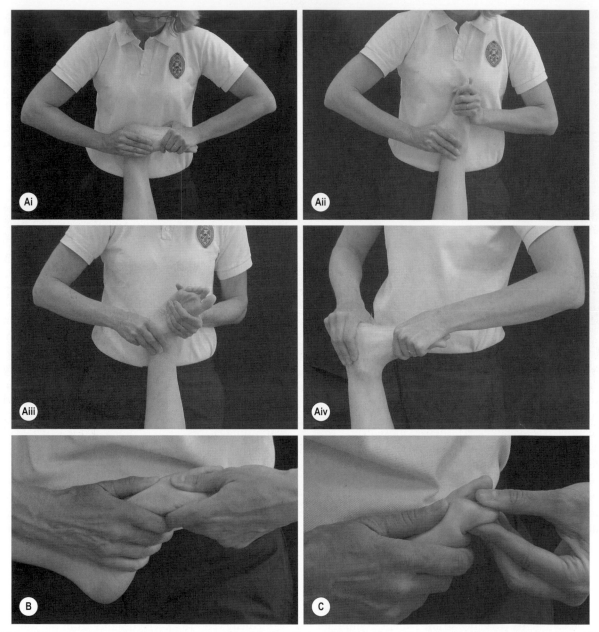

FIG. 16.6 ■ Overpressures to the foot and ankle. (Ai) Dorsiflexion. The right hand tips the calcaneus into dorsiflexion while the left hand and forearm apply overpressure to dorsiflexion through the forefoot. (Aii) Plantarflexion. The left hand grips the forefoot and the right hand grips the calcaneus and together they move the foot into plantarflexion. (Aiii) Inversion. The right hand adducts the calcaneus and reinforces the plantarflexion movement while the left hand plantarflexes the hindfoot and adducts, supinates and plantarflexes the midfoot and forefoot. (Aiv) Eversion. The right hand abducts the calcaneus and reinforces the dorsiflexion while the left hand dorsiflexes the hindfoot and abducts, pronates and dorsiflexes the midfoot and forefoot. (B) Metatarsophalangeal joint flexion and extension. The right hand stabilizes the metatarsal while the left hand flexes and extends the proximal phalanx. (C) Interphalangeal joint flexion and extension. The right hand stabilizes the proximal phalanx while the left hand flexes and extends the distal phalanx.

TABLE 16.2

Active Physiological Movements and Possible Modifications

Active Physiological Movements	Modifications
Ankle dorsiflexion	Repeated
Ankle plantarflexion	Speed altered
Inversion	Combined, e.g.
Eversion	■ Inversion with plantarflexion
Metatarsophalangeal	Compression or distraction
■ Flexion	Sustained
■ Extension	Injuring movement
Interphalangeal joints:	Differentiation tests
■ Flexion	Function
■ Extension	

test to detect true patient change in range of motion (Powden et al. 2015).

Passive Physiological Movements

All of the active movements described above can be examined passively with the patient in prone with the knee at 90° flexion, or supine with the knee flexed over a pillow, comparing the left and right sides. Comparison of the response of symptoms to the active and passive movements can help to determine whether the structures contributing to symptoms are non-contractile (articular) or contractile (extraarticular, e.g. myogenic) (Cyriax 1982). If the lesion is non-contractile, such as ligament or joint capsule, then active and passive movements will be painful and/or restricted in the same direction. If the lesion is in a contractile tissue (i.e. muscle), then active and passive movements are painful and/or restricted in opposite directions (see Chapter 3). Metatarsophalangeal and interphalangeal abduction/adduction and rotation can also be tested (Fig. 16.8).

Muscle Tests

Muscle tests include examining muscle strength, length, isometric muscle testing and some other muscle tests. Selection should be clinically reasoned based on the patient's subjective examination as well as observations of posture and movement (Kendall et al. 2010). See Chapter 3 for details of muscle testing.

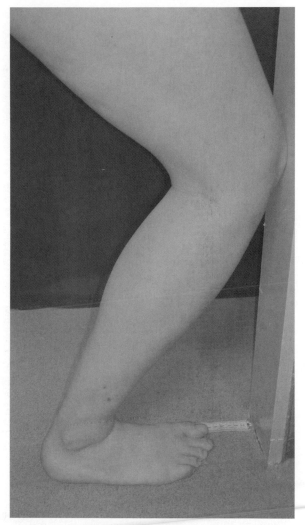

FIG. 16.7 ■ Weight-bearing lunge test. Ankle fully dorsiflexed and knee against the wall. Note the heel is firmly on the floor and perpendicular to the wall, with measurement of the distance of the big toe from the wall.

Muscle Strength

For a true appreciation of a muscle's strength, the clinician tests the muscle isotonically through the available range. Manual muscle testing may be carried out for the following muscle groups:

- ankle dorsiflexors, plantarflexors
- foot inverters, everters
- toe flexors, extensors, abductors and adductors.

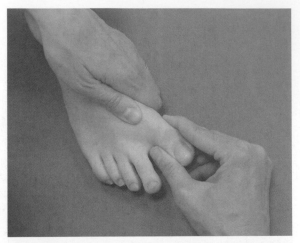

FIG. 16.8 ■ Metatarsophalangeal joint abduction and adduction. The left hand stabilizes the metatarsal while the right hand moves the proximal phalanx into abduction and adduction.

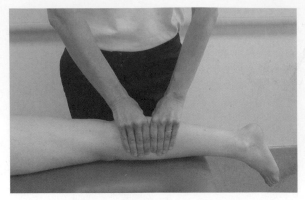

FIG. 16.9 ■ Thompson's test. The therapist's hands squeeze the calf while observing plantarflexion movement of the foot.

For details of these tests readers are directed to Kendall et al. (2010). The strength of proximal muscles should be considered when deviations are observed during testing of functional movements which cannot be solely explained by the foot and ankle. Please refer to the relevant chapters and Kendall et al. (2010) for further details.

Muscle Length

The clinician tests the length of muscles that may have an impact on lower-limb function, in particular those thought prone to shorten (Janda 1994, 2002); that is, piriformis, iliopsoas, rectus femoris, tensor fasciae latae, hamstrings, gastrocnemius and soleus (Jull & Janda 1987). Testing the length of these muscles is described in Chapter 3.

Isometric Muscle Testing

The clinician tests the ankle dorsiflexors and plantar-flexors and any other relevant muscle group in a resting position and, if indicated, in different parts of the physiological range. The clinician observes the quality of the muscle contraction to hold this position, the adoption of substitution strategies as well as the reproduction of the patient's symptoms. Muscles are palpated for trigger points (see Chapter 3).

Other Muscle Tests

Thompson's Test for Achilles Tendon Rupture. With the patient prone and the feet over the end of the plinth or kneeling with the foot unsupported, the clinician squeezes the calf muscle; the absence of ankle plantarflexion indicates a positive test, suggesting rupture of tendocalcaneus (Fig. 16.9). Maffulli (1998) reported a sensitivity of 96% and a specificity of 93% for Thompson's test to detect a subcutaneous Achilles tendon rupture.

Matles Test for Achilles Tendon Rupture. The patient is positioned in prone lying and is asked to actively flex the knees to 90°. The position of the ankles and feet is observed during flexion of the knee. If the foot on the affected side falls into neutral or into dorsiflexion, an Achilles tendon tear is diagnosed. On the uninjured side, the foot remains in slight plantarflexion when the knee is flexed to 90° (Matles 1975). Maffulli (1998) reported a sensitivity of 88% and a specificity of 85% for Matles test to detect subcutaneous Achilles tendon rupture.

Neurological Tests

This incorporates neurological examination and includes neurological integrity testing, sensorimotor tests and other nerve tests.

Integrity of the Nervous System

Using the onset, description and distribution of symptoms the clinician will use clinical reasoning to justify a neurological examination to assess if symptoms are emanating from neural tissue in the spine or from peripheral nerves.

Dermatomes/Peripheral Nerves. Light touch and pain sensation of the lower limb are tested using cotton wool and pinprick, respectively, as described in Chapter 3. Knowledge of the cutaneous distribution of nerve roots (dermatomes) and peripheral nerves enables the clinician to distinguish sensory loss due to a root lesion from that due to a peripheral nerve lesion. The cutaneous nerve distribution and dermatome areas are shown in Chapter 3.

Myotomes/Peripheral Nerves. The following myotomes may be tested and are shown in Chapter 3:

- L2: hip flexion
- L3: knee extension
- L4: foot dorsiflexion and inversion
- L5: extension of the big toe
- S1: eversion of the foot, contract buttock, knee flexion
- S2: knee flexion, toe standing
- S3–S4: muscles of pelvic floor, bladder and genital function.

A working knowledge of the muscular distribution of nerve roots (myotomes) and peripheral nerves enables the clinician to distinguish motor loss due to a root lesion from that due to a peripheral nerve lesion. The peripheral nerve distributions are shown in Chapter 3.

Reflex Testing. The following deep tendon reflexes can be tested (see Chapter 3):

- L3–L4: knee jerk
- S1: ankle jerk.

Neurodynamic Tests

Neurodynamic tests may be carried out in order to test neural sensitivity to movement and ascertain the degree to which neural tissue is responsible for the production of the patient's ankle and foot symptom(s). These tests are described in detail in Chapter 3:

- passive neck flexion
- straight-leg raise

- passive knee bend
- slump.

Variations in foot position have been suggested to stress different peripheral nerves. For example, ankle plantarflexion/inversion may bias the common peroneal nerve, ankle dorsiflexion/eversion may bias the tibial (and consequently the medial and lateral plantar nerves and the medial calcaneal nerve), whilst dorsiflexion/inversion may bias the sural nerve (Pahor & Toppenberg 1996; Butler 2000; Alshami et al. 2008).

Nerve Palpation

- Palpable nerves in the lower limb are as follows:

  - The tibial nerve can be palpated behind the medial malleolus, which may be more noticeable with the foot in dorsiflexion and eversion.
  - The common peroneal nerve can be palpated medial to the tendon of biceps femoris and also around the head of the fibula.
  - The superficial peroneal nerve can be palpated on the dorsum of the foot along an imaginary line over the fourth metatarsal; it is more noticeable with the foot in plantarflexion and inversion.
  - The deep peroneal nerve can be palpated between the first and second metatarsals, lateral to the extensor hallucis tendon.
  - The sural nerve can be palpated on the lateral aspect of the foot behind the lateral malleolus, lateral to the Achilles.

Tests for Circulation and Swelling

Vascular Tests

The vascular evaluation of the foot and ankle includes palpation of the dorsalis pedis and posterior tibial pulses and peripheral testing of capillary refill (Thordarson 2013; King et al. 2014). The state of the vascular system can also be determined by the response of symptoms to positions of dependence and elevation of the lower limbs and response to exercise, e.g. intermittent claudication.

Wells Score for Suspected Deep-Vein Thrombosis. If a patient presents with signs or symptoms of deep-vein thrombosis (DVT), clinicians are advised to carry out an assessment of their general medical history and a physical examination to exclude other causes. National Institute for Health and Care Excellence (NICE) guidelines currently recommend the use of a two-level DVT Wells score to estimate the clinical probability of DVT (NICE 2015). From this the patient is given a score of between −2 and +9. A simplified scoring system of 2 points or more indicates a likely DVT, whilst a score of 1 point or less indicates this is unlikely. In both situations further investigation is required; this may include a D-dimer blood test, proximal leg vein ultrasound or parenteral anticoagulant. Readers are referred to the most current NICE guidelines for further information on this topic, including details of the two-level Wells score (Wells et al. 2003; NICE 2015).

Figure-of-Eight Ankle Measurement. This test measures the size and swelling of an ankle. The patient is positioned in long sitting with both feet extended over the end of a plinth. The ankle should be in approximately 20° of plantarflexion (Rohner-Spengler et al. 2007). A 6-mm (1/4-inch)-wide plastic tape measure is placed midway between the tendon of the tibialis anterior and the lateral malleolus. The tape is pulled medially toward the instep, just distal to the tuberosity of the navicular. The tape is then drawn across the arch of the foot to just proximal to the base of the fifth metatarsal, then continues across the tibialis anterior tendon, around the ankle joint just distal to the medial malleolus and then across the Achilles tendon. From here the tape circles around the ankle, ending just distal to the lateral malleolus, before returning to the start position (Fig. 16.10). The figure-of-eight method has been demonstrated to be a reliable and valid indirect method of measuring ankle oedema in individuals with oedema secondary to sprains or other lower-extremity musculoskeletal disorders (Mawdsley et al. 2000).

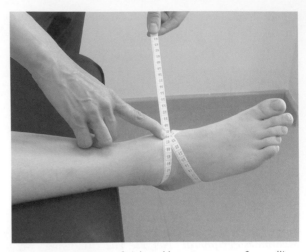

FIG. 16.10 ■ Figure-of-eight ankle measurement for swelling.

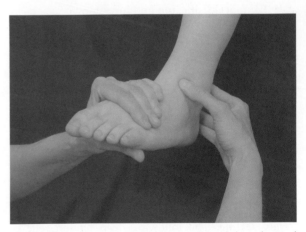

FIG. 16.11 ■ Anterior impingement sign of the talocrural joint. The thumb of the right hand palpates the anterolateral aspect of the ankle joint, applying a localized pressure whilst the left hand moves the ankle from a plantarflexed to dorsiflexed position.

Miscellaneous Tests of the Foot and Ankle

Anterior Impingement Sign of the Talocrural Joint

This is a pain provocation test for anterior impingement of the talocrual joint (bony/soft tissue). The patient is usually positioned in sitting with 90° of knee flexion, with the leg relaxed and unsupported. The test can also be performed with the patient supine or prone. One hand of the examiner is placed with the thumb palpating the anterolateral ankle and applying localized pressure whilst the other hand moves the ankle from a plantarflexed to dorsiflexed position (Fig. 16.11). Reproduction of symptoms signifies a positive test. Research suggests a sensitivity of 95% and a specificity of 88% for this sign (Molloy et al. 2003).

Mulders Click Test for Morton's Neuroma

This is a pain provocation test for Morton's neuroma between the metatarsal heads. The patient is normally positioned in supine with the foot relaxed. This test is performed with the thumb and index finger on the plantar and dorsal aspect of the painful intermetatarsal space, exerting local pressure. The forefoot is then further compressed with the opposite hand by squeezing together the metatarsal heads. The test is considered positive if a palpable click is felt with reproduction of pain. Mahadevan et al. (2015) report a sensitivity of 62% and a specificity of 100% for this test compared with ultrasonography.

Star Excursion Balance Test (SEBT)

This is a measurement of impairment of balance and voluntary movement function. The SEBT layout consists of eight lines set out from a central point, arranged at 45° angles (Fig. 16.12). The patient is asked to maintain balance on the lower limb to be tested while reaching as far as possible in eight different directions with the other foot, lightly touching the ground with that foot and then returning to centre. The distance achieved is measured in centimetres along each line. Patients should not move their supporting foot and keep their hands on their hips. The patient is allowed six practice and three test trials in each of the eight directions.

The SEBT has been shown to be a valid and reliable measure which can predict risk of lower-extremity injury, identify dynamic balance deficits in patients with a variety of lower-extremity conditions, and is responsive to training programmes in healthy and injured populations (Gribble et al. 2012). Modifications to the test include reduction of the number of practice tests to four (Robinson & Gribble 2008) and simplifying the SEBT to three directions only (anterior, posterolateral and posteromedial); this is known as the Y-balance test (Hertel et al. 2006).

Palpation

The clinician palpates the foot and ankle and any other relevant areas. It is useful to record palpation findings on a body chart (see Fig. 2.3) and/or palpation chart (see Fig. 3.35).

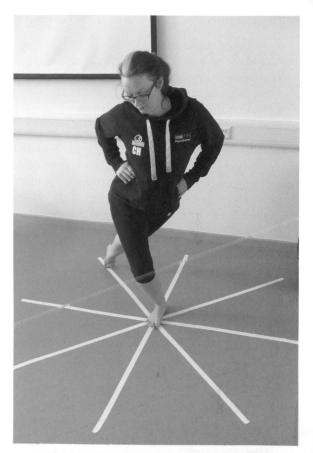

FIG. 16.12 ■ Star excursion balance test (SEBT).

The clinician notes the following:

- the temperature of the area
- localized increased skin moisture
- the presence of oedema
- mobility and feel of superficial tissues, e.g. ganglions, nodules, scar tissue
- the presence or elicitation of any muscle spasm
- tenderness of bone, ligament, muscle, tendon, tendon sheath, trigger points (shown in Fig. 3.36) or nerve
- increased or decreased prominence of bones
- pain provoked or reduced on palpation.

Accessory Movements

It is useful to use the palpation chart and movement diagrams (or joint pictures) to record findings. These are explained in detail in Chapter 3.

The clinician notes the:

■ quality of movement
■ range of movement
■ resistance through the range and at the end of the range of movement
■ behaviour of pain through the range
■ provocation of any protective muscle spasm.

A selection of accessory movements for the foot and ankle joints are shown in Fig. 16.13 and listed in Table 16.3; however it will not be necessary to test all of those listed, as selection will be based on clinical reasoning. For example, if ankle dorsiflexion is limited then examination may initially primarily focus on the talocrural joint, where the majority of dorsiflexion occurs. Accessory tests will be selected in order to refine the clinician's working hypothesis. For example, Kaltenborn's 10 point test can be used to explore the foot and ankle joints in more detail, although it may not be necessary to complete all parts of the test. If the patient's symptoms were focused around the medial aspect of the midfoot the clinician may choose to explore parts 3, 4 and 5 of the Kaltenborn test (Table 16.4).

Accessory movements can then be tested for other regions suspected to be a source of, or contributing to, the patient's symptoms. Again, following accessory movements to any one region, the clinician reassesses all the asterisks. Regions likely to be examined are the lumbar spine, sacroiliac joint, hip and knee.

Symptom Modification and Mobilizations With Movements

Mobilizations with movements are accessory movements applied during an active movement and were developed by physiotherapist Brian Mulligan. These techniques can be used to assess changes in symptoms /ROM and if cause a noticeable range, this may strengthen hypotheses relating to the structures contributing to symptoms and hence be considered as treatment options.

Inferior Tibiofibular Joint

The patient lies supine and is asked actively to invert the foot while the clinician applies an anteroposterior glide to the fibula (Fig. 16.14). An increase in range and no/reduced pain are positive examination findings indicating a possible mechanical joint problem.

Plantarflexion of the Ankle Joint

The patient lies supine with the knee flexed and the foot over the end of the plinth. With one hand the clinician applies an anteroposterior glide to the lower end of the tibia and fibula and with the other hand rolls the talus anteriorly while the patient is asked actively to plantarflex the ankle (Fig. 16.15A). An increase in range and no/reduced pain are positive examination findings potentially indicating a possible mechanical joint problem.

Dorsiflexion of the Ankle Joint

The patient lies supine with the foot over the end of the plinth, and knee slightly flexed over a rolled towel. The clinician uses one hand to hold the calcaneus, whilst the web space of the other hand contacts the anterior talus. Both hands contribute to the anteroposterior glide of the talus, while the patient is asked actively to dorsiflex the ankle (Fig. 16.15B). Since the extensor tendons lift the examiner's hand away from the talus, the patient is asked to contract repetitively and then relax. With relaxation, the clinician moves the ankle into the further range of dorsiflexion gained during the contraction.

For further guidance on the use of mobilizations with movements, see Mulligan (2010) and Hing et al. (2015).

COMPLETION OF THE EXAMINATION

Once the above tests have been carried out, the basic examination of the foot and ankle is complete. The subjective and physical examinations produce a large amount of information which needs to be recorded accurately and quickly. The outline subjective and physical examination charts in Chapters 2 and 3 may be useful for some clinicians. It is important, however, that the clinician does not examine in a rigid manner. Each patient presents differently and this needs to be reflected in the examination process. It is vital at this stage to highlight with an asterisk (*) important findings from the examination. These findings are reassessed at, and within, subsequent treatment

Text continued to page 446

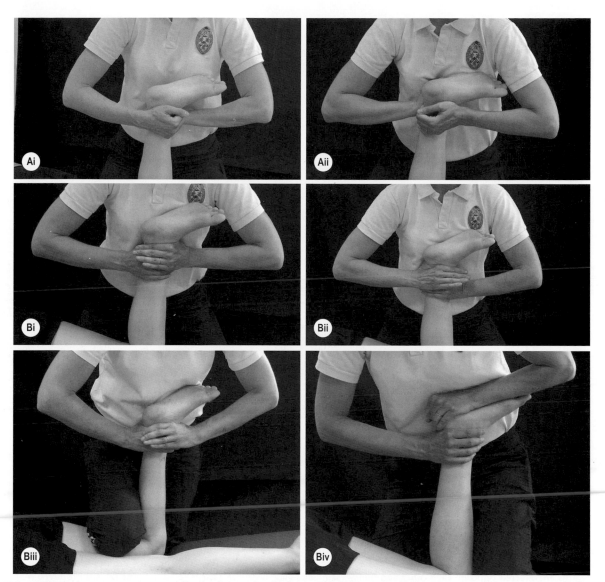

FIG. 16.13 ■ Accessory movements for the foot and ankle joints. (A) Inferior tibiofibular joint. (Ai) Anteroposterior. The heel of the right hand applies a posteroanterior force to the tibia while the left hand applies an anteroposterior force to the fibula. (Aii) Posteroanterior. The left hand applies an anteroposterior force to the tibia while the right hand applies a posteroanterior force to the fibula. (B) Talocrural joint. (Bi) Anteroposterior. The right hand stabilizes the calf while the left hand applies an anteroposterior force to the anterior aspect of the talus. (Bii) Posteroanterior. The left hand stabilizes the tibia/fibula while the right hand applies a posteroanterior force to the posterior aspect of the talus. (Biii) Longitudinal caudad. The clinician lightly rests the leg on the posterior aspect of the patient's thigh to stabilize and then grasps around the talus to pull upwards. (Biv) Longitudinal cephalad. The right hand supports the foot in dorsiflexion while the left hand applies a longitudinal cephalad force through the calcaneus. *Continued*

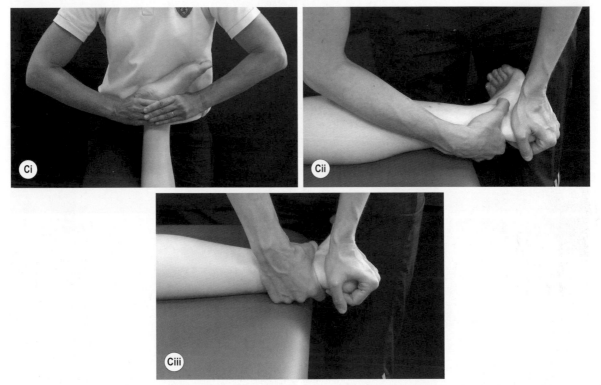

FIG. 16.13, cont'd ■ (C) Subtalar joint. (Ci) Longitudinal caudad. The clinician lightly rests her leg on the posterior aspect of the patient's thigh to stabilize it and then grasps around the calcaneus with the right hand and the forefoot with the left hand, and pulls the foot upwards. (Cii) Transverse medial glide. The patient is in side-lying. The therapist's right hand stabilizes the talus and distal tibia with the second and third fingers in a 'V' formation, while the left hand cups around the calcaneus. The forearms are directed opposite each other and transverse medial glide of the calcaneus relative to the talus is produced mainly via the left hand whilst the right hand maintains the position of the talus. (Ciii) Transverse lateral glide. The patient is in side-lying. The therapist's right hand stabilizes the talus and distal tibia with the second and third fingers in a 'V' formation, while the left hand cups around the calcaneus. The forearms are directed opposite each other and movement is produced mainly via the left hand whilst the right hand maintains the position of the talus.

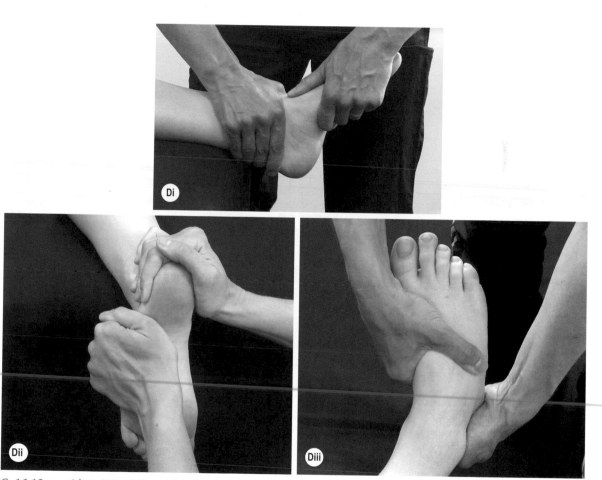

FIG. 16.13, cont'd ■ (D) Midfoot. (Di) Anteroposterior to the navicular. Pressure is applied to the anterior aspect of the navicular through a key grip or the thenar eminence. The other hand stabilizes the talus. (Dii) Posteroanterior to the cuboid. Pressure is applied to the posterior aspect of the cuboid through the thenar eminence whilst the other hand stabilizes the calcaneum. (Diii) Abduction/adduction. The left hand grasps and stabilizes the heel while the right hand grasps the forefoot. The right hand then applies an abduction force to the foot. The foot does not evert. Hands swapped over for adduction.

Continued